Thoracic Malignancies

European Respiratory Monograph 44
June 2009

Editor in Chief
K. Larsson

This book is one in a series of European Respiratory Monographs. Each individual issue provides a comprehensive overview of one specific clinical area of respiratory health, communicating information about the most advanced techniques and systems needed to investigate it. It provides factual and useful scientific detail, drawing on specific case studies and looking into the diagnosis and management of individual patients. Previously published titles in this series are listed at the back of this book with details of how they can be purchased.

Thoracic Malignancies

Edited by
S.G. Spiro, R.M. Huber and S.M. Janes

European Respiratory Society

Published by European Respiratory Society Journals Ltd ©2009
June 2009
Hardback ISBN: 978-1-904097-68-6
Paperback ISBN: 978-1-904097-69-3
ISSN: 1025-448x
Printed by Latimer Trend & Co. Ltd, Plymouth, UK

Managing Editors: Pippa Powell, Fiona Marks and Catherine Pumphrey,
European Respiratory Society Journals Ltd, Publications Office,
442 Glossop Road, Sheffield, S10 2PX, UK.
Tel: 44 114 2672860; Fax: 44 114 2665064; E-mail: Monograph@ersj.org.uk

The European Respiratory Monograph

Number 44 June 2009

CONTENTS

The Guest Editors

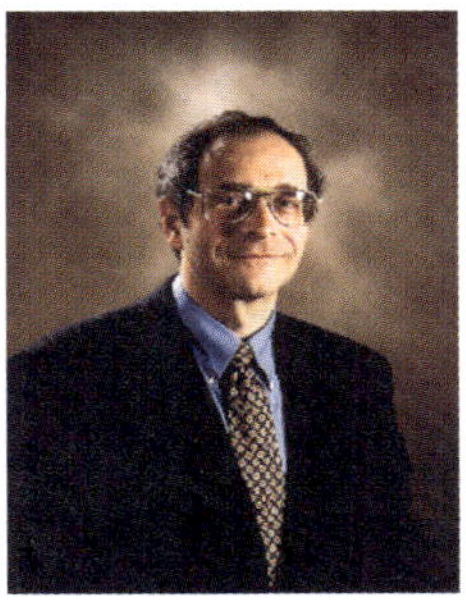
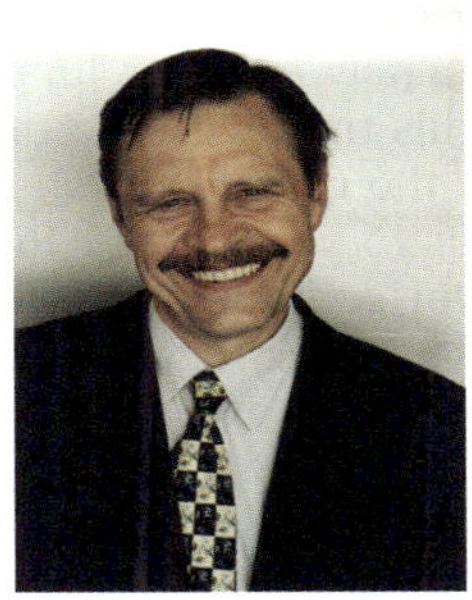
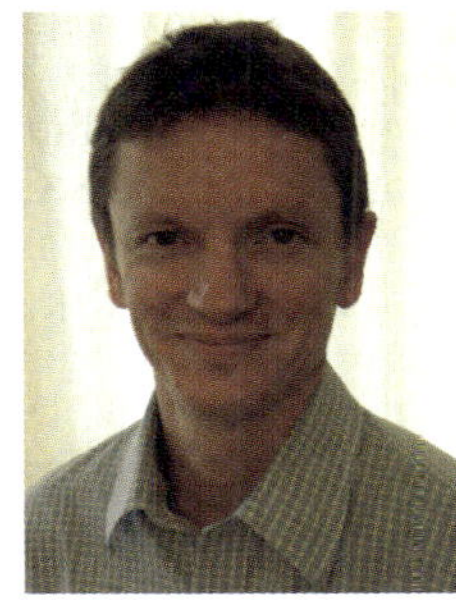

S.G. Spiro R.M. Huber S.M. Janes

S.G. Spiro was Head of the Dept of Thoracic Medicine at University College London Hospitals (London, UK) until December 2008; from 2001–2002 he was Medical Director. During 1996–1997 he was the President of the European Respiratory Society (ERS), and served as a member of the *European Respiratory Journal* Editorial Board for many years. He is also a former editor of *Thorax* and was Chair of the Royal College of Physicians Subcommittee on Respiratory Medicine (1997–2001). In 2004 he was President of the British Thoracic Society. His major interests include clinical trials in lung cancer and he was Co-Chair of the London Lung Cancer Group, a national clinical trials group in the UK. He also participates on other international bodies concerned with the treatment of lung cancer. His other research interests include respiratory physiology and sleep-disordered breathing.

R.M. Huber is Professor of Medicine at the Medical School at the Ludwig Maximilian University of Munich, and Head of the Division of Respiratory Medicine at the University Hospital of Munich, (Munich, Germany). He is also Chair of Thoracic Oncology section of the Cancer Centre of Munich. His research is focused on local endoscopic therapy, detection and treatment of early lung cancer, reactions of the bronchial wall (organ cultures, co-cultures and lung slices) and radiochemotherapy of locally advanced cancer, as well as integration of new systemic therapies in the management of lung cancer. He is the principal investigator of several multicenter studies on the treatment of lung cancer. R.M. Huber is Head of the ERS Thoracic Oncology Assembly and a member of the Arbeitsgemeinschaft Internistische Onkologie of the German Cancer Society. He was a board member of the Deutsche Gesellschaft für Pneumologie and co-chair of its Thoracic Oncology section. He is also the Secretary of the Süddeutsche Gesellschaft für Pneumologie. He has been, and is currently, a member of several national and international Task Forces covering all aspects of respiratory medicine.

S.M. Janes is a Consultant in respiratory and general medicine at University College London Hospitals. In 2006, he co-organised the British Association for Lung Research meeting on Stem Cells. He also co-organised the 2009 ERS Lung Science Conference in Estoril, Portugal. He was Guest Editor for a review issue of *International Journal of Biochemistry & Cell Biology* on respiratory epithelial biology. S.M. Janes is also Chair of the Lung Head and Neck and Neurology group, which is currently planning a new cancer centre. He is currently running the BOOST trial (a new pathway with BronchOscopic or Oesophageal ultrasound for lung cancer diagnosis and STaging), which is run by a Medical Research Council Clinical Training Fellow. He is also co-principle investigator of the lung-SEARCH trial: a randomised controlled trial of surveillance for early lung cancer in a high-risk group.

Preface

In 1995, the very first issue of the *European Respiratory Monograph* (*ERM*) was published, an issue that was dedicated to carcinoma of the lung. Six years later, in 2001, the topic was again in focus and a new *ERM* on lung cancer appeared. Now it is time for the third *ERM* on the subject, this time with the title *Thoracic Malignancies*. As in the two former issues, S.G. Spiro is the Guest Editor, this time together with R.M. Huber and S.M. Janes. Within less than 15 years lung cancer is estimated to be the fifth most common cause of death in the world. This makes the subject of certain importance and, as there has been significant progress as regards diagnosis and treatment of malignant thoracic conditions, there are good reasons for continuous updates.

It is therefore a pleasure to introduce a new and extended *ERM* covering most types of thoracic malignancies. In this issue, a chapter on pre-malignant diseases of the lung has been added, as have three chapters on epidemiology, diagnosis, staging and treatment of mesothelioma. A chapter on functional evaluation for treatment will most likely be useful and much appreciated by physicians who are actively involved in pre-operative evaluation of patients with thoracic malignancies. Adjuvant therapy and novel techniques regarding endobronchial diagnosing and management of neoplasms have been addressed and new achievements in lung cancer biology are presented. I am convinced that this third *ERM* on thoracic malignancies will supply a felt demand and that it will be very useful for a great number of physicians working in the field.

Editor in Chief,
K. Larsson

Eur Respir Mon, 2009, 44, viii. Printed in UK - all rights reserved. Copyright ERS Journals Ltd 2009; European Respiratory Monograph; ISSN 1025-448x.

INTRODUCTION

S.G. Spiro, R.M. Huber#, S.M. Janes¶*

**Dept of Thoracic Medicine, University College London Hospitals, ¶Centre for Respiratory Research, University College London, London, UK. #Pneumologie, Dept of Medicine, University of Munich – Campus Innenstadt, Munich, Germany.*

Correspondence: S.M. Janes, Centre for Respiratory Research, University College London, Rayne Building, 5 University Street, London, WC1E 6JJ, UK. Fax: 44 2073809476; E-mail: s.janes@ucl.ac.uk

This is the third *European Respiratory Monograph* (*ERM*) on lung cancer. The first in 1990 and the second in 2001 concentrated on just lung cancer; however, the current *ERM* now includes mesothelioma, which is reaching the peak of its epidemic within Europe. The *ERM* has been significantly updated from previous issues with a wide variety of contributors who have generously submitted cutting-edge research. This *ERM* is both scientific and educational, and provides readers with an updated and comprehensive educational tool to use in everyday clinical practice.

Lung cancer remains an alarming disease with high mortality and social cost. In Europe it remains the most common killing cancer in both males and females. Over the last 30 yrs there has been little improvement in the survival of lung cancer patients and its management remains a major challenge for respiratory physicians, surgeons and oncologists. However, since 2001, huge steps have been made in understanding the biology of lung cancer, as well as great improvements in diagnostic staging and the introduction to the therapeutic armory of new molecularly targeted therapies. Indeed, comparing the last *ERM* on lung cancer to the current *ERM*, it is surprising how much more is known and how clinical practice has altered in the last 8 yrs.

Thus, while the disease remains unconquered we hope this issue of the *ERM* illustrates that there have been major advances over the last 8 yrs which we will continue to build upon.

We hope this issue of the *ERM* is of interest to all our colleagues and helps to improve the understanding of this most serious of all cancers.

Eur Respir Mon, 2009, 44, ix. Printed in UK - all rights reserved. Copyright ERS Journals Ltd 2009; European Respiratory Monograph; ISSN 1025-448x.

CHAPTER 1

Lung cancer: oncogenesis and prevention

N. van Zandwijk

Correspondence: N. van Zandwijk, Asbestos Diseases Research Institute, Bernie Banton Centre, University of Sydney, Hospital Road, Concord NSW 2139, Australia. E-mail: zwk@med.usyd.edu.au

Lung cancer is by far the leading cause of cancer-related death worldwide [1]. Median survival in all stages of disease has improved during the last decades but the likelihood of obtaining a cure, even with optimal modern therapy, is low, largely due to the fact that symptoms of respiratory cancer occur when the disease is in an advanced stage. Late diagnosis is almost certainly related to a covert carcinogenesis phase that evolves over 10–20 yrs and requires multiple molecular genetic changes before the development of invasive lung cancer [2, 3]. Consequently, there exists a strong rationale for intervening in those stages of lung carcinogenesis that could result in arrest or delay of disease progression to invasive cancer. Tobacco smoking accounts for >80% of the attributable risk for lung cancer [4]. At the same time other aetiological factors are being uncovered and it has become evident that more than one pre-neoplastic pathway exists. Despite smoking cessation, lung cancer risk remains elevated for many years and never reaches the level of never-smokers [4]. A significant percentage of newly diagnosed lung cancer occurs in former smokers [5]. Thus, in certain individuals, the carcinogenic process elicited by tobacco smoke continues to evolve despite smoking cessation. These observations underline why strategies to slow, halt or even reverse the carcinogenic process continue to gain great interest. Traditional prevention studies with vitamins, micronutrients and cancer incidence as the primary endpoint required many years of follow-up and thousands of participants to detect a significant impact. The interpretation of results has been complicated by the fact that in many of these studies a significant percentage of participants continued smoking [6]. Moreover these studies with cancer incidence as the end-point have shown how critical it is to select a population significantly at risk. Individuals with a 20 pack-yr history do not have a >10–15% lifetime risk for developing lung cancer. Recent studies have therefore focused on intermediate marker end-points to identify potential useful prevention strategies.

Epidemiology

As mentioned above, lung cancer is strongly associated with direct consumption of tobacco products. In fact, 87% of all lung cancers are detected in individuals who are active or former smokers, with an additional 6–7% composed of partners of smokers or their offspring. The second and third most common known causes of lung cancer are radon and asbestos [7, 8]. Despite the high degree of certainty that currently exists over the link between tobacco smoke and lung cancer, the understanding of these facts took several decades to clarify. It was finally discovered that tobacco smoke was capable of producing the identical p53 mutations found in lung cancer patients and in smoke-exposed mice, adding biological evidence to a strong, incontrovertible epidemiological association [9].

Eur Respir Mon, 2009, 44, 1–14. Printed in UK - all rights reserved. Copyright ERS Journals Ltd 2009; European Respiratory Monograph; ISSN 1025-448x.

Oncogenesis

The original description of "field cancerisation" dates back to SLAUGHTER *et al.* [10], who showed that multiple foci of epithelial hyperplasia, hyperkeratinisation, atypia, dysplasia and carcinoma *in situ* occurred in otherwise normal appearing epithelium adjacent to cancers of the oral pharynx in smokers. This empirical evidence strongly suggested that carcinogen exposure has widespread effects throughout the entire carcinogen-damaged epithelial field. AUERBACH *et al.* [11] observed the same pattern of heterogeneous, multi-focal histological changes in the bronchial epithelium of smokers, many of whom had lung cancer. Thus, the concept of field cancerisation was coined to describe the diffuse damage elicited by chronic exposure to carcinogens. Field carcinogenesis also forms the basis for the observation that individuals who survive a first cancer are likely to develop a second malignancy in the region of the condemned epithelium [12–14]. As these findings have been validated over the last several decades, increasing evidence has come to bear explaining the molecular genetic abnormalities that ultimately lead to the stepwise development of clonal invasion-competent cancer of the airway. Among the earliest findings in the aerodigestive tract of chronic smokers are loss of heterozygosity in chromosomes 3p, 9p and 17p [2, 15–19]. Clonal genetic abnormalities seen in normal histological regions of the tobacco smoke-exposed airway were further evidence that damage was scattered throughout the entire field. It also brought to bear the limitations of modern histological techniques in detecting the extent of the tobacco smoke-induced damage. The importance of these losses of heterozygosity are crystallised in the fact that, for example, the short arm of chromosome 3, which is often the earliest loss and is demonstrated on occasion even in early hyperplasia [15], results in the loss of a region rich in tumour suppressor genes. There is also evidence for losses of the short arms of chromosomes 9 and 17, resulting in loss of tumour suppressor genes in p16 and p53, both of which are important to the cell's ability to repair DNA damage elicited by tobacco smoke. p53 in particular acts as a transcription factor in the control of G1 arrest and apoptosis, or programmed cell death, thereby allowing the cell to repair existing DNA damage or make the determinant decision to push a cell into the apoptotic process once it is too far damaged for repair. p16, found on chromosome 9p, negatively controls cyclin-dependent kinase (CDK) activity by overexpression of cyclin-D1. By inhibiting cyclin-D1/CDK, the damaged cell is also prevented from entering into mitosis and proliferating with damaged DNA.

The loss of these and other tumour suppressor genes in lung cancer seems to be augmented by the activation of several critical proto-oncogenes. For example, RAS, c-MYC and the epidermal growth factor receptors (EGFR) are all tumour-promoting genes that are activated progressively during lung carcinogenesis. K-ras mutations are particularly common in adenocarcinomas of the lung, with some studies showing 30% of lung adenocarcinomas in smokers containing K-ras mutations [20]. The EGFR is frequently found amplified in lung carcinogenesis [21]. Mutations have been detected in the EGFR tyrosine kinase binding domain conferring sensitivity to small molecule EGFR-tyrosine kinase inhibitors [22–24]. Interestingly, both K-ras mutations and EGFR mutations have been found in the airways of smokers and nonsmokers in regions distant from the primary tumour, suggesting that both play a role in field carcinogenesis [20, 25].

Gene silencing

Loss of function of tumour suppressor genes and more prominent function of oncogenes through mutations or gene activations are not the only mechanisms by which carcinogenesis is augmented in lung cancer patients. A growing body of evidence suggests that gene silencing through epigenetic means can be crucial in lung carcinogenesis. For example, in nonsmall cell lung cancer (NSCLC), some tumour suppressor genes, such as RASSF1A, which is also located in the tumour suppressor gene-rich chromosome 3p, encodes a protein that heterodimerises with Nore-1, an important Ras effector with pro-apoptotic effect [26]. Evidence from several groups suggests that in NSCLC, RASSF1A can be inactivated by hypermethylation [27, 28]. Another important gene that can be inactivated by epigenetic means is the retinoic acid receptor (RAR)-β, which also maps to chromosome 3p. RAR-β is a nuclear retinoid receptor with vitamin A-dependent transcriptional activity [29]. RAR-β is a gene that has been shown to be gradually lost during lung carcinogenesis [30], and this may be caused by either loss or hypermethylation [31, 32]. Interestingly, the maintenance of RAR-β in mature tumours is a factor for poor prognosis [33], and it is differentially regulated in current *versus* former smokers. For example, a recent retrospective study on methylation status and occurrence of second primary tumours (SPTs) in completely resected NSCLC patients revealed an association between RAR-β2 hypermethylation in the development of SPTs only in former smokers [34]. In current smokers, hypermethylation was associated with a protective effect, pointing to the critical value of context with regard to smoking status in understanding the biological effects of retinoid receptors in lung cancer [34, 35].

Lung cancer susceptibility

There is progressive evidence that the risk of developing lung cancer, even among the heaviest smokers, varies widely according to genetic and perhaps even dietary factors. This is reinforced by the fact that 85% of heavy smokers will not develop lung cancer, implicating important differences in lung cancer susceptibility. Accumulating evidence suggests that genetic and epigenetic factors are critical in modulating individual susceptibility to lung cancer [36]. A recent support for this statement is found in the identification of a susceptibility locus for lung cancer at 15q25 in a large genome-wide association study [37, 38]. 15q25 contains nicotinic acetylcholine receptor subunit genes and seems to be involved in carcinogen metabolism. The two major carcinogens from cigarette smoke, benzo[a]pyrene and 4-(methylnitrosamino)-1-(3-pyridyl)-1-butanone (NNK) require metabolic activation before they can exert full carcinogenic effects. Various activation pathways compete with detoxification pathways and the balance between the two is critical in modulating cancer risk. Cytochrome P-450s serve as carcinogen-metabolising enzymes, while glutathione transferases serve as detoxification enzymes. Both sets of these important genes are known to have significant polymorphisms correlating with variations in lung cancer risk [39–41]. Moreover, DNA repair capacity most probably plays a significant role in lung cancer susceptibility [42].

Other modulators of risk in lung cancer include diet and gender. Dietary factors play an important role as epigenetic modulators of lung cancer susceptibility. In several case-controlled studies, defective detoxification and defective repair of genetic damage have been shown to be associated with increased individual susceptibility to lung cancer [43, 44]. Food constituents, such as fruits and specific vegetables, appear to afford a significant degree of protection to individuals with limitations to their detoxification capacity [40]. This relationship between diet and lung cancer has been extensively explored and is being used as a basis for the development of preventive approaches to lung cancer.

Vitamins and micronutrients

As several dietary adjustments and micronutrients have been associated with lower risks of lung cancer, including vitamin E, selenium, isothiocyanates and polyphenols, several large randomised trials have sought to delineate which compounds in complex human diets are most responsible for the protective effects seen [45, 46]. Initially, the greatest degree of evidence existed around the potency of carotenoids and retinoids and the broad epidemiologic indications implicating them in reduction of cancer risk in general, and in particular in lung cancer risk. In fact, the original definition of chemoprevention as "attempts to reverse, suppress, and prevent carcinogenic progression to overt cancer" [47] is based on experimental work showing that vitamin A analogues are capable of reversing or preventing epithelial carcinogenesis in animal experiments.

Consequently, the identification of populations at risk for development of this disease followed suit. For example, target populations in many of the early prevention studies included broad populations of individuals at risk due to their exposure to tobacco and/ or asbestos. Others sought to develop strategies for uranium miners, a population known to be at an enhanced risk for developing lung cancer. Thus, with several decades of epidemiological and dietary investigation, augmented by various experimental systems a number of compounds, including retinoids and carotenoids, were found capable of reversing cell damage and a strong drive to develop this approach in human populations was born. The trials focused on broad patient populations, including those of individuals at even higher risk, in other words, individuals with known pre-malignancy of the airway, or those patients who had already developed a primary tobacco-related cancer, and thus were at the greatest risk for developing an SPT.

Chemoprevention trials

As risk categories were different across carcinogen-exposed individuals, *i.e.* individuals with pre-malignancy and those who already had tobacco smoke-related cancer, the three categories of chemoprevention were defined as primary, secondary and tertiary prevention. Primary prevention involved intervening in patient populations only at increased risk. The end-point here was reduction in incidence of, and death from lung cancer. Secondary prevention involved attempts in individuals with evidence of lung pre-malignancy to prevent progression of that pre-malignancy or, ideally, to reverse it to an earlier stage of carcinogenesis. Finally, studies in the highest risk population, *i.e.* in those who had already developed tobacco-related malignancy, focused on the prevention of development of SPTs. Many of the early trials focused on using retinoids and carotenoids as the chemoprevention agents of choice, given that the weight of epidemiological and experimental evidence for these compounds was significantly greater than that for other classes of compounds.

Primary chemoprevention

Several large randomised studies were undertaken in populations deemed to be at increased risk of lung cancer due to exposure to tobacco smoke or asbestos, or their occupation as uranium miners. Three major studies, the ATBC, CARET and the US Physician Study, were carried out using increasingly high doses of the carotenoid, β-carotene (table 1). None of the three studies showed any reduction of lung cancer risk

Table 1. – Primary randomised chemoprevention trials in lung cancer

Study [ref.]	Intervention	End-point	Patients n	Outcome
ATBC [48]	β-Carotene/α-tocopherol	Lung cancer	29133	Negative/harmful
CARET [49]	β-Carotene/retinol	Lung cancer	18314	Negative/harmful
Physicians' Health Study [50]	β-Carotene	Lung cancer	22071	Negative

utilising these compounds, and two of these studies, the Alpha-Tocopherol, Beta-Carotene Cancer (ATBC) study and the beta-Carotene and Retinol Efficacy Trial (CARET) had surprising findings, both showing significant increases in lung cancer risk associated with supplementation with β-carotene. Both of these studies, which were 2 plus 2 factorial studies, also involved a second agent as an intervention. In these cases, neither the second agent nor vitamin A itself was found to be associated with an increased risk of lung cancer, but neither were they protective against lung cancer incidence. Interestingly, both of these studies showed that the risk of lung cancer was increased only in populations that were smokers.

The ATBC cancer prevention study was a randomised 2 by 2 factorial, double-blind, placebo-controlled, primary prevention study, in which 29,133 Finnish male smokers received either α-tocopherol (50 mg·day^{-1} alone), β-carotene (20 mg·day^{-1}), both α-tocopherol and β-carotene, or a placebo. The participants, aged 50–69 yrs, all of whom smoked ≥5 cigarettes·day^{-1}, were enrolled on the study and received follow-up observation for 5–8 yrs. While lung cancer incidence, the primary end-point, was not modified by the addition of α-tocopherol alone, both groups who received β-carotene supplementation, either alone or with α-tocopherol, had an 18% increase in the incidence of lung cancer and a significant increase in lung cancer mortality. This study showed a stronger adverse effect from β-carotene in males who smoked >20 cigarettes·day^{-1}, and was the first to raise the concern that pharmacological doses of β-carotene could be harmful in active smokers. A recent update suggested that the excess risk for β-carotene recipients was no longer evident 4–6 yrs after any intervention and, at that point, morbidity was largely due to cardiovascular diseases [48, 51].

The CARET confirmed the results of the ATBC trial. This was also a randomised, double-blind, placebo-controlled trial testing the combination of 30 mg·day^{-1} of β-carotene and 25,000 IU of retinyl palmitate in 18,314 male and female subjects aged 50–69 yrs who were considered at increased risk for lung cancer. The majority of participants had a smoking history of ≥20 pack-yrs, and were either current smokers or recent former-smokers. Significant and even extensive occupational exposure to asbestos was noted in 4,060 men in this trial [52]. The trial was stopped early because of evidence of possible harm, consistent with the ATBC study. In fact, lung cancer incidence, the primary end-point, increased by 28% in the active intervention group, with an increase in overall mortality of 17% in this group [49].

By contrast, the Physicians' Health Study [50], a randomised, double-blind, placebo-controlled trial studied 22,071 healthy male physicians, half of whom received 50 mg·day^{-1} of β-carotene on alternate days and the other half received placebo. The use of supplemental β-carotene in this study comprising a majority of nonsmokers showed no adverse or beneficial effects on cancer incidence or overall mortality rate during a 12-yr follow-up [50].

Subsequent subgroup analyses of the ATBC study and the CARET have indicated that β-carotene had a harmful effect only in the high-risk heavy smokers, or those with previous exposure to asbestos [53].

Secondary prevention

While there has been dispute over which are the optimal pre-malignant markers of lung cancer to follow, the success in developing studies with patients with pre-malignancy has been rather limited. To date, eight randomised trials have used various end-points, including reversal of sputum atypia, reduction in DNA micronuclei, and reversal of dysplasia or hyperplasia (table 2). Some of these trials have used retinoids, and have shown that in the absence of smoking cessation, retinoids are incapable of reversing pre-malignant lesions. While some biomarker-driven studies utilising novel pen-retinoids, such as 9-*cis*-retinoic acid, or atypical retinoids, such as fenretinoid, have shown that these agents can modulate biomarkers, such as RAR-β or human telomerase reverse transcriptase (hTERT) expression, respectively, there is little evidence to suggest that any of the compounds listed in table 2 are capable of consistently reversing pre-malignant lesions. To date, one of the most positive studies has been one that utilised folate and vitamin B12, which showed some improvement in bronchial epithelial metaplasia in smokers. Given the difficulty in validation of the end-points, even these positive results must be viewed with caution. Larger trials using biological end-points are needed to confirm efficacy.

The findings by LEE *et al.* [54] are important; they indicated that retinoids could be effective in the presence of smoking cessation, but were highly ineffective in active (continuing) smokers. Recent studies employing novel retinoids have indicated that they may have significant promise. One such trial by KURIE *et al.* [55] reported the results of a randomised controlled trial in former smokers who received either 9-*cis*-retinoic acid or 13-*cis*-retinoic acid with α-tocopherol. The end-point of the trial by KURIE *et al.* [55] was upregulation of RAR-β, the loss of which is gradually seen in pulmonary carcinogenesis. Of 177 evaluable patients, those treated with 9-*cis*-retinoic acid were found to have restoration of RAR-β expression ($p<0.03$) and reduction of metaplasia ($p<0.01$) [55]. There was no significant effect in the 13-*cis*-retinoic acid with α-tocopherol arm, encouraging this group of investigators to move forward with 9-*cis*-retinoic acid, a pan-retinoid agonist, targeting former smokers.

Table 2. – Secondary randomised chemoprevention trials in lung cancer

First author [ref.]	Intervention	End-point	Patients n	Outcome
LEE *et al.* [54]	Isotretinoin	Metaplasia	40	Negative
KURIE *et al.* [55]	Fenretinide	Metaplasia	82	Negative
ARNOLD *et al.* [56]	Etretinate	Metaplasia	150	Negative
MCLARTY *et al.* [57]	β-Carotene/retinol	Sputum atypia	755	Negative
HEIMBURGER *et al.* [58]	Vitamin B12/folic acid	Sputum atypia	73	Positive
VAN POPPEL *et al.* [59]	β-Carotene	Micronuclei sputum	114	Positive
KURIE *et al.* [55]	9-*cis*-Retinoic acid	RAR-β expression/ metaplasia	149	Positive
MAO *et al.* [60]	Celecoxib	Ki-67 expression	20	Positive
VAN SCHOOTEN *et al.* [61]	*N*-Acetylcysteine	DNA adducts	41	Positive
LAM *et al.* [62]	ADT	Dysplasia	101	Positive
SORIA *et al.* [63]	Fenretinide	hTERT expression	57	Positive
LAM *et al.* [64]	Budesonide	Dysplasia	112	Negative
VAN DEN BERG *et al.* [65]	Fluticasone	Dysplasia	108	Negative

RAR: retinoic acid receptor; ADT: anethole dithiolethione; hTERT: telomerase reverse transcriptase.

Tertiary prevention

Patients with tobacco-related cancers remain at a substantially elevated risk for developing subsequent tumours in the tobacco-damaged epithelium [12, 13, 66–70]. While the treatment for the initial cancer can often be successful, these patients are at significantly increased risk for developing an SPT [71]. The lifetime risk of developing an SPT in the head and neck region is ~20%, with a similar incidence in the lung. While estimates have varied between 3–7% per year, evidence remains incontrovertible that SPTs are the major cause of death after curative surgery in head and neck cancer [69–74].

Due to the high likelihood of both recurrence and SPTs in patients with advanced oral, oropharyngeal, or laryngeal squamous cell cancers, HONG *et al.* [75] launched a randomised, placebo-controlled study of 103 patients with stage I–IV head and neck squamous cell cancer. The patients were randomised to receive either high dose 13-*cis*-retinoic acid (100 $mg \cdot m^{-2} \cdot day^{-1}$) or placebo for 1 yr after definitive local therapy. The dosage of 13-*cis*-retinoic acid was reduced to 50 $mg \cdot m^{-2} \cdot day^{-1}$ after 13 of the first 44 patients experienced intolerable side-effects. The primary end-points were primary tumour recurrence and SPT development. In the two treatment arms, there was no difference in local recurrence or distant metastases. However, the patients treated with 13-*cis*-retinoic acid had a dramatically lower incidence of SPTs. Of the 103 patients followed for a median of 42 months, SPTs developed in 6% (three out of 49) of those in the 13-*cis*-retinoic acid arm, whereas 28% (14 out of 51) of the patients on the placebo arm developed SPTs.

A large scale follow-up to this trial using a much lower dose of 13-*cis*-retinoic acid was completed and presented a few years ago. In this trial, a randomised, double-blind, placebo-controlled study, launched in 1991, over 1,382 patients were registered and 1,192 were randomised to either low dose 13-*cis*-retinoic acid at 30 $mg \cdot day^{-1}$ *versus* placebo. These patients were definitively treated for stage I or II head and neck squamous cell cancer. With a median follow-up of 7 yrs, no effect was seen of the low dose retinoid on reducing the incidence of SPT in the lung or aerodigestive tract [76].

Several phase III trials have been launched in lung cancer in an attempt to prevent SPTs. The first of these was a trial by PASTORINO *et al.* [77] that randomised >300 patients with early-stage lung cancer to retinyl palmitate or placebo. This study showed a significant reduction in the development of second primary lung cancers on the retinyl palmitate arm. A subsequent study by BOLLA *et al.* [78] using a different synthetic retinoid, etretinate, failed to show a reduction in SPTs.

Two large phase III trials reported in the last decade include the EUROSCAN and the US Intergroup National Cancer Institute trial (table 3). EUROSCAN, a randomised adjuvant chemoprevention study by the European Organization for Research and Treatment of Cancer (EORTC), head and neck and lung groups, studied the effects of vitamin A (retinyl palmitate) and *N*-acetylcysteine in patients with early-stage head and neck and lung cancer [79]. In this trial, 2,592 patients with cancers of the larynx, TIS–T3 and 0–N1; oral cavity, TIS–T2 and 0–N1; and NSCLC, T1–T2 and 0–N1, received retinyl palmitate, 300,000 $IU \cdot day^{-1}$ in year 1 and 150,000 $IU \cdot day^{-1}$ in year 2, *N*-acetylcysteine 600 $mg \cdot day^{-1}$ for 2 yrs, both drugs, or placebo. No significant differences were seen between the three active treatment arms and the placebo group in terms of recurrence rates, SPT development, or survival. Of the patient population, >90% were regular smokers, with 43 median pack-yrs of tobacco exposure.

The US Intergroup National Cancer Institute 91-0001 trial was a randomised, double-blind, placebo-controlled study utilising the same low dose of 30 mg 13-*cis*-retinoic acid after complete resection of stage I NSCLC [80]. This trial was completed in 1997, having accrued 1,486 participants. The study objectives were to evaluate the efficacy of

Table 3. – Lung and aerodigestive second primary tumour (SPT) prevention studies (tertiary chemoprevention)

First author [ref.]	Intervention	End-point	Patients n	Outcome
PASTORINO [77]	Retinyl palmitate	SPT	307	Positive
VAN ZANDWIJK [79]	Retinyl palmitate/*N*-acetylcysteine	SPT	2592	Negative
LIPPMAN [80]	13-*cis*-Retinoic acid	SPT	1304	Negative
KHURI [76]	13-*cis*-Retinoic acid	SPT	1190	Negative
HONG [75]	Isotretinoin	SPT	130	Positive

low-dose daily 13-*cis*-retinoic acid for 3 yrs at 30 mg·day^{-1} *versus* placebo in the prevention of SPTs. Patients were required to have complete resection of primary, stage I NSCLC (post-operative T1 or T2 and 0) and to be registered between 6 weeks and 3 yrs after completion of therapy. After a median follow-up of 3.5 yrs, no statistically significant differences were seen between the placebo and 13-*cis*-retinoic acid arms with respect to time to SPT development, recurrence rate, or mortality. Multivariate analyses showed that the rate of SPT development was not affected by any stratification factor, with recurrence rate affected only by treatment stage, and evidence for a treatment-by-smoking interaction (hazard ratio for treatment-by-current *versus* never-smoking status=3.11; 95% confidence interval, 1.00–9.71). Therefore, 13-*cis*-retinoic acid was not shown to affect overall survival rates or development of SPTs, recurrences, or mortality in stage I NSCLC. Subsequent subset analyses have indicated that 13-*cis*-retinoic acid was potentially harmful in current smokers and beneficial in never-smokers.

Future strategies

After more than two decades of unsuccessful interventions in NSCLC, evidence has now accumulated to suggest that approaches relying exclusively on the development of epidemiological guidance for selection of compounds are unlikely to lead to effective interventions across broad and disparate populations. While clues continue to emerge from the epidemiological literature showing that dietary constituents, such as phyto-oestrogens, appear to significantly reduce lung cancer risk [81], few have suggested moving prevention approaches forward without further testing of the concept in well-designed, biomarker-driven trials.

To date, significant evidence exists to show that over-expression of the EGFR occurs throughout lung carcinogenesis [21, 82, 83], and that mutations of the EGFR-tyrosine kinase (EGFR-TK) binding domain can be seen diffusely across the normal-appearing airway in patients with resected adenocarcinomas who are nonsmokers and harbour an EGFR-TK binding domain mutation in their primary tumour. This discovery [25] of a novel field effect in which EGFR-TK mutations are seen in apparently normal-appearing, nontobacco-damaged airways suggests that despite the absence of an identifiable carcinogen leading to EGFR mutations, this represents a new and as yet not understood type of field effect. Several investigators have proposed novel chemopreven-tion approaches using the EGFR-TK inhibitors, erlotinib and gefitinib, in high-risk patient populations. Given the fact that the incidence of EGFR-TK mutation-bearing adenocarcinoma of the lung is most frequently seen in Asian, female nonsmokers [84, 85], the identification of individuals at greatest risk would likely lead to the recognition of a target population, thereby enhancing the chances of successful intervention.

Important data also implicate the progressive upregulation of cyclooxygenase (COX)-2 in lung carcinogenesis, and trials targeting both suppression of COX-2 with selective COX-2 inhibitors have shown promising preliminary results [60, 86]. Another approach has sought to upregulate prostacycline, thereby downregulating PGE-2, potentially the critical downstream effector pathway for COX-2 [87].

Another targeted approach is based on epidemiological data. GOVINDARAJAN *et al.* [88] showed that thiazolidinediones, peroxisome proliferator-activated receptor stimulators, are able to induce cell cycle arrest. These investigators examined a large cohort study in 87,678 male veterans aged >40 yrs, and showed a 33% reduction of lung cancer risk among the 11,289 thiazolidinedione users. A caveat is formed by the fact that this study failed to account for variations by smoking status.

Others have utilised corticosteroids, both inhaled and oral, or inhaled retinoids, all of which have shown promise. Unfortunately, two randomised phase II studies in high risk patients have failed to show a trend in favour of inhalational corticoids [64, 65].

In the meantime, a surprising trial that sought to prevent SPT skin cancer in a selenium-poor population in Arizona, USA, showed a 34% reduction in lung cancer incidence [46]. This observation formed the basis for a (tertiary) phase III prevention study (Eastern Cooperative Oncologic Group (ECOG)-5597) that randomises patients in a 2:1 ratio to receive selenium methionine at 200 $\mu g \cdot day^{-1}$ *versus* placebo. The ECOG study [46] was initiated without preliminary studies and the recommendation must be to continue to build biomarker-driven, targeted, phase II approaches that appropriately pursue modulation of a critical biomarker, and confirm it prior to proceeding with large-scale studies.

Conclusions

Notwithstanding the negative outcome of several large comparative trials, a significant number of epidemiological, experimental and also clinical observations continue to provide evidence that antioxidants, anti-inflammatory agents, tyrosine kinase inhibitors of the EGFR and phytochemicals have modes to inhibit the carcinogenic process. However, the mode of action of several of these agents at the gene transcription level is not yet completely understood. Thanks to new molecular biological techniques, this insight is rapidly increasing and after many years with meagre results from chemoprevention studies, we may have entered a more positive era in this area of research.

Summary

Lung cancer is the leading cause of cancer mortality for males and females, and has grown into a worldwide problem over the last 50 yrs.
Cigarette smoking elicits >80% of all lung cancers. Although the prevalence of smoking is declining, the risk of lung cancer after smoking cessation persists and remains elevated in comparison to never-smokers.
Despite a rapid increase in insight into carcinogenesis, the accurate identification of high-risk groups has remained difficult; attempts to decrease lung cancer risk by preventive measures other than smoking cessation have so far been unsuccessful.
However, strategies to slow, halt or even reverse the carcinogenic process continue to gain great interest. It is very likely that further identification of the different molecular steps of carcinogenesis will finally translate into effective preventive strategies.

Keywords: Carcinogenesis, chemoprevention, lung cancer, micronutrients.

Statement of interest
None declared.

References

1. Jemal A, Siegel R, Ward E, *et al.* Cancer statistics, 2008. *CA Cancer J Clin* 2008; 58: 71–96.
2. Mao L, Lee JS, Kurie JM, *et al.* Clonal genetic alterations in the lungs of current and former smokers.[see comment]. *J Natl Cancer Inst* 1997; 89: 857–862.
3. Bartsch H, Petruzzelli S, De Flora S, *et al.* Carcinogen metabolism in human lung tissues and the effect of tobacco smoking: results from a case–control multicenter study on lung cancer patients. *Environ Health Perspect* 1992; 98: 119–124.
4. Peto R, Darby S, Deo H, *et al.* Smoking, smoking cessation, and lung cancer in the UK since 1950: combination of national statistics with two case–control studies. *BMJ* 2000; 321: 323–329.
5. Tong L, Spitz MR, Fueger JJ, *et al.* Lung carcinoma in former smokers. *Cancer* 1996; 78: 1004–1010.
6. van Zandwijk N, Mulshine JL. Chemoprevention. *In*: Francis T, ed. Prevention and Early Detection of Lung Cancer. IASLC, Oxford, 2006; pp. 341–360.
7. Al-Zoughool M, Krewski D. Health effects of radon: a review of the literature. *Int J Radiat Biol* 2009; 85: 57–69.
8. Boffetta P. Human cancer from environmental pollutants: the epidemiological evidence. *Mutat Res* 2006; 608: 157–162.
9. Denissenko MF, Pao A, Tang M, *et al.* Preferential formation of benzo[a]pyrene adducts at lung cancer mutational hotspots in P53. *Science* 1996; 274: 430–432.
10. Slaughter DP, Southwick HW, Smejkal W. Field cancerization in oral stratified squamous epithelium; clinical implications of multicentric origin. *Cancer* 1953; 6: 963–968.
11. Auerbach O, Hammond EC, Garfinkel L. Changes in bronchial epithelium in relation to cigarette smoking, 1955–1960 vs. 1970–1977. *N Engl J Med* 1979; 300: 381–385.
12. Boice JD Jr, Fraumeni JF Jr. Second cancer following cancer of the respiratory system in Connecticut, 1935–1982. *Natl Cancer Inst Monogr* 1985; 68: 83–98.
13. de Vries N, Snow GB. Multiple primary tumours in laryngeal cancer. *J Laryngol Otol* 1986; 100: 915–918.

14. Vikram B, Strong EW, Shah JP, *et al.* Second malignant neoplasms in patients successfully treated with multimodality treatment for advanced head and neck cancer. *Head Neck Surg* 1984; 6: 734–737.
15. Hung J, Kishimoto Y, Sugio K, *et al.* Allele-specific chromosome 3p deletions occur at an early stage in the pathogenesis of lung carcinoma. *JAMA* 1995; 273: 1908.
16. Mao L. Tumor suppressor genes: does FHIT fit? *J Natl Cancer Inst* 1998; 90: 412–414.
17. Wistuba II, Lam S, Behrens C, *et al.* Molecular damage in the bronchial epithelium of current and former smokers. *J Natl Cancer Inst* 1997; 89: 1366–1373.
18. Kishimoto Y, Sugio K, Hung JY, *et al.* Allele-specific loss in chromosome 9p loci in preneoplastic lesions accompanying non-small-cell lung cancers. *J Natl Cancer Inst* 1995; 87: 1224–1229.
19. Kishimoto Y, Murakami Y, Shiraishi M, *et al.* Aberrations of the p53 tumor suppressor gene in human non-small cell carcinomas of the lung. *Cancer Res* 1992; 52: 4799–4804.
20. Westra WH, Slebos RJ, Offerhaus GJ, *et al.* K-ras oncogene activation in lung adenocarcinomas from former smokers. Evidence that K-ras mutations are an early and irreversible event in the development of adenocarcinoma of the lung. *Cancer* 1993; 72: 432–438.
21. Hirsch FR, Varella-Garcia M, Bunn PA Jr, *et al.* Epidermal growth factor receptor in non-small-cell lung carcinomas: correlation between gene copy number and protein expression and impact on prognosis. *J Clin Oncol* 2003; 21: 3798–3807.
22. Lynch TJ, Bell DW, Sordella R, *et al.* Activating mutations in the epidermal growth factor receptor underlying responsiveness of non-small-cell lung cancer to gefitinib. *N Engl J Med* 2004; 350: 2129–2139.
23. Paez JG, Janne PA, Lee JC, *et al.* EGFR mutations in lung cancer: correlation with clinical response to gefitinib therapy. *Science* 2004; 304: 1497–1500.
24. van Zandwijk N, Mathy A, Boerrigter L, *et al.* EGFR and KRAS mutations as criteria for treatment with tyrosine kinase inhibitors: retro- and prospective observations in non-small-cell lung cancer. *Ann Oncol* 2007; 18: 99–103.
25. Tang X, Shigematsu H, Bekele BN, *et al.* EGFR tyrosine kinase domain mutations are detected in histologically normal respiratory epithelium in lung cancer patients. *Cancer Res* 2005; 65: 7568–7572.
26. Ortiz-Vega S, Khokhlatchev A, Nedwidek M, *et al.* The putative tumor suppressor RASSF1A homodimerizes and heterodimerizes with the Ras-GTP binding protein Nore1. *Oncogene* 2002; 21: 1381–1390.
27. Agathanggelou A, Honorio S, Macartney DP, *et al.* Methylation associated inactivation of RASSF1A from region 3p21.3 in lung, breast and ovarian tumours. *Oncogene* 2001; 20: 1509–1518.
28. Burbee DG, Forgacs E, Zochbauer-Muller S, *et al.* Epigenetic inactivation of RASSF1A in lung and breast cancers and malignant phenotype suppression. *J Natl Cancer Inst* 2001; 93: 691–699.
29. Leid M, Kastner P, Chambon P. Multiplicity generates diversity in the retinoic acid signalling pathways. *Trends Biochem Sci* 1992; 17: 427–433.
30. Xu XC, Sozzi G, Lee JS, *et al.* Suppression of retinoic acid receptor-β in non-small-cell lung cancer *in vivo*: implications for lung cancer development. *J Natl Cancer Inst* 1997; 89: 624–629.
31. Berard J, Laboune F, Mukuna M, *et al.* Lung tumors in mice expressing an antisense RARβ2 transgene. *FASEB J* 1996; 10: 1091–1097.
32. Toulouse A, Morin J, Dion PA, *et al.* RARβ2 specificity in mediating RA inhibition of growth of lung cancer-derived cells. *Lung Cancer* 2000; 28: 127–137.
33. Khuri FR, Lotan R, Kemp BL, *et al.* Retinoic acid receptor-β as a prognostic indicator in stage I non-small-cell lung cancer. *J Clin Oncol* 2000; 18: 2798–2804.
34. Kim JS, Lee H, Kim H, *et al.* Promoter methylation of retinoic acid receptor β2 and the development of second primary lung cancers in non-small-cell lung cancer. *J Clin Oncol* 2004; 22: 3443–3450.
35. Khuri FR, Lotan R. Retinoids in lung cancer: friend, foe, or fellow traveler? *J Clin Oncol* 2004; 22: 3435–3437.

36. Xu H, Spitz MR, Amos CI, *et al.* Complex segregation analysis reveals a multigene model for lung cancer. *Hum Genet* 2005; 116: 121–127.
37. Hung RJ, McKay JD, Gaborieau V, *et al.* A susceptibility locus for lung cancer maps to nicotinic acetylcholine receptor subunit genes on 15q25. *Nature* 2008; 452: 633–637.
38. Amos CI, Wu X, Broderick P, *et al.* Genome-wide association scan of tag SNPs identifies a susceptibility locus for lung cancer at 15q25.1. *Nat Genet* 2008; 40: 616–622.
39. Spitz MR, Wu X, Wang Y, *et al.* Modulation of nucleotide excision repair capacity by XPD polymorphisms in lung cancer patients. *Cancer Res* 2001; 61: 1354–1357.
40. Spitz MR, Duphorne CM, Detry MA, *et al.* Dietary intake of isothiocyanates: evidence of a joint effect with glutathione *S*-transferase polymorphisms in lung cancer risk. *Cancer Epidemiol Biomarkers Prev* 2000; 9: 1017–1020.
41. Wang L-E, Cheng L, Spitz MR, *et al.* Fas A670G polymorphism, apoptotic capacity in lymphocyte cultures, and risk of lung cancer. *Lung Cancer* 2003; 42: 1–8.
42. Wu X, Zhao H, Wei Q, *et al.* XPA polymorphism associated with reduced lung cancer risk and a modulating effect on nucleotide excision repair capacity. *Carcinogenesis* 2003; 24: 505–509.
43. Wei Q, Cheng L, Amos CI, *et al.* Repair of tobacco carcinogen-induced DNA adducts and lung cancer risk: a molecular epidemiologic study. *J Natl Cancer Inst* 2000; 92: 1764–1772.
44. Hecht SS. Tobacco smoke carcinogens and lung cancer. *J Natl Cancer Inst* 1999; 91: 1194–1210.
45. Block G, Patterson B, Subar A. Fruit, vegetables, and cancer prevention: a review of the epidemiological evidence. *Nutr Cancer* 1992; 18: 1–29.
46. Clark LC, Combs GF Jr, Turnbull BW, *et al.* Effects of selenium supplementation for cancer prevention in patients with carcinoma of the skin. A randomized controlled trial. Nutritional Prevention of Cancer Study Group. *JAMA* 1996; 276: 1957–1963.
47. Sporn MB, Dunlop NM, Newton DL, *et al.* Prevention of chemical carcinogenesis by vitamin A and its synthetic analogs (retinoids). *Fed Proc* 1976; 35: 1332–1338.
48. The effect of vitamin E and beta carotene on the incidence of lung cancer and other cancers in male smokers. The Alpha-Tocopherol, Beta Carotene Cancer Prevention Study Group. *N Engl J Med* 1994; 330: 1029–1035.
49. Omenn GS, Goodman GE, Thornquist MD, *et al.* Effects of a combination of beta carotene and vitamin A on lung cancer and cardiovascular disease. *N Engl J Med* 1996; 334: 1150–1155.
50. Hennekens CH, Buring JE, Manson JE, *et al.* Lack of effect of long-term supplementation with beta carotene on the incidence of malignant neoplasms and cardiovascular disease. *N Engl J Med* 1996; 334: 1145–1149.
51. Virtamo J, Pietinen P, Huttunen JK, *et al.* Incidence of cancer and mortality following alpha-tocopherol and beta-carotene supplementation: a postintervention follow-up. *JAMA* 2003; 290: 476–485.
52. Goodman M, Morgan RW, Ray R, *et al.* Cancer in asbestos-exposed occupational cohorts: a meta-analysis. *Cancer Causes Control* 1999; 10: 453–465.
53. Cullen MR, Barnett MJ, Balmes JR, *et al.* Predictors of lung cancer among asbestos-exposed men in the beta-carotene and retinol efficacy trial. *Am J Epidemiol* 2005; 161: 260–270.
54. Lee JS, Lippman SM, Benner SE, *et al.* Randomized placebo-controlled trial of isotretinoin in chemoprevention of bronchial squamous metaplasia. *J Clin Oncol* 1994; 12: 937–945.
55. Kurie JM, Lotan R, Lee JJ, *et al.* Treatment of former smokers with 9-*cis*-retinoic acid reverses loss of retinoic acid receptor-β expression in the bronchial epithelium: results from a randomized placebo-controlled trial. *J Natl Cancer Inst* 2003; 95: 206–214.
56. Arnold AM, Browman GP, Levine MN, *et al.* The effect of the synthetic retinoid etretinate on sputum cytology: results from a randomised trial. *Br J Cancer* 1992; 65: 737–743.
57. McLarty JW, Holiday DB, Girard WM, *et al.* Beta-carotene, vitamin A, and lung cancer chemoprevention: results of an intermediate endpoint study. *Am J Clin Nutr* 1995; 62: Suppl. 6, 1431S–1438S.

58. Heimburger DC, Alexander CB, Birch R, *et al.* Improvement in bronchial squamous metaplasia in smokers treated with folate and vitamin B12. Report of a preliminary randomized, double-blind intervention trial. *JAMA* 1988; 259: 1525–1530.
59. van Poppel G, Kok FJ, Hermus RJ. Beta-carotene supplementation in smokers reduces the frequency of micronuclei in sputum. *Br J Cancer* 1992; 66: 1164–1168.
60. Mao JT, Fishbein MC, Adams B, *et al.* Celecoxib decreases Ki-67 proliferative index in active smokers. *Clin Cancer Res* 2006; 12: 314–320.
61. Van Schooten FJ, Besaratinia A, De Flora S, *et al.* Effects of oral administration of *N*-acetyl-L-cysteine: a multi-biomarker study in smokers. *Cancer Epidemiol Biomarkers Prev* 2002; 11: 167–175.
62. Lam S, MacAulay C, Le Riche JC, *et al.* A randomized phase IIb trial of anethole dithiolethione in smokers with bronchial dysplasia. *J Natl Cancer Inst* 2002; 94: 1001–1009.
63. Soria JC, Moon C, Wang L, *et al.* Effects of *N*-(4-hydroxyphenyl)retinamide on hTERT expression in the bronchial epithelium of cigarette smokers. *J Natl Cancer Inst* 2001; 93: 1257–1263.
64. Lam S, leRiche JC, McWilliams A, *et al.* A randomized phase IIb trial of pulmicort turbuhaler (budesonide) in people with dysplasia of the bronchial epithelium. *Clin Cancer Res* 2004; 10: 6502–6511.
65. van den Berg RM, van Tinteren H, van Zandwijk N, *et al.* The influence of fluticasone inhalation on markers of carcinogenesis in bronchial epithelium. *Am J Respir Crit Care Med* 2007; 175: 1061–1065.
66. Decker J, Goldstein JC. Risk factors in head and neck cancer. *N Engl J Med* 1982; 306: 1151–1155.
67. Wynder EL, Stellman SD. Impact of long-term filter cigarette usage on lung and larynx cancer risk: a case-control study. *J Natl Cancer Inst* 1979; 62: 471–477.
68. Gluckman JL, Crissman JD. Survival rates in 548 patients with multiple neoplasms of the upper aerodigestive tract. *Laryngoscope* 1983; 93: 71–74.
69. Yellin A, Hill LR, Benfield JR. Bronchogenic carcinoma associated with upper aerodigestive cancers. *J Thorac Cardiovasc Surg* 1986; 91: 674–683.
70. Vokes EE, Weichselbaum RR, Lippman SM, Hong WK. Head and neck cancer. *N Engl J Med* 1993; 328: 184–194.
71. Vikram B. Changing patterns of failure in advanced head and neck cancer. *Arch Otolaryngol* 1984; 110: 564–565.
72. Lippman SM, Hong WK. Not yet standard: retinoids *versus* second primary tumors. *J Clin Oncol* 1993; 11: 1204–1207.
73. Lippman SM, Hong WK. Second malignant tumors in head and neck squamous cell carcinoma: the overshadowing threat for patients with early-stage disease. *Int J Radiat Oncol Biol Phys* 1989; 17: 691–694.
74. Larson JT, Adams GL, Fattah HA. Survival statistics for multiple primaries in head and neck cancer. *Otolaryngol Head Neck Surg* 1990; 103: 14–24.
75. Hong WK, Lippman SM, Itri LM, *et al.* Prevention of second primary tumors with isotretinoin in squamous-cell carcinoma of the head and neck. *N Engl J Med* 1990; 323: 795–801.
76. Khuri FR, Lee JJ, Lippman SM, *et al.* Randomized phase III trial of low-dose isotretinoin for prevention of second primary tumors in stage I and II head and neck cancer patients. *J Natl Cancer Inst* 2006; 98: 441–450.
77. Pastorino U, Infante M, Maioli M, *et al.* Adjuvant treatment of stage I lung cancer with high-dose vitamin A. *J Clin Oncol* 1993; 11: 1216–1222.
78. Bolla M, Lefur R, Ton Van J, *et al.* Prevention of second primary tumours with etretinate in squamous cell carcinoma of the oral cavity and oropharynx. Results of a multicentric double-blind randomised study. *Eur J Cancer* 1994; 30A: 767–772.
79. van Zandwijk N, Dalesio O, Pastorino U, *et al.* EUROSCAN, a randomized trial of vitamin A and *N*-acetylcysteine in patients with head and neck cancer or lung cancer. For the European Organization for Research and Treatment of Cancer Head and Neck and Lung Cancer Cooperative Groups. *J Natl Cancer Inst* 2000; 92: 977–986.

80. Lippman SM, Lee JJ, Karp DD, *et al.* Randomized phase III intergroup trial of isotretinoin to prevent second primary tumors in stage I non-small-cell lung cancer. *J Natl Cancer Inst* 2001; 93: 605–618.
81. Schabath MB, Hernandez LM, Wu X, *et al.* Dietary phytoestrogens and lung cancer risk. *JAMA* 2005; 294: 1493–1504.
82. Kurie JM, Shin HJ, Lee JS, *et al.* Increased epidermal growth factor receptor expression in metaplastic bronchial epithelium. *Clin Cancer Res* 1996; 2: 1787–1793.
83. Rusch V, Baselga J, Cordon-Cardo C, *et al.* Differential expression of the epidermal growth factor receptor and its ligands in primary non-small cell lung cancers and adjacent benign lung. *Cancer Res* 1993; 53: Suppl. 10, 2379–2385.
84. Shepherd FA, Rodrigues Pereira J, Ciuleanu T, *et al.* Erlotinib in previously treated non-small-cell lung cancer. *N Engl J Med* 2005; 353: 123–132.
85. Thatcher N, Chang A, Parikh P, *et al.* Gefitinib plus best supportive care in previously treated patients with refractory advanced non-small-cell lung cancer: results from a randomised, placebo-controlled, multicentre study (Iressa Survival Evaluation in Lung Cancer). *Lancet* 2005; 366: 1527–1537.
86. Kim ES, Hong WK, Lee JJ, *et al.* A randomized double-blind study of the biological effects of celecoxib as a chemopreventive agent in current and former smokers. *J Clin Oncol* 2008; 26S: 1501.
87. Keith RL, Miller YE, Hudish TM, *et al.* Pulmonary prostacyclin synthase overexpression chemoprevents tobacco smoke lung carcinogenesis in mice. *Cancer Res* 2004; 64: 5897–5904.
88. Govindarajan R, Ratnasinghe L, Simmons DL, *et al.* Thiazolidinediones and the risk of lung, prostate, and colon cancer in patients with diabetes. *J Clin Oncol* 2007; 25: 1476–1481.

CHAPTER 2

Pathology and immunohistochemistry of lung cancer

E. Brambilla, S. Lantuejoul

Institut Albert Bonniot, INSERM U823, Université Joseph Fourier Grenoble 1, CHU Albert Michallon, Dept of Pathology, Grenoble, France.

Correspondence: E. Brambilla, CHU Albert Michallon, Dept of Pathology, BP 217, 38043 Grenoble Cedex 09, France. Fax: 33 476765949; E-mail: EBrambilla@chu-grenoble.fr

With 169,500 new cases per year in the USA and 182,000 new cases per year in Europe, lung cancer is the most common worldwide diagnosed cancer and the major cause of mortality [1], with 157,400 cancer deaths [2] in the USA and 190,000 cancer deaths in the European Union in 2001. Although cancer incidence began to decline in males in the USA from 1980, its rate is increasing in females as a consequence of the increasing proportion of smoking females [2].

The international standard for histological classification of lung tumours is that proposed by the World Health Organization (WHO) and the International Association for the Study of Lung Cancer (IASLC) in 1999 [3]; the standard was further documented with molecular characteristics in 2004 [4] (table 1). The four major histological types of lung cancer are as follows: squamous cell carcinoma (SCC); adenocarcinoma, the incidence of which is increasing at the expense of SCC; small cell lung carcinoma (SCLC); and large cell carcinoma. These major types have been subclassified into subtypes, the clinical significance of which might be extremely important, *e.g.* bronchioloalveolar carcinoma (BAC) as a variant of adenocarcinoma [3].

While lung cancer can be divided into many subtypes, the most important distinction is not only between SCLC and nonsmall cell lung carcinoma (NSCLC). Clinical importance has been given to this distinction because of the major clinical differences in presentation, metastatic spread and response to therapy of SCLC. However, this is an extremely simplistic way of distinguishing between these subtypes that is not recommended because it may override the clinical significance of specific subtypes like BAC and because the chemotherapeutical decisions are, more than ever, based on histological typing (*e.g.* nonsquamous adenocarcinoma *versus* squamous). There is a strong distribution bias of histology between smokers developing all categories and nonsmokers presenting mostly with adenocarcinoma. Histological heterogeneity is an important feature of the pathology of lung cancer that often consists of a mixture of histological types representing a derivation of lung cancer from a pluripotent stem cell [5, 6]. This histological heterogeneity is apparent on light microscopic examination in $\geq 30\%$ of lung cancers, and is even more frequently seen by electron microscopy.

Squamous cell carcinoma

SCC is a malignant epithelial tumour showing keratinisation and/or intercellular bridges that arises from bronchial epithelium [4]. It is divided into the following

Eur Respir Mon, 2009, 44, 15–35. Printed in UK - all rights reserved. Copyright ERS Journals Ltd 2009; European Respiratory Monograph; ISSN 1025-448x.

Table 1. – World Health Organization histological classification of tumours of the lung[#]

Malignant epithelial tumours		
Squamous cell carcinoma		8070/3
Papillary	8052/3	
Clear cell		8084/3
Small cell		8073/3
Basaloid	8083/3	
Small cell carcinoma		8041/3
Combined small cell carcinoma		8045/3
Adenocarcinoma		8140/3
Adenocarcinoma, mixed subtype		8255/3
Acinar adenocarcinoma		8550/3
Papillary adenocarcinoma		8260/3
Bronchioloalveolar carcinoma		8250/3
Nonmucinous		8252/3
Mucinous		8253/3
Mixed nonmucinous and mucinous or indeterminate		8254/3
Solid adenocarcinoma with mucin production	8230/3	
Fetal adenocarcinoma		8333/3
Mucinous ("colloid") carcinoma		8480/3
Mucinous cystadenocarcinoma		8470/3
Signet ring adenocarcinoma	8490/3	
Clear cell adenocarcinoma	8310/3	
Large cell carcinoma		8012/3
Large cell neuroendocrine carcinoma	8013/3	
Combined large cell neuroendocrine carcinoma	8013/3	
Basaloid carcinoma		8123/3
Lymphoepithelioma-like carcinoma		8082/3
Clear cell carcinoma		8310/3
Large cell carcinoma with rhabdoid phenotype	8014/3	
Adenosquamous carcinoma	8560/3	
Sarcomatoid carcinoma		8033/3
Pleomorphic carcinoma		8022/3
Spindle cell carcinoma		8032/3
Giant cell carcinoma		8031/3
Carcinosarcoma		8980/3
Pulmonary blastoma		8972/3
Carcinoid tumour	8240/3	
Typical carcinoid		8240/3
Atypical carcinoma	8249/3	
Salivary gland tumours		
Mucoepidermoid carcinoma	8430/3	
Adenoid cystic carcinoma		8200/3
Epithelial–myoepithelial carcinoma		8562/3
Pre-invasive lesions		
Squamous carcinoma *in situ*	8070/2	
Atypical adenomatous hyperplasia		
Diffuse idiopathic pulmonary neuroendocrine cell hyperplasia		
Mesenchymal tumours		
Epithelioid haemangioendothelioma	9133/1	
Angiosarcoma		9120/3
Pleuropulmonary blastoma	8973/3	
Chondroma		9220/0
Congenial peribronchial myofibroblastic tumour	8827/1	
Diffuse pulmonary lymphangiomatosis		
Inflammatory myofibroblastic tumour	8825/1	
Lymphangioleiomyomatosis	9174/1	
Synovial sarcoma	9040/3	
Monophasic		9041/3
Biphasic	9043/3	
Pulmonary artery sarcoma	8800/3	
Pulmonary vein sarcoma		8800/3

Table 1. – Continued

Benign epithelial tumours		
Papillomas		
Squamous cell papilloma		8052/0
Exophytic		8052/0
Inverted		8053/0
Glandular papilloma		8260/0
Mixed squamous cell and glandular papilloma	8560/0	
Adenomas		
Alveolar adenoma	8251/0	
Papillary adenoma	8260/0	
Adenomas of the salivary gland type		
Mucous gland adenoma		8140/0
Pleomorphic adenoma		8940/0
Others		
Mucinous cystadenoma		8470/0
Lymphoproliferative tumours		
Marginal zone B-cell lymphoma of the MALT type		9699/3
Diffuse large B-cell lymphoma		9680/3
Lymphomatoid granulomatosis		9766/1
Langerhans cell histiocystosis		9751/1
Miscellaneous tumours		
Harmatoma		
Sclerosing haemangioma		8832/0
Clear cell tumour		8005/0
Germ cell tumours		
Teratoma, mature	9080/0	
Immature		9080/3
Other germ cell tumours		
Intrapulmonary thymoma		8590/1
Melanoma		8720/3
Metastatic tumours		

#: the second and third columns show the morphology code of the International Classification of Diseases for Oncology (ICD-O) [6] and the Systematized Nomenclature of Medicine (http://snomed.org). Behaviour is coded /0 for benign tumours, /3 for malignant tumours, and /1 for borderline or uncertain behaviour.

subtypes: 1) papillary subtype; 2) clear cell subtype; 3) small cell subtype; and 4) basaloid subtype.

SCC accounts for ~30% of all lung cancers in the USA and 45% in Europe. 20 yrs ago, it was the most frequent histological type of lung cancer in Europe; incidence progressively decreased, while adenocarcinoma increased in incidence. >90% of SCCs occur in cigarette smokers. An undefined proportion of SCCs develop from invasive lesions collectively called squamous dysplasia. The rate of progression from pre-invasive to invasive lesion is unpredictable, although a higher risk parallels a higher grade of dysplasia. Most carcinoma *in situ* are believed to evolve in lung cancer after local treatment [7]. Two-thirds of SCCs present as central tumours, whereas one-third present as peripheral tumours, although the primary bronchial site may be easily detected at histology [8]. The morphological features that characterise squamous differentiation include intercellular bridges and keratinisation (or individual cell keratinisation or squamous pearl formation). These differentiated features are readily apparent in well-differentiated and difficult to detect in poorly differentiated tumours. However, this spectrum of differentiation has not been demonstrated to correlate with prognosis in lung SCC. Segmental bronchi more often than lobar and mainstem bronchi are the primary site of SCC.

Variants described in the WHO classification include papillary, clear cell, small cell and basaloid subtypes [3, 9]. The last variant, basaloid carcinoma, has a dismal prognosis compared with poorly differentiated SCC [10, 11]. In a recent evaluation of a large series of cases where those with basaloid carcinoma appear to have a shorter survival time than those cases with other types of NSCLCs ($p=0.005$), the basaloid variant of SCC did not differ from pure basaloid cases with respect to survival [12]. Papillary SCCs often show a pattern of exophytic endobronchial growth. Although a small cell variant has been described, it is still an ill-defined entity that should not be used.

Immunohistochemistry

SSC diagnosis does not rely on immunohistochemical markers on surgical or large samples; it shows obvious squamous differentiation signs in small biopsies. However, in the context of a specific targeted chemotherapy (pemetrexed, bevacizumab), where survival benefit or safety has been shown to be restricted to nonsquamous carcinoma, one may question the use of immunohistochemical markers on poorly differentiated carcinoma. Thyroid transcription factor (TTF)-1 and mucin-positive stainings may be used as exclusion markers, characteristic of adenocarcinoma and cytokeratins (CKs) of certain isoforms, such as CKs 1, 5, 10 and 14 (collectively recognised by antibodies CK903 and CK34βE12), CK 5–6 and p63, as inclusion markers, although none of these positive markers disclose a 100% sensitivity or specificity. A panel of negative and positive markers will be highly recommended for this distinction between squamous and nonsquamous carcinoma in the next revision of the WHO lung cancer classification.

Adenocarcinoma

Adenocarcinoma is a malignant epithelial tumour with glandular differentiation or mucin production, showing acinar, papillary, bronchioloalveolar or solid with mucin growth patterns or a mixture of these patterns. It is divided into the following subtypes. 1) Adenocarcinoma, 2) adenocarcinoma mixed subtype, 3) acinar adenocarcinoma, 4) papillary adenocarcinoma, and 5) BAC, of which there are the following: i) nonmucinous, ii) mucinous, iii) mixed nonmucinous and mucinous, and iv) solid adenocarcinoma with mucin production. The variants of adenocarcinoma are as follows: 1) fetal adenocarcinoma; 2) mucinous ("colloid") carcinoma; 3) mucinous cystadenocarcinoma; 4) signet ring adenocarcinoma; and 5) clear cell adenocarcinoma.

Adenocarcinomas account for 50–60% of lung cancer in Europe and the USA [13]. Most primary pulmonary adenocarcinomas, in contrast with metastases, are highly heterogeneous and consist of a mixture of histological subtypes. Adenocarcinomas are histologically the most heterogeneous lung tumours, with sarcomatoid carcinoma consisting of two or more of the histological subtypes; most of lung adenocarcinomas diagnosed today are classified into the mixed subtype. For this reason, the adenocarcinoma mixed subtype was moved to the top of the list of adenocarcinoma subtypes in the 2004 WHO classification, despite not being recognised in the 1981 WHO classification [14]. The acinar and papillary subtypes are recognised by their architectural pattern of tumour cell growth and, together with solid type, represent invasive adenocarcinoma. The solid type is a poorly differentiated carcinoma presenting intracytoplasmic mucins that should consist of at least of five mucin droplets at two different high-power fields. Periodic acid–Schiff with diastase digestion and Kreyberg staining with Alcian blue are the recommended mucin stains. A substantially different definition has been given for BAC subtype, which should be restricted to tumours that grow in a purely lepidic fashion without invasion of stroma, blood vessels or pleura.

Several additional unusual variants were also recognised, such as well-differentiated fetal adenocarcinoma [15], mucinous ("colloid") adenocarcinoma [16], mucinous cystadenocarcinoma [17], signet ring carcinoma, and clear cell adenocarcinoma [3]. Two unusual gross patterns of adenocarcinoma include the endobronchial polypoid adenocarcinoma [18] and pseudomesotheliomatous adenocarcinoma [19].

BAC is uncommon in its pure type, and probably restricted to <3% of all lung malignancies [13]. In the new 1999 WHO/IASLC classification, BAC is defined as a tumour showing lepidic growth along respected alveolar septa with intact elastic and basal lamina frames, without invasive growth. It should be noticed that some increased fibrotic collagen deposit of alveolar walls is accepted, as long as no myofibroblastic proliferation is visible. Invasive growth includes alveolar lumens with papillary and micropapillary structures. The lack of invasive growth is added as an essential criterion [3], based on clinicopathological data indicating that BAC may be curable by economic surgical resection in patients with <2 cm growth [20]. As a result of the narrow criteria for BAC, the term adenocarcinoma, mixed subtype is used for tumours that have both BAC and an invasive component. In such cases, the invasive patterns present (acinar, papillary or solid) should be mentioned. It is common to observe central scars in pulmonary adenocarcinoma that contain invasive components and a focal BAC-like pattern at the periphery of the tumour. As a consequence of this revised definition of BAC, the literature dealing with these tumours needs complete re-evaluation. Indeed, previously to the last classification, BAC included tumours with obvious invasive growth [14, 21], especially papillary components. Those tumours with a predominantly lepidic growth pattern (as a dominant component over the others) behave differently to other mixed invasive adenocarcinomas, with longer survival at stage I–II [22]. Of carcinomas previously defined as BACs, >50% present with focal central desmoplastic scaring tissue or intra-alveolar complex papillary growth, while the lepidic growth starts around the edge of the scar. The diagnosis for those tumours with predominant lepidic (BAC) growth pattern showing malignant tumour cell nests in a desmoplastic stromal reaction is adenocarcinoma mixed subtype, and the percentage of subtypes present should be mentioned (such as acinar, papillary or BAC) and measured in quartiles (at 10% intervals). These are no longer considered to be pure BAC, and filling of alveolar lumens by papillary or micropapillary structures is also considered to be papillary adenocarcinoma but not BAC. The extent of micropapillary or papillary component in stage I adenocarcinoma with BAC lepidic growth pattern is an important prognostic factor [23].

BACs have two major cytological subtypes, nonmucinous and mucinous [3], and are rarely mixed, *i.e.* consisting of an association of mucinous and nonmucinous cells [3]. The majority of BACs are mucin-producing, followed by nonmucinous type, while ~12% are a mixture of both. Nonmucinous BACs consist of Clara cells and type II pneumocytes, which is a common stem cell for distal bronchioles and alveoli identified in fetal lung and nowadays considered to be the lung adenocarcinoma stem cell [24]. Nonmucinous BACs are more likely to be solitary than the mucinous type. These tumours are composed of cuboidal cells proliferating along alveolar septa and show a hobnail appearance. Specific nuclear inclusions are patent in half of the nonmucinous tumour cells that are stained with diastase-digested periodic acid–Schiff and immunohistochemically for surfactant apoprotein. On electron microscopy, these inclusions form a network of 40-nm diameter microtubules [25, 26]. Nonmucinous BAC may be epidermal growth factor receptor (EGFR) mutant or Ras mutant.

The mucin-producing BACs tend to be more multicentric and characteristically have mucin production. They may cause lobar consolidation resembling pneumonia on gross examination. Histologically, these tumours consist of tall columnar cells with abundant apical cytoplasmic mucin and small basally oriented regular bland nuclei lining thin alveolar septa. Their stem cell is likely to be a mucinous metaplastic bronchiolar cell. Alveolar and bronchiolar spaces are filled with abundant mucin. They are more often Ras mutant and not EGFR mutant.

According to the 1999 WHO/IASLC classification, a final diagnosis of BAC can only be achieved at examination of a surgical resection specimen. Small biopsies obtained by bronchoscopy or fine needle sampling may show a lepidic growth pattern, suggesting the possibility of BAC, but are not sufficient to exclude the presence of an invasive growth.

Papillary adenocarcinomas include several papillary patterns, usually papillae with wide fibrovascular cores lined by high cuboidal to cylindrical nonmucinous tumour cells, complex secondary and tertiary papillary pattern filling alveolar lumen in the background on preserved alveolar walls and micropapillary pattern, the last of which is possibly associated with any invasive histological type: acinary, papillary, solid and BAC. These micropapillary components are important as adverse prognostic factors in mixed adenocarcinoma [23, 27].

Papillary adenocarcinoma is the most frequent adenocarcinoma associated with EGFR mutations [28], followed by acinar pattern.

Pathoradiological correlations

There are several growth presentations for the most common adenocarcinoma mixed subtype with BAC: 1) a solitary nodule, 2) multiple nodules with 3) lobar consolidation, and 4) pseudopneumonic diffuse infiltration.

The typical radiological appearance of BAC (pure BAC or BAC component) is the ground-glass opacity by computed tomography (CT) and an ill-defined aerated spongy density at gross examination. In contrast, a grossly circumscribed nodule at growth examination and a pure solid appearance by CT is typical of purely invasive adenocarcinoma (acinar, papillary, solid). In between, a mixture of these growth and CT appearances is seen in mixed subtype adenocarcinoma with both invasive (often centrally located) components and BAC component (often peripheral). When BAC and other adenocarcinoma present with multiple nodules, they can be unilateral or bilateral. Unilateral nodules (classified T4 according to TNM classification) or multiple nodules in another lobe (classified as M1). Lobar consolidation and diffuse pseudopneumonic condensation patterns are difficult to distinguish either grossly or radiologically from infective pneumonia. All cases of adenocarcinoma presenting with diffuse or pseudopneumonic consolidation pattern have been shown to correspond to mixed subtype adenocarcinoma with BAC component, more frequently of mucinous type, and a varying amount of acinar, papillary and solid components.

Prognostic correlations with solitary small peripheral lung nodules

Several important clinicopathological studies have shown the clinical significance of BAC [20, 29, 30]. NOGUCHI *et al.* [20] reported on a large series of 236 patients with peripheral lung adenocarcinomas of <2 cm with a 100% 5-yr survival rate. These were pure BAC, and patient survival rates contrast sharply with those of patients with "invasive BAC", who experienced higher mortality and reduced 5-yr survival rate of 75%, while purely invasive form had a 5-yr survival rate of 52%. In a series of 100 patients with peripheral adenocarcinoma <3 cm, SUZUKI *et al.* [29] demonstrated that a fibrotic scar size of ≤5 mm was correlated with a 100% 5-yr survival rate, which was in contrast with a 70% 5-yr survival rate for patients with larger scars (5–15 mm) and a 40% 5-yr survival rate for patients with a central scar >15 mm in size. In this study [29], the size of central fibrosis was an independent prognostic factor on multivariate analysis (p=0.01) that was as significant as vascular invasion (p=0.024) and lymph node metastasis (p=0.024). Later, YOKOSE *et al.* [30] studied multiple pathological factors for prognostic assessment in 200 patients: 100% 5-yr survival was associated with at least one of the following features: 1) a pattern of lepidic growth of >75%, 2) a central scar measuring ≤5 mm, and 3) a lack of destruction of the elastic fibre framework by tumour cells [30]. The most significant determinants of shorter survival in the multivariate analysis were vascular invasion (p<0.001) and >25% papillary or invasive growth (p=0.043). Size and grade/pattern of stromal invasion [22, 31] are also influencing survival. Recently, confirmation was given in a series in the USA [32, 33] showing the significant survival differences in stage I–II adenocarcinoma based on proportion of BAC component (<5 mm or >5 mm invasive scar). This has practical consequences: all small (≤3 cm) tumours with a predominant BAC component should be serially entirely sampled and included so that potential foci of invasion are detected, providing the prognostic importance of invasion, size and proportion.

Immunohistochemistry

TTF-1 is the stem cell marker and hallmark of all peripheral respiratory unit proliferations characterised by Clara cell-type II histogenesis. TTF-1 expression, CK7 expression, surfactant AB and/or Clara cell antigen CC10, are the usual phenotype of peripheral adenocarcinoma, including nonmucinous BAC, mixed-type adenocarcinoma with BAC component, and papillary adenocarcinoma, the two last being less commonly used for differential diagnosis. TTF-1 is negative in 25% of adenocarcinomas comprising of central/derived tumours arising from a bronchial ill-defined stem cells. Mucinous BAC presents no TTF-1 expression, positive CK-7 and/or CK-20 expression, and abundant mucin production.

Acinar adenocarcinoma shows usually, and papillary always, TTF-1 expression. Solid-type adenocarcinoma is typically mucin producing with at least five droplets in two independent high-power fields. TTF-1 is expressed in the majority, but not all.

There are contrasting phenotypic features between peripheral-type adenocarcinoma and those of bronchioloalveolar origin in TTF-1 expression and nonmucin and EGFR (nonsmokers) or Ras mutation and central-type adenocarcinoma of mucinous or cells origin with no TTF-1 expression but exclusive Ras mutation (smokers).

Central adenocarcinoma may display P53 and KRas and/or LKB1 (STK11) mutation but no EGFR mutation. They may show EML4-ALK translocation and fusion transcript linked with ALK4 expression [34].

Small cell lung carcinoma

SCLC is a malignant epithelial tumour consisting of small cells with scant cytoplasm, ill-defined cell borders, finely granular nuclear chromatin, and absent or inconspicuous nucleoli. The cells are round, oval and spindle-shaped. Its variant is the combined SCLC.

SCLC accounts for 25% of all lung cancers in the USA, as well as in Europe [13]. Two-thirds of SCLC are proximal and present as a perihilar tumour. They occur in bronchial locations infiltrating the bronchial submucosa and subsequently lead to bronchial obstruction by circumferential compression. SCLC is not commonly observed on a surgical specimen as extensive lymph node metastasis is common and the tumour is not surgically curable. Macroscopically the tumour is soft, friable, white-tan in colour and extensively necrotic. Extensive lymph node metastasis is common and <5% of cases present as a solitary coin lesion [35].

The 1999 WHO/IASLC classification presents only two types of SCLC, SCLC (with pure SCLC histology) and combined SCLC (combined with any nonsmall cell type; see table 1) [3]. The two subtypes are oat cell carcinoma and intermediate cell type, which were proposed in the 1981 WHO classification, as well as the category of mixed small cell, large cell proposed in 1988 by IASLC recommendation, were discarded from the new classification because of difficulties in reproducibility of these subtypes and lack of confirmation that these patients had a different prognosis [36].

SCLC has a distinctive histological appearance. Tumour cells have a small size, not exceeding that of three lymphocytes. They have a round or fusiform shape, scant cytoplasm with a nuclear to cytoplasmic ratio of 9:10, a finely granular nuclear chromatin (salt and pepper appearance) and either absent or inconspicuous nucleoli [13]. Nuclear moulding and smearing of nuclear chromatin is frequent, caused by crush artefact. There is usually an extensive necrosis and mitotic rate exceeding 20 and reaching 100 mitosis per 2 mm^2 area. Most often, the growth pattern consists of diffuse sheets, although endocrine differentiations with rosettes, palisading, ribbons and organoid nesting might be seen. In necrotic areas, basophilic encrustation of vessel walls is known as the Azzopardi effect.

Depending on the biopsy specimens, the tumour cell size of SCLC might appear larger, which is often the case in well-fixed open biopsies, for example, on surgical resection or mediastinoscopy obtained material.

Fine-needle aspiration (FNA) biopsy and core biopsy may provide excellent material for assessment of the diagnosis of SCLC, essentially because cytological features of SCLC have a high diagnosis value, although architecture is not critical for the diagnosis. The small cell proliferation, with nuclear moulding, the very high nuclear to cytoplasmic ratio, and the "salt and pepper" quality of chromatin are extremely useful for this diagnosis on FNA. The diagnostic markers (neuroendocrine (NE) markers, TTF-1, absence of CK34βE12 expression) are of primary help in the diagnosis of SCLC. There is an excellent yield of these markers on FNA and/or biopsy [37].

Combined SCLC

The frequency of combined SCLC depends on the extent of histological sampling, and the extent of the associated component. Combined SCLC represents about 10% of SCLC if small biopsies are considered. However, in a recent study on surgically treated SCLC and using a conservative estimate of 10% of tumours showing NSCLC associated for subclassifying a tumour as a combined variant of SCLC, 20% of the cases of SCLC showed a combination with NSCLC, more commonly with large cell lung carcinoma followed by adenocarcinoma and SCC [36, 38–40]. SCLC can also be associated, albeit rarely, with spindle cell carcinoma [41, 42], giant cell carcinoma [41], and carcinosarcoma [43]. Immunohistochemistry that tends to stain NSCLC components, *e.g.* CK antibody cocktails, might help to recognise associated components; CKs 1, 5, 10 and 14 are a good example, being recognised by 34βE12 [44]. However, evidence is lacking that pure SCLC combined SCLC behaved differently regarding prognosis and response to therapy [38]. Following chemotherapy, a mixture of large cells, squamous cells, adenocarcinoma or giant cells with SCLC may be seen in 15–45% of the cases [39, 45–47]; this is likely to be due to selection by chemotherapy of multipotent stem cells of the proliferation. This favours the hypothesis of a common stem cell for derivation of NSCLC and SCLC.

Immunohistochemistry. The most useful and specific neuroendocrine markers for distinction of SCLC in formalin-fixed, paraffin-embedded tissue sections are chromo-

Table 2. – Light microscopic features for distinguishing small cell carcinoma and large cell neuroendocrine carcinoma

Histological feature	Small cell carcinoma	Large cell neuroendocrine carcinoma
Cell size	Smaller (less than the diameter of three lymphocytes)	Larger
Nuclear/cytoplasmic ratio	Higher	Lower
Nuclear chromatin	Finely granular, uniform	Coarsely granular or vesicular; less uniform
Nucleoli	Absent or faint	Often (not always) present; may be prominent or faint
Nuclear moulding	Characteristic	Less prominent
Fusiform shape	Common	Uncommon
Polygonal shape with ample pink cytoplasm	Uncharacteristic	Characteristic
Nuclear smear	Frequent	Uncommon
Basophilic staining of vessels and stroma	Occasional	Rare

Reproduced from [48], with permission from the publisher.

granin A, synaptophysin, and the neural cell adhesion molecule CD56 [48, 49]. Keratin (AE1/AE3) and epithelial membrane antigen , as well as TTF-1, stain virtually all SCLC in open lung biopsy and transbronchial biopsy specimens [44, 48, 50]. However, TTF-1 has a yield of no more than 75–85%. In contrast, a specific set of CKs never expressed in neuroendocrine proliferations (CK 1, 5, 10 and 14) called 34βE12 is always absent in pure SCLC [37]. In cases where common CKs are negative in a suspected SCLC, especially in small biopsy specimens with crush artefact, the pathologist should exclude other possibilities, such as lymphoma (CD45 positive), primitive neuroectodermal tumour, or small cell round sarcoma. One difficulty resides in the fact that ~25% of SCLC express the antigen CD99/MIC-2, as do primitive neuroectodermal tumours and small round cell sarcoma. It is important to recognise that this distinction is based primarily on light microscopy (table 2) [3]. Since no single monoclonal antibody can reliably distinguish SCLC from NSCLC [49], a set of reliable markers should be considered (table 3).

Differential diagnosis. As SCLC has distinctive clinical properties with aggressive clinical course, frequent widespread metastasis of presentation, common paraneoplastic syndrome and responsiveness to chemotherapy, histological classification of lung cancer is often simplified into SCLC *versus* NSCLC. A plethora of criteria is applied for the distinction between SCLC and large cell neuroendocrine carcinoma (LCNEC), including cell size, nucleoli, nuclear-to-cytoplasmic ratio, nuclear chromatin pattern, nuclear moulding, cell shape (fusiform *versus* polygonal), and Azzopardi phenomenon (table 2) [3, 14, 48, 51].

Table 3. – Histochemical differential diagnosis between small cell lung carcinoma, basaloid carcinoma and large cell neuroendocrine carcinoma

	Neuroendocrine markers	Thyroid transcription factor-1	Cytokeratins 1, 5, 10 and 14
Small cell lung cancer	+	+	-
Basaloid carcinoma	-	-	+
Large cell neuroendocrine carcinoma	+	±	-

Disagreement among expert lung cancer pathologists over this distinction occurs in up to 10% of cases [6, 52], owing to the fact that LCNEC may sometimes adopt the nuclear features of SCLC. With the new description of LCNEC, the main differential resides in the distinction of SCLC from LCNEC (table 2).

Large cell carcinoma

Large cell carcinoma comprises large cell neuroendocrine carcinoma and basaloid carcinoma, and the following rare variants: lymphoepithelioma-like carcinoma, clear cell carcinoma and carcinoma with rhabdoid phenotype. It is a tumour that shows no differentiation pattern allowing classification into SCC, adenocarcinoma or SCLC. These poorly differentiated tumours most often arise in the lung periphery, although they may be located centrally. They frequently appear on gross examination as large, necrotic tumours. Histologically, these consist of sheets or nests of large polygonal cells with vesicular nuclei and prominent nucleoli [14]. Although, they are undifferentiated by light microscopy, features of squamous cell or adenocarcinoma might be found at electron microscopy examination [53, 54].

There are several variants of large cell carcinoma, some of which have high clinical significance, recognised in the new WHO/IASLC histological classification of lung cancer (table 1) [3]. These include LCNEC [3, 55], basaloid carcinoma [10, 11, 56], lymphoepithelial-like carcinoma [57], clear cell carcinoma [58], and large cell carcinoma with rhabdoid phenotype [59]. Lymphoepithelial-like carcinoma is described as an Epstein–Barr virus-dependent epithelial proliferation more commonly seen in upper respiratory tract.

As lung cancers are classified according to the best-differentiated component, and areas of large cell carcinoma are frequently observed in poorly differentiated adenocarcinoma or SCC, it is difficult to specifically and appropriately classify many lung cancers in which only small pieces of tissue are available and owing to the common heterogeneity of these cancers. In such cases, the best diagnosis might be "NSCLC" and specification of the most obvious component [60, 61]. A strategy for histological markers differentiating poorly differentiated squamous carcinoma from poorly differentiated adenocarcinoma has been proposed above.

Large cell neuroendocrine carcinoma

LCNEC is a variant of large cell carcinoma. It is a high-grade nonsmall cell neuroendocrine carcinoma that differs from atypical carcinoid and SCLC. Histological criteria include: 1) neuroendocrine morphology (organoid, palisading, trabecular, or rosette-like growth patterns); 2) nonsmall cell cytological features (large size, polygonal shape, low nuclear-to-cytoplasmic ratio, coarse or vesicular nuclear chromatin, and obvious nucleoli); 3) high mitotic rate (≥ 11 per 2 mm^2) with a mean of 60 mitoses per 2 mm^2; 4) frequent necrosis; and 5) at least one positive neuroendocrine immunohistochemical specific marker or neuroendocrine granules by electron microscopy [3]. It is difficult to diagnose LCNEC based on small biopsy specimens because of frequent lack of neuroendocrine morphology without a substantial sampling of the tumours. Some criteria have been proposed based on cytology [62].

The term combined LCNEC is used for tumours associated with other histological types of NSCLC, such as adenocarcinoma or SCC (table 1) [3]. Any combination of LCNEC with SCLC is diagnosed as SCLC combined [3]. A variety of criteria must be used to separate SCLC from LCNEC (table 2).

Immunohistochemistry. By definition, LCNEC diagnosis rests on the expression of NE markers, and at least one of the majority of tumour cells of those considered as specific for NE differentiation. As in SCLC, CKs 1, 5, 10 and 14 are not expressed, except in the combined cases in the NSCLC component. TTF-1 is expressed in 40% of LCNEC, especially in all those cases combined with an adenocarcinoma [37].

In 10% of the cases of NSCLC lacking neuroendocrine morphology, immunohistochemical neuroendocrine markers or neuroendocrine granules by electron microscopy can be demonstrated. Such tumours are called NSCLCs (adenocarcinoma, SCC, or large cell carcinoma) with neuroendocrine differentiation (NSCLC-NED) [3, 48]. IYODA *et al.* [63] found that the tumour size of large cell carcinoma with neuroendocrine differentiation was significantly larger than that for LCNEC and that, in their series, the survival rate was not different from patients with LCNEC. At the present time, the clinical significance of the diagnosis of NSCLC-NED is not known. Whether these tumours are responsive to SCLC chemotherapy regimens [64, 65], or whether expression of neuroendocrine markers may be an unfavourable prognostic factor remains to be determined [66–73].

Basaloid carcinoma

Basaloid carcinoma is the most prominent variant of large cell carcinoma after LCNEC [3, 10, 56]. Basaloid carcinomas represent 3–4% of NSCLC in Europe, almost always occur in males and most of these tumours develop in proximal bronchi where they frequently have an endobronchial component. Two-thirds of these tumours arise from long areas on bronchial mucosa and show prolonged and laterally extended carcinoma *in situ*. About half of the tumours present with a pure basaloid pattern that belong to a variant of large cell carcinoma. The remaining cases have a minor (<50%) component of SCC or, more rarely, adenocarcinoma and are thus classified as SCC (basaloid variant) or adenocarcinoma, respectively. These tumours consist of a lobular, trabecular or palisading gross pattern of relatively small monomorphic cuboidal to fusiform cells with moderately hyperchromatic nuclei, finely granular chromatin, absent or only focally conspicuous nucleoli, scant cytoplasm but a nuclear to cytoplasmic ratio lower than that of SCLC, and a high mitotic rate of 20–100 mitosis per 2 mm^2. Neither intercellular bridges nor individual cell keratinisation are present, which allows them to be distinguished from poorly differentiated SCC. However, abrupt keratin pearls are occasionally encountered and do not rule out the diagnosis of pure basaloid carcinoma. Patients with basaloid carcinoma have a significantly shorter survival than those with poorly differentiated SCC, which deserves this differential diagnosis [10–12, 56].

Immunohistochemistry and differential diagnosis. Since comedo-type-necrosis is common, palisading is a characteristic feature of basaloid carcinoma, and rosettes can be identified in about one-third of cases, the main differential diagnosis resides in separation from LCNEC. Immunohistochemical stains for neuroendocrine markers are negative in basaloid carcinoma and positive in LCNEC. No secretory granules have been seen by electron microscopy in BC. Two antibodies are helpful to make the distinction on small biopsies between basaloid carcinoma, SCLC and LCNEC. The specific CKs 1, 5, 10 and 14 recognised by 34βE12 show no staining in small cell, large cell and LCNEC, while almost all basaloid carcinoma is stained. TTF-1 is never present in basaloid carcinoma, but is present in the majority of SCLC and LCNEC (table 3) [44, 74]. P63 is expressed in most cells of all basaloid carcinoma.

Adenosquamous carcinoma

Adenosquamous carcinoma accounts for 0.6–2.3% of all lung cancers [75–79] and is defined as a lung carcinoma having at least 10% of squamous cell or adenocarcinoma components [3]. Adenosquamous carcinoma should not be confused with mucoepidermoid carcinoma, a malignant epithelial tumour characterised by the presence of squamoid cells, mucin-secreting cells and cells having intermediate type, identical to the same tumours encountered in the salivary glands. Mucoepidermoid carcinoma of high-grade malignancy is differentiated from adenocarcinoma by a variety of features including a mixture of mucin containing cells and squamoid cells, transition areas from classical low-grade mucoepidermoid carcinoma and lack of keratinisation.

Sarcomatoid carcinoma

Sarcomatoid cancinamas include the following: pleomorphic carcinoma, giant cell carcinoma, spindle cell carcinoma, carcinosarcoma and pulmonary blastoma.

This group of lung carcinomas is poorly differentiated and expresses a spectrum of pleomorphic, sarcomatoid and sarcomatous elements. They include pleomorphic carcinoma, giant cell and spindle cell carcinoma, carcinosarcoma and pulmonary blastoma. They express the features and the biological behaviour of epithelial cells that adopt an epithelial-to-mesenchymal transition in certain conditions of cultures *in vitro*. Sarcomatoid carcinomas tend to be large peripheral tumours invading bronchial lumens forming endobronchial growth. They often invade the chest wall and are associated with a poor prognosis [41]. Due to the characteristic histological heterogeneity of this tumour, adequate sampling is required and should consist of at least one section per centimetre of the tumour diameter.

Pleomorphic carcinoma

A pleomorphic carcinoma should have at least a 10% component of a spindle or giant cells associated but be distinctly identifiable with another histological type, such as adenocarcinoma or SCC [3]. A few giant cells disseminated in an otherwise recognisable squamous cell adenocarcinoma or SCLC have no value for classification in the category of sarcomatoid carcinoma.

Giant cell and spindle cell carcinoma

Rarely, carcinomas present with a pure giant cell or spindle cell pattern and thus are termed either giant cell or spindle cell carcinoma, respectively. Giant cell carcinoma consists of huge, bizarre pleomorphic and multinucleated tumour cells that engulf numerous inflammatory cells, particularly polymorphonuclear leukocytes in their cytoplasm [80–82]. They are discohesive and separated by important infiltration of inflammatory cells. This tumour is defined as a carcinoma by light microscopy, but immunohistochemical and epithelial markers, such as keratins, are also quite helpful in confirming their epithelial nature [3].

Carcinosarcoma

Carcinosarcoma is a tumour composed of a mixture of carcinoma and sarcoma. An heterologous component should be demonstrated, such as cartilage, bone and skeletal muscle sarcomatous heterologous elements, which does not display CK staining [3]. Experience proves that these cases are extremely rare, while observation of pseudochondromatous or pseudo-osseous patterns in sarcomatoid carcinoma are frequent: in these cases, the pseudosarcomatous component also expresses keratins.

Immunohistochemistry. The diagnosis of pleomorphic carcinoma does not rely on the immunohistochemical demonstration of CK in the sarcomatoid component, owing to the evidence of a well-differentiated NSCLC component. In contrast, giant cell and spindle cell carcinoma (pure types) requires the demonstration of CKs expression to be distinguished from sarcoma; cocktails of CK and CK18 are recommended [83].

Pulmonary blastoma

Pulmonary blastoma are defined as biphasic tumours consisting of an associated glandular component that resembles well-differentiated fetal adenocarcinoma and a primitive sarcomatous or mesenchymal component [3]. Well-differentiated fetal adenocarcinoma is no longer regarded as the epithelial pattern of monophasic pulmonary blastoma but rather as a variant of adenocarcinoma [3].

Immunohistochemical characteristics of pulmonary blastoma are TTF-1-positive epithelial components, which also express CKs, whereas the primitive mesenchymal component does not. Neuroendocrine markers are often expressed on the epithelial component. Pulmonary blastoma may express neuroendocrine markers in the epithelial component.

Typical and atypical carcinoid

Carcinoid tumours accounts for 1–2% of all invasive lung malignancies [13]. The majority of patients are asymptomatic at presentation [84]. Symptoms include haemoptysis, postobstructive pneumonitis, dyspnoea, paraneoplastic syndromes including carcinoid, Cushing's syndrome [84–86], and acromegaly [87]. There is no sex predilection [84, 88]. There is no association with smoking, as 40% of patients with carcinoid are nonsmokers, which is the proportion within the normal population. The mean age for presentation is 55 yrs, with a range up to 82 yrs [84]. This is also the most common lung tumour in childhood [89].

The treatment of choice for pulmonary carcinoids is surgical resection [84, 90]. Patients with typical carcinoid have an excellent prognosis and rarely die from their tumours [84, 91]. However, metastases do not disqualify the diagnosis of typical carcinoid. 5–10% of typical carcinoids have regional lymph node involvement [92]. Compared with typical carcinoids, atypical carcinoids present with a larger tumour size, a higher rate of metastases and a significantly reduced survival. Most series where the diagnosis was based on actual accepted criteria reported a mortality of 27–47% [84, 93–95].

Carcinoid tumours are most often centrally located with a polypoid endobronchial obstructive component. When peripheral carcinoids occur they are more often of the spindle cell type. Both typical and atypical carcinoids are characterised histologically by an endocrinoid, organoid growth pattern and uniform cytological features, consisting of moderate eosinophilic, finely granular cytoplasm, a nucleus with a finely granular chromatin (table 4), and having inconspicuous nucleoli that can be discretely more prominent in atypical carcinoid. A variety of histological patterns may occur in atypical carcinoid and typical carcinoid, including trabecular, palisading, rosette-like, papillary, sclerosing papillary, glandular, paragangliomatous, spindle cell and follicular patterns

Table 4. – Typical and atypical carcinoid: distinguishing features

Histological or clinical feature	Typical carcinoid	Atypical carcinoid
Histological patterns: organoid, trabecular, palisading and spindle cell	Characteristic	Characteristic
Mitoses	Absent or < 2 per 2 mm^2 area of viable tumour (10 high-power fields on some microscopes)	2–10 per 2 mm^2 area of viable tumour (10 high-power fields on some microscopes)
Necrosis	Absent	Characteristic, usually focal or punctate
Nuclear pleomorphism, hyperchromatism	Usually absent, not sufficient by itself for diagnosis of aypical carcinoid	Often present
Regional lymph node metastases at presentation	5–15%	40–48%
Distant metastases at presentation	Rare	20%
Survival at 5 yrs	90–95%	58%
Disease-free survival at 10 yrs	90–95%	35%

[48]. More rarely the tumour cells of pulmonary carcinoid tumours may have oncocytic, acinic cell-like, signet ring, mucin-producing or melanocytic features [48].

The most distinguishing feature between typical carcinoid and atypical carcinoid is the rate of mitosis and the presence or absence of necrosis. Typical carcinoids show fewer than two mitosis per 2 mm^2 area of viable tumour (10 high-power field) and no necrosis. The presence of mitosis of between 2–10 per 2 mm^2 or the presence of necrosis [55] defines the diagnosis of atypical carcinoids. The presence of features such as cell pleomorphism, vascular invasion and increased cellularity are of no help in separating typical carcinoid from atypical carcinoid and in allowing stratification of patients for prediction of survival [55]. Typical carcinoid may well show focal cytological pleomorphism, as do paraganglioma in the head and neck area [48, 93]. The necrosis in atypical carcinoid usually consists of small foci centrally located within organoid nests of tumour cells.

Immunohistochemistry

Nearly 80% of typical and atypical carcinoids stain for pan-CKs and, as in other pulmonary neuroendocrine tumours, they always express CKs 8, 18 and 19 [96]. From a more practical point of view, the expression of CKs 1, 5, 10 and 14 has never been observed along the whole spectrum of neuroendocrine tumours of the lung [37].

Neuroendocrine markers are present in all carcinoids. Chromogranin A is present in neurosecretory granules and synaptophysin contained in synaptic vesicles [97]. All carcinoids express CD 56/NCAM, which belongs to the immunoglobulin superfamily of transmembrane adhesion molecules and, to date, as for other neuroendocrine tumours of the lung, NCAM remains the most useful immunohistochemical marker, even on crushed biopsies or small specimens, in the differential diagnosis with papillary adenocarcinoma and sclerosing haemangioma. In contrast, as widely reported, neuron-specific enolase immunostaining is of little help in the diagnosis of neuroendocrine tumours, in general because of its lack of specificity [98, 99].

TTF-1 expression was demonstrated to be negative in the spectrum of neuroendocrine hyperplasia, tumourlets, and typical and carcinoid tumours [74]. However, other authors have reported some TTF-1 expression in nearly one-third of typical carcinoid and atypical carcinoid [100, 101], predominantly in peripheral location [102]. This discrepancy could be related to differences in immunohistochemical techniques or in assessing the threshold of positivity. TTF-1 expression has not been demonstrated in cDNA expression profiling, whereas it is in high-grade NE tumours of poor prognosis [103].

If the proliferation antigen Ki67 is used in carcinoids, staining is observed in <10%; an index >4% is more frequently observed in atypical carcinoids, and seems to be related to a shorter survival rate [104].

Differential diagnosis

Carcinoids differ from tumourlets by the size of the latter which is >5 mm in diameter. Sclerosing haemangioma may resemble carcinoids, especially with papillary or pseudoglandular pattern. The demonstration of neuroendocrine markers and the absence of TTF-1 expression distinguish carcinoids from sclerosing haemangioma [105]. Carcinoids may be confused with paraganglioma, but this lesion remains very rare in the lung, and the lack of CK expression in the latter is a discriminative feature. Glomus tumours and other smooth muscle tumours may mimic carcinoids; they are distinguished from these by the presence of smooth muscle actin and the absence of neuroendocrine markers. Adenocarcinoma enters the differential diagnosis because gland-like pattern occurs in carcinoids. Mucin production is not a definitive distinguishing feature, as carcinoids may disclose mucin formation. TTF-1 and the absence of NE markers in adenocarcinoma are of great help. The solid-type adenoid cystic carcinoma may be mistaken for carcinoid, but is negative for neuroendocrine markers.

Salivary gland-type carcinoma includes adenoid cystic carcinoma, mucoepidermoid tumours and rare pleomorphic carcinoma. They are not discussed in this section as there is no difference from their location in upper airways tracts.

Conclusions

Histological subclassification of lung tumours is essentially based on light microscopy in order to achieve the widest application worldwide and assume comparability and consistency of data. However, techniques including immunohistochemistry, electron microscopy, tissue culture and molecular biology might provide valuable information on carcinogenesis, histogenesis and differentiation. It is highly recognised that either immunohistochemistry or electron microscopy may detect differentiation, specifically regarding histological heterogeneity of lung cancer that cannot be seen by routine light microscopy. However, these techniques are occasionally required for precise classification. An example of this is LCNEC and malignant mesothelioma, which requires appropriate immunohistochemical and/or electron microscopy findings to confirm the diagnosis. Molecular biomarkers are not helpful for histopathological classification, but are for therapeutic decisions, especially in adenocarcinoma where EGFR mutation and gene copy number by fluorescent *in situ* hybridisation *versus* Ras mutation may indicate the potential for response to tyrosine kinase inhibitors.

Summary

Lung cancer is the most commonly diagnosed cancer and the first cause of mortality worldwide. The clinical importance of a standard international classification is increasing, since therapeutic decisions and treatment response are more than ever based on histological typing. The international standard for histological classification of lung tumours is that proposed by the World Health Organization in 1999, revised with further molecular characteristics in 2004. The four major histological classes, squamous cell carcinoma, adenocarcinoma (the highest in frequency), small cell carcinoma and large cell carcinoma, are distinguished by objective criteria on surgical samples and rarely by immunohistochemical markers. However, differentiation signs required for classification may not be present in small biopsies in the context of extended late-stage nonsurgical disease and classification will then rely on a panel of immunohistochemical markers, in order to keep minimal the diagnosis of nonsmall cell or large cell carcinoma, which is of no help in the specific or targeted therapy indications.

Histological heterogeneity is an important feature of lung cancer, as is the strong distribution bias of histology, with smokers developing all categories and nonsmokers presenting mostly with adenocarcinoma.

Keywords: Adenocarcinoma, immunohistochemistry, lung cancer, pathology, small cell, squamous cell.

Statement of interest

None declared.

References

1. Parkin DM, Pisani P, Ferlay J. Global cancer statistics. *CA Cancer J Clin* 1999; 49: 33–64.
2. Greenlee RT, Hill-Harmon MB, Murray T, *et al.* Cancer statistics, 2001. *CA Cancer J Clin* 2001; 51: 15–36.
3. Travis WD, Colby TV, Corrin B, *et al.* Histological Typing of Lung and Pleural Tumors. In Collaboration with L.H. Sobin and Pathologists from 14 Countries. World Health Organization. International Histological Classification of Tumors, 3rd Edn. Berlin, Heidelberg, New York, Springer, 1999.
4. Travis W, Brambilla E, Muller-Hermelink HK, *et al.* World Health Organization Classification of Tumours. Pathology and Genetics of Tumours of the Lung, Pleura, Thymus and Heart. Lyon, IARC Press, 2004.
5. Mooi WJ, Dingemans KP, Wagenaar SS, *et al.* Ultrastructural heterogeneity of lung carcinomas: representativity of samples for electron microscopy in tumor classification. *Hum Pathol* 1990; 21: 1227–1234.
6. Roggli VL, Vollmer RT, Greenberg SD, *et al.* Lung cancer heterogeneity: a blinded and randomized study of 100 consecutive cases. *Hum Pathol* 1985; 16: 569–579.
7. Moro-Sibilot D, Fievet F, Jeanmart M, *et al.* Clinical prognostic indicators of high-grade pre-invasive bronchial lesions. *Eur Respir J* 2004; 24: 24–29.
8. Tomashefski JF Jr, Connors AF Jr, Rosenthal ES, *et al.* Peripheral *vs.* central squamous cell carcinoma of the lung. A comparison of clinical features, histopathology, and survival. *Arch Pathol Lab Med* 1990; 114: 468–474.

9. Churg A, Johnston WH, Stulbarg M. Small cell squamous and mixed small cell squamous–small cell anaplastic carcinomas of the lung. *Am J Surg Pathol* 1980; 4: 255–263.
10. Moro D, Brichon PY, Brambilla E, *et al.* Basaloid bronchial carcinoma. A histologic group with a poor prognosis. *Cancer* 1994; 73: 2734–2739.
11. Brambilla E, Moro D, Veale D, *et al.* Basal cell (basaloid) carcinoma of the lung: a new morphologic and phenotypic entity with separate prognostic significance. *Hum Pathol* 1992; 23: 993–1003.
12. Moro-Sibilot D, Lantuejoul S, Diab S, *et al.* Lung carcinomas with a basaloid pattern: a study of 90 cases focusing on their poor prognosis. *Eur Respir J* 2008; 31: 854–859.
13. Travis WD, Travis LB, Devesa SS. Lung cancer. *Cancer* 1995; 75: Suppl. 1, 191–202.
14. World Health Organization. Histological Typing of Lung Tumours. Geneva, World Health Organization, 1981.
15. Kodama T, Shimosato Y, Watanabe S, *et al.* Six cases of well-differentiated adenocarcinoma simulating fetal lung tubules in pseudoglandular stage. Comparison with pulmonary blastoma. *Am J Surg Pathol* 1984; 8: 735–744.
16. Moran CA, Hochholzer L, Fishback N, *et al.* Mucinous (so-called colloid) carcinomas of lung. *Mod Pathol* 1992; 5: 634–638.
17. Higashiyama M, Doi O, Kodama K, *et al.* Cystic mucinous adenocarcinoma of the lung. Two cases of cystic variant of mucus-producing lung adenocarcinoma. *Chest* 1992; 101: 763–766.
18. Kodama T, Shimosato Y, Koide T, *et al.* Endobronchial polypoid adenocarcinoma of the lung. Histological and ultrastructural studies of five cases. *Am J Surg Pathol* 1984; 8: 845–854.
19. Koss M, Travis W, Moran C, *et al.* Pseudomesotheliomatous adenocarcinoma: a reappraisal. *Semin Diagn Pathol* 1992; 9: 117–123.
20. Noguchi M, Morikawa A, Kawasaki M, *et al.* Small adenocarcinoma of the lung. Histologic characteristics and prognosis. *Cancer* 1995; 75: 2844–2852.
21. World Health Organization. Histological Typing of Lung Tumours. Geneva, World Health Organization, 1967.
22. Terasaki H, Niki T, Matsuno Y, *et al.* Lung adenocarcinoma with mixed bronchioloalveolar and invasive components: clinicopathological features, subclassification by extent of invasive foci, and immunohistochemical characterization. *Am J Surg Pathol* 2003; 27: 937–951.
23. Kamiya K, Hayashi Y, Douguchi J, *et al.* Histopathological features and prognostic significance of the micropapillary pattern in lung adenocarcinoma. *Mod Pathol* 2008; 21: 992–1001.
24. Kim CF, Jackson EL, Woolfenden AE, *et al.* Identification of bronchioalveolar stem cells in normal lung and lung cancer. *Cell* 2005; 121: 823–835.
25. Clayton F. Bronchioloalveolar carcinomas. Cell types, patterns of growth, and prognostic correlates. *Cancer* 1986; 57: 1555–1564.
26. Singh G, Scheithauer BW, Katyal SL. The pathobiologic features of carcinomas of type II pneumocytes. An immunocytologic study. *Cancer* 1986; 57: 994–999.
27. Miyoshi T, Satoh Y, Okumura S, *et al.* Early-stage lung adenocarcinomas with a micropapillary pattern, a distinct pathologic marker for a significantly poor prognosis. *Am J Surg Pathol* 2003; 27: 101–109.
28. Motoi N, Szoke J, Riely GJ, *et al.* Lung adenocarcinoma: modification of the 2004 WHO mixed subtype to include the major histologic subtype suggests correlations between papillary and micropapillary adenocarcinoma subtypes, EGFR mutations and gene expression analysis. *Am J Surg Pathol* 2008; 32: 810–827.
29. Suzuki K, Yokose T, Yoshida J, *et al.* Prognostic significance of the size of central fibrosis in peripheral adenocarcinoma of the lung. *Ann Thorac Surg* 2000; 69: 893–897.
30. Yokose T, Suzuki K, Nagai K, *et al.* Favorable and unfavorable morphological prognostic factors in peripheral adenocarcinoma of the lung 3 cm or less in diameter. *Lung Cancer* 2000; 29: 179–188.
31. Sakurai H, Maeshima A, Watanabe S, *et al.* Grade of stromal invasion in small adenocarcinoma of the lung: histopathological minimal invasion and prognosis. *Am J Surg Pathol* 2004; 28: 198–206.

32. Yim J, Zhu LC, Chiriboga L, *et al.* Histologic features are important prognostic indicators in early stages lung adenocarcinomas. *Mod Pathol* 2007; 20: 233–241.
33. Borczuk AC, Qian F, Kazeros A, *et al.* Invasive size is an independent predictor of survival in pulmonary adenocarcinoma. *Am J Surg Pathol* 2009; 33: 462–469.
34. Inamura K, Takeuchi K, Togashi Y, *et al.* EML4-ALK fusion is linked to histological characteristics in a subset of lung cancers. *J Thorac Oncol* 2008; 3: 13–17.
35. Kreisman H, Wolkove N, Quoix E. Small cell lung cancer presenting as a solitary pulmonary nodule. *Chest* 1992; 101: 225–231.
36. Fraire AE, Johnson EH, Yesner R, *et al.* Prognostic significance of histopathologic subtype and stage in small cell lung cancer. *Hum Pathol* 1992; 23: 520–528.
37. Sturm N, Rossi G, Lantuejoul S, *et al.* 34BetaE12 expression along the whole spectrum of neuroendocrine proliferations of the lung, from neuroendocrine cell hyperplasia to small cell carcinoma. *Histopathology* 2003; 42: 156–166.
38. Mangum MD, Greco FA, Hainsworth JD, *et al.* Combined small-cell and non-small-cell lung cancer. *J Clin Oncol* 1989; 7: 607–612.
39. Sehested M, Hirsch FR, Osterlind K, *et al.* Morphologic variations of small cell lung cancer. A histopathologic study of pretreatment and posttreatment specimens in 104 patients. *Cancer* 1986; 57: 804–807.
40. Nicholson SA, Beasley MB, Brambilla E, *et al.* Small cell lung carcinoma (SCLC): a clinicopathologic study of 100 cases with surgical specimens. *Am J Surg Pathol* 2002; 26: 1184–1197.
41. Fishback NF, Travis WD, Moran CA, *et al.* Pleomorphic (spindle/giant cell) carcinoma of the lung. A clinicopathologic correlation of 78 cases. *Cancer* 1994; 73: 2936–2945.
42. Tsubota YT, Kawaguchi T, Hoso T, *et al.* A combined small cell and spindle cell carcinoma of the lung. Report of a unique case with immunohistochemical and ultrastructural studies. *Am J Surg Pathol* 1992; 16: 1108–1115.
43. Summermann E, Huwer H, Seitz G. Carcinosarcoma of the lung, a tumour which has a poor prognosis and is extremely rarely diagnosed preoperatively. *Thorac Cardiovasc Surg* 1990; 38: 247–250.
44. Sturm N, Lantuejoul S, Laverriere MH, *et al.* Thyroid transcription factor 1 and cytokeratins 1, 5, 10, 14 (34betaE12) expression in basaloid and large-cell neuroendocrine carcinomas of the lung. *Hum Pathol* 2001; 32: 918–925.
45. Bepler G, Neumann K, Holle R, *et al.* Clinical relevance of histologic subtyping in small cell lung cancer. *Cancer* 1989; 64: 74–79.
46. Begin P, Sahai S, Wang NS. Giant cell formation in small cell carcinoma of the lung. *Cancer* 1983; 52: 1875–1879.
47. Brambilla E, Moro D, Gazzeri S, *et al.* Cytotoxic chemotherapy induces cell differentiation in small-cell lung carcinoma. *J Clin Oncol* 1991; 9: 50–61.
48. Travis WD, Linnoila RI, Tsokos MG, *et al.* Neuroendocrine tumors of the lung with proposed criteria for large-cell neuroendocrine carcinoma. An ultrastructural, immunohistochemical, and flow cytometric study of 35 cases. *Am J Surg Pathol* 1991; 15: 529–553.
49. Brambilla E, Veale D, Moro D, *et al.* Neuroendocrine phenotype in lung cancers. Comparison of immunohistochemistry with biochemical determination of enolase isoenzymes. *Am J Clin Pathol* 1992; 98: 88–97.
50. Ordonez NG. Value of thyroid transcription factor-1 immunostaining in distinguishing small cell lung carcinomas from other small cell carcinomas. *Am J Surg Pathol* 2000; 24: 1217–1223.
51. Vollmer RT. The effect of cell size on the pathologic diagnosis of small and large cell carcinomas of the lung. *Cancer* 1982; 50: 1380–1383.
52. Vollmer RT, Ogden L, Crissman JD. Separation of small-cell from non-small-cell lung cancer. The Southeastern Cancer Study Group pathologists' experience. *Arch Pathol Lab Med* 1984; 108: 792–794.

53. Churg A. The fine structure of large cell undifferentiated carcinoma of the lung. Evidence for its relation to squamous cell carcinomas and adenocarcinomas. *Hum Pathol* 1978; 9: 143–156.
54. Yesner R. The dynamic histopathologic spectrum of lung cancer. *Yale J Biol Med* 1981; 54: 447–456.
55. Travis WD, Rush W, Flieder DB, *et al.* Survival analysis of 200 pulmonary neuroendocrine tumors with clarification of criteria for atypical carcinoid and its separation from typical carcinoid. *Am J Surg Pathol* 1998; 22: 934–944.
56. Brambilla E. Basaloid of the lung. *In:* Corrin B, ed. Pathology of Lung Tumors. New York, Edinburgh, London, Melbourne, San Francisco, Tokyo, Churchill Livingstone, 1997.
57. Pittaluga S, Wong MP, Chung LP, *et al.* Clonal Epstein–Barr virus in lymphoepithelioma-like carcinoma of the lung. *Am J Surg Pathol* 1993; 17: 678–682.
58. Katzenstein AL, Prioleau PG, Askin FB. The histologic spectrum and significance of clear-cell change in lung carcinoma. *Cancer* 1980; 45: 943–947.
59. Cavazza A, Colby TV, Tsokos M, *et al.* Lung tumors with a rhabdoid phenotype. *Am J Clin Pathol* 1996; 105: 182–188.
60. Auerbach O, Frasca JM, Parks VR, *et al.* A comparison of World Health Organization (WHO) classification of lung tumors by light and electron microscopy. *Cancer* 1982; 50: 2079–2088.
61. Chuang MT, Marchevsky A, Teirstein AS, *et al.* Diagnosis of lung cancer by fibreoptic bronchoscopy: problems in the histological classification of non-small cell carcinomas. *Thorax* 1984; 39: 175–178.
62. Wiatrowska BA, Krol J, Zakowski MF. Large-cell neuroendocrine carcinoma of the lung: proposed criteria for cytologic diagnosis. *Diagn Cytopathol* 2001; 24: 58–64.
63. Iyoda A, Hiroshima K, Toyozaki T, *et al.* Clinical characterization of pulmonary large cell neuroendocrine carcinoma and large cell carcinoma with neuroendocrine morphology. *Cancer* 2001; 91: 1992–2000.
64. Gazdar AF, Kadoyama C, Venzon D, *et al.* Association between histological type and neuroendocrine differentiation on drug sensitivity of lung cancer cell lines. *J Natl Cancer Inst Monogr* 1992; 13: 191–196.
65. Graziano SL, Mazid R, Newman N, *et al.* The use of neuroendocrine immunoperoxidase markers to predict chemotherapy response in patients with non-small-cell lung cancer. *J Clin Oncol* 1989; 7: 1398–1406.
66. Berendsen HH, de Leij L, Poppema S, *et al.* Clinical characterization of non-small-cell lung cancer tumors showing neuroendocrine differentiation features. *J Clin Oncol* 1989; 7: 1614–1620.
67. Carles J, Rosell R, Ariza A, *et al.* Neuroendocrine differentiation as a prognostic factor in non-small cell lung cancer. *Lung Cancer* 1993; 10: 209–219.
68. Kibbelaar RE, Moolenaar KE, Michalides RJ, *et al.* Neural cell adhesion molecule expression, neuroendocrine differentiation and prognosis in lung carcinoma. *Eur J Cancer* 1991; 27: 431–435.
69. Kiriakogiani-Psaropoulou P, Malamou-Mitsi V, Martinopoulou U, *et al.* The value of neuroendocrine markers in non-small cell lung cancer: a comparative immunohistopathologic study. *Lung Cancer* 1994; 11: 353–364.
70. Linnoila RI, Piantadosi S, Ruckdeschel JC. Impact of neuroendocrine differentiation in non-small cell lung cancer. The LCSG experience. *Chest* 1994; 106: Suppl. 6, 367S–371S.
71. Schleusener JT, Tazelaar HD, Jung SH, *et al.* Neuroendocrine differentiation is an independent prognostic factor in chemotherapy-treated nonsmall cell lung carcinoma. *Cancer* 1996; 77: 1284–1291.
72. Skov BG, Sorensen JB, Hirsch FR, *et al.* Prognostic impact of histologic demonstration of chromogranin A and neuron specific enolase in pulmonary adenocarcinoma. *Ann Oncol* 1991; 2: 355–360.
73. Pujol JL, Simony J, Demoly P, *et al.* Neural cell adhesion molecule and prognosis of surgically resected lung cancer. *Am Rev Respir Dis* 1993; 148: 1071–1075.
74. Sturm N, Rossi G, Lantuejoul S, *et al.* Expression of thyroid transcription factor-1 in the spectrum of neuroendocrine cell lung proliferations with special interest in carcinoids. *Hum Pathol* 2002; 33: 175–182.

75. Fitzgibbons PL, Kern WH. Adenosquamous carcinoma of the lung: a clinical and pathologic study of seven cases. *Hum Pathol* 1985; 16: 463–466.
76. Ishida T, Kaneko S, Yokoyama H, *et al.* Adenosquamous carcinoma of the lung. Clinicopathologic and immunohistochemical features. *Am J Clin Pathol* 1992; 97: 678–685.
77. Naunheim KS, Taylor JR, Skosey C, *et al.* Adenosquamous lung carcinoma: clinical characteristics, treatment, and prognosis. *Ann Thorac Surg* 1987; 44: 462–466.
78. Sridhar KS, Raub WA Jr, Duncan RC, *et al.* The increasing recognition of adenosquamous lung carcinoma (1977–1986). *Am J Clin Oncol* 1992; 15: 356–362.
79. Takamori S, Noguchi M, Morinaga S, *et al.* Clinicopathologic characteristics of adenosquamous carcinoma of the lung. *Cancer* 1991; 67: 649–654.
80. Addis BJ, Dewar A, Thurlow NP. Giant cell carcinoma of the lung – immunohistochemical and ultrastructural evidence of dedifferentiation. *J Pathol* 1988; 155: 231–240.
81. Chejfec G, Candel A, Jansson DS, *et al.* Immunohistochemical features of giant cell carcinoma of the lung: patterns of expression of cytokeratins, vimentin, and the mucinous glycoprotein recognized by monoclonal antibody A-80. *Ultrastruct Pathol* 1991; 15: 131–138.
82. Ginsberg SS, Buzaid AC, Stern H, *et al.* Giant cell carcinoma of the lung. *Cancer* 1992; 70: 606–610.
83. Rossi G, Cavazza A, Sturm N, *et al.* Pulmonary carcinomas with pleomorphic, sarcomatoid, or sarcomatous elements: a clinicopathologic and immunohistochemical study of 75 cases. *Am J Surg Pathol* 2003; 27: 311–324.
84. McCaughan BC, Martini N, Bains MS. Bronchial carcinoids. Review of 124 cases. *J Thorac Cardiovasc Surg* 1985; 89: 8–17.
85. Pass HI, Doppman JL, Nieman L, *et al.* Management of the ectopic ACTH syndrome due to thoracic carcinoids. *Ann Thorac Surg* 1990; 50: 52–57.
86. Ricci C, Patrassi N, Massa R, *et al.* Carcinoid syndrome in bronchial adenoma. *Am J Surg* 1973; 126: 671–677.
87. Scheithauer BW, Carpenter PC, Bloch B, *et al.* Ectopic secretion of a growth hormone-releasing factor. Report of a case of acromegaly with bronchial carcinoid tumor. *Am J Med* 1984; 76: 605–616.
88. el-Naggar AK, Ballance W, Karim FW, *et al.* Typical and atypical bronchopulmonary carcinoids. A clinicopathologic and flow cytometric study. *Am J Clin Pathol* 1991; 95: 828–834.
89. Lack EE, Harris GB, Eraklis AJ, *et al.* Primary bronchial tumors in childhood. A clinicopathologic study of six cases. *Cancer* 1983; 51: 492–497.
90. Stamatis G, Freitag L, Greschuchna D. Limited and radical resection for tracheal and bronchopulmonary carcinoid tumour. Report on 227 cases. *Eur J Cardiothorac Surg* 1990; 4: 527–532.
91. Warren WH, Gould VE. Long-term follow-up of classical bronchial carcinoid tumors. Clinicopathologic observations. *Scand J Thorac Cardiovasc Surg* 1990; 24: 125–130.
92. Colby TV, Koss M, Travis WD. Tumors of the Lower Respiratory Tract. Washington, Armed Forces Institute of Pathology, 1995.
93. Arrigoni MG, Woolner LB, Bernatz PE. Atypical carcinoid tumors of the lung. *J Thorac Cardiovasc Surg* 1972; 64: 413–421.
94. Bonato M, Cerati M, Pagani A, *et al.* Differential diagnostic patterns of lung neuroendocrine tumours. A clinico-pathological and immunohistochemical study of 122 cases. *Virchows Arch A Pathol Anat Histopathol* 1992; 420: 201–211.
95. Paladugu RR, Benfield JR, Pak HY, *et al.* Bronchopulmonary Kulchitzky cell carcinomas. A new classification scheme for typical and atypical carcinoids. *Cancer* 1985; 55: 1303–1311.
96. Brambilla E, Brambilla C. Heterogeneity of malignant bronchial tumors. Problems of histogenesis. *Rev Mal Respir* 1986; 3: 235–245.
97. Lantuejoul S, Moro D, Michalides RJ, *et al.* Neural cell adhesion molecules (NCAM) and NCAM-PSA expression in neuroendocrine lung tumors. *Am J Surg Pathol* 1998; 22: 1267–1276.
98. Linnoila RI, Mulshine JL, Steinberg SM, *et al.* Neuroendocrine differentiation in endocrine and nonendocrine lung carcinomas. *Am J Clin Pathol* 1988; 90: 641–652.

99. Bergh J, Esscher T, Steinholtz L, *et al.* Immunocytochemical demonstration of neuron-specific enolase (NSE) in human lung cancers. *Am J Clin Pathol* 1985; 84: 1–7.
100. Folpe AL, Gown AM, Lamps LW, *et al.* Thyroid transcription factor-1: immunohistochemical evaluation in pulmonary neuroendocrine tumors. *Mod Pathol* 1999; 12: 5–8.
101. Oliveira AM, Tazelaar HD, Myers JL, *et al.* Thyroid transcription factor-1 distinguishes metastatic pulmonary from well-differentiated neuroendocrine tumors of other sites. *Am J Surg Pathol* 2001; 25: 815–819.
102. Du EZ, Goldstraw P, Zacharias J, *et al.* TTF-1 expression is specific for lung primary in typical and atypical carcinoids: TTF-1-positive carcinoids are predominantly in peripheral location. *Hum Pathol* 2004; 35: 825–831.
103. Jones MH, Virtanen C, Honjoh D, *et al.* Two prognostically significant subtypes of high-grade lung neuroendocrine tumours independent of small-cell and large-cell neuroendocrine carcinomas identified by gene expression profiles. *Lancet* 2004; 363: 775–781.
104. Costes V, Marty-Ane C, Picot MC, *et al.* Typical and atypical bronchopulmonary carcinoid tumors: a clinicopathologic and KI-67-labeling study. *Hum Pathol* 1995; 26: 740–745.
105. Devouassoux-Shisheboran M, Hayashi T, Linnoila RI, *et al.* A clinicopathologic study of 100 cases of pulmonary sclerosing hemangioma with immunohistochemical studies: TTF-1 is expressed in both round and surface cells, suggesting an origin from primitive respiratory epithelium. *Am J Surg Pathol* 2000; 24: 906–916.

CHAPTER 3

Pre-invasive diseases of the lung

D.T. Merrick[*,¶], *F.R. Hirsch*[*,#]

*Depts of *Pathology and #Oncology, University of Colorado Cancer Center, and ¶Dept of Pathology, Denver Veteran's Administration Medical Center, Denver, CO, USA.*

Correspondence: F.R. Hirsch, University of Colorado Cancer Center, P.O. Box 6511, Mail Stop 8117, Aurora, CO 80045, USA. E-mail: Fred.Hirsch@UCHSC.edu

Pre-malignant diseases of the lung are represented by a complex, diverse set of lesions that are as yet only incompletely understood. However, they may well hold the key to achieving significant reduction in mortality and morbidity from lung cancer. It is well known that lung cancer is the number one cause of death due to malignancy [1]. Furthermore, the poor prognosis associated with this malignancy appears to be directly related to the fact that lung cancer is often advanced at the time of diagnosis and is notoriously difficult to treat when discovered at the invasive stage. Thus, detection and elimination of this disease before the development of invasive carcinoma may represent the most effective method for reducing the devastating toll exacted by lung cancer. Prevention of cancer is a very promising approach for reducing the impact of malignant neoplasms as has been dramatically demonstrated in cancer of the uterine cervix. Similar benefits are now beginning to be developed in other malignancies, such as those of the breast, colon and oesophagus, for which surveillance for detection and methods for the treatment of pre-malignant lesions are being established. Pre-malignant lung lesions include squamous dysplasia, atypical adenomatous hyperplasia (AAH) and diffuse idiopathic pulmonary neuroendocrine hyperplasia (DIPNECH), which are postulated precursor lesions of squamous cell carcinoma, adenocarcinoma and carcinoid tumours of the lung, respectively. However, there are significant issues that complicate the characterisation and clinical management of pre-malignant lung disease. One such issue is the scale of the tissue that can be involved by this disease. Indeed, it has been stated that the surface area of the bronchial airways and alveolar spaces is equivalent to the area covered by a tennis court. In addition, by virtue of its location within the thorax and the extremely complex branching organisation of lung tissue, the pulmonary system is relatively difficult to access. This creates problems in respect to efficient detection and follow-up of pre-invasive disease. Finally, the large area that can be involved in pre-malignant disease has significant implications for the methods by which preventive treatment can be applied. Despite these challenges, extensive analyses have provided an abundance of information about pre-malignant lung disease and numerous groups are rapidly accumulating important data central to defining the behaviour of these lesions and establishing therapeutic strategies for the prevention of lung cancer. The present chapter will begin with a description of the pre-malignant lesions of the lung and a brief discussion of the technologies employed to detect them. This will be followed by a review of the natural history of pre-malignant lung disease and a discussion of its relationship to risk for the development of invasive lung cancer. This will include a description of the molecular and genetic alterations that underlie the development and progression of pre-malignant disease. Finally, we will explore current strategies for

Eur Respir Mon, 2009, 44, 36–56. Printed in UK - all rights reserved. Copyright ERS Journals Ltd 2009; European Respiratory Monograph; ISSN 1025-448x.

prevention of lung cancer and the methods by which the efficacy of these prevention studies may best be evaluated.

Histology of pre-malignant lesions of the lung

Putative precursor lesions for each of the primary types of lung cancer have been proposed and are at various levels of characterisation. The most thoroughly studied pre-malignant pulmonary lesion is bronchial dysplasia (BD), a metaplastic squamous proliferation that develops in the central airways of the lung. Initially, these lesions were primarily studied by analysis of sputa from subjects at high risk for the development of lung cancer in which keratinised epithelial cells with varying degrees of nuclear atypia were described [2]. Saccomano and co-workers (reviewed in [2]) followed a large cohort of patients with tobacco smoking histories and uranium exposure documenting a temporal increase in cytological atypia and correlating this with incidence of invasive lung cancer. The subsequent development of bronchoscopic techniques provided tissue specimens that could be used to characterise the *in situ* histological features of BD. From these analyses it was shown that chronic injury from irritants, such as tobacco smoke, can lead to inflammation associated airway damage and the development of basal cell hyperplasia with expansion of the basal layer of bronchial epithelium. Such injury may also cause metaplastic change from glandular to squamous epithelial morphology. These alterations have been considered to be reversible, but repetitive injury can lead to the development of lesions with significant pre-malignant potential. These lesions are characterised by the development of cellular atypia in metaplastic foci and are designated BD. They are classified, in order of increasing atypia, as mild, moderate or severe dysplasia and carcinoma *in situ* (CIS) (fig. 1). A series of publications have helped to establish the microscopic features that distinguish these lesions [2, 3]. The stroma underlying dysplastic foci may also demonstrate morphological alterations, the most prominent of which may be a vascular proliferation with characteristic papillary stromal projections extending into overlying epithelium (fig. 1f). Lesions with these structures have been termed angiogenic squamous dysplasias (ASD) and can be seen in a subset of metaplastic lesions of all degrees of atypia [4]. Given the importance of relating clinical features, molecular characteristics and other parameters to increased risk in BD, the development of a standardised classification of these lesions has been a primary goal of the lung cancer community. Recent World Health Organization (WHO) diagnostic guidelines have been published and one study has demonstrated relatively satisfactory reproducibility in pathologist classification of these lesions [5, 6].

AAH is the putative precursor lesion for adenocarcinoma of the lung (fig. 2). This lesion is found in the peripheral lung and is thought to represent the pre-malignant stage of the nonmucinous type of bronchioloalveolar carcinoma (BAC). Its relationship, if any, to mucinous BAC or invasive adenocarcinoma is less clear. Additionally, given that BACs are not invasive by definition, the distinction between AAH and early BAC is ill-defined. Differentiation of AAH from reactive type II pneumocyte hyperplasia may be difficult, but the latter process is associated with significant inflammation and septal thickening that is composed of true fibrosis and is more extensive than the mild collagenous thickening of AAH [7, 8]. At the other end of the spectrum, separation of AAH and early BAC is often determined by size criteria that were arbitrarily established in some of the earliest publications describing AAH. The diagnosis of AAH has been assigned to those lesions measuring ≤ 0.5 cm and BAC to those over this threshold. Conversely, histological criteria to distinguish AAH and BAC have been described in which the presence of stratification of epithelium, and formation of papillary structures

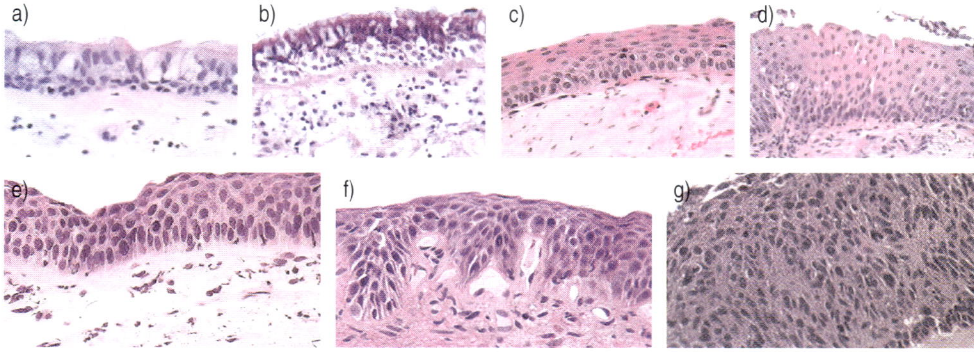

Fig. 1. – Histological features of pre-invasive bronchial lesions. b) Basal cell hyperplasia shows an increase of small round basal cells in comparison to a) normal. c) Squamous metaplasia can progress to d) mild, e) moderate and f) severe dysplasia and g) carcinoma *in situ* (CIS). Atypia and mitotic activity are restricted to lower and mid-levels of mild and moderate dysplasia respectively. Nuclear enlargement and irregularity become prominent in moderate dysplasia. Severe dysplasia shows prominent nucleoli, coarse chromatin and greater nuclear pleomorphism. CIS shows full-thickness atypia and absence of nuclear orientation. CIS also demonstrates the property that inversion of the epithelium would not change its appearance. Magnification: a) ×600; b–g) ×400.

indicate a diagnosis of BAC. This distinction is further complicated by the fact that a number of cellular alterations that distinguish AAH from normal tissue are found predominantly in lesions that are classified as high grade. The features that have been described to define high-grade AAH include high cellular density, cytological atypia, stratification and increased fibrosis. It is likely this overlap between definitions for high-grade AAH and BAC that led a recent WHO panel to recommend that grading of AAH not be applied at this time. When morphological criteria are employed, some AAH may greatly exceed 0.5 cm in diameter and other very small lesions may demonstrate worrisome histology. If it is accepted that these early BAC lesions correspond to the type A or possibly some type B lesions as defined in the benchmark study of NOGUCHI *et al.* [9], it can be argued that the clinical impact of differentiating these lesions is negligible. The 5-yr survival of Naguchi type A and B lesions was 100%, and none were associated with metastases [9]. However, in order to establish the natural history of adenocarcinoma and the pre-malignant potential of AAH, a reproducible classification of these lesions is paramount.

DIPNECH is considered to be a precursor lesion of neuroendocrine tumours of the lung. It is characterised by proliferative foci of neuroendocrine cells in the central and

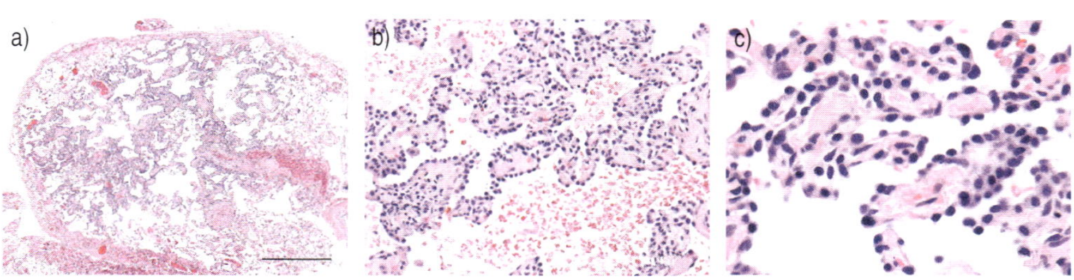

Fig. 2. – a) Atypical adenomatous hyperplasia (AAH) is well circumscribed and usually small in size. b) The pre-invasive cells grow in a single layer along only slightly thickened alveolar septae in a "lepidic" fashion. c) The cells of AAH show mild atypia with enlarged nuclei, hyperchromasia and some apical "hobnail" cytoplasmic snouts. Stratification and papillae (not present) are seen in progression to bronchioloalveolar carcinoma. a) Scale bar=1 mm. Magnification: a) ×40; b) ×400; c) ×1000. Images provided courtesy of W.A. Franklin, University of Colorado, Denver, CO, USA.

peripheral airways that are confined within bronchial epithelium on the luminal side of the basement membrane (fig. 3) [7]. In contrast, carcinoid tumourlets refer to small neuroendocrine lesions (<0.5 cm) that extend beyond the basement membrane of the airways. The precursor nature of DIPNECH has been inferred from their frequent association with tumourlets and carcinoids of both typical and atypical varieties in resection specimens. Although not fully explored, an association between DIPNECH and the development of the more aggressive neuroendocrine lung tumours, small cell lung carcinoma (SCLC) and large cell neuroendocrine carcinoma (LCNEC), appears to be unlikely. Of note, is the well-documented relationship between DIPNECH and obstructive pulmonary disease, which can be associated with significant morbidity and mortality [5]. DIPNECH lesions in these cases show extensive peri-bronchiolar fibrosis and may be associated with mild-to-moderate chronic inflammation.

Detection of pre-invasive lesions of the lung

A critical factor that has allowed for in-depth study of pre-invasive lesions is the development of new technologies for their detection. The study of BD has been greatly advanced by new bronchoscopic techniques. These lesions have no corresponding radiographic abnormality. AAH, conversely, is now detectable in many cases by high resolution computed tomography. DIPNECH may occasionally be discovered by bronchoscopic or radiographic techniques. Autofluorescence bronchoscopy has provided increased sensitivity for the detection of BD in comparison to traditional white light techniques [10]. Autofluorescence bronchoscopy is also very sensitive for the detection of ASD, but this sensitivity may be significantly increased by adding the more recently developed technique of narrow band imaging or confocal laser scanning microscopy to bronchoscopic examinations [11]. Another exciting new bronchoscopic technique is optical coherence tomography. This technology produces a cross-sectional image of bronchial tissue providing a method by which to assess epithelial thickness. It has been reported to accurately distinguish simple metaplasia or hyperplasia from dysplasia as well as invasive carcinoma from CIS [12]. The important implication of these advances is that we can now more sensitively identify dysplasia and can more accurately characterise their outcome on repeat bronchoscopies. These features are essential for the description of the natural history of these lesions and the evaluation of the effects of chemopreventive agents.

The application of spiral/high-resolution computed tomography (HRCT) has led to the frequent detection of lung nodules measuring <10 mm. Removal of such lesions has demonstrated that they may on occasion represent AAH. However, these lesions can

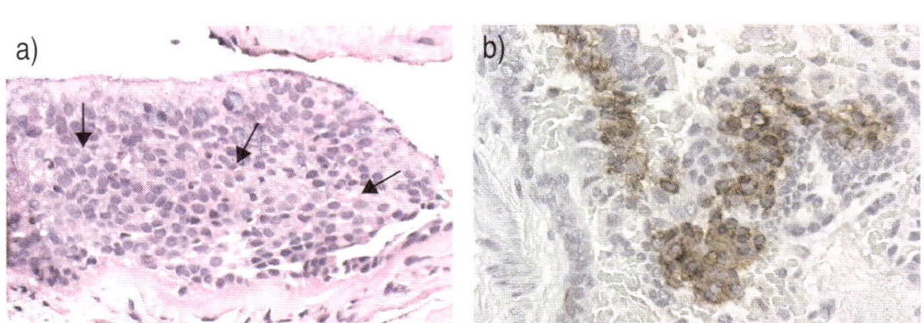

Fig. 3. – a) Diffuse idiopathic pulmonary neuroendocrine hyperplasia are usually nodular and are confined between the basal layer (arrows) and the basement membrane of bronchial epithelium. b) They may also form a single layer of neuroendocrine cells that are best detected on chromogranin immunostains. Magnification: ×400. Chromogranin immunostain provided courtesy of C. Cool, University of Colorado, Denver, CO, USA.

also represent BAC, invasive adenocarcinoma, lymphoproliferative disease or non-neoplastic fibrosis and organising pneumonia. Thus, improved specificity is needed to employ HRCT as a primary screening tool. Indeed, the positive predictive value for adenocarcinoma or BAC with the finding of a small nodule on HRCT can be as low as 12% [13]. With respect to the characterisation of AAH, the finding and removal of such small lesions has provided invaluable tissue for analyses. Although these lesions are too small to be reliably targeted by current biopsy or aspiration methods, the ability to perform such sampling might substantially increase the ability to characterise the natural history of AAH [13]. It must be noted though, that even biopsy sampling of these lesions would likely leave some uncertainty because AAH type histological features can be seen within BAC or even invasive adenocarcinoma. Indeed, it is generally accepted that in biopsies demonstrating features of BAC, reports should indicate that invasive adenocarcinoma cannot be ruled out.

Interestingly, some cases of DIPNECH have been reported to show characteristic mosaic perfusion due to air trapping on HRCT [14]. Airway thickening and small nodules may also be found with the latter likely representing tumourlets. Although central location may be less frequent in DIPNECH, the lesions that do develop in this location would be accessible by bronchoscopy. The few reports documenting bronchoscopic findings have shown either no detection of these lesions on biopsies from cases with resection proven disease or only nonspecific bronchoalveolar lavage results [15]. It seems likely that the infrequent sampling of neuroendocrine hyperplasia on biopsy may be due to their rarity and to a lack of visible associated epithelial or autofluorescent changes.

Biology of pre-malignant lesions

Establishment of an association between putative lesions and malignant potential is the central defining feature of pre-invasive disease. Documenting progression of a pre-malignant lesion to invasive carcinoma is the ultimate proof of this concept, but this appears to be a relatively infrequent event and one that can often take many years to occur. As a result, very high-risk populations (*i.e.* subjects with concurrent or previous carcinoma, exposure to known carcinogens, *etc.*) are often used in an effort to document enough of these events to suggest a correlation. Such studies have been critical to the identification of pre-malignant potential but are often confounded by a multitude of potential risk factors making it difficult to establish an independent relationship or identify the key biological changes leading to malignant progression. Although documentation of histological progression is generally unfeasible in animals, such models allow for the tight control of confounding genetic and environmental variables and are invaluable for establishing relationships between such variables and the development of disease. Some of these models are also associated with putative corresponding pre-malignant lesions. Although infrequently employed in the study of pre-malignant lung lesions, cultured cells provide an *in vitro* tool that can be powerful in respect to establishing a direct relationship between altered gene expression or effects of external stimuli and the development of pre-malignant cellular characteristics. Finally, some of the most important observations are made by studying the features of these lesions *in situ*. Tissue derived directly from human pre-invasive lesions allows for the longitudinal study of these lesions and for the correlation of the outcome in such lesions with clinical factors, histological features and molecular alterations. In the following sections, we will present a thorough review of benchmark studies and recent developments encompassing all of these areas of research for each of the three primary types of pre-malignant lesions of the lung.

Bronchial dysplasia

Longitudinal evaluation of bronchial sites in subjects at high risk for lung cancer has been performed by several groups and has consistently documented progression of these lesions to higher grade dysplasia or invasive carcinoma [16–18]. Progression from CIS to invasive carcinoma has been reported frequently with rates ranging from 17 to 56%. In addition, progression to CIS or invasive carcinoma has been shown to be more frequent with severe dysplasia than with lesser grades of dysplasia or in nondysplastic epithelium [18, 19]. The risk of progression with mild dysplasia is less clear and, in some studies, has not been shown to be different than that observed in sites with normal or hyperplastic histology. The demonstration of an increase in the incidence of severe dysplasia and CIS in patients who are current smokers or who have histories of exposure to asbestos, radiation or other known lung carcinogens in comparison to those without these exposures also supports the pre-malignant nature of BD [19]. The fact that progression of these lesions has not been correlated with current tobacco use is noteworthy. Other clinical parameters that have been associated with increased incidence of BD include male sex, and an increase in the development of BD with increasing severity of chronic obstructive pulmonary disease [20]. Another important finding is that some carcinomas have been shown to arise in sites with previous normal or low-grade diagnoses. Overall, the data from these longitudinal studies provide compelling support for the pre-malignant character of BD, but it should also be pointed out that interpretation of virtually all of these studies is complicated by a few prominent factors. In most cases, the dysplastic lesions were not compared with non-dysplastic sites in control groups with similar lung cancer risk. Furthermore, most of the patients included in these analyses had current or prior lung carcinomas and many of the dysplastic lesions received therapy. The implications of these variations in protocol have been well documented and thoroughly in a recent review [21]. Thus, it is not yet possible to make definitive conclusions regarding the true risk associated with a given bronchial lesion. We have recently presented preliminary analyses of multiply biopsied sites from patients who have not received treatment that reveal increased persistence of high-grade lesions in comparison to lower grade foci. In addition, we have found that the frequency of persistence is higher in cases associated with prior or incident invasive small cell carcinoma (SCC) compared with those without cancer. It is hoped that further characterisation of these types of persistent and progressive lesions will allow for the identification of cellular alterations that may help predict the course of BD.

Genetic abnormalities in BD. Indeed, the most compelling question raised by these *in situ* characterisations of the natural course of BD may be "how do we determine which of these lesions has the most significant risk for progression to invasive carcinoma?" Some of the first strong lines of evidence used to establish a role for BD as a pre-malignant lesion for squamous cell carcinoma documented cellular changes in these lesions that corresponded to similar changes in invasive lung cancer. Genetic abnormalities including loss of heterozygosity (LOH), gene amplification and chromosomal aneusomy are common in invasive carcinomas and have also been detected in BD [2]. LOH can contribute to tumorigenesis by inactivating tumour suppressor genes for which the uninvolved allele has sustained a mutational event or promoter hypermethlyation inhibiting normal activity. Amplification generally leads to increased expression of oncogenes. Aneusomy refers to numeric gains in chromosomal content and is thought to contribute to tumorigenesis primarily *via* changes in gene dosage. Early studies showed that LOH on the short arm of chromosome 3 (3p) was detectable in BD, and that these alterations increased in size and frequency with increasing grade of atypia. In addition, other regions of loss including portions of chromosomes 9p, 17p and 5q have been shown to demonstrate LOH. Importantly, recent studies have correlated the accumulation of such genetic abnormalities with progression of dysplastic lesions (table 1) [22]. It has also been suggested that some of these alterations are more frequent in different stages of tumorigenesis with, for instance, detection of 5q abnormalities being found only in the final step of progression to invasive cancer. Aneusomy, as characterised by scoring of signal from four representative chromosomal loci, has been demonstrated to be more advanced with increasing grade of dysplasia and more frequent in cases associated with carcinoma *versus* those without [24]. A recent analysis of several severe dysplasia and CIS lesions showed that 3p LOH with or without 9p LOH was predictive of progression and that either of these alterations was more common in lesions that persisted than those that regressed [23]. It is worth noting however, that in most studies in which the important association between the presence of a genetic alteration and progression of BD has been demonstrated, several chromosomal abnormalities must be characterised in order to detect this relationship. In addition to supporting a multistep model of carcinogenesis in lung, this feature also hints at a common theme in many of the findings presented herein, namely that characterisation of multiple abnormalities may often be necessary in order to accurately predict the behaviour of pre-malignant lesions of the lung.

Table 1. – Predictive features in bronchial dysplasia (BD)

	Onset in BD#	Predictive change¶	Frequency+	[Ref.]
Morphological features				
Histological atypia	Progressive	Progression to CIS or CA	++ (HGD)	[16,17]
ASD	LGD	Persistence of BD	++	[4]
Genetic changes				
3p LOH	Progressive	Persistence of BD	++	[23]
5q LOH	CIS	Progression to CA	+	[22]
Aneusomy	HGD	Increased in CA associated lesions	++	[24]
Proliferation, apoptosis and differentiation				
Cyclin D1	HGD	Progression to CIS or CA	+	[25]
Cyclin E	Progressive	Progression to CIS or CA	++	[25]
p53	HGD	Progression to CIS or CA	++	[25,26]
Bax/Bcl2 (BBR) <1	HGD	Progression to CIS or CA	++	[25]
hTERT activity	Progressive	Persistence of BD	+	[26]
Ki-67	Progressive	Persistence of BD	+	[26]
Inflammation and other				
C-reactive protein plasma	Not evaluated	Progression of BD	+	[27]
CC10-lavage fluid	Not evaluated	Persistence of BD	+	[28]
Blood group Ag loss	Progressive	Progression to CA	++	[29]
Panels				
Multiple LOH (3p or 9p)	Progressive	Persistence of BD	+++	[23]
Cyc D1/E/p53/BBR (>2)	Progressive	Progression to CIS or CA	+++	[25]

Morphological, genetic and molecular alterations associated with persistence and progression of BD. CIS: carcinoma *in situ*; CA: carcinoma; HGD: high-grade dysplasia; ASD: angiogenic squamous dysplasia; LGD: low-grade dysplasia; LOH: loss of heterozygosity; hTERT: human telomerase reverse transcriptase. #: degree of atypia for which change in parameter becomes significantly different *versus* normal; ¶: change in BD lesion that was associated with predictive feature; +: approximate frequency of predictive feature in persistent/progressive lesions: + <50%; ++ 50–75%; +++ >75%.

Altered proliferation and differentiation in BD. In addition to correlation with the biological behaviour of pre-malignant lesions, the chromosomal regions identified in the characterisation of genetic alterations associated with BD have pointed to specific genes for which targeted analysis has been performed in order to help elucidate their roles in promoting progression of these lesions to invasive carcinoma. Many of these biomarkers are directly involved in the control of cellular proliferation. Epidermal growth factor receptor (EGFR) overexpression, as indicated by full thickness epithelial staining on immunohistochemistry (IHC), is increasingly frequent with increasing grade of dysplastic change [30]. EGFR overexpression also correlates with increased levels of Ki-67 expression, one of several general proliferation markers, such as proliferating cell nuclear antigen, mini-chromosome maintenance protein 2 (MCM2) and others, that have also been correlated with degree of atypia [31]. However, elevation of some the latter markers also correlate with current tobacco use, whereas EGFR does not show this association, indicating it is an independent marker of dysplastic change. Altered expression of tumour suppressor genes are frequently found in BD. Several of these, including p53 and fragile histidine triad tumor suppressor (FHIT), are associated with loci that demonstrate LOH in BD. FHIT is located at 3p14.2, a site that is known to be extremely sensitive to genetic damage. Loss of FHIT expression has been described in clean-up workers from the Chernobyl nuclear reactor accident and was correlated with radiation exposure, tobacco use and presence of dysplasia in that study [32]. Among other tumour suppressors, a correlation between decreased expression of p16, the microtubule associated protein TPX2 and Bax with increasing grades of dysplasia have been demonstrated. In addition, increased expression of cell cycle related proteins cyclins D1 and E, p63, fatty acid synthase and cycloxygenase-2 were similarly associated with progressive atypia [33, 34]. Aberrant expression of p53 has been demonstrated to increase in frequency with increasing grade of dysplasia, and its expression in these lesions has been associated with an increased risk for the development of invasive carcinoma [25]. In more recent studies of the biomarkers associated with proliferative capacity, several have been demonstrated to display a relationship between their altered expression profiles and persistence or progression of BD [25, 26]. While frequency of altered expression patterns for p53, cyclin D1, cyclin E or Bax/Bcl-2 ratio alone were not statistically different in lesions showing progression of dysplasia to CIS or invasive carcinoma compared to those that did not, a combination of any two of these abnormalities was predictive of progression. When persistence or progression was compared to regression in another analysis, levels of p53 and ki67 expression were higher in the former *versus* the latter groups.

Mutational changes in several of these tumour suppressors or oncogenes are often found in invasive carcinoma. The exploration of this aspect of deregulation of these genes in BD is not as extensive but has led to the description of some mutations occurring at the stage of pre-malignant change in p53 and K-ras. Given its prominent role as a tumour suppressor gene, the counterintuitive association of increased p53 expression with increased risk of progression to invasive carcinoma is thought to be best explained by altered p53 activity for which mutation is the most frequently described mechanism. In BD, p53 mutation has been detected with this finding being more common in high-grade lesions and frequently associated with overexpression of the protein by IHC [35]. Anecdotally, the development of p53 mutations have been demonstrated in dysplasias that were associated with the development of invasive squamous cell carcinomas and after the progression of CIS to invasive disease. Increased p53 protein expression is detected more frequently and at lower grades of dysplasia than p53 mutation and is most often found in the absence of demonstrable mutations in the less atypical lesions. Activating mutations in codon 12 of the K-ras oncogene have been shown to be more frequent in dysplastic *versus* normal foci in the airways of subjects exposed to high levels of radiation, although no association with progression of dysplasia was demonstrated for these K-ras mutation positive lesions [32]. Mutations in the EGFR gene have been found with relatively common frequency in adenocarcinoma of the lung, but are distinctly uncommon in squamous cell carcinoma. Interestingly, EGFR overexpression is more common in SCC than in other types of lung carcinoma and amplification of the EGFR gene is also relatively frequent in this subtype. To date, no analysis of EGFR amplification or mutation in BD has been performed.

Another important mechanism in the inactivation of tumour suppressor genes involves inhibition of expression by hypermethylation of gene promoter regions [36]. Proteins p16 and p14 are encoded by the CDKN2A gene and act to inhibit cell cycle progression by blocking CDK4 and CDK6 inactivation of the retinoblastoma gene product, Rb. The CDKN2A gene has been shown to be frequently hypermethylated in nonsmall cell lung cancer (NSCLC) and may also be altered in pre-malignant airway lesions. Hypermethylation of CDKN2A, however, is not frequent in these pre-malignant lesions and, when present, is usually detected in advanced lesions demonstrating severe dysplasia or CIS. Because of its relatively infrequent occurrence in BD, it has not as yet been possible to demonstrate a relationship between this hypermethylation event and persistence or progression of dysplastic sites [25]. Corroborating the later role of promoter hypermethylation in progression of NSCLC is the finding of rare or absent hypermethylation of RASSF1A and DAPK in BD despite their relatively frequent presence in invasive SCC. It is noteworthy that hypermethlyation has been shown to be an important mechanism for the silencing of other genes involved in epithelial differentiation and apoptosis, cellular functions that are also important in the development and progression of BD as discussed below. The methylation of such genes in BD has not been extensively studied.

Epithelial differentiation and apoptosis represent normal cellular processes that antagonise proliferation. Patterns of cytokeratin expression indicate commitment of epithelial cells to terminal differentiation. BD demonstrates cytokeratin expression profiles that reflect the metaplastic change to a squamous epithelium, but also show expression of cytokeratin 6 or other epithelial proteins that are not expressed in terminal squamous differentiation [37]. Cell to cell interactions are mediated by E-cadherin in squamous epithelium and this protein, through interactions with catenins, can have effects on the activity of membrane associated factors such as EGFR with implications on the differentiation and proliferation of epithelial cells. Progressive loss of E-cadherin and α- and β-catenin has been demonstrated with increasing degrees of atypia in BD [38]. Proteins such as telomerase and survivin are involved in cellular senescence and control of apoptosis. Human telomerase reverse transcriptase (hTERT), the catalytic subunit of telomerase shows increased expression of RNA and protein at early stages of dysplasia as compared to normal bronchial epithelium and, additionally, levels of telomerase activity have been shown to directly correlate with persistence or progression of dysplastic lesions [26]. Survivin inhibits apoptosis and has been demonstrated by IHC to increase in expression as degree of atypia increases [39]. This appears to be mediated by inhibition of the deactivating interaction between survivin and the mammalian target of rapamycin (mTOR) protein. Furthermore, this increase in survivin can be inhibited by deguelin, a naturally occurring substance that acts through mTOR mediated actions and is thus postulated to have potential applications in the chemoprevention of lung cancer.

Angiogenesis and inflammation in BD. Angiogenesis, the formation of new blood vessels, has been long accepted to be a critical activity in invasive tumours, but we and others have also now demonstrated angiogenic activity in BD. Vascular endothelial growth factor (VEGF) is expressed in higher levels in BD than in normal bronchial epithelium or basal cell hyperplasia, and levels of VEGF correlate with increased microvessel density, a histological parameter used to estimate angiogenic activity [40, 41]. Both VEGF and microvessel density levels are maximally expressed in the morphologically distinct ASD described above [4]. VEGF expression has been demonstrated by IHC in the bronchial epithelium of these lesions. In BD, there is a preponderance of expression of the VEGF121 isoform, a biologically available isoform that preferentially interacts with the VEGFR2 (KDR) VEGF receptor and appears to direct angiogenesis toward a predominantly proliferative state. This pattern of VEGF isoform expression is also seen in early but not late stage invasive carcinoma. Furthermore, in comparison to advanced stage invasive carcinoma, BD lacks significant increases in expression of angiopoietin-1, an angiogenic factor that promotes vascular differentiation and a decrease in endothelial proliferation [41]. These findings have suggested that the robust proliferation of microvessels is a key process in the development of pre-malignant bronchial lesions. A lack of vascular maturation might also be postulated to be important to the progression of these lesions *via* unchecked delivery of pro-oncogenic substances to these pre-malignant epithelial foci. In addition, ASDs frequently persist and are more common in patients with invasive carcinomas as compared to those without invasive lesions [4]. Altered expression of other angiogenic factors, such as inducible nitric oxide synthase and hypoxia inducible factor-1a, have also been found in BD. Thus, angiogenesis and increases in production of VEGF and possibly other angiogenic factors occur early in the development of lung cancer and may be central to the incidence and progression of BD.

Inflammatory processes are thought to contribute to carcinogenesis in several organ systems, and recent work in lung cancer has suggested a potential application for the analysis of inflammatory mediators as indicators of risk for progression in BD [27]. Plasma levels of C-reactive protein have been demonstrated to be significantly higher in subjects with bronchial lesions that progressed to higher grades of dysplasia compared to C-reactive protein levels in patients without progressive lesions. CC10, an anti-inflammatory protein secreted by Clara cells, was found to be expressed at higher levels in bronchoalveolar lavage fluid from patients with regression of BD as compared to those without change in their baseline level of dysplasia [28]. The relationship between inflammatory changes in the airways and the development and progression of BD is difficult to evaluate. It is possible that these changes are simply secondary phenomena, but, as such, still hold value for predictive purposes. Indeed, an analysis of the effect of the inhaled steroid, fluticasone, on dysplastic lesions showed no increase in the regression of these lesions or alteration in the expression of intermediate end-point biomarkers p53 and Ki-67 [42]. Nonetheless, the informative potential of inflammatory marker analysis for predictive purposes and potential insight into the natural history of BD appears promising.

Proteomic profiles and other changes. Proteomic characterisation of BD is a potential tool that could be valuable for identifying high-risk lesions. Indeed the discriminatory power of this technique has been demonstrated in invasive tumours for which specific profiles can be used to differentiate tumour types and tumours with associated lymph node metastasis. Studies that have undertaken this type of analysis in BD are limited, but there has been the demonstration of unique proteomic profiles that distinguish between normal, low-grade dysplasia, high-grade dysplasia and invasive carcinoma [43]. Perhaps due to limitations in sample sizes and the extent of the proteome analysed, it was not possible to use these profiles to differentiate pre-malignant lesions from normal tissue in a predictive manner. Furthermore, features that were unique to non-normal histology generally were found in significantly <50% of dysplastic lesions. A relationship to persistence or progression of specific lesions has not been evaluated. Nonetheless, there appears to be significant promise in using proteomic analyses to identify a profile that could provide predictive data for the characterisation of a given BD. It may also be possible to characterise unique dysplasia-associated peaks, such that specific protein factors with informative value could be identified.

Mouse models of SCC tumorigenesis have only recently been developed and thus have not yet contributed significantly to the characterisation of the natural history of BD. These models are being employed in the evaluation of chemopreventive agents in BD and thus will be discussed in the upcoming section on treatment of these lesions. Some additional interesting observations have been made regarding features of BD that do not easily fit into the categories described above. Loss of expression of blood group antigens in dysplasias has been associated with frequent progression to invasive lung carcinoma and interestingly has also been noted in high-grade AAH [29]. Heterogenous ribonucleoprotein A2/B1 has been detected in the sputum of patients with NSCLC, and its expression has also been demonstrated in the majority of BD [44]. Whether these hnRNPA2/B1 positive lesions have an increased propensity to progress has not been determined. Maspin, a protease inhibitor, has also been shown to be associated with increased expression in BD as compared to normal tissue [30].

Atypical adenomatous hyperplasia

Demonstrating longitudinal histological progression of AAH to an invasive carcinoma in a manner similar to that employed to provide support for the pre-malignant nature of BD has not been feasible because of the sampling problems associated with the peripheral location of AAH, and their frequent detection only as incidental lesions discovered at resection for another reason. Therefore, associative histological and molecular parameters have been the primary methods employed to provide support for the association between AAH and adenocarcinoma of the lung. AAH has been found in the uninvolved lung tissue of <40% of patients with resected adenocarcinoma *versus* ~10% of those with SCC and, when multiple, is almost exclusively associated with adenocarcinoma [8]. Clonality of these lesions has been proven by characterisation of X-chromosome inactivation in which identical clones were also demonstrated in two BACs and their adjacent AAHs. AAH is frequently associated with tobacco use and also shows other classic features of pre-malignant change including increased cellular proliferation and a progressive increase in nuclear karyometric parameters, such as mean nuclear area and DNA content [7]. However, some of these changes, such as proliferative activity, are relatively unimpressive and may only be of note when analyses are concentrated on high-grade AAH lesions. Observations in these high-grade lesions have been made by groups with extensive experience in the classification of AAH and are very informative, but it should be noted that this group of lesions is probably associated with the greatest difficulty in respect to differentiation from early BAC as discussed above.

Molecular analyses have provided great insight into the biology of AAH and have also produced important supporting evidence for the pre-malignant nature of these lesions (table 2). Again many, though not all, of these alterations have been detected primarily in high-grade AAH. High-grade AAH shows LOH at 3p, 9p and 17p that, while less frequently than seen in BD, may be present in ~20% of lesions [7]. The chromosomal regions involved are similar to those implicated in BD, thus implicating some of the same tumour suppressor genes and cellular mechanisms. Similarly, p53 overexpression is only found in ~10% of AAHs overall, but, when present, is usually

Table 2. – Observations indicating pre-malignant nature of atypical adenomatous hyperplasia (AAH) and features of AAH that are cited as evidence for role as precursor lesion for adenocarcinoma

	Change *versus* normal	Onset in AAH	Adenocarcinoma *versus* AAH	[Ref.]
Karyometric features				
Mean nuclear area	Increased	Progressive	Increased	[7][#]
DNA content	Increased	Progressive	Increased	[7][#]
Genetic changes				
LOH (3p, 9p, 17p)	Increased	HG-AAH	Increased	[7][#]
Oncogenes				
K-ras mutation	Increased	LG-AAH	Decreased	[45]
EGFR mutation	Increased	LG-AAH	Increased	[45]
EGFR amplification	Increased	HG-AAH	Increased	[46]
Cyclin D1 expression	Increased	LG-AAH	Similar	[47][#]
Tumour suppressors				
p53 expression	Increased	HG-AAH	Increased	[8][#]
p16 expression	Decreased	LG-AAH	Similar	
LKB1 expression	Decreased	Progressive	Similar	[47][#]
Apoptosis				
Survivin expression	Increased	HG-AAH	Similar	[47][#]
hTERT expression	Increased	Progressive	Increased	[48]
Differentiation markers				
CEA expression	Increased	Progressive	Increased (BAC)	[7][#]
SAP expression	Increased	HG-AAH	Increased (BAC)	[7][#]
Blood group Ag expressing	Decreased	HG-AAH	Increased	[7][#]

LOH: loss of heterozygosity; HG: high grade; LG: low grade; Progressive: increased change from normal to LG-AAH to HG-AAH; EGFR: epidermal growth factor receptor; LKB: liver kinase B1; hTERT: human telomerase reverse transcriptase; CEA: carcinoembryonic antigen; BAC: bronchioloalveolar carcinoma; SAP: surfactant apoprotein A. [#]: reviewed.

seen in high-grade AAH [7]. Mutations in the p53 gene have been documented but are very uncommon in AAH. CEA and surfactant apoprotein A show progressive increases in expression from normal tissue to low- and high-grade AAH and invasive adenocarcinoma. Increased survivin expression is associated with high-grade AAH, while increased cyclin D1 and decreased p16 are seen frequently in AAH of all grades [47]. Increased levels of hTERT and loss of expression of tumour suppressor gene LKB1 are predominantly seen in high-grade AAH [48]. An interesting aspect of AAH is its frequent association with mutation in the K-ras and EGFR genes. Although the rates vary somewhat from study to study, a recent analysis of 40 AAHs found that 33% demonstrated K-ras mutation and 25% EGFR mutation with no overlap in the presence of these mutations [45]. Also noteworthy is the recent finding of much more frequent EGFR amplification in invasive adenocarcinoma as compared to AAH, suggesting that this is a late change the development of adenocarcinoma [46]. While the presentation of certain molecular abnormalities in the high-grade *versus* low-grade types of AAH has led to the suggestion that these alterations may be related to progression of AAH, the need for a longitudinal model of this stepwise progression has been repeatedly recognised.

Mouse models of AAH-adenocarcinoma sequence. Very robust mouse models of lung adenocarcinoma have been developed and have provided an important tool for the characterisation of the hyperplasia-carcinoma sequence. Morphological lesions equivalent to AAH have been described in mice that develop adenocarcinomas (fig. 4). Recently published guidelines outline the features that distinguish mouse AAH from benign glandular proliferations and invasive adenocarcinomas [49]. Transgenic mouse models have shown that expression of mutant oncogenic K-ras or stabilised cyclin E can lead to AAH development [50]. Furthermore, conditional expression of mutant K-ras showed that AAH lesions appeared in mice earlier than adenocarcinomas, and that removal of stimuli for expression could be associated with regression of AAH. These studies lend strong support for the pre-malignant nature of AAH and also provide an invaluable model for analyses of the role of numerous other factors in the establishment and progression of these lesions.

AAH relationship to subclasses of lung adenocarcinoma. An important unresolved question in respect to the pre-malignant nature of AAH centres on the possibility that only a subset of adenocarcinomas are directly derived from this lesion. Indeed, a gathering amount of evidence supports the concept that adenocarcinoma can be derived from central or peripheral tissues of the lung with the latter group often referred to as terminal respiratory unit-type adenocarcinoma. When rigorous morphological definitions are employed, these terminal respiratory unit-type adenocarcinomas are distinguished from central adenocarcinomas by thyroid transcription factor-1 (TTF-1) positivity and frequent EGFR mutations [51]. TTF-1 is expressed in alveolar cells and Clara cells of the terminal bronchioles, and is also positive in nonmucinous BAC, the tumour that is believed to develop directly from AAH. AAH displaying K-ras mutations are often associated with a smoking history and may represent a unique pathway as compared to the AAH nonmucinous BAC sequence. However, a significant number of adenocarcinomas are associated with neither K-ras nor EGFR mutations. A possible association between BD and the development of this subset of adenocarcinomas could be postulated. In fact, gene expression analyses have indicated that lung adenocarcinomas are a heterogenous group of neoplasms [52], and up to 30% of these tumours lack expression of TTF-1. These findings suggest that some adenocarcinomas may be derived from more proximal locations with as yet undetermined precursor lesions.

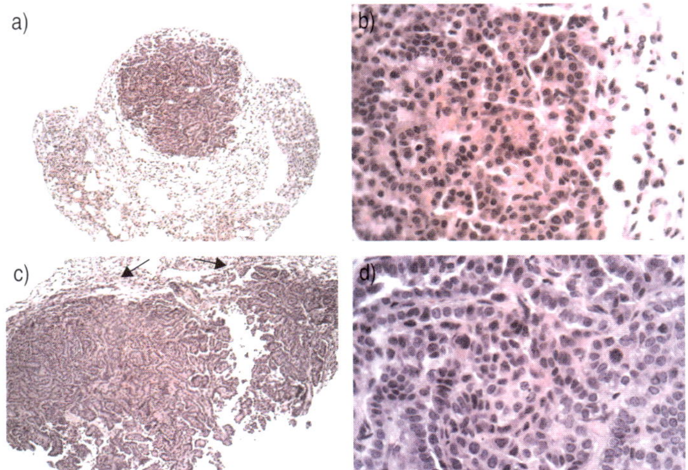

Fig. 4. – Atypical adenomatous hyperplasia in mice at magnification of a) × 100 and b) × 600 are well circumscribed and show uniform cellular features. Invasive adenocarcinoma at magnification of c) × 100 and d) × 600 is infiltrative (arrows) and composed of cells with nuclear pleomorphism that stratify and demonstrate papillary growth.

DIPNECH

Neuroendocrine cells of normal lung are found as single cells that elaborate regulatory paracrine factors and small collections of cells, referred to as neuroendocrine bodies, which act as chemoreceptors for monitoring hypoxia and hypercapnia. The putative pre-neoplastic lesion, DIPNECH, is presumably derived from a hyperplastic process involving these structures. Although only small series of patients have been studied, these have uniformly documented a lack of association between the development of these lesions and tobacco use and have shown an ~3.5:1 predominance of incidence in females [5, 7]. In addition to the concurrent presence of carcinoid tumours in patients with DIPNECH, a few studies have characterised TTF-1 expression patterns in these lesions in an effort to correlate cellular characteristics between DIPNECH and neuroendocrine tumours. While the results of these studies have been somewhat discordant, they have generated interesting hypotheses regarding potential differences in central *versus* peripheral neuroendocrine tumorigenesis. STURM *et al.* [53] reported no TTF-1 expression in DIPNECH, a pattern similar to that found in the carcinoid tumours of their series. The majority of SCLC and LCNEC tumours showed TTF-1 expression. In addition, a previous study by this group showed a cytokeratin expression profile that was identical in DIPNECH and carcinoid tumours (typical or atypical), but was absent in SCLC and LCNEC [53]. Alternatively, DU *et al.* [54] found frequent, albeit sometimes weak, TTF-1 expression in the DIPNECH lesions they studied, but also noted that nearly all of their cases were associated with peripheral carcinoid tumours that frequently demonstrated spindle cell features. DU *et al.* [54] hypothesised that central and peripheral carcinoid tumours represent fundamentally different entities with the peripheral tumours being derived from TTF-1 positive DIPNECH lesions and frequently demonstrating spindle cell morphology.

The molecular basis of tumorigenesis *via* this putative DIPNECH-carcinoid pathway has not been extensively studied. A report in a German publication has documented high expression of EGFR in these lesions, suggesting a role for this receptor in the development of DIPNECH [55]. Interestingly, EGFR expression was variable in carcinoid tumours. More extensive characterisation of production of fibrogenic factors in DIPNECH has been completed, and elaboration of a number of fibrogenic substances, such as bombesin, has been documented. To this point, no compelling evidence for a precursor lesion to SCLC has been identified. In fact, given that extensive genetic abnormalities have been described in histologically normal airway epithelium of patients with SCLC, it has been proposed that these lesions may arise rapidly without development of an intervening morphologically atypical pre-malignant lesion [47].

Therapeutic approaches in pre-invasive lung disease

The previous data reviewed herein have provided strong evidence for the pre-malignant nature of BD, AAH and DIPNECH. With accumulating information indicating that we will be able to identify features that can be used to predict the behaviour of these lesions, an increasingly important focal point in the study of pre-invasive lung disease is the identification of effective methods for preventing their progression to invasive carcinoma. There is already significant activity in the field of lung cancer prevention. These techniques can be generally categorised as localised or systemic approaches to prevention. The following sections will review advances in localised therapy, models for evaluating potential agents for use in systemic therapy, and a review of recent and ongoing chemoprevention trials.

Localised therapy for pre-invasive lung lesions

As described above, newly developed techniques have greatly increased our ability to detect pre-malignant lesions. Some of these techniques are now being explored as methods by which treatment for pre-malignant lesions can be delivered. Autofluorescent bronchoscopy and other new methods of evaluating the airways of the lung are important for follow-up in patients with cytological abnormalities or known pre-invasive disease. Recent recommendations for the employment of these techniques in the assessment and follow-up of patients at risk for the development of lung cancer have been published [56]. In addition, this article [56] discusses the use of five bronchoscopically applied therapeutic modalities in the treatment of BD. The most extensively studied of these is photodynamic therapy (PDT), which uses a photo-sensitiser and direction of narrow bandwidth light at the target lesion to induce cell death. A number of studies have documented complete initial response rates in 50–90% of lesions treated by PDT with frequent documentation of lack of recurrence at the site of treatment for periods of up to $\geq$4 yrs. However, recurrence can occur and is sometimes associated with nodal metastases. Therefore, the current guidelines suggest use of such localised therapy primarily in patients with high-grade lesions who have contraindications for surgery. Nonetheless, this can be a significant population. Indeed, patients who have undergone previous resections for invasive lung cancers frequently demonstrate high-grade BD and are at very high risk for recurrence or development of a second primary invasive carcinoma. Electrocautery, cryotherapy and brachytherapy methods have all been shown to have efficacy similar to that of PDT and can be used for localised therapy. Neodymium yttrium-aluminium-garnet laser therapy is also effective in eliminating these lesions. However, because of possible airway perforation associated complications, it is not a currently recommended method for localised therapy. Given the frequently widespread nature of BD in the airways of high-risk patients, the use of localised therapy for primary prevention purposes is controversial. AAH and DIPNECH may also be widespread in creating difficulties in the development of preventive treatment for these lesions. Currently, the only method of therapy for AAH that has been employed is resection, although definitive diagnosis prior to surgical resection is difficult. The impact of resection of these lesions in preventing subsequent development of invasive carcinoma is unknown.

Models of chemoprevention

The concept of field cancerisation postulates that cells throughout an entire organ system will harbour early alterations that, given adequate accumulation of additional cellular abnormalities, can progress to invasive carcinoma. Tobacco-related damage creates a classic example of this situation in the airways of the lung. ~10% of resected or bronchoscopically sampled lungs with known carcinoma harbour a synchronous invasive lesion [2]. Furthermore, patients that develop invasive SCC of the lung generally exhibit more widespread pre-malignant changes than those that do not [56]. Therefore, it is desirable to apply a systemic or pan-pulmonary chemopreventive treatment, such that potentially pre-invasive lesions can be eliminated throughout the lungs. Prerequisites for effective chemoprevention include the ability to identify a high-risk population in which economically feasible screening can be employed, and the discovery of agents with acceptably minimal side-effects for use in prevention [57]. The preceding data reviewed in the present chapter has established an appropriate population that could benefit from chemoprevention for lung cancer. Yet there are challenges associated with identifying worthy targets and evaluating the efficacy of chemopreventive agents. The latter point requires adequate pre-clinical evaluation and employment of informative end-points that can sensitively demonstrate benefit in clinical chemoprevention trials. The obvious end-point is reduction of cancer incidence, but because progression to carcinoma is a relatively infrequent event in target populations of interest, it often is associated with inadequate sensitivity as a marker of efficacy. Thus, trials of potential chemopreventive agents in lung cancer have often evaluated effects by using reduction of BD as a histological end-point. Efforts are also being made to evaluate the potential use of molecular markers, referred to as intermediate end-point biomarkers, in the characterisation of chemoprevention efficacy.

Pre-clinical evaluation of chemoprevention agents has been performed using mouse models of lung cancer. One such model has used transgenic-mediated overexpression of prostacyclin synthase to demonstrate a reduction of tumour formation in the presence of tobacco carcinogens. Prostacyclin is associated with cellular effects that are anti-tumorigenic, and based on the findings in this pre-clinical mouse study, a multi-centre chemoprevention trial using iloprost, a prostacyclin analogue, is currently underway. Similar to the large majority of mouse models, this model was characterised by the formation of adenocarcinoma. A significant recent development is a mouse model of SCC in which bronchial lesions with histological features equivalent to human BD are also seen (fig. 5) [58]. This could provide a model in which the effect of a chemopreventive agent on the incidence of BD and invasive SCC could be evaluated. Given the common use of these markers as end-points in human trials, the increased relevance of this model is associated with obvious advantages. *In vitro* assays utilising cultured bronchial cells have been less frequently employed in pre-clinical studies but may of substantial worth. Soft agar colony formation can be helpful in characterising cellular pathways that are central to tumorigenesis, but the relationship of findings in this assay to *in vivo* tumorigenesis is difficult to ascertain. Organotypic culture, a technique that uses culture of epithelial cells on an underlying stromal equivalent and growth at the air liquid interface, can be used to produce stratified epithelium in which the state of differentiation can be histologically evaluated. Recently it has been shown that features of BD can be produced by expressing hTERT and Cdk4 in normal bronchial epithelial cells grown in organotypic culture [59]. We have also been able to reproduce normal and dysplastic histology from unaltered primary cultures of bronchial epithelial cells derived from normal and dysplastic sites *in vivo* (fig. 6). Furthermore, these cultures closely recapitulate the *in vivo* expression of biomarkers such as Ki-67 and EGFR, and preliminary studies of potential chemopreventive agents suggest that there application to these cultures can reverse expression patterns of such biomarkers. Given the past unexpected harmful effects of some proposed chemopreventive agents, such as β-carotene, which had not been thoroughly evaluated in assays such as these, it seems

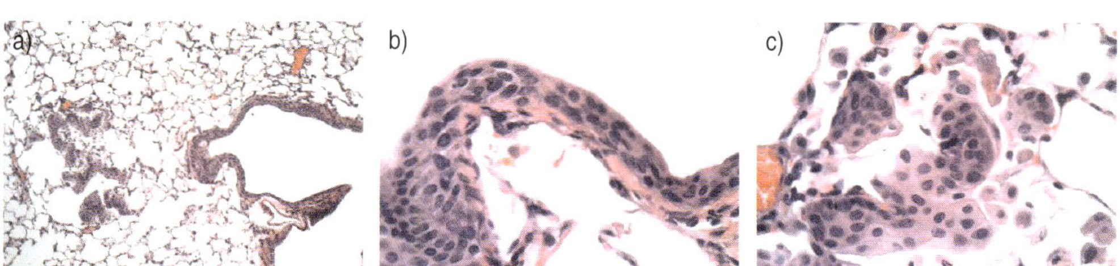

Fig. 5. – a) Dysplastic airway and associated invasive squamous cell carcinoma in *N*-nitroso-tris-chloroethylurea treated mouse. b) Histology consistent with moderate dysplasia is seen in the airway. c) The invasive carcinoma is composed of keratinised cells forming early keratin pearls. Magnification: a) ×100; b) ×600; c) ×600.

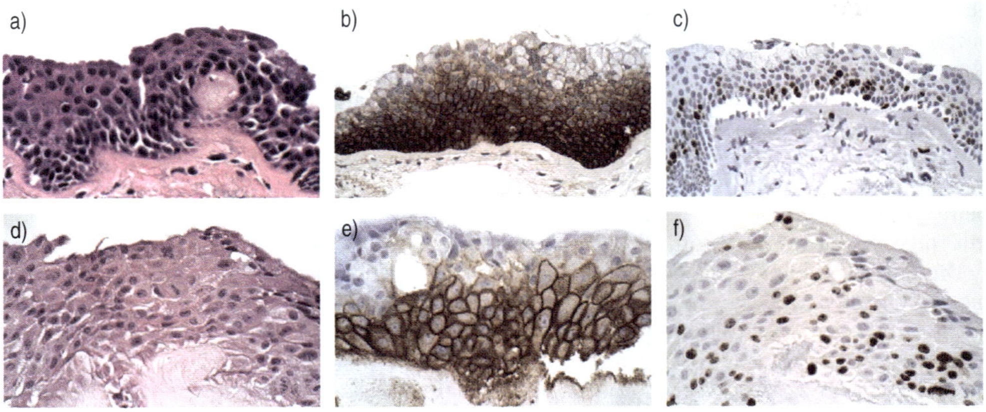

Fig. 6. – Organotypic culture (d–f) of cells derived from tissue immediately adjacent to an *in situ* moderate dysplasia (a–c). Organotypic culture shows d) histological atypia (haematoxylin and eosin stain), e) expansion of epidermal growth factor receptor (EGFR) staining into upper layers of the epithelium, and f) an increase in the percentage of Ki-67-positive cells identical to that seen in the *in situ* lesion (see corresponding panels: a) biopsy, b) EGFR staining and c) Ki-67-positive cells). Magnification: all ×400.

likely that more rigorous pre-clinical evaluation can greatly expedite the discovery of effective agents and informative intermediate end-point biomarkers.

Chemoprevention trials

A number of agents that have been tested in pre-clinical mouse models are now being evaluated in preliminary chemoprevention trials in humans. The organosulfur compound anethole dithiolethione has chemopreventive effects that are thought to be related to its antioxidant activity. It has been shown to reduce the progression rate of BD in humans in significantly larger numbers than for similar lesions followed in a placebo arm [60]. Nuclear morphometry index, a computerised categorisation based on nuclear morphological detail was used as a secondary biomarker end-point in this trial and was associated with more frequent progression when abnormal in the placebo group *versus* the treatment group, although this difference was not statistically significant. Myoinositol is a glucose isomer that has chemoprotective effects in mice *via* an undetermined mechanism. It was evaluated in a small clinical trial, in which treated subjects showed more frequent regression of dysplastic bronchial lesions in comparison to the placebo arm [61]. Noteworthy, however, was the inclusion of only one site in the treatment arm of this study, in which moderate or higher degree of dysplasia was found at baseline. Of importance in both of these studies was the documentation of infrequent side-effects that consisted primarily of minor gastrointestinal complaints. The use of differing methods for determining effect at bronchial sites may make it difficult to compare results from these various trials, but the inclusion of potential intermediate end-point biomarkers in their design should be informative. The ultimate interpretation of results from these and future trials will require a more thorough characterisation of how these end-points reflect the natural history of BD. In order to accomplish this, studies that correlate changes in these end-point markers with persistence of BD or progression to lung cancer in populations with clinical parameters of risk, age, sex, prior cancer history and other factors that are similar to those for subjects included in these chemoprevention trials must be completed.

Conclusion

The development of increasingly sensitive methods for the detection and sampling of pre-invasive lung lesions along with detailed histological classification schemes has led to recent advances in defining their natural history. Characterisation of the genetic and molecular alterations associated with the development of pre-malignancy in the lung is paramount to identifying markers of risk for progression and targets for chemoprevention. Successful lung cancer prevention must be associated with a favourable cost–benefit ratio, and will therefore depend on an accurate definition of high-risk populations and identification of effective therapeutic options. In order to achieve prevention in patients before the onset of their first primary lung cancer, more refined high-risk profiles must be developed. This will require characterisation of lesion outcome in less overtly high-risk populations and must include comparisons to appropriate matched control groups. Importantly, these studies should also identify markers of risk that can be employed as surrogate end-point biomarkers in clinical chemoprevention trials. Successful identification of efficacious targets for chemoprevention will be greatly benefited by employing robust pre-clinical testing in increasingly relevant mouse models and potentially useful *in vitro* systems. While difficulties related to the observation and complexity of pre-invasive lung lesions present challenging obstacles, recent progress in our understanding and recognition of the enormous potential for reduction of lung cancer related mortality associated with the study of pre-invasive disease provide great hope for the future.

Summary

Bronchial dysplasia, atypical adenomatous hyperplasia and diffuse idiopathic pulmonary neuroendocrine hyperplasia are putative pre-invasive lesions for squamous cell carcinoma, adenocarcinoma and carcinoid tumours of the lung, respectively.

Recent improvements in our ability to detect and sample these lesions along with detailed histological classification schemes have led to numerous advances in our understanding of their natural history. Importantly, many molecular and genetic alterations can now be associated with the development of these lesions and, in some instances, are being related to their progression. These findings are leading to the description of biomarkers that will have applications in the early detection of pre-invasive lung lesions and can be used as indicators of their malignant potential.

In addition, new techniques and therapies are being developed for the prevention of lung cancer. The evaluation of these potential therapeutic strategies are being tested in increasingly relevant pre-clinical models of pre-invasive disease, and the findings from these studies are being used to efficiently evaluate potential preventive therapies in ongoing clinical trials.

In the present chapter, we present new findings related to the detection, molecular characterisation and evaluation of diagnostic and therapeutic intervention for pre-invasive lesions of the lung.

Keywords: Biology, chemoprevention, dysplasia, lung cancer, pre-neoplasia.

Statement of interest
D.T. Merrick has previously participated in and received a fee for speaking at a symposium sponsored by AstraZeneca.

References

1. Jemal A, Murray T, Ward E, *et al.* Cancer Statistics, 2005. *CA Cancer J Clin* 2005; 55: 10–30.
2. Franklin WA. The biology of bronchial premalignancy. *Semin Respir Crit Care Med* 1996; 17: 309–321.
3. Colby TV, Wistuba II, Gazdar A. Precursors to pulmonary neoplasia. *Adv Anat Pathol* 1998; 5: 205–215.
4. Keith RL, Miller YE, Gemmill RM, *et al.* Angiogenic squamous dysplasia in bronchi of individuals at high risk for lung cancer. *Clin Cancer Res* 2000; 6: 1616–1625.
5. Brambilla E, Travis WD, Colby TV, *et al.* The new World Health Organization of lung cancers. *Eur Respir J* 2001; 18: 1059–1068.
6. Nicholson AG, Perry LJ, Cury PM, *et al.* Reproducibility of the WHO/IASLC grading system for pre-invasive squamous lesions of the bronchus: a study of inter-observer and intra-observer variation. *Histopathology* 2001; 38: 202–208.
7. Kerr KM. Pulmonary preinvasive neoplasia. *J Clin Pathol* 2001; 54: 257–271.
8. Westra WH. Early glandular neoplasia of the lung. *Respir Res* 2000; 1: 163–169.
9. Noguchi M, Morikawa A, Kawasaki M, *et al.* Small adenocarcinoma of the lung. Histologic characteristics and prognosis. *Cancer* 1995; 75: 2844–2852.
10. Hirsch FR, Prindiville SA, Miller YE, *et al.* Fluorescence *versus* white-light bronchoscopy for detection of preneoplastic lesions: a randomized study. *J Natl Cancer Inst* 2001; 93: 1385–1391.
11. Shibuya K, Hoshino H, Chiyo M, *et al.* High magnification bronchovideoscopy combined with narrow band imaging could detect capillary loops of angiogenic squamous dysplasia in heavy smokers at high risk for lung cancer. *Thorax* 2003; 58: 989–995.
12. Lam S, Standish B, Baldwin C, *et al. In vivo* optical coherence tomography imaging of preinvasive bronchial lesions. *Clin Cancer Res* 2008; 14: 2006–2011.
13. McWilliams A, MacAulay C, Gazdar AF, *et al.* Innovative molecular and imaging approaches for the detection of lung cancer and its precursor lesions. *Oncogene* 2002; 21: 6949–6959.
14. Lee JS, Brown KK, Cool C, *et al.* Diffuse pulmonary neuroendocrine hyperplasias: radiologic and clinical features. *J Comput Assist Tomogr* 2002; 26: 180–184.
15. Reyes LJ, Majo J, Perich D, *et al.* Neuroendocrine cell hyperplasia as an unusual form of interstitial lung disease. *Respir Med* 2007; 101: 1840–1843.
16. Venmans BJW, van Boxem TJM, Smit EF, *et al.* Outcome of bronchial carcinoma *in situ. Chest* 2000; 117: 1572–1576.
17. Bota S, Auliac JB, Paris C, *et al.* Follow-up of bronchial precancerous lesions and carcinoma *in situ* using fluorescence endoscopy. *Am J Respir Crit Care Med* 2000; 164: 1688–1693.
18. Breuer RH, Pasic A, Smit EF, *et al.* The natural course of preneoplastic lesions in bronchial epithelium. *Clin Cancer Res* 2005; 11: 537–543.
19. Paris C, Benichou J, Bota S, *et al.* Occupational and nonoccupational factors associated with high grade bronchial lesions. *Eur Respir J* 2003; 21: 332–341.
20. Lam S, LeRiche JC, Zheng Y, *et al.* Sex-related differences in bronchial epithelial changes associated with tobacco smoking. *J Natl Cancer Inst* 1999; 91: 691–696.
21. Bannerjee AK. Pre-invasive lesions of the bronchus. *J Thorac Oncol* 2008; 4: 545–551.
22. Thiberville L, Payne P, Vielkinds J, *et al.* Evidence of cumulative gene losses with progression of premalignant epithelial lesions to carcinoma of the bronchus. *Cancer Res* 1995; 55: 5133–5139.
23. Salaun M, Sesboue R, Moreno-Swirc S, *et al.* Molecular predictive factors for progression of high-grade bronchial lesions. *Am J Respir Crit Care Med* 2008; 177: 880–886.
24. Jonsson S, Varell-Garcia M, Miller YE, *et al.* Chromosomal aneusomy in bronchial high-grade lesions is associated with invasive lung cancer. *Am J Respir Crit Care Med* 2008; 177: 342–347.
25. Jeanmart M, Lantuejoul S, Fievet F, *et al.* Value of immunohistochemical markers in preinvasive bronchial lesions in risk assessment of lung cancer. *Clin Cancer Res* 2003; 9: 2195–2203.

26. Hoshino H, Shibuya K, Chiyo M, *et al.* Biological features of bronchial squamous dysplasia followed up by AFB. *Lung Cancer* 2004; 46: 187–196.
27. Sin DD, Man SF, McWilliams A, *et al.* Progression of airway dysplasia and C-reactive protein in smokers at high risk of lung cancer. *Am J Respir Crit Care Med* 2006; 173: 535–539.
28. Chen J, Lam S, Pilon A, *et al.* Higher levels of the anti-inflammatory protein CC10 are associated with improvement in dysplasia and sputum cytometric assessment in individuals at high risk for lung cancer. *Clin Cancer Res* 2008; 14: 1590–1597.
29. Sanchez-Mora N, Cebollero Presmanes M, Monroy V, *et al.* Expression of histo-blood group antigens in bronchial metaplasia *Eur Respir J* 2007; 29: 268–272.
30. Chanin T, Merrick DT, Franklin WA, *et al.* Recent developments in biomarkers for the early detection of lung cancer: perspectives on publications 2003 to present. *Curr Opin Pulm Med* 2004; 10: 242–247.
31. Merrick DT, Kittelson J, Winterhalder R, *et al.* Analysis of C-erb-B1/epidermal growth factor receptor and C-erb-B2/HER2 in bronchial dysplasia: evaluation of potential targets for chemprevention. *Clin Cancer Res* 2006; 12: 2281–2288.
32. Chizikhov V, Chikina S, Gasparian A, *et al.* Molecular follow-up of preneoplastic lesions in bronchial epithelium of former Chernobyl clean-up workers. *Oncogene* 2002; 21: 2398–2405
33. Mascaux C, Martin B, Verdebout JM, *et al.* COX-2 expression during early lung squamous cell carcinoma oncogenesis. *Eur Respir J* 2005; 26: 198–203.
34. Orita H, Coulter J, Tully E, *et al.* Inhibiting fatty acid synthase for chemoprevention of chemically induced lung tumors. *Clin Cancer Res* 2008; 14: 2458–2464.
35. Nishisaka T, Takeshima Y, Inai K. Evaluation of p53 gene mutation and loss of heterozygosity of 3p, 9p and 17p in precancerous lesions of 29 lung cancer patients. *Hiroshima J Med Sci* 2000; 49: 109–116.
36. Belinsky S. Gene-promoter hypermethylation as a biomarker in lung cancer. *Nat Rev Cancer* 2004; 4: 707–717.
37. Merrick DT, Sugita M, Bemis L, *et al.* Affymetrix gene expression profiles in premalignant bronchial mucosa. *Lung Cancer* 2005; 49: Suppl. 2, S19–S20.
38. Kato Y, Hirano T, Yoshida K, *et al.* Frequent loss of E-cadherin and/or catenins in intrabronchial lesions during carcinogenesis of the bronchial epithelium. *Lung Cancer* 2005; 48: 323–330.
39. Jin Q, Feng L, Behrens C, *et al.* Implication of AMP-activated protein kinase and Akt-regulated surviving in lung cancer chemopreventive activities of deguelin. *Cancer Res* 2007; 67: 11630–11639.
40. Merrick DT, Haney J, Petrunich S, *et al.* Overexpression of vascular endothelial growth factor and its receptors in bronchial dysplasia demonstrated by quantitative RT-PCR analysis. *Lung Cancer* 2005; 48: 31–45.
41. Merrick DT, Petrunich S, Miller YE, *et al.* Characterization of angiogenic activity and identification of mediators in bronchial dysplasia and invasive lung cancer: role of vascular endothelial growth factor and angiopoietins. *In:* New Research on Precancerous Lesions, Ch. 10. Litchfield JE, ed. Hauppauge, NOVA Editorials, 2007.
42. van den Berg RM, van Tinteren H, van Zandwijk N, *et al.* The influence of fluticasone inhalation on markers of carcinogenesis in bronchial epithelium. *Am J Respir Crit Care Med* 2007; 175: 1061–1065.
43. Rahman SMJ, Shyr Y, Yidiz PE, *et al.* Proteomic patterns of preinvasive bronchial lesions. *Am J Respir Crit Care Med* 2006; 172: 1556–1562.
44. Hirsch FR, Merrick DT, Franklin WA. Role of biomarkers for early detection of lung cancer and chemoprevention. *Eur Respir J* 2002; 19: 1151–1158.
45. Sakamoto H, Shimizu J, Horio Y, *et al.* Disproportionate representation of KRAS gene mutation in atypical adenomatous hyperplasia, but even distribution of EGFR gene mutation from preinvasive to invasive adenocarcinomas. *J Pathol* 2007; 212: 287–294.

46. Soh J, Toyooka S, Ichihara S, *et al.* Sequential molecular changes during multistage pathogenesis of small peripheral adenocarcinomas of the lung. *J Thorac Oncol* 2008; 3: 340–347.
47. Wistuba II, Gazdar AF. Lung cancer preneoplasia. *Annu Rev Pathol* 2006; 1: 331–348.
48. Nakanashi K, Kawai T, Kumaki F, *et al.* Expression of human telomerase RNA component and telomerase reverse transcriptase mRNA in atypical adenomatous hyperplasia of the lung. *Hum Pathol* 2002; 33: 697–702.
49. Nikitin AY, Alcaraz A, Anver MR, *et al.* Classification of proliferative pulmonary lesions of the mouse: recommendations of the mouse models of human cancers consortium. *Cancer Res* 2004; 64: 2307–2316.
50. Ma Y, Fiering S, Black C, *et al.* Transgenic cyclin E triggers dysplasia and multiple pulmonary adenocarcinomas. *Proc Natl Acad Sci USA* 2007; 104: 4089–4094.
51. Yatabe Y, Kosaka T, Takahashi T, *et al.* EGFR mutation is specific for terminal respiratory unit type adenocarcinoma. *Am J Surg Pathol* 2005; 29: 633–639.
52. Batterjee A, Richards WG, Staunton J, *et al.* Classification of human lung carcinomas by mRNA expression profiling reveals distinct adenocarcinoma classes. *Proc Natl Acad Sci USA* 2001; 98: 13790–13795.
53. Sturm N, Rossi G, Lantuejoul S, *et al.* 34BetaE12 expression along the whole spectrum of neuroendocrine proliferations of the lung, from neuroendocrine cell hyperplasia to small cell carcinoma. *Histopathology* 2003; 42: 156–166.
54. Du EZ, Goldstraw P, Zacharias J, *et al.* TTF-1 expression is specific for lung primary in typical and atypical carcinoids: TTF-1 positive carcinoids are predominantly in peripheral location. *Hum Pathol* 2004; 35: 825–831.
55. Kuhnen C, Winter BU. [EGFR expression in pulmonary neuroendocrine cell hyperplasia]. *Pathologe* 2006; 27: 147–151.
56. Kennedy TC, McWilliams A, Edell E, *et al.* Bronchial intraepithelial neoplasia/early central airways lung cancer. ACCP evidence-based clinical practice guidelines (2nd edition). *Chest* 2007; 132: 221S–233S.
57. Keith RL, Miller YE. Lung cancer: genetics of risk and advances in chemoprevention. *Curr Opin Pulm Med* 2005; 11: 265–271.
58. Ye B, Zhang YX, Yang F, *et al.* Induction of lung lesions in Wistar rats by 4-(methylnitrosamino)-1-(3-pyridyl)-1-butanone and its inhibition by aspirin and phenethyl isothiocyanate. *BMC Cancer* 2007; 7: 90.
59. Ramirez RD, Sheridan S, Girard L, *et al.* Immortalization of human bronchial epithelial cells in the absence of viral oncoproteins. *Cancer Res* 2004; 64: 9027–9034.
60. Lam S, MacAulay C, leRiche J, *et al.* A randomized phase IIb trial of anethole dithiolethione in smokers with bronchial dysplasia. *J Natl Cancer Inst* 2002; 94: 1001–1009.
61. Lam S, McWilliams A, leRiche J, *et al.* A phase I study of myo-inositol for lung cancer prevention. *Cancer Epidemiol Biomarkers Prev* 2006; 15: 1526–1531.

CHAPTER 4

Screening for lung cancer

D.E. Midthun, J.R. Jett

Mayo Clinic, Rochester, MN, USA.

Correspondence: J.R. Jett, Mayo Clinic, Rochester, MN 55905, USA. E-mail: Jett.James@mayo.edu

Detection of lung cancer currently centres on the patient presenting with clinical symptoms. Earlier detection is preferred but no test has proven efficacy in lives saved as a screening test for lung cancer. Chest radiography and sputum cytology showed the ability to identify more cancers, to identify more cancers in early stage, and to improve survival, but failed to show a reduction in deaths from lung cancer. Advances in computed tomography (CT) technology allow for scanning of the entire chest in <15 s and in a single breath-hold. Prospective single-arm studies of low-dose spiral CT (LDSCT) screening have created considerable excitement about the potential to effectively screen for lung cancer. Usual clinical practice identifies only ~20% of lung cancer in stage I. CT screening series report 58–93% of prevalence cancers and 25–100% of incidence cancers identified were stage I [1–13]. These findings suggest an ability of CT to shift the diagnosis from late-stage detection to early stage detection when compared with historical clinical practice. However, at this point in time we do not know that CT screening reduces deaths from lung cancer. The present chapter will examine the problem of lung cancer, the issues presented by screening, and the results of past and recent studies of lung cancer screening.

The problem

Although the role of screening in lung cancer management is a subject of considerable controversy, there is no controversy as to the devastation of this disease. Overstating the gravity of the problem of lung cancer is difficult to do. More females and males die of lung cancer annually worldwide than any other cancer [14]. More people die of lung cancer than from breast, colon and prostate cancer combined [15].

Prevention through smoking avoidance or cessation remains key, but improving outcomes for patients with lung cancer will result from early detection and effective treatment. The 5-yr survival of 16% for lung cancer pales in comparison to 88% of breast cancer, 65% for colon cancer and 100% for prostate cancer [15]. Part of the reason that lung cancer lags so far behind in survival is that there is no established screening test. As has been shown with mammography for breast cancer and with faecal occult blood testing for colon cancer, proving mortality reduction with a test for lung cancer would lead to application among those at risk. In the absence of screening, the majority of lung cancers are found on symptomatic presentation and are incurable. The persistence of smoking prevalence rates and the fact that more lung cancers are diagnosed annually in former smokers than in current smokers suggests that the problem of lung cancer will have a secure hold on mortality for a number of decades. An effective screening tool is desired.

Eur Respir Mon, 2009, 44, 57–70. Printed in UK - all rights reserved. Copyright ERS Journals Ltd 2009; European Respiratory Monograph; ISSN 1025-448x.

Screening: the issues

The American Cancer Society (ACS) Guidelines for the early detection of cancer state that: "At present neither the ACS, nor any other medical/scientific organisation, recommends testing for early lung cancer detection in asymptomatic individuals." [16]. Why are we not screening when we know that screening with chest radiography or CT leads to the detection of more cancers and more early-stage cancers and indicates a marked improvement in survival? The answer lies within issues introduced by screening: each of those measures are necessary outcomes but together are insufficient to show efficacy from screening.

Use of a screening test introduces biases that are inherent in screening. The most significant of these include lead time, length time and overdiagnosis bias. Lead-time bias occurs when a cancer is detected earlier than it would have been in the absence of screening; intervention occurs earlier, but the natural history of the disease is not changed. Apparent survival, the measure of time between detection and death, is lengthened, which suggests benefit, but true survival (time from disease onset to eventual death, whether it be due to lung cancer or not) is something we cannot measure. As a result of applying a screening test, though apparent survival is improved, mortality may remain unchanged. A patient with cancer would appear to live longer because the disease was detected earlier; this would be expected even if the natural history of the disease has not been changed by intervention. For example, an aggressive cancer that originates from a single cell at time zero and leads to the patient's death in 5 yrs might be detected at the onset of symptoms in year 4. Survival from diagnosis would be 1 yr. Applying a screening tool in this situation might lead to detection and intervention at year 2. Even if intervention did not change the course of the cancer and death occurred at year 5, survival is 3 yrs from diagnosis. Survival has tripled with screening yet death resulted at the same time it would have without screening. Although lengthening apparent survival is attractive and necessary, it is not sufficient proof of benefit.

Length-time bias shows an apparent improvement in survival when that improvement is actually due to the selective detection of cancers with a less progressive course and missing of cancers that have the most rapidly progressive course. Application of a screening tool at specified intervals would have a higher likelihood of detecting a cancer with a more indolent course than one with a more rapid course that may present with symptoms between screenings. The result is to show an apparent improvement in survival through the better outcome of the more indolent cancers found with screening. CT screening is most likely to detect peripheral nodular cancers; these are more likely to be adenocarcinomas and may have a more favourable outcome than small cell lung cancer (SCLC), which is central and likely to be missed by screening CT.

Overdiagnosis bias is an extreme form of length-time bias in which indolent lung cancers are detected. These are cancers that would not have altered the expected survival when compared with the normal population. Patients with overdiagnosed lung cancers would have died of a cause other than lung cancer and the lung cancer may have gone undetected. People die *with* rather than die *from* these cancers. The natural history of these cancers does not need to be altered with detection and treatment.

Due to these biases inherent in screening, survival would be expected to be more favourable, even if earlier detection and intervention did not alter the course of the disease. For this reason, mortality reduction rather than survival improvement is the ultimate measure of a screening tool's effectiveness and this requires performance of randomised controlled trials. The randomised, controlled trial has long been accepted as the best scientific method for determining the effectiveness of medical practice and for screening [17].

Chest radiography and sputum cytology

In the 1970s and early 1980s, the National Cancer Institute in the USA supported three prospective randomised trials screening for lung cancer involving Johns Hopkins, Baltimore, MD; Memorial Sloan-Kettering, New York, NY; and the Mayo Clinic, Rochester, MN [18–24]. These studies involved >30,000 males aged >45 yrs who were either current or former smokers. The screening algorithm at Johns Hopkins and Memorial Sloan-Kettering investigated the addition of sputum cytology every 4 months to annual chest radiographs. These two trials showed that adding sputum cytology every 4 months to annual chest radiographs did not improve mortality rates of lung cancer when compared with the use of annual chest radiographs alone. The 5-yr survival in these two studies was nearly 35% and considerably above the historical average at the time of 13% [19–22].

The Mayo Lung Project (MLP) compared chest radiograph and sputum cytology to standard care. After prevalence screening, those without cancer were randomised to a group that received chest radiograph and sputum cytology every 4 months or to a group that was advised to have yearly chest radiograph and sputum cytology. In the screened group, 206 cancers were detected, and 160 were detected in the control group [23]. Resection was feasible in 46% of the cancers in the intervention group compared with 32% of cancers in the control group. However, a stage shift from advanced stage to earlier stage was not seen. There were 112 participants with unresectable lung cancer identified in the group screened every 4 months compared with 109 unresectable cancers identified in the control group. The MLP showed that the screened group had a 5-yr survival of nearly 35%, whereas the 5-yr survival in the nonscreening group was 15% [24]. However, the mortality from lung cancer in the screen group was 3.2 per 1,000 person-yrs and not statistically different from the 3.0 per 1,000 person-yrs in the control group [24]. Lack of improvement in mortality in all three of the National Cancer Institute sponsored studies failed to prove that screening for lung cancer was appropriate. Considerable controversy has resulted from the interpretation of these trials [17]. From the clinical standpoint, it would have been most helpful to have a no-screen control group. The MLP came closest to this, but over half of the control group had a chest radiograph in the last year of the study and 75% in the last 2 yrs. The lack of reduction in mortality has been interpreted as showing that screening was of no benefit, but these studies evaluated screening at different frequencies rather than screening *versus* no screening. A meta-analysis showed that more frequent screening with chest radiograph led to an increase in mortality when compared with less frequent screening. In other words, screening did more harm than good [25].

Although the chest radiograph is easy to perform, of low risk and well accepted by patients, it is not very sensitive. From the results of the National Cancer Institute trials, Flehinger and Melamed [26] estimated that the probability of detecting the presence of a stage I lung cancer by chest radiograph was only 16%. Within the MLP, 90% of the peripheral lung cancers detected using every 4-month chest radiographs were evident in retrospect, despite the fact that three radiologists had interpreted the previous radiographic findings as normal [27]. These studies were not designed to evaluate screening with chest radiograph and or sputum cytology *versus* no screening, yet the results stopped reimbursement for any screening for lung cancer.

CT screening

The most sensitive image modality currently available for detecting pulmonary nodules is CT. Conventional chest CT requires radiation dosage and image-acquisition time that is impractical for screening purposes. The development of low-dose, fast spiral (LDS)CT greatly reduced the radiation dose and the scan time, making screening feasible. Conventional CT images are obtained at 140–300 mA and are performed over many minutes using multiple breath-holds. In contrast, LDSCT images may be obtained at 20–50 mA and the entire scan completed in 15 s during a single breath-hold. LDSCT is comparable in sensitivity and specificity of lung nodule detection when compared with conventional CT mode.

Initial studies from Japan created excitement in suggesting the viability of LDSCT as a tool for early lung cancer detection. The first report was from KANEKO *et al.* [1] comparing LDSCT scanning with chest radiography in screening a high-risk population for lung cancer [1]. CT scans and chest radiographs were obtained every 6 months in 1,369 participants who were aged >50 yrs and had a >20-pack-yr history of smoking. CT detected 15 cases of peripheral lung cancer and 11 of these were missed on chest radiography (fig. 1). An incredible 93% of the nonsmall cell lung carcinomas (NSCLCs) identified were stage I. The second report in the literature was from SONE *et al.* [2], who screened 3,958 participants with LDSCT. A total of 19 lung cancers were detected by CT, and only four of these were seen on chest radiograph. Remarkably, 16 out of the 19 (84%) were stage I at resection (table 1).

In the USA, CT screening efforts were led by HENSCHKE *et al.* [3] with the Early Lung Cancer Action Project (ELCAP). They enrolled 1,000 current or former smokers aged ≥60 yrs and screened with LDSCT and chest radiograph. Prevalence results were reported in 1999. CT detected a total of 27 prevalence lung cancers, and only seven were also seen by chest radiograph. CT detected four times as many lung cancers and six times the number of stage I lesions than did chest radiography. At surgery, 23 out of the 27 (85%) malignancies were stage IA.

In the CT screening study by SWENSEN *et al.* [4], 1,520 participants aged ≥50 yrs who were current or former smokers of ≥20 pack-yrs were enrolled and screened within 1 yr [4]. Chest radiograph was not performed as part of the study. There were 31 prevalence cancers and 22 (71%) were surgical stage I. DIEDERICH *et al.* [7] reported further prevalence data of CT screening in Germany. LDSCT of the chest was performed in 817 participants aged 40–78 yrs who had at least a 20-pack-yrs smoking history. A prevalence of cancer was detected in 11 out of 817 (1.3%) subjects, and seven out of 12 (58%) cancers detected were surgical stage I lesions.

Cancers detected that are not present on the baseline scan are incidence cancers (found subsequent screens; table 2). SOBUE *et al.* [5] reported 22 incidence cancers

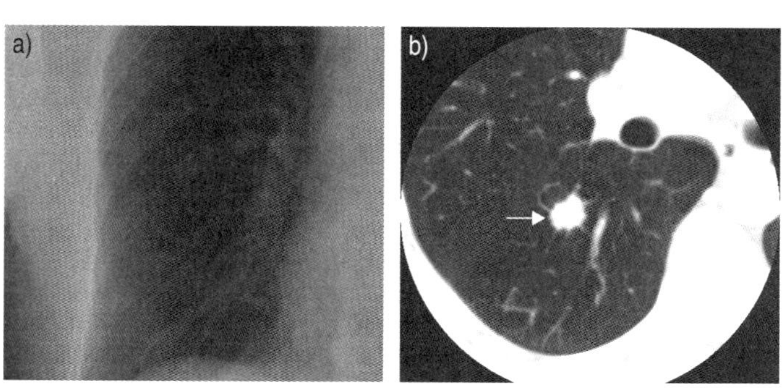

Fig. 1. – A 58-yr-old former smoker. a) Negative chest radiograph taken the same day as computed tomography. b) Spiculated 15 mm nodule in the right lower lobe (arrow); this manifested itself as an adenocarcinoma (T1N1M0) at resection.

Table 1. – Prevalence nodules and cancers detected: prospective, single-arm observational low-dose spiral computed tomography (CT) screening studies

First author [ref.]	Subjects n	Participants with noncalcified nodules	CT collimation mm	CT-detected lung cancers	Missed on chest radiograph	Surgical stage I A/B
KANEKO [1]	1369	588[#] (17)	10	15	11 (73)	14 (93)
SONE [2]	3967	217[¶] (5)	10	19	15 (79)	16 (84)
HENSCHKE [3]	1000	233 (23)	10	27	20 (74)	23 (85)
SWENSEN [4]	1520	782 (51)	5	31	Not done	22 (71)
DIEDERICH [7]	817	350 (43)	5	12	Not done	7 (58)
NAWA [8]	7956	2099 (26)	10	36	Not done	31 (86)
MCWILLIAMS [9]	561	431 (46)	7 (36) 1.25 (60)	10	Not done	7 (70)
IELCAP [11]	31,567	4186 (13)[+]	1.25–10	405	Not done	85%[§]
ROBERTS [12]	1000	256 (26)[+]	1–1.25	20	Not done	15 (75)
WILSON [13]	3642	1477 (41)	2.5	53	Not done	31 (58)

Data are presented as n or n (%), unless otherwise indicated. IELCAP: International Early Lung Cancer Action Program. [#]: CT findings described as abnormal shadows; [¶]: CT findings described as suspicious or indeterminate; [+]: not reported for nodules <5 mm; [§]: only pooled prevalence and incidence clinical stage information reported.

detected among 7,891 examinations. Surgical stage was IA in 82% and mean tumour diameter was 14.6 mm. Of the participants, >40% had five or more semi-annual scans after baseline. CT detected 19 of the 22 cancers and the other three were detected by sputum cytology alone. In the ELCAP study, 84% of the individuals underwent a first repeat screen and another 34% underwent subsequent screenings [6]. CT detected seven cancers, one of which was a limited-stage SCLC. Of the six NSCLCs, three were surgical IA lesions, one was stage IIIA and two were clinical IA lesions that were not resected because of medical contraindications. In the by study SWENSEN *et al.* [4], at the end of 5 yrs of screening, 34 incidence cancers were detected, 17 (61%) were stage I, and three were interval carcinomas (fig. 2).

The largest single-arm, observational report of CT screening is a combination of the results of ELCAP combined with those of the International Early Lung Cancer Action

Table 2. – Incidence cancers detected: prospective, single-arm observational low-dose, spiral computed tomography (CT) screening studies

First author [ref.]	Subjects	Scans	Scans with newly detected noncalcified nodules	CT-detected lung cancers	Surgical stage I	Interval cancers
SOBUE [5]	1611	7891	721 (9)	22	18 (82)	N/A
HENSCHKE [6]	841	1184	63 (5)	7	3 (43)[#]	2
SWENSEN [4]	1478		9–13%	34	17 (61)	3
DIEDERICH [7]	668		13%	10	7 (70)	5
NAWA [8]	5568	5568	148 (3)[¶]	4	4 (100)	N/A
GOHAGAN [10]	1398		18%	8	2 (25)	2
IELCAP [11]	27456		1460 (5)[+]	74	85%[§]	5
WILSON [13]	3423		256 (7.5)	27	9 (33)	3

Data are presented as n or n (%), unless otherwise indicated. N/A: not available; IELCAP: International Early Lung Cancer Action Program. [#]: two cancers were clinical stage IA but not resected due to medical reasons, and therefore not surgically staged; [¶]: only nodules ≥8 mm reported; [+]: not reported for nodules <5 mm; [§]: only pooled prevalence and incidence clinical stage information reported.

Program (IELCAP) [11]. The 31,567 participants received a baseline scan and 27,456 repeat scans were performed. A total of 484 cancers were found, 412 (85%) of these were clinical stage I NSCLCs, and 375 (77%) were surgical stage I. Actuarial 10-yr, lung cancer survival was 80% overall. The actuarial survival for those with clinical stage I was 88%; median follow-up in this study was only 40 months [11]. The high percentage of cancer found in stage I suggests that LDSCT may have the potential to shift identification of a lung cancer to stage I from a more advanced stage. Though the calculated survival results are impressive, in the absence of a control arm, one cannot be certain that screening is not simply identifying more cancers in early stage while not changing the number of advanced cancers or the number of deaths from lung cancer. Note also that the IELCAP study results should be interpreted in the light of significant conflicts of interest [28].

A subsequent report raises concern that despite earlier diagnosis, CT may not result in lives saved with screening. Investigators applied a validated lung cancer prediction model to three prospective single-arm observational studies of CT screening combining 3,246 participants [29]. CT screening found three times the number of expected cancers, resulted in 10 times the expected number of resections (109 out of 144 cancers were resectable), and identified more than the expected number of advanced stage cancers. Despite have a 94% actual 4-yr survival for participants with clinical stage 1 cancers who underwent surgery, CT screening did not result in a reduction in the expected number of deaths from lung cancer. These results emphasise the need to evaluate the effectiveness of screening by mortality rather than survival.

Problems with CT screening

Although low-dose screening CT shows promise, with problems being quickly identified, a few of the major concerns raised include the following: false positives, whether earlier detection is early enough and overdiagnosis.

In the study by Swensen *et al.* [4], baseline scanning revealed one or more noncalcified nodules in 51% of the participants and after four annual scans, 74% of the

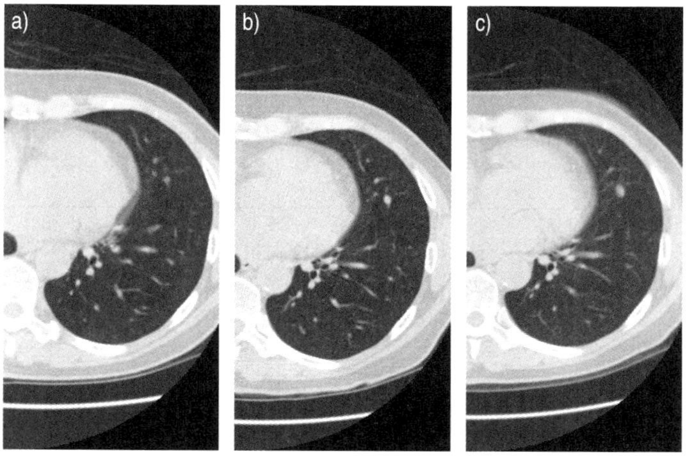

Fig. 2. – A 63-yr-old current smoker had a solid nodule, found to be a 6-mm (T1N0M0) adenocarcinoma, in the lingula and first noted a) in January 2004 and shown to enlarge on follow-up (b and c).

participants had one or more nodules. In the ELCAP study, a total of 559 noncalcified nodules were detected in 233 participants (23%) at baseline and, of the 1,184 annual repeat screenings, noncalcified nodules were newly detected in 63 participants (5.3%) [6]. The ELCAP study used a single-detector scanner with 10-mm collimation (slice thickness) and increments of 5 mm of overlap (table 1). The study by SWENSEN *et al.* [4] used a multidetector scanner with 5-mm slice width and a 3.75-mm reconstruction interval. In the study by DIEDERICH *et al.* [7], noncalcified pulmonary nodules were detected in 43% of the participants. DIEDERICH *et al.* [7] also used 5-mm collimation with 5-mm reconstruction interval and the rate of nodule detection was similar to the study by SWENSEN *et al.* [4]. In the study by MCWILLIAMS *et al.* [9] in Vancouver, the number of participants with one or more nodules detected increased from 36% to 60% when scan-slice thickness was reduced from 7 mm to 1.25 mm. The prevalence of data from these prospective, single-arm CT studies show a rate of nodule detection among participants of between 23% and 60%. Frequency of nodule detection appears to be a function of slice thickness rather than the geographical location of screening. To reduce the number of false positives, researchers decided to call a scan negative if the largest nodule detected is <5 mm [11]. This approach will increase the number of false negatives; in the study by MCWILLIAMS *et al.* [30], 18% of the cancers identified were first detected when <4 mm.

Potential harm from screening would include the as yet unmeasured impact of knowing that one has an abnormality on CT. Another potential harm is unnecessary surgery. In the study by CRESTANELLO *et al.* [31], 10 out of of 55 participants (18%) underwent resection for benign disease [31]. Similarly, in a German study [7], benign nodules represented 20% of resections. BACH *et al.* [29] found that as a result of CT screening, there were 10 times the number of surgeries expected and only three times the number of cancers expected. Careful evaluation of detected nodules with old images, serial exams, positron emission tomography or needle biopsy may allow avoiding removal of benign nodules in most, but not all, circumstances. The expensive and invasive interventions need to be considered in addition to the emotional and financial costs of screening.

CT relies on the radiologist's ability to identify cancers. The goal is to detect them when they are smaller and, therefore, detect them earlier, and at a time when intervention leads to cure. Current CT techniques identify nodules as small as 2–3 mm. In the IELCAP study [11], the median stage I tumour size was 13 mm at baseline and 9 mm for incidence stage I cancers. In the study by SWENSEN *et al.* [4], the median diameter of incidence NSCLCs at the time of resection was 10 mm. Screening with chest radiography identifies cancers when they are an average size of 30 mm [32]. Identifying a cancer that is <15 mm in diameter is undoubtedly earlier in its life than when it is 30 mm. The screening studies show that few lung cancers are detected at a size of ≤5 mm, and by the time their evaluation leads to resection, they are considerably larger. By the time a lung cancer has reached the size of 5 mm, it is estimated to be 10^8 cells [33]. By the time a cancer reaches 10 mm, it is estimated to have gone through 30 doublings in volume and to contain approximately one billion cells. Detection of lung cancer with CT appears to be earlier than that detected by chest radiograph but is not necessarily early in the life of the cancer. With traditional estimates of lung cancer doubling times of between 21 and 400 days, a 10-mm tumour would have been in existence for at least 20 months if not many years [34]. The question is whether or not a cancer will have progressed beyond the critical point of metastasis by time of visual detection by CT. That some lung cancers have already metastasised by the time they are 5 mm in size is supported by current data. In the ELCAP study [6], a prevalence lung cancer detected when it was 6–10 mm in size was already stage IIIB at resection; in addition, an incidence cancer had a diameter of 5 mm lesion at detection and was already stage IIIA at surgery [6]. Smaller implies earlier, and earlier is better, but may not be early enough for some cancers, as size may not reflect the biological aggression or differentiation of the tumour.

Contrary to the concern that spiral CT might not be able to identify lung cancers early enough in their course is the notion of overdiagnosis. Although the issue of overdiagnosis may initially raise eyebrows in the context of lung cancer, clinicians are quite familiar with it in prostate cancer and breast ductal carcinoma *in situ*. Support for the presence of overdiagnosis in lung cancer was found within an extended follow-up of the MLP. MARCUS *et al.* [35] reported on participant follow-up through 1996 (median follow-up time 20.5 yrs). The median survival for patients with resected early-stage cancer was 16.0 yrs in the intervention arm *versus* 5.0 yrs in the control arm. However, lung cancer mortality was 4.4 deaths per 1,000 person-yrs in the intervention arm and 3.9 in the control arm (p=0.09). The improvement in survival and the lack of reduction in mortality for participants in the screening arm suggested that some cancers with limited clinical significance were identified; in other words, some cancers were overdiagnosed. A corollary to the existence of overdiagnosis would be the anticipated finding of insignificant lung cancers at autopsy. The findings of MCFARLANE *et al.* [36] that 73% of the lung cancers identified at autopsy were early stage lesions (stage 0, I or II) would support this notion.

CT data regarding tumour-doubling times lend further evidence that overdiagnosis is a factor in the apparent survival improvement with LDSCT screening. AOKI *et al.* [37] reported on 34 patients with peripheral adenocarcinoma <3 cm in size who had undergone CT and chest radiography before surgery, but also had chest radiograph or CT >6 months before surgery. Tumour doubling times were calculated based on the tumour growth pattern in comparing the films. Those with bronchoalveolar cell carcinomas had tumour doubling times ranging from 662 to 1,486 days with a mean of 880 days. A mean doubling time of 880 days would take a 10 mm bronchoalveolar cell cancer 19 yrs to grow to a size of 20 cm. Adding to the concern of overdiagnosis is the report from NAWA *et al.* [8], which found 23 out of 40 (58%) prevalence cancers in a CT-screened population were never-smokers. Further support for overdiagnosis with CT screening came from an analysis of the cancers identified in the Mayo CT screening study [4]. Volume doubling times were retrospectively calculated for 48 screen-detected cancers; 13 (27%) were slow growing cancers with doubling times over 400 days (fig. 3) [38].

Other methods of screening

Advances in molecular biology have led to new insights regarding lung cancer biology. Sputum and serum are sources for the identification of tumour DNA with genetic alterations, such as loss of heterozygosity, identification of hypermethylation of tumour suppressor genes, and expression of telomerase detected in most cancers and rarely in normal tissue. The development of gene expression arrays now allows the assessment of thousands of genes simultaneously. Similarly, proteomics, the detection of novel proteins, may identify proteins associated with the early presence of lung cancer in serum or sputum. Identification of these molecular genetic alterations present in lung cancers provides potential for identifying these changes in sputum or serum as an indication of presence or high risk of cancer.

ZHONG *et al.* [39] reported a study using NSCLC cDNA libraries to test serum for tumour-associated antibodies in order to predict the presence of cancer in participants of the Mayo screening trial. In 32 out of 40 participants with CT screening-detected incidence cancers, the serum test predicted cancer 1–5 yrs prior to diagnosis [39]. Similar

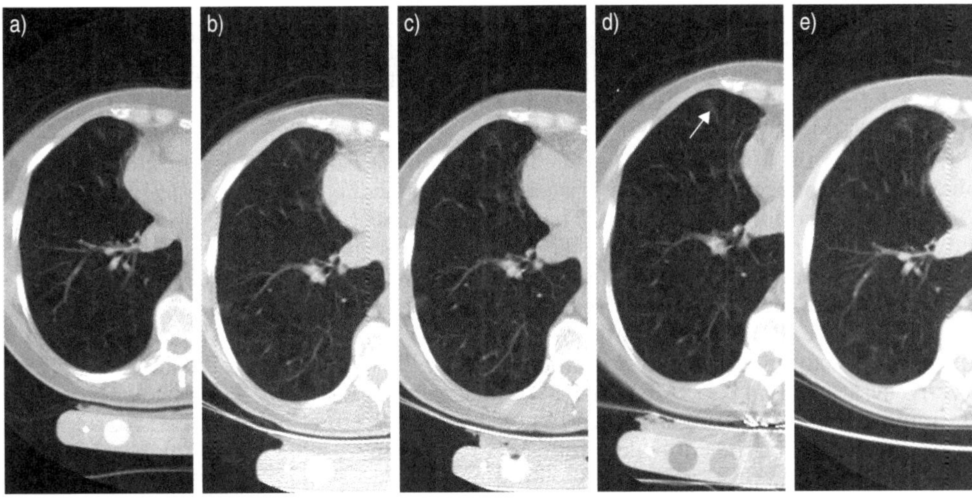

Fig. 3. – Probable overdiagnosis cancer shown at periods of b, c and d) 1-yearly and e) 6-monthly intervals. The slowly growing ground-glass opacity (arrow) was d) first noted, although a) present in retrospect on the baseline image. Resection revealed a 15 mm (T1N0M0) bronchoalveolar cell carcinoma.

results were reported by Chapman *et al.* [40], who studied the sera from patients with lung cancer compared with normal controls. One of seven autoantibodies (p53, c-myc, HER2, NY-ESO-1, CAGE, MUC1 and GBU4-5) was identified by enzyme-linked immunoassay in 89% of node-negative patients with lung cancer for a specificity of 92%; only one normal control showed more than one antibody response. Using the presence of four serum proteins (carcinoembryonic antigen, retinol-binding protein, α_1-anti-trypsin and squamous cell carcinoma antigen), Patz *et al.* [41] correctly classified sera from lung cancer cases *versus* controls with sensitivity of 89% and specificity of 85%. To date, none of these techniques is ready for clinical application, but these or similar methods may be used as primary screen or to evaluate those with abnormalities identified at CT screening.

Advances in bronchoscopy have improved the detection of airway neoplasia by the bronchoscopist. Studies have shown improved detection of intraepithelial neoplasia with autofluorescence bronchoscopy and narrow band imaging when compared with standard white-light inspection [42, 43]. The only study using bronchoscopy as a primary screening modality with CT reported detection of 28 cancers, of which seven were identified by bronchoscopy [30]. This was a single-arm observational study and so, similar to the CT only studies, the significance of the findings in regard to mortality from lung cancer is unknown. Further studies may show that bronchoscopic techniques have a role in the surveillance of patients with a history of lung cancer, evaluating those with dysplastic cells in their sputum, or in screening those at high risk for lung cancer.

Conclusions

Reports of the single-arm prospective studies have resulted in a great deal of interest among physicians and the public. Popularity of the notion that lung cancers could be found early led to screening CT offerings in physician offices and shopping malls. Many experts in the field feel that the issues of screening bias, concern of over diagnosis and the lack of mortality reduction for any screening test for lung cancer demand that CT be held to the standard of mortality reduction [44–46]. Some feel that the results from currently available screening studies are indication enough of benefit and that a randomised controlled trial is unnecessary [47, 48].

Results of the nonrandomised trials appear to be insufficient evidence to move CT screening from the realm of personal choice for those of means to a matter of public policy. A randomised controlled trial is the only available method to demonstrate mortality reduction from screening. The National Cancer Institute has sponsored such a study. The National Lung Screening Trial (NLST) has enrolled over 50,000 participants aged 55–74 yrs and current or former smokers of $\geq$30 pack-yrs [49]. Participants were randomised between LDSCT and chest radiograph at baseline, and 1 and 2 yrs with follow-up. There is great anticipation that this study [49] will show mortality reduction with LDSCT scanning and that this effectiveness will be at a cost that is not prohibitive. Effectiveness needs to be demonstrated before accurate cost-effectiveness can be determined. If CT screening is shown to achieve a 20% reduction in mortality from lung cancer, this would be the equivalent in lives saved of eliminating mortality from prostate cancer. A 25% reduction in mortality would have the equivalency of eliminating deaths from breast cancer. Given the number of lives lost to lung cancer each year, the stakes are high. However, the stakes are even higher if we pursue with time and money a screening test that does not reduce mortality and further delays the pursuit of one that does. The only randomised trial data concerning CT *versus* chest radiograph detection of cancer come from three studies [46–48], one reported from the USA, one from France and the other from Italy (table 3). In the Lung Screening Study, 1,660 participants were randomised to low-dose spiral CT and 1,658 to chest radiography [50]. After the baseline and one annual follow-up scan, 40 lung cancers were diagnosed in the CT arm and 20 in the chest radiograph arm. Similarly, in the Depiscan study [51], there were eight lung cancers among 336 participants randomised to LDSCT and one cancer among 285 in the chest radiograph arm [51]. The high resection rate of screening-detected patients suggests a possible increase in cure rate. Somewhat to the contrary are the baseline results of the DANTE trial [52]; in this trial [52], the stage I detection rate was four-times higher for spiral CT *versus* chest radiograph, although more cancers in an advanced stage were also detected by CT. A multicentre study in the Netherlands and Belgium (Nederlands Leuvens Longkanker Screeningsonderzoek; NELSON) [53] is also underway comparing LDSCT to no screening.

Table 3. – Cancers detected: randomised, controlled low-dose spiral computed tomography (CT) screening studies

Study [ref.]	Subjects	Noncalcified nodules %	CT collimation mm	Cancers detected	Surgical stage I %
Lung Screening study [46]					
CT	1660	25.8#	5	40	48
Chest radiograph	1658	8.7#		20	40
Depiscan [47]					
CT	336	45.2	1–1.5	8	37.5
Chest radiograph	285	7.4		1	100
DANTE [48]					
CT	1276	15.6¶	N/A	28	68
Chest radiograph	1196	3.1¶		8	50

Data are presented as n, unless otherwise indicated. N/A: not available. #: reported as positive if a nodule $\geq$4mm was detected; ¶: reported as positive only if a nodule was $\geq$10 mm or spiculated.

Results of the NLST, Depiscan, DANTE and NELSON studies will not be available for a few years and it is not known when results of the Prostate, Lung, Colorectal and Ovarian (PLCO) study [54] screening with a chest radiograph *versus* no screening will be available. Until a positive effect by mortality reduction from either of these studies is demonstrated, it is unlikely that screening for lung cancer will be covered by health insurance plans. What is a clinician to do in the mean time? The answer is not clear. Screening with a chest radiograph or LDSCT has been shown to find more lung cancers, more cancers at an early stage, and to improve survival, but neither has demonstrated a benefit in the number of lives saved. In the absence of clearly demonstrated benefits, the decision to case-find lung cancer with screening requires a discussion between the physician and the patient of the risks and potential benefits. Given the potential harm in unnecessary biopsies and surgery, increasing survival in the absence of mortality reduction suggests that screening benefit may not outweigh the risk.

Summary

Currently, the diagnosis of lung cancer is made primarily in the pursuit of symptoms. Screening is not being widely applied in patients at risk for lung cancer because no screening test (chest radiography, sputum cytology or computed tomography (CT)) has been shown to reduce mortality from lung cancer.

The most sensitive image modality currently available for detecting pulmonary nodules is CT. Conventional chest CT requires radiation dosage and image-acquisition time that is impractical for screening purposes. However, the development of low-dose, fast-spiral CT has greatly reduced the radiation dose and the scan time, making screening feasible.

Prospective, single-arm observational studies have shown that screening with CT detects a large percentage of lung cancer in early stage and with favourable prognosis for those cancers detected, but the apparent survival improvement may be due to the biases inherent with screening. Screening introduces inherent biases of lead time, length time and overdiagnosis; it is not clear if the calculated survival is true improvement or just apparent improvement due to bias.

Randomised controlled trials of CT screening are currently under way in the USA and Europe that will hopefully definitively show mortality reduction with CT screening.

Keywords: Noncalcified nodules, overdiagnosis, screening, serum markers.

Statement of interest
None declared.

References

1. Kaneko M, Eguchi K, Ohmatsu H, *et al.* Peripheral lung cancer: screening and detection with low-dose spiral CT *versus* radiography. *Radiology* 1999; 201: 798–802.
2. Sone S, Takashima S, Li F, *et al.* Mass screening for lung cancer with mobile spiral computed tomography scanner. *Lancet* 1998; 351: 1242–1245.
3. Henschke CI, McCauley DI, Yankelevitz DF, *et al.* Early lung cancer action project: overall design and findings from baseline screening. *Lancet* 1999; 354: 99–105.

4. Swensen SJ, Jett JR, Hartman TE, *et al.* CT screening for lung cancer: five-year prospective experience. *Radiology* 2005; 235: 259–265.
5. Sobue T, Moriyama N, Kaneko M, *et al.* Screening for lung cancer with low-dose helical computed tomography: Anti-Lung Cancer Association project. *J Clin Oncol* 2002; 20: 911–920.
6. Henschke CI, Naidich DP, Yankelevitz DF, *et al.* Early lung cancer action project: initial findings on repeat scanning. *Cancer* 2001; 92: 153–159.
7. Diederich S, Wormanns D, Semik M, *et al.* Screening for early lung cancer with low-dose spiral CT: prevalence in 817 asymptomatic smokers. *Radiology* 2002; 222: 773–781.
8. Nawa T, Nakagawa T, Suzushi S, *et al.* Lung cancer screening using low-dose spiral CT: results of baseline and 1-year follow-up studies. *Chest* 2002; 122: 15–20.
9. McWilliams A, Mayo J, MacDonald S, *et al.* Lung cancer screening: A different paradigm. *Am J Respir Crit Care Med* 2003; 168: 1167–1173.
10. Gohagan J, Marcus P, Fagerstrom R, *et al.* Baseline findings of a randomized feasibility trial of lung cancer screening with spiral CT scan vs chest radiograph: the Lung Screening Study of the National Cancer Institute. *Chest* 2004; 126: 114–121.
11. The International Early Lung Cancer Action Program Investigators. Survival of patients with stage I lung cancer detected on CT screening. *N Engl J Med* 2006; 355: 1763–1771.
12. Roberts HC, Patsios D, Paul NS, *et al.* Lung cancer screening with low-dose computed tomography: Canadian experience. *Can Assoc Radiol J* 2007; 58: 225–235.
13. Wilson DO, Weissfeld JL, Fuhrman CR, *et al.* The Pittsburgh Lung Screening Study (PLuSS): Outcomes within 3 years of a first CT Scan. *Am J Respir Crit Care Med* 2008; 178: 956–961.
14. Parkin DM, Bray F, Ferlay J, Pisani P. Global cancer statistics, 2002. *CA Cancer J Clin* 2005; 55: 74–108.
15. Jemal A, Siegel R, Ward E, *et al.* Cancer statistics, 2008. *CA Cancer J Clin* 2008; 58: 71–96.
16. Smith RA, Cokkinides V, Brawley OW. Cancer screening in the United States, 2008: a review of current American Cancer Society guidelines and cancer screening issues. *CA Cancer J Clin* 2008; 58: 161–179.
17. Strauss GM. Screening for lung cancer. *Surg Oncol Clin N Am* 1999; 8: 747–774.
18. Frost JK, Ball WC, Levin ML, *et al.* Early lung cancer detection: results of the initial (prevalence) radiologic and cytologic screening in the Johns Hopkins Study. *Am Rev Respir Dis* 1984; 130: 549–554.
19. Tockman MS. Survival and mortality from lung cancer in a screened population: The Johns Hopkins Study. *Chest* 1986; 89: 324S–326S.
20. Johns Hopkins Medical Institutions Final Report. Lung Cancer Control, Detection and Therapy. Phase II, NCI-PHS Contract No. N01-CN-4537. December 31, 1984. Bethesda, MD, National Cancer Institute, 1984.
21. Flehinger BJ, Melamed MR, Zaman MB, *et al.* Early lung cancer detection: results of the initial (prevalence) radiologic and cytologic screening in the Memorial Sloan-Kettering study. *Am Rev Respir Dis* 1984; 130: 555–560.
22. National Lung Program, Memorial Sloan-Kettering Cancer Center: Final report and data summary. December 31, 1984. Bethesda, MD, National Cancer Institute, 1984.
23. Fontana RS, Sanderson DR, Taylor WF, *et al.* Early lung cancer detection: results of the initial (prevalence) radiologic and cytologic screening in the Mayo Clinic Study. *Am Rev Respir Dis* 1984; 130: 561–565.
24. Fontana RS, Sanderson DR, Woolner LB, *et al.* Screening for lung cancer: A critique of the Mayo Lung Project. *Cancer* 1991; 67: 1155–1164.
25. Manser R, Wright G, Hart D, *et al.* Surgery for early stage non-small cell lung cancer. *Cochrane Database Syst Rev* 2005; 1: CD004699.
26. Flehinger BJ, Melamed MR. Current status of screening for lung cancer. *Chest Surg Clin N Am* 1994; 4: 1–15.
27. Muhm JR, Miller WE, Fontana RS, *et al.* Lung cancer detected during a screening program using four-month chest radiographs. *Radiology* 1983; 148: 609–615.

28. Chabner BA. Smoke, then fire: lung cancer screening studies under further scrutiny. *Oncologist* 2008; 13: 348–349.
29. Bach PB, Jett JR, Pastorino U, *et al.* Computed tomography screening and lung cancer outcomes. *JAMA* 2007; 297: 953–961.
30. McWilliams AM, Mayo JR, Ahn MI, *et al.* Lung cancer screening using multi-slice thin-section computed tomography and autofluorescence bronchoscopy. *J Thorac Oncol* 2006; 1: 61–68.
31. Crestanello JA, Allen MS, Jett JR, *et al.* Thoracic surgical operations in patients enrolled in a computed tomographic screening trial. *J Thorac Cardiovasc Surg* 2004; 128: 254–259.
32. Quekel LG, Kessels A, Goei R, *et al.* Miss rate of lung cancer on the chest radiograph in clinical practice. *Chest* 1999; 115: 720–724.
33. DeVita VT, Young RC, Canellos GP. Combination *versus* single-agent chemotherapy: a review of the bases for selection of drug treatment of cancer. *Cancer* 1975; 35: 98–110.
34. Nathan MH, Collins VP, Adams RA. Differentiation of benign and malignant pulmonary nodules by growth rate. *Radiology* 1962; 79: 221–231.
35. Marcus PM, Bergstralh EJ, Fagerstrom RM, *et al.* Lung cancer mortality in the Mayo Lung Project: the impact of extended follow-up. *J Natl Cancer Inst* 2000; 92: 1308–1316.
36. McFarlane MJ, Feinstein AR, Wells CK, Chan CK. The "epidemiologic necropsy," unexpected detections, demographic selections, and changing rates of lung cancer. *JAMA* 1987; 258: 331–338.
37. Aoki T, Nakata H, Watanabe H, *et al.* Evolution of peripheral lung adenocarcinomas: CT findings correlated with histology tumor doubling time. *AJR Am J Roentgenol* 2000; 174: 763–768.
38. Lindell RM, Hartman TE, Swensen SJ, *et al.* Five-year lung cancer screening experience: CT appearance, growth rate, location, and histologic features of 61 lung cancers. *Radiology* 2007, 242: 555–562.
39. Zhong L, Coe SP, Stromberg AJ, *et al.* Profiling tumor-associated antibodies for early detection of non-small cell lung cancer. *J Thorac Oncol* 2006; 1: 513–519.
40. Chapman CJ, Murray A, McElveen JE, *et al.* Autoantibodies in lung cancer: possibilities for early detection and subsequent cure. *Thorax* 2008; 63: 228–233.
41. Patz EF Jr, Campa MJ, Gottlin EB, *et al.* Panel of serum biomarkers for the diagnosis of lung cancer. *J Clin Oncol* 2007; 25: 5578–5583.
42. Lam S, Kennedy T, Unger M, *et al.* Localization of bronchial intraepithelial neoplastic lesions by fluorescence bronchoscopy. *Chest* 1998; 113: 696–702.
43. Vincent BD, Fraig M, Silvestri GA. A pilot study of narrow-band imaging compared to white light bronchoscopy for evaluation of normal airways and premalignant and malignant airways disease. *Chest* 2007; 131: 1794–1799.
44. Aberle DR, Gamsu G, Henschke CI, *et al.* A consensus statement of the Society of Thoracic Radiology: screening for lung cancer with helical computed tomography. *J Thorac Imaging* 2001; 16: 65–68.
45. Black WC, Baron JA. CT screening for lung cancer: spiraling into confusion? *JAMA* 2007; 297: 995–997.
46. Bach PB, Silvestri GA, Hanger M, *et al.* Screening for lung cancer: ACCP evidence-based clinical practice guidelines (2nd edition). *Chest* 2007; 132: 69S–77S.
47. Strauss GM, Gleason RE, Sugarbaker DJ. Screening for lung cancer: another look; a different view. *Chest* 1997; 111: 754–768.
48. Miettinen OS. Screening for lung cancer. *Radiol Clin North Am* 2000; 38: 479–486.
49. Hillman BJ. Economic, legal, and ethical rationales for the ACRIN National Lung Screening Trial of CT screening for lung cancer. *Acad Radiol* 2003; 10: 349–350.
50. Gohagan JK, Marcus PM, Fagerstrom RM, *et al.* Final results of the Lung Screening Study, a randomized feasibility study of spiral CT *versus* chest X-ray screening for lung cancer. *Lung Cancer* 2005; 47: 9–15.
51. Blanchon T, Brechot JM, Grenier PA, *et al.* Baseline results of the Depiscan study: a French randomized pilot trial of lung cancer screening comparing low dose CT scan (LDCT) and chest X-ray (CXR). *Lung Cancer* 2007; 58: 50–58.

52. Infante M, Lutman FR, Cavuto S, *et al.* Lung cancer screening with spiral CT: baseline results of the randomized DANTE trial. *Lung Cancer* 2008; 59: 355–363.
53. Xu DM, Gietema H, de Koning H, *et al.* Nodule management protocol of the NELSON randomized lung cancer screening trial. *Lung Cancer* 2006; 54: 177–184.
54. Oken MM, Marcus PM, Hu P, *et al.* Baseline chest radiograph for lung cancer detection in the randomized Prostate, Lung, Colorectal and Ovarian Cancer Screening Trial. *J Natl Cancer Inst* 2005; 97: 1832–1839.

CHAPTER 5

Symptoms and signs of lung cancer

N. Navani*, S.G. Spiro#

*Centre for Respiratory Research, University College London, and #Dept of Thoracic Medicine, University College London Hospitals, London, UK.

Correspondence: N. Navani, Centre for Respiratory Research, University College London, Rayne Building, 5 University Street, London, WC1E 6JJ, UK. E-mail: n.navani@ucl.ac.uk

Lung cancer remains the leading cause of cancer mortality in both males and females. Recognising the symptoms and signs of lung cancer is an important first step in establishing the diagnosis and may also provide information on disease stage and prognosis. Unfortunately, lung cancer is usually recognised late in its natural history, so that curative treatment is often not possible. This reflects the fact that the presentation of lung cancer suffers with two main problems. First, the anatomy of the thorax allows a tumour to grow for a considerable period of time before symptoms arise and, secondly, the symptoms of lung cancer, when they do occur, are often nonspecific (*e.g.* cough). Lung parenchyma (and visceral pleura) are equipped with afferent C fibres that relay stretch sensations only and so intraparenchymal lesions often remain asymptomatic, since there are no pain fibres within the lungs. The doubling time of untreated lung cancer ranges from 29 days for the small cell type to 161 days for adenocarcinoma (table 1) [1]. Assuming the model that lung cancer originates as a single cell, by the time a tumour has doubled 20 times, it is 1 mm in diameter, yet usually presents on average at 3–4 cm in diameter on chest radiograph. Therefore, lung cancers are often asymptomatic for much of their natural history and, by the time they cause symptoms and signs, the patient often has advanced disease that is beyond cure. These observations explain why the curative surgery rate for lung cancer in Europe is only between 10 and 20% and overall 5-yr survival is as low as 7%.

The presentation of lung cancer may predict survival. Given the insidious and late presentation of the disease, patients who have lung cancer detected incidentally have improved survival. Increasingly, imaging with chest radiography or computed tomography (CT) is carried out for other reasons, without a clinical suspicion of lung cancer. An asymptomatic lung cancer detected by chance is less likely to have spread and, therefore, may be more amenable to curative treatment. CARBONE *et al.* [2] found that in 678 patients with lung cancer only 6% of patients were asymptomatic at presentation. Another study of 1,277 consecutive lung cancer patients from a single centre observed 154 (13%) patients who were asymptomatic at diagnosis [3]. The 5-yr survival for these patients was higher, at 18%, when compared with those with nonspecific symptoms (6% 5-yr survival).

The majority of patients who present with lung cancer, therefore, do have symptoms or signs of the underlying disease. However, these clinical features are often nonspecific and insidious in their onset. This contributes to delay from the patient first experiencing symptoms to seeking medical attention. A Swedish study of 134 patients found that the mean delay from first symptom to presentation was 43 days with a range of 0–256 days [4]. The vague nature of most presenting symptoms and the fact that they are more usually attributable to benign causes often results in further delay in diagnosis.

Eur Respir Mon, 2009, 44, 71–87. Printed in UK - all rights reserved. Copyright ERS Journals Ltd 2009; European Respiratory Monograph; ISSN 1025-448x.

Table 1. – Natural history of untreated lung cancer

Cell type	Doubling time days	Time from malignant change to diagnosis yrs	Time from malignant change to death yrs
Small cell	20–50	2.8	3.2
Squamous cell	80–100	8.4	9.6
Adenocarcinoma	150–175	15.4	17.6

Data taken from [1].

The clinical features of lung cancer therefore occur late in the natural history of the disease and when they do occur are often nonspecific, causing further delay in diagnosis. The symptoms and signs of lung cancer may arise from: 1) the growth of the primary tumour; 2) intrathoracic metastasis of the tumour; 3) extrathoracic metastasis; 4) paraneoplastic syndromes; and 5) constitutional effects of cancer. The frequency of symptoms and signs of lung cancer and their underlying pathology are summarised in table 2.

Symptoms and signs of the primary tumour

Cough

Cough is the most common symptom associated with lung cancer and may be present in up to 75% of patients with the disease. However, cough is a feature of many other respiratory diseases and in particular chronic obstructive pulmonary disease (COPD), which may commonly co-exist with lung cancer. OKKES *et al.* [12] retrospectively analysed patient attendance to primary care physicians in the Netherlands from 1985 to 1995. Cough was a presenting complaint in 11,092 patient encounters, but lung cancer was not specifically included in the top 20 diagnoses.

Table 2. – Presenting symptoms and signs of lung cancer

Symptom or sign	Range of frequency %	Underlying pathology
Cough	8–75	Airway obstruction, compression, infiltration or infection
Weight loss	0–68	Cancer cachexia syndrome, liver metastases
Dyspnoea	3–60	Airway obstruction, pleural effusion, diaphragmatic paralysis, superadded infection
Chest pain	20–49	Invasion of thoracic nerves, chest wall, brachial plexus, mediastinal lymphadenopathy
Haemoptysis	6–35	Airway involvement by tumour
Bone pain	6–25	Bone metastases
Clubbing	0–20	New bone formation along inner periosteum of fingers and toes
Fever	0–20	Host–tumour response resulting in cytokine production
Hoarseness	2–18	Recurrent laryngeal nerve compression
Weakness	0–10	Cancer cachexia syndrome, myasthenic syndrome
Superior vena cava obstruction	0–4	Direct obstruction of superior vena cava by tumour
Dysphagia	0–2	Compression of the oesophagus by tumour
Wheezing and stridor	0–2	Intrinsic or extrinsic compression of trachea or main bronchus by tumour

Data adapted from [5–11].

Cough occurs with both central and peripheral lesions, but is more common with centrally located tumours. It may result from an endobronchial tumour causing irritation to the airway or by submucosal infiltration. Although a nonspecific symptom in itself, a sustained change in quality or quantity of cough should raise suspicion of underlying lung cancer. Copious sputum production of more than 100 cm^3 per day (bronchorrhea) is a typical but very infrequent symptom of bronchoalveolar cell carcinoma [13].

Haemoptysis

Although most cases of haemoptysis are not caused by lung cancer, this symptom most commonly alerts patients and physicians to the possibility. As a presenting feature it usually causes streaking of the sputum. Larger amounts of haemoptysis without sputum may signal vascular invasion of the tumour and more commonly occur in the terminal phase. At various degrees of severity, it may occur in up to 35% of patients with lung cancer.

The differential diagnosis for haemoptysis may be wide but the symptom always warrants further investigation, particularly in patients over the age of 40 yrs. A recent prospective analysis of 184 patients admitted to a university hospital in Greece with haemoptysis demonstrated that 13% of cases were due to lung cancer [14]. Most patients with haemoptysis have an abnormal chest radiograph but even if the radiograph is within normal limits, lung cancer may still be discovered in 5–10% of patients at bronchoscopy [15]. Even CT scanning may occasionally fail to detect small endobronchial tumours [16].

Recurrent or unresolved pneumonia

A recurrent focal pneumonia or one that fails to resolve in a timely fashion prompts the investigation for an underlying malignancy and is an important presentation of lung cancer. Several factors may determine the ability of the host to clear infection, including age, underlying lung disease and pathogen sensitivity to treatment, such that it may take at least 8 weeks for pneumonia to resolve radiographically. However, should the pneumonia persist or recur in the same territory, bronchoscopy and CT scan should be performed to exclude a proximal obstructing lesion.

Dyspnoea, wheeze and stridor

Dyspnoea is a distressing symptom that occurs in up to 60% of patients. In patients with proximal tumours, airway narrowing may result in monophonic unilateral wheeze as well as breathlessness. As the tumour progresses, this may result in complete occlusion of a main airway either by intraluminal tumour or external compression. Complete occlusion of a major airway may result in distal lung collapse and the accompanying signs of reduced expansion and dullness to percussion over the collapsed area. Breathlessness may be compounded by the fact that patients with lung cancer often have limited respiratory reserve due to co-existing COPD, pulmonary fibrosis or heart failure.

Encroachment of the tumour into the trachea or proximal main bronchi may result in stridor. This is an important sign, since it is often misdiagnosed as asthma or COPD initially. The peak expiratory flow (PEF) is disproportionately reduced in patients with tracheal obstruction when compared to the forced expiratory volume in 1 s (FEV_1), such that the ratio of the FEV_1 (in mL) to the PEF (in $L \cdot min^{-1}$) is greater than 10 (Empey index) [17]. This simple bedside assessment may identify impending upper airway obstruction due to lung cancer.

Breathlessness in the patient with lung cancer may also result from pleural or pericardial effusion, pulmonary embolic disease, lymphangitis carcinomatosa or compression of the major pulmonary vessels.

Chest pain

Chest pain in the form of a vague, central discomfort may persist for many weeks before the patient seeks medical attention. More severe pain may be caused by direct extension of the primary tumour into the parietal pleura, chest wall and intercostal nerves.

Symptoms and signs of intrathoracic metastasis

Bronchogenic carcinoma may spread *via* lymphatics, blood vessels or direct invasion. Any of the structures within the thoracic cage may be involved and this results in a wide range of symptoms and signs.

Superior vena cava obstruction

Up to 75% of cases of superior vena cava obstruction (SVCO) are due to lung cancer, with small cell being the most frequent histological subtype. Right upper lobe tumours or adjacent metastatic right paratracheal nodes compress or invade the superior vena cava. The patient complains of headaches, blurred vision, facial fullness on bending over, and breathlessness due to extrinsic tracheal compression. Examination may reveal facial plethora and oedema, persistently elevated jugular venous pressure and dilated superficial collateral veins over the upper chest, arms, rib cage and abdomen [18]. The symptoms and signs may develop relatively swiftly over the course of a few weeks and, unless a collateral circulation develops, sudden death can occur.

The development of SVCO implies mediastinal invasion of the tumour and therefore a poor prognosis in patients with nonsmall cell lung cancer. However, a French prospective series of 724 patients with small cell lung cancer had an incidence of SVCO of 12% and showed that the presence of SVCO was not associated with higher mortality, when treatment for the underlying condition with chemotherapy was applied promptly [19].

Pancoast's tumour and Horner's syndrome

5% of nonsmall cell lung cancers present as superior sulcus or Pancoast's tumours (fig. 1). They arise in the apex of the lung and may invade the second and third ribs, the brachial plexus, the subclavian vessels, the stellate ganglion and adjacent vertebral bodies. The Pancoast syndrome is characterised by pain, which may arise in the shoulder or chest wall or radiate to the neck. Patients are commonly treated for arthritis or bursitis of the shoulder before the correct diagnosis is determined and, in many cases, the diagnosis is delayed for 6–9 months before the tumour is discovered. In addition, weakness and wasting of the small muscles of the hand and pain and paraesthesiae on the ulnar surface are important clinical findings, resulting from invasion into the C8 and T1 roots of the brachial plexus. Horner's syndrome, which is composed of unilateral

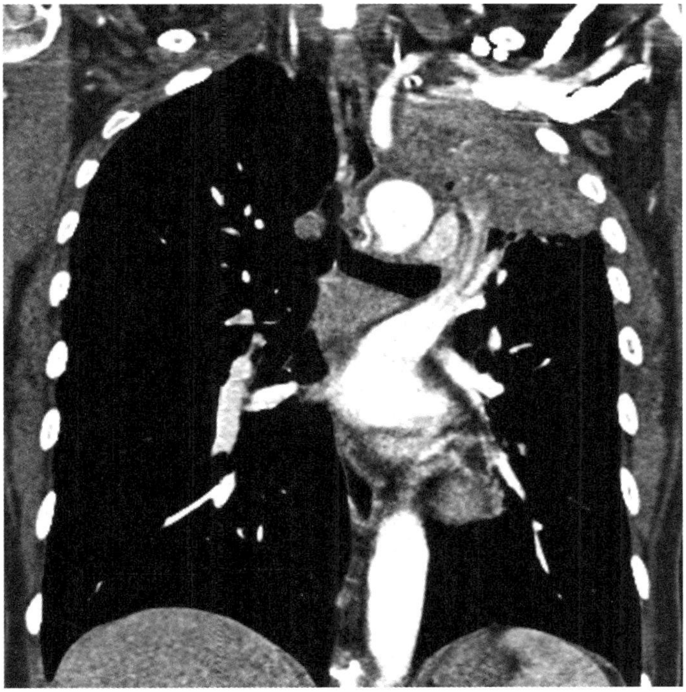

Fig. 1. – Coronal computed tomography image of left Pancoast tumour.

enopthalmos, ptosis, meiosis and anhydrosis, results from invasion of the paravertebral sympathetic chain. This group of patients with superior sulcus tumours also have a high incidence of brain metastases of up to 17% [20], and many centres employ routine magnetic resonance imaging (MRI) of the brain in this scenario, prior to any treatment with curative intent.

Recurrent laryngeal nerve palsy

Palsy of the recurrent laryngeal nerve may result from superior sulcus tumours on the right, but more commonly from tumours at the left hilum, resulting in hoarseness. The left recurrent laryngeal nerve hooks under the arch of the aorta before ascending between the trachea and oesophagus to supply the muscles of the larynx. A left vocal palsy due to neoplastic lesions in the subaortic fossa is more common than a right-sided lesion, since the right recurrent laryngeal only loops around the subclavian artery at the lung apex. The chest radiograph often shows a left upper lobe mass or collapsed left upper lobe. A vocal cord palsy causes hoarseness, which may be present in up to 18% of lung cancer patients during the natural history of the disease, and direct vision at nasendoscopy or bronchoscopy will confirm an adducted, relatively immobile vocal cord. Vocal cord paralysis may also increase the risk of aspiration.

Phrenic nerve palsy

Malignant infiltration of either phrenic nerve usually occurs due to metastatic mediastinal lymphadenopathy. Interruption of the phrenic nerve along its intrathoracic course results in an ipsilateral raised hemidiaphragm. Decreased, absent or paradoxical diaphragmatic movement decreases the vital capacity and breathlessness may dramatically worsen, particularly in patients with co-existing COPD.

Dysphagia

Although posterior mediastinal lymph nodes are commonly involved early in lung cancer, dysphagia is a relatively uncommon presenting symptom. LE ROUX [21] reported that 1–2% of lung cancer patients had dysphagia at presentation, about the same proportion as those with wheeze or stridor. When the full clinical course of the disease is considered, the percentage experiencing dysphagia rises to 6–7%, usually due to lesions extending from the left main bronchus. In addition to external compression of the middle third of the oesophagus, dysphagia may occur due to cervical lymph nodes compressing the upper third of the oesophagus, secondary achalasia, hypercalcaemia and metastatic brainstem lesions resulting in bulbar or pseudo-bulbar palsy [22].

Cardiac involvement

Primary bronchogenic carcinoma or its metastatic deposits may invade the pericardium, myocardium or (rarely) endocardium, resulting in a variety of clinical features. Although rarely a presenting symptom, cardiac involvement is reported in 25% of patients at autopsy [23]. The pericardium is the most common site of metastasis due to direct invasion or lymphatic drainage, rather than haemtogenous spread [24]. Cardiac involvement may manifest clinically with supraventricular arrhythmias (especially atrial fibrillation) that are resistant to conventional therapy. Asymptomatic pericardial effusions are relatively common, with an enlarged cardiac silhouette on chest radiography the only evidence. Life-threatening cardiac tamponade does also occur and, in one retrospective series of 51 cases of malignant pericardial effusions from a tertiary Japanese centre, 45 patients had tamponade. Of those patients, cardiac tamponade was the presenting manifestation of lung cancer in three patients [25].

Chest wall invasion

Chest wall invasion by the primary tumour causes localised pain, a common presenting symptom. It is often dull in nature at the site of the lesion and does not alter with respiration. Metastatic hilar or mediastinal nodal involvement may manifest with retrosternal discomfort. Severe pain may result from intercostal nerve involvement and may be referred to the corresponding dermatome. Rib metastases are often identified by discrete areas of tenderness and occasionally a soft tissue mass may be palpable. It is worth noting that chest wall invasion is not an exclusion criterion for surgical treatment of the primary lung cancer, in the absence of other metastatic disease.

Pleural disease

Peripheral lung cancers, particularly adenocarcinoma, may directly invade visceral pleura, resulting in pain and pleural effusion. Other lung cancers also commonly metastasise to the pleura and up to 15% of patients have pleural involvement. The parietal pleura is equipped with pain fibres that are sensitive to tumour invasion, and pleuritic pain (worse on inspiration) may be a particularly debilitating symptom. Chest pain may improve, however, with development of pleural effusion, which occurs due to direct pleural invasion or mediastinal lymphadenopathy causing lymphatic obstruction.

A large blood-stained pleural effusion is most commonly due to malignancy, particularly in a patient over the age of 40 yrs, and represents a poor prognosis. A transudative effusion may develop in patients with trapped lung due to endobronchial obstruction by the tumour and is also associated with a poor prognosis. Approximately 10% of patients present with a pleural effusion. Breathlessness may progress over weeks and months and is associated with signs of stony dull percussion note, reduced breath sounds over the effusion and reduced vocal resonance.

Symptoms and signs of extrathoracic metastasis

Extrathoracic disease is commonly detected by CT or positron emission tomography (PET) scans in asymptomatic patients, but most patients have symptoms, signs or laboratory findings that suggest extrathoracic metastasis. *Post mortem* studies performed in the post-operative period before CT was routinely available suggested a prevalence of distant metastases of between 18 and 36% [26]. Bronchogenic carcinoma, however, does not follow a set pattern of metastasis. Adenocarcinoma is more likely to have extrathoracic deposits than squamous cell carcinoma but the likelihood of discovering metastatic disease does not correlate with primary tumour or nodal staging [27]. The commonest sites of extrathoracic metastatic disease are the supraclavicular lymph nodes, liver, adrenal glands, brain, bone, kidneys, skin and abdominal lymph nodes.

Supraclavicular lymph nodes

The examination of the supraclavicular and anterior cervical lymph node stations is an important part of the initial evaluation of the patient with suspected lung cancer. Cervical or supraclavicular lymph nodes may be present in 20% of patients at presentation and sampling them may provide crucial diagnostic and staging information. Physical examination is relatively crude when compared with ultrasound examination of the neck. One single-centre UK study suggested that over 40% of patients with enlarged mediastinal nodes on CT may have lung cancer diagnosed by ultrasound lymph node aspiration [28].

Liver

The development of liver metastases is an adverse prognostic event in the natural history of lung cancer. Most liver metastases are, initially at least, asymptomatic. The symptoms and signs of more advanced liver involvement are weight loss, anorexia, epigastric pain and nodular hepatomegaly. Jaundice and ascites are even later features. Organ-specific indicators, for example raised liver enzymes, are found in less than 50% of cases.

Adrenal glands

Metastatic deposits to the adrenal glands are not usually suspected clinically and adrenal insufficiency is rarely observed. However, retrospective studies have demonstrated that the adrenal glands are a common site of extrathoracic metastasis, being the site in approximately 6% of patients [29].

Brain

Lung cancer is the commonest cause of malignant tumours of the brain, accounting for 50% of all brain parenchymal deposits. The incidence of brain metastases in patients with lung cancer depends upon the imaging modality, tumour tissue type, TN stage and the presence or absence of symptoms. In one series of 809 lung cancer patients, 181 (22%) had brain metastases and, of these patients, 61 were asymptomatic [30]. In the same series, 30.9% of patients had no other extrathoracic disease. The study confirmed previous findings that patients with adenocarcinoma, large cell carcinoma, small cell carcinoma or upper lobe tumours have a high incidence of brain metastases at presentation, even in the absence of nodal disease [30].

The frontal lobes and cerebellum are the most common sites of cerebral metastases. Headaches, nausea and vomiting, seizures, hemiplegia, cranial nerve palsies, confusion and changes in personality are the most common clinical features. Obstruction of cerebrospinal fluid is a feature of cerebellar deposits and may result in ataxia and other features of raised intracranial pressure.

Spinal cord

Metastases to the spinal cord may cause spinal cord compression. The onset of symptoms is often insidious, with back pain present up to 4 months before spinal cord compression. The recumbent position may worsen pain from vertebral metastasis, in contrast to degenerative joint disease. The emergence of leg weakness, paraesthesiae in the lower extremities, and/or bowel or bladder dysfunction should evoke immediate concern for cord compression. Examination may reveal spasticity, hyperreflexia and loss of pinprick, temperature, position and vibratory sensation. Sensation may be preserved above a particular dermatome, which is referred to as the sensory level. Percussion tenderness over the affected spinal region may be also present. Deep-tendon reflexes may be initially absent and the Babinski sign (upward movement of the toe in response to plantar stimulation) is also often absent early in the course of compression. Lax rectal sphincter tone is a late sign of spinal cord compression.

Spinal involvement is usually extra-dural and compression results from tumour involvement of the vertebral body. Analysis of 102 cases of spinal cord compression secondary to lung cancer demonstrated that 40% of cases were due to small cell carcinoma, with adenocarcinoma the next most common cell type [31]. Early recognition of spinal cord compression remains the key to preventing permanent sphincter or gait dysfunction. An MRI scan should be the immediate investigation, regardless of normal plain lumbar spine radiographs.

Bone

Bone metastases commonly occur in the axial skeleton, with the spine, pelvis, ribs, skull and femora being the most common sites. They commonly cause pain, pathological fractures and reduced mobility. They may also be associated with raised alkaline phosphatase or hypercalcaemia. Approximately a quarter of bone metastases are asymptomatic on presentation and are only detected on isotope bone or PET scanning.

Skin

Cutaneous metastases are a rare presentation of lung cancer but may occur in up to 15% of patients with advanced disease. They occur most commonly with large cell carcinoma [32] and appear as painless, purplish and rapidly growing masses. Biopsy of the skin lesion provides diagnostic and staging information and confers a poor prognosis.

Coeliac lymph nodes

Metastases to coeliac lymph nodes are increasingly recognised as important extrathoracic deposits that imply advanced disease. They are usually asymptomatic and may be suspected on staging CT or endoscopic ultrasound examination. SINGH *et al.* [33] examined the coeliac lymph nodes in 93 consecutive patients with suspected lung cancer using endoscopic ultrasound and diagnosed extrathoracic coeliac axis disease in 11% of cases, half of which had not been identified on prior CT scan.

Uncommon sites

Metastases to kidneys, gastrointestinal tract and pancreas are relatively uncommon and usually asymptomatic. Choroidal metastases are also well recognised and may cause blurred vision and spots before the eyes.

Symptoms and signs that predict extrathoracic metastasis

Initial evaluation of the patient with suspected lung cancer should include an assessment of the probability of extrathoracic disease. HOOPER and co-workers [34, 35] showed that a selection of symptoms, signs and blood tests could reliably predict the presence of extrathoracic disease (table 3). The more factors that were present, the higher the likelihood of metastatic disease and, moreover, if no factors were present, extrathoracic disease was very improbable. SILVESTRI *et al.* [36] carried out a meta-analysis of the performance of the clinical evaluation in detecting extrathoracic disease. Over 3,000 bone scans and CT scans of the brain and abdomen were evaluated following clinical assessment. The study confirmed the high negative predictive value of clinical assessment. Therefore, in patients with little evidence of extrathoracic disease on clinical grounds, routine scanning for metastatic disease may not be justified. This currently remains the case for the assessment of brain metastases, but highly sensitive PET scanning has now become a standard tool in the pre-operative assessment of lung cancer patients.

Paraneoplastic syndromes

Paraneoplastic syndromes refer to a constellation of symptoms and signs that are not due to any physical effect of the tumour, but due to the secretion of a compound or compounds from the primary site and any metastases. They may occur prior to the diagnosis of malignant disease or herald tumour recurrence. 10% of patients with bronchogenic carcinoma may have evidence of a paraneoplastic syndrome, which represents a diagnostic and therapeutic challenge but also an opportunity to diagnose an otherwise asymptomatic malignancy. The mechanism by which the syndrome occurs is

Table 3. – Symptoms, signs and laboratory tests that indicate extrathoracic metastases of lung cancer

Symptoms	Signs	Laboratory tests
Weight loss >4.5 kg (10 lb)	Lymphadenopathy	Haematocrit <40% in males
Focal skeletal pain	Hoarseness, SVCO	Haematocrit <35% in females
Neurological: headaches, syncope, weakness, confusion	Bone tenderness, hepatomegaly, focal neurological signs, soft tissue mass	Elevated ALP and γGT

Data taken from [11]. SVCO: superior vena cava obstruction; ALP: alkaline phosphatase; γGT: γ-glutamyltransferase.

not understood in all cases but is often due to cytokine or hormone production by the tumour itself or an abnormal host reaction to the cancer resulting in antibody production. A wide range of syndromes may be found in patients with lung cancer (table 4), and those affecting the skeletal, endocrine, neurological and haematological systems are most common.

Clubbing and hypertrophic pulmonary osteoarthropathy

Digital clubbing is one of the most common paraneoplastic syndromes associated with lung cancer and more than 80% of cases of clubbing occur in adults with lung cancer. It may affect both fingers and toes. The process is characterised by bulbous uniform swelling of the soft tissue of the terminal phalanx of a digit with subsequent loss of the normal nail angle and the nail bed. Obliteration of the diamond-shaped window when the distal phalanges of corresponding fingers are opposed confirms the diagnosis (Schamroth's sign). Clubbing is usually noticed by the physician rather than the patient

Table 4. – Paraneoplastic syndromes found in lung cancer

	Common	Rare
General	Anorexia, cachexia, weight loss	Fever, marantic endocarditis
Musculoskeletal	Clubbing, HPOA	
Endocrine	Hypercalcaemia, SIADH, ectopic ACTH production	Acromegaly, carcinoid syndrome, hypokalaemic alkalosis, gynaecomastia, lactic acidaemia, hypophosphataemia, hypoglycaemia, hyperthyroidism, elevated LH and FSH
Haematological	Anaemia, polycythaemia	Amyloidosis, leukoerythroblastic reaction, eosinophilia, thrombocytopenia
Neurological	Peripheral neuropathy, cerebellar degeneration, LEMS	Mononeuritis multiplex, encephalomyelitis, necrotising myelopathy, cancer-associated retinopathy
Cutaneous	Acanthosis nigricans	Acquired hypertrichosis languinosa, erythema gyratum repens, erythema multiforme, tylosis, erythroderma, exfoliative dermatitis, pruritus, urticaria
Connective tissue	Dermatomyositis	Systemic lupus erythematosus, vasculitis
Renal		Glomerulonephritis, nephrotic syndrome
Coagulopathy	Venous thromboembolism	Thrombophlebitis, disseminated intravascular coagulation

HPOA: hypertrophic pulmonary osteoarthropathy; SIADH: syndrome of inappropriate antidiuretic hormone; ACTH: adrenocorticotrophic hormone; LH: luteinising hormone; FSH: follicle stimulating hormone; LEMS: Lambert–Eaton myasthenic syndrome.

and is associated with all stages of lung cancer. It occurs most commonly with squamous cell and adenocarcinoma and only rarely in small cell bronchogenic carcinoma.

Hypertrophic pulmonary osteoarthropathy (HPOA) may be considered a systemic disorder and occurs with or without clubbing. It involves a symmetrical arthropathy of wrists and ankles and periosteal new bone formation of the fibula, tibia, radius and ulnar. Patients may experience a deep-seated aching pain due to periostitis. Joints are often painful and hyperaemic. Although the pathogenesis of clubbing and HPOA has not been fully elucidated, vascular endothelial growth factor (VEGF) and platelet-derived growth factor have been implicated [37]. After resection of the cancer, serum VEGF levels have been noted to fall and analysis of the primary tumour suggested it was the source of ectopic VEGF production [38]. This would support anecdotal observations that resection of the primary tumour results in regression of clubbing and HPOA. Recent evidence suggests that mutations in 15-hydroxyprostaglandin dehydrogenase result in primary hypertrophic osteoarthropathy, implicating raised prostaglandin E2 levels in the pathogenesis of HPOA [39].

Endocrine

Lung cancers commonly secrete hormones such as adrenocorticotrophic hormone (ACTH), antidiuretic hormone (ADH), calcitonin, oxytocin and parathyroid hormone related peptide (PTH-rP). Elevated levels may be detected but only a proportion of patients develop the syndromes with which they are associated.

Hypercalcaemia (corrected serum calcium $>2.8\ \text{mmol}\cdot\text{L}^{-1}$) is found in up to 25% of patients with lung cancer at some point in their clinical course and may arise from osteolytic bone destruction or from PTH-rP secreted by squamous cell carcinomas. PTH-rP is a 141-amino-acid protein that stimulates osteoclast bone resorption as well as renal tubular calcium resorption, resulting in hypercalcaemia [40]. Raised serum calcium levels cause negative feedback on endogenous PTH, making serum levels of PTH undetectable by traditional assay in malignant hypercalcaemia. Symptoms of hypercalcaemia may mimic cerebral metastases and include confusion, headache, drowsiness, seizures and coma. Other symptoms include polyuria, polydipsia and gastrointestinal effects resulting in constipation, nausea and abdominal pain. Failure of hypercalcaemia to respond to intravenous fluid therapy and bisphosphonates represents a poor prognosis.

The syndrome of inappropriate ADH (SIADH) occurs in approximately 10% of patients with small cell lung cancer. A retrospective review of 350 patients with small cell lung cancer revealed a sodium level of $<130\ \text{mEq}\cdot\text{L}^{-1}$ due to SIADH in 40 (11%) patients, and hyponatraemia was severe in most cases with a mean sodium level of $117\ \text{mEq}\cdot\text{L}^{-1}$ [41]. In this series, SIADH resolved promptly (in <3 weeks) with initiation of combination chemotherapy in 80% of patients [41]. In patients with lung cancer and hyponatraemia, half of the cases are attributable to ectopic ADH production from the tumour and the remainder occur due to excess ADH production from the posterior pituitary. Clinical manifestations usually only occur when the serum sodium falls below $125\ \text{mEq}\cdot\text{L}^{-1}$ and may include anorexia, nausea, vomiting, confusion, altered mental status, seizures and coma. The diagnosis is confirmed in a euvolaemic patient by finding an inappropriately increased urine concentration and osmolarity ($>500\ \text{mOsm}\cdot\text{kg}^{-1}$) in the setting of serum hyponatraemia and reduced serum osmolality ($<280\ \text{mOsm}\cdot\text{kg}^{-1}$).

ACTH is the most commonly produced ectopic hormone and elevated levels are found in up to 50% of lung cancer patients. However, the clinical features of Cushing's syndrome are only seen in up to 10% of individuals and appear before, simultaneously with or after the diagnosis of lung cancer is established. The classic symptoms of

Cushing's syndrome are rarely observed in their entirety. Peripheral oedema, proximal myopathy and moon facies are most commonly reported, along with weight loss, hypokalaemic alkalosis and hyperglycaemia [42]. Small cell lung cancer is the most common ectopic source of ACTH but it may also be produced by carcinoid and nonsmall cell lung cancers. As with other paraneoplastic syndromes, the pathophysiology is not well understood; however, normal lung produces a small amount of pro-opiomelanocortin (POMC), a precursor of ACTH. Malignant transformation may result in the over-expression of the gene responsible for POMC production [43] and result in ectopic ACTH secretion. A diagnosis is achieved by finding an elevated 24-h urinary free cortisol level and a raised serum ACTH that does not decrease with a high-dose dexamethasone suppression test. Ectopic Cushing's syndrome in small cell carcinoma is associated with a reduction in responsiveness to chemotherapy, increased incidence of opportunistic infection and decreased survival [42].

Neurological

The tumour, particularly small cell carcinoma, and the nervous system have common antigens. A host immune response to the tumour may, therefore, result in antibodies that cross-react with antigens in the nervous system resulting in a spectrum of paraneoplastic syndromes. Table 5 summarises the antibodies associated with para-neoplastic neurological syndromes observed in small cell carcinoma that may be present in the serum or cerebrospinal fluid. Neurological disease and, particularly, metastases must be excluded before a paraneoplastic syndrome can be diagnosed.

A subacute peripheral neuropathy is the most common paraneoplastic neurological finding in small cell lung cancer. This may be sensory, motor or combined and progresses rapidly over weeks to months. Inflammation of the dorsal root ganglion results in loss of proprioception, sensation and deep tendon reflexes. The motor neuropathy may also cause weakness and wasting, particularly in the lower limb extremities. Serum anti-Hu antibodies may aid the diagnosis in previously unexplained peripheral neuropathy.

Paraneoplastic cerebellar degeneration (PCD) is characterised by ataxia, nystagmus, dysarthria and diplopia that is progressive over weeks and months and due to diffuse loss of Purkinje cells. The prognosis of small cell carcinoma is worse when PCD also occurs. Periventricular white matter changes and abnormal T2 signal on MRI may be observed. Treatment of the tumour does not alter the course of PCD. One study of 57 patients with PCD showed that 25 (44%) were associated with the anti-Hu antibody [45]. Patients with the antibody were more likely to develop other neurological features, in particular neuropathy and encephalomyelitis.

Table 5. – Antibodies associated with neurological paraneoplastic syndromes

Paraneoplastic syndrome	Antibodies
Peripheral neuropathy and encephalomyelitis	Anti-Hu (ANNA-1) Anti-anphiphysin Anti-CV2
Cerebellar degeneration	Anti-Hu
Cancer-associated retinopathy	Anti-CAR
Lambert–Eaton myasthenic syndrome	Anti-voltage-gated calcium channel antibodies

Data taken from [44].

The Lambert–Eaton myasthenic syndrome (LEMS) is one of the most well studied neurological paraneoplastic syndromes and occurs in 3% of patients with small cell lung cancer [46]. Voltage-gated calcium channel antibodies are present in nearly all patients with LEMS and the clinical presentation is of proximal weakness affecting the lower extremities, fatigue, dry mouth and ptosis. It usually manifests before the small cell lung cancer is evident. Facilitation (strength improvement after exercise) allows LEMS to be distinguished clinically from myasthenia gravis, in which muscles demonstrate fatiguability (weakness after exercise). Preliminary data from a recent prospective study adds weight to previous data suggesting that clinical evidence of LEMS confers a survival advantage in patients with small cell lung cancer [47].

Cutaneous

Acanthosis nigricans is characterised by the presence of pigmented, velvety plaques most often seen on the sides and nape of the neck and other intertriginous areas. It is a rare feature of adenocarcinoma of the lung. Dermatomyositis may be recognised by the heliotrope periorbital erythema and the progressive weakness of tender extensor muscles. In one review of 24 cases of dermatomyositis and lung cancer, the paraneoplastic syndrome commonly pre-dated the discovery of malignancy and small cell lung cancer was the most common cell type [48].

Constitutional symptoms

Anorexia and cachexia of lung cancer are common and may predict the presence of metastatic disease and a poor prognosis. However, these symptoms may be present in patients without distant spread and therefore be considered as a paraneoplastic syndrome. The resting energy expenditure is raised in patients with lung cancer [49]. Evidence exists that proteolysis-inducing factor and lipid-mobilising factor are produced by the tumour and result in weight loss. Host–tumour interaction results in the excess production of tumour necrosis factor (TNF)-α, interleukin (IL)-1, interferon-γ and IL-6 cytokines, which contribute to cachexia by inhibiting lipoprotein lipase and therefore preventing adipocytes from storing fatty acids. C-reactive protein is an indirect measure of IL-6 levels and may correlate with symptoms. Anorexia is mediated by the inability of the hypothalamus to respond appropriately to peripheral signals that indicate an energy deficit. The neuropeptide Y pathway in the hypothalamus stimulates food intake. Cytokines, including IL-1 and TNF-α, appear to mediate this "hypothalamic resistance", by inhibiting the neuropeptide Y pathway in animal models [50]. The cancer cachexia syndrome can have a large impact on quality of life and can lower performance status and worsen outcome.

As with other paraneoplastic syndromes, symptoms may pre-date the discovery of the primary lung cancer. In most cases their occurrence does not reflect stage or prognosis and so it is important that patients should not be precluded from potentially curative therapy on the basis of these syndromes alone.

Risk factors for lung cancer

The predictive value of presenting symptoms and signs may be improved by considering them in the context of risk factors for lung cancer. Given that the presenting symptoms of lung cancer are often nonspecific, establishing the patient's risk of developing the disease is important in determining which patients to investigate further.

Those patients with multiple risk factors for developing lung cancer may warrant investigations even though initial presentation may be unimpressive, for example a dry cough.

Smoking is the most important aetiological agent in patients with lung cancer, accounting for 90% of cases in males and 80% in females. The relationship between smoking and lung cancer mortality was first established by DOLL and HILL [51] in their cohort study of 40,000 medical practitioners. Subsequently, it has been demonstrated that smoking exposure is linearly related to lung cancer risk, so that those patients with a heavy smoking history are at higher risk. COPD has been implicated as an independent risk factor for lung cancer. Therefore, patients with airflow limitation are more likely to develop lung cancer than those with normal airway function [52]. Although the vast majority of patients who develop lung cancer (and COPD) have a significant smoking history, the converse is not true. The majority of smokers do not develop lung cancer. Approximately 5% of smokers develop lung cancer, whereas 20% will develop COPD.

Asbestos exposure is a critical risk factor for lung cancer. Asbestos was used for its remarkable heat-resistant properties and is found in insulation, pipe lagging and brake pads. Lung cancer is estimated to develop in 20–25% of heavily exposed asbestos workers. Smoking has a cumulative effect, further increasing the risk of lung cancer to a factor of 90 *versus* a factor of 5 in exposed nonsmokers. The synergistic effect of smoking and asbestos exposure may be explained by the fact that cigarette smoke enhances the retention of asbestos fibres [53]. Often, asbestos-related interstitial disease (asbestosis) is associated; however, no correlation exists between the severity of asbestosis and the development of lung cancer. Furthermore, lung cancer is seen in individuals without interstitial lung disease who are exposed to asbestos. A latency period of 25–35 yrs is usual. Histologically, the predominant subtype is bronchoalveolar cell carcinoma, but adenocarcinoma and squamous cell carcinoma also occur.

The incidence of lung cancer is also higher in patients that have previously had head and neck malignancy. Other factors that may predispose to bronchogenic lung cancer include pulmonary fibrosis (of any aetiology) and exposure to radon, chromium, arsenic and beryllium. Patients who have previously had lymphoma treated with thoracic radiotherapy also appear to be at increased risk. A family history of lung cancer has also been implicated in conferring a higher risk [54].

Summary

Lung cancer presents late in its natural history and its symptoms and signs are often nonspecific. Spread of the disease within the chest may result in pleural effusion and mediastinal involvement. Extrathoracic metastases commonly occur to bone, brain and liver. Distant effects of lung cancer, termed paraneoplastic syndromes, produce a varied constellation of symptoms and signs with musculoskeletal, endocrine and neurological abnormalities predominating. Paraneoplastic syndromes do not imply metastatic spread and may manifest prior to the discovery of the underlying tumour.

Keywords: Cough, haemoptysis, nonsmall cell lung cancer, paraneoplastic syndrome, small cell lung cancer.

Statement of interest
None declared.

References

1. Geddes DM. The natural history of lung cancer: a review based on rates of tumour growth. *Br J Dis Chest* 1979; 73: 1–17.
2. Carbone PP, Frost JK, Feinstein AR, *et al.* Lung cancer: perspectives and prospects. *Ann Intern Med* 1970; 73: 1003–1024.
3. Buccheri G, Ferrigno D. Lung cancer: clinical presentation and specialist referral time. *Eur Respir J* 2004; 24: 898–904.
4. Koyi H, Hillerdal G, Branden E. A prospective study of a total material of lung cancer from a county in Sweden 1997-1999: gender, symptoms, type, stage, and smoking habits. *Lung Cancer* 2002; 36: 9–14.
5. Scagliotti GV. Symptoms, signs and staging of lung cancer. *In*: Spiro SG, ed. Lung Cancer. *Eur Respir Mon* 2001; 17: 86–119.
6. Andersen HA, Prakash UBS. Diagnosis of symptomatic lung cancer. *Semin Respir Med* 1982; 3: 165–175.
7. Grippi MA. Clinical aspects of lung cancer. *Semin Roentgenol* 1990; 25: 12–24.
8. Hyde L, Hyde CI. Clinical manifestations of lung cancer. *Chest* 1974; 65: 299–306.
9. Cromartie RS, Parker EF, May JE, *et al.* Carcinoma of the lung. *Ann Thorac Surg* 1980; 68: 288–296.
10. Karsell PR, McDougall JC. Diagnostic tests for lung cancer. *Mayo Clin Proc* 1993; 68: 288–296.
11. Spiro SG, Gould MK, Colice GL. Initial evaluation of the patient with lung cancer: Symptoms, signs, laboratory tests and paraneoplastic syndromes: ACCP evidenced-based clinical practice guidelines (2nd edition). *Chest* 2007; 132: 149–160.
12. Okkes IM, Oskam SK, Lamberts H. The probability of specific diagnoses for patients presenting with common symptoms to Dutch family physicians. *J Fam Pract* 2002; 51: 31–36.
13. Garfield DH, Cadrenel JL, Wislez M, *et al.* The bronchioloalveolar carcinoma and peripheral adenocarcinoma spectrum of diseases. *J Thorac Oncol* 2006; 1: 344–359.
14. Tsoumakidou M, Chrysofakis G, Tsiligianni I, *et al.* A prospective analysis of 184 hemoptysis cases: diagnostic impact of chest X-ray, computed tomography, bronchoscopy. *Respiration* 2006; 73: 808–814.
15. Lederle FA, Nichol KL, Parenti CM. Bronchoscopy to evaluate hemoptysis in older men with nonsuspicious chest roentgenograms. *Chest* 1989; 95: 1043–1047.
16. Aristizabal JF, Young KR, Nath H. Can chest CT decrease the use of preoperative bronchoscopy in the evaluation of suspected bronchogenic carcinoma? *Chest* 1998; 113: 1244–1249.
17. Empey DW. Assessment of upper airways obstruction. *Br Med J* 1972; 3: 503–505.
18. Wilson LD, Detterbeck FC, Yahalom J. Superior vena cava syndrome with malignant causes. *N Engl J Med* 2007; 356: 1862–1869.
19. Urban T, Lebeau B, Chastang C, *et al.* Superior vena cava syndrome in small-cell lung cancer. *Arch Intern Med* 1993; 153: 384–387.
20. Komaki R, Roth JA, Walsh GL, *et al.* Outcome predictors for 143 patients with superior sulcus tumors treated by multidisciplinary approach at the University of Texas MD Anderson Cancer Center. *Int J Radiat Oncol Biol Phys* 2000; 48: 347–354.
21. Le Roux BT. The presentation of bronchial carcinoma. *Scott Med J* 1968; 13: 31–37.
22. Camidge DR. The causes of dysphagia in carcinoma of the lung. *J R Soc Med* 2001; 94: 567–572.
23. Strauss BL, Matthews MJ, Cohen MH, *et al.* Cardiac metastases in lung cancer. *Chest* 1977; 71: 607–611.
24. Tamura A, Matsubara O, Yoshimura N, *et al.* Cardiac metastasis of lung cancer. A study of metastatic pathways and clinical manifestations. *Cancer* 1992; 70: 437–442.
25. Okamoto H, Shinkai T, Yamakido M, *et al.* Cardiac tamponade caused by primary lung cancer and the management of pericardial effusion. *Cancer* 1993; 71: 93–98.
26. Quint LE, Francis IR. Radiologic staging of lung cancer. *J Thorac Imaging* 1999; 14: 235–246.

27. Salvatierra A, Baamonde C, Llamas JM, *et al.* Extrathoracic staging of bronchogenic carcinoma. *Chest* 1990; 97: 1052–1058.
28. Kumaran M, Benamore RE, Vaidhyanath R, *et al.* Ultrasound guided cytological aspiration of supraclavicular lymph nodes in patients with suspected lung cancer. *Thorax* 2005; 60: 229–233.
29. Eggesbø HB, Hansen G. Clinical impact of adrenal expansive lesions in bronchial carcinoma. *Acta Radiol* 1996; 37: 242–247.
30. Shi AA, Digumarthy SR, Temel JS, *et al.* Does initial staging or tumor histology better identify asymptomatic brain metastases in patients with non-small cell lung cancer? *J Thorac Oncol* 2006; 1: 205–210.
31. Bach F, Agerlin N, Sorensen JB, *et al.* Metastatic spinal cord compression secondary to lung cancer. *J Clin Oncol* 1992; 10: 1781–1787.
32. Terashima T, Kanazawa M. Lung cancer with skin metastasis. *Chest* 1994; 106: 1448–1450.
33. Singh P, Camazine B, Jadhav Y, *et al.* Endoscopic ultrasound as a first test for diagnosis and staging of lung cancer: a prospective study. *Am J Respir Crit Care Med* 2007; 175: 345–354.
34. Hooper RG, Tenholder MF, Underwood GH, *et al.* Computed tomographic scanning of the brain in the initial staging of bronchogenic carcinoma. *Chest* 1984; 85: 774–776.
35. Hooper RG, Beechler CR, Johnson MC. Radioisotope scanning in the initial staging of bronchogenic carcinoma. *Am Rev Respir Dis* 1978; 118: 279–286.
36. Silvestri GA, Littenberg B, Colice GL. The clinical evaluation for detecting metastatic lung cancer. A meta-analysis. *Am J Respir Crit Care Med* 1995; 152: 225–230.
37. Atkinson S, Fox SB. Vascular endothelial growth factor (VEGF)-A and platelet-derived growth factor (PDGF) play a central role in the pathogenesis of digital clubbing. *J Pathol* 2004; 203: 721–728.
38. Olan F, Portela M, Navarro C, *et al.* Circulating VEGF in a case of pulmonary hypertrophic osteoarthropathy. *J Rheumatol* 2004; 31: 614–616.
39. Uppal S, Diggle CP, Carr IM, *et al.* Mutations in 15-hydroxyprostaglandin dehydrogenase cause primary hypertrophic osteoarthropathy. *Nat Genet* 2008; 40: 789–793.
40. Miyake Y, Yamaguchi K, Honda S, *et al.* Production of parathyroid hormone related protein in tumour xenografts in nude mice presenting with hypercalcaemia. *Br J Cancer* 1991; 63: 252–256.
41. List AF, Hainsworth JD, Davis BW, *et al.* The syndrome of inappropriate secretion of antidiuretic hormone (SIADH) in small-cell lung cancer. *J Clin Oncol* 1986; 4: 1191–1198.
42. Shepherd FA, Laskey J, Evans WK, *et al.* Cushing's syndrome associated with ectopic corticotropin production and small cell lung cancer. *J Clin Oncol* 1992; 10: 21–27.
43. Stewart PM, Gibson S, Crosby SR, *et al.* ACTH precursors characterize the ectopic ACTH syndrome. *Clin Endocrinol* 1994; 40: 199–204.
44. Gerber RB, Mazzone P, Arroliga AC. Paraneoplastic syndromes associated with bronchogenic carcinoma. *Clin Chest Med* 2002; 23: 257–264.
45. Mason WP, Graus F, Lang B, *et al.* Small-cell lung cancer, paraneoplastic cerebellar degeneration and the Lambert–Eaton myasthenic syndrome. *Brain* 1997; 120: 1279–1300.
46. Elrington GM, Murray NM, Spiro SG, *et al.* Neurological paraneoplastic syndromes in patients with small cell lung cancer. A prospective survey of 150 patients. *J Neurol Neurosurg Psychiatry* 1991; 54: 764–767.
47. Maddison P, Lang B. Paraneoplastic neurological autoimmunity and survival in small-cell lung cancer. *J Neuroimmunol* 2008; 201: 159–162.
48. Fujita J, Tokuda M, Bandoh S, *et al.* Primary lung cancer associated with polymyositis/dermatomyositis, with a review of the literature. *Rheumatol Int* 2001; 20: 81–84.
49. Jatoi A, Daly BD, Hughes VA, *et al.* Do patients with nonmetastatic non-small cell lung cancer demonstrate altered resting energy expenditure? *Ann Thorac Surg* 2001; 72: 348–351.
50. Laviano A, Russo M, Freda F, *et al.* Neurochemical mechanisms for cancer anorexia. *Nutrition* 2002; 18: 100–105.
51. Doll R, Hill AB. The mortality of doctors in relation to their smoking habits; a preliminary report. *Br Med J* 1954; 1: 1451–1455.

52. Purdue MP, Gold L, Jarvholm B, *et al.* Impaired lung function and lung cancer incidence in a cohort of Swedish construction workers. *Thorax* 2007; 62: 51–56.
53. Churg A, Stevens B. Enhanced retention of asbestos fibers in the airways of human smokers. *Am J Respir Crit Care Med* 1995; 151: 1409–1413.
54. Matakidou A, Eisen T, Houlston RS. Systematic review of the relationship between family history and lung cancer risk. *Br J Cancer* 2005; 93: 825–833.

CHAPTER 6

The biology of lung cancer

M.H. Lawson*,#, T. Eisen*

*Dept of Oncology, University of Cambridge and Addenbrooke's Hospital, and #CRUK Cambridge Research Institute, Li Ka Shing Centre, Cambridge, UK.

Correspondence: T. Eisen, Dept of Oncology, University of Cambridge and Addenbrooke's Hospital, Cambridge CB2 0QQ, UK. E-mail: tim.eisen@medschl.cam.ac.uk

Lung cancer remains the leading cause of cancer deaths in the UK [1], and data suggest that 5-yr survival in Europe has not significantly improved since the early 1990s [2]. Recent major public health initiatives banning smoking are likely to have a future impact on lung cancer incidence, but this may take >30 yrs to become evident [3]. In contrast to the static survival rates in lung cancer, significant progress in clinical and laboratory techniques has occurred over recent years, with increasing use of positron electron tomography, computed tomography, autofluorescence bronchoscopy and genomic technology. Although nihilism in management still exists, this progress has revitalised the drive to improve resection rates and overall survival.

An understanding of basic cancer biology underpins much of the progress that has been made; for example, understanding angiogenesis has helped in the development of targeted therapies. However, there are several fundamental questions about lung cancer biology that remain to be answered.

The present chapter will summarise recent progress in basic lung cancer biology in the key areas of genetics, carcinogenesis, progression of disease and development of chemoresistance. The chapter concludes with a summary of how this knowledge may lead to clinical advances.

Genetics

Lung cancer susceptibility

Smoking is the single most important risk factor for the development of lung cancer and 90% of lung cancer cases are attributable to smoking [1]. However, only <16% of male smokers develop lung cancer by the age of 75 yrs [4]. Whilst the individual risk is influenced by duration of smoking, age at starting and level of cigarette consumption, it seems likely that genetic susceptibility factors may also have an important role in determining which smokers develop cancer, and this has been an area of active research.

Since the 1960s there have been many case-control and cohort studies published that demonstrate familial aggregation of lung cancer in the absence of recognised, rare cancer syndromes. These are well summarised in a recent meta-analysis that showed an overall relative risk of lung cancer in individuals with a family history of the disease of 1.84 (95% CI 1.64–2.05) [5]. However, the authors also demonstrated the inherent difficulty in this type of research where the dominant risk factor, smoking, is environmental, when they reported a relative risk of lung cancer associated with a history of lung cancer in a spouse of 1.58 (95% CI 1.30–1.92). Overall, they concluded

Eur Respir Mon, 2009, 44, 88–105. Printed in UK - all rights reserved. Copyright ERS Journals Ltd 2009; European Respiratory Monograph; ISSN 1025-448x.

that there appears to be a genetic component to lung cancer risk associated with having an affected relative, and this risk is increased with earlier onset of disease and multiple affected family members, but that inability to control for smoking precludes strong conclusions being drawn.

Advances in genomic analysis have allowed investigators to search the whole genome for mutations associated with lung cancer. BAILEY-WILSON *et al.* [6] performed a genome-wide linkage analysis in 52 families with at least three individuals affected by upper or lower airway cancers. They were able to identify a putative susceptibility locus at 16q23-25 associated with these cancer types under an autosomal dominant model. This locus was only significantly linked to cancer in a subset of families with ≥ 5 affected individuals, and attempting to control for smoking reduced the logarithm of the odds favouring genetic linkage below the critical threshold of significance.

The use of single nucleotide polymorphisms (SNPs) has allowed rapid and accurate mapping of the genome at high resolution. SNPs are single base pair variations (giving two possible alleles) that occur with a minor allele frequency of >1% at evolutionarily conserved loci throughout the genome. Once the genome is mapped, SNPs can be identified that are associated with the characteristic of interest, and this method can be used to detect low-penetrance alleles or alleles associated with a small increase in relative risk. This type of genome-wide association study has been used to identify a susceptibility locus for nonsmall cell lung cancer (NSCLC) at 15q25.1 in current or former smokers of European descent [7]. The two SNPs within this locus each conferred an odds ratio of NSCLC of 1.32 and the effect of the SNPs on lung cancer risk appeared to be independent of smoking. 15q25.1 contains two nicotinic acetylcholine receptor subunit genes, and these are suggested as candidates for the increased risk although no conclusions about the mechanism of the association can be made from this type of study. Independently, another large, genome-wide association study also found the 15q25 locus to be strongly associated with lung cancer [8]. The population attributable risk for lung cancer of carrying the variant allele was ~15% and the prevalence of the allele in the population was 34%. HUNG *et al.* [8] note that the risk allele has different frequencies in different ethnic groups, but the risk it confers appears to be independent of lung cancer histology, age and sex of the patients. The risk was increased in smokers, former smokers and nonsmokers, but the allele was not associated with smoking-related head and neck cancers in two separate studies that were re-analysed, leading to the conclusion that the risk is not related to tobacco addiction. The authors also identify the nicotinic acetylcholine receptor subunit genes within the risk locus as being the most likely candidate effectors of the risk. The independent identification of the same locus as conferring lung cancer risk by two groups in large and scientifically powerful studies adds to the weight of the finding. Whilst more studies looking for genes that increase the susceptibility to lung cancer are ongoing, work can begin to try to understand the mechanism behind the 15q25 locus susceptibility.

Knowing that a single, common, low-penetrance allele confers risk has limited clinical use, and is unlikely to improve the efficiency of population-based screening programmes. However, taking breast cancer as a model, it is clear that knowledge of several of these genes does have the potential to form the basis of a risk stratification model for screening [9]. This may in turn make screening programmes for lung cancer more acceptable both economically and scientifically.

Smoking dependency

Starting and maintaining a smoking habit is known to be influenced by social factors, such as having parents who smoke and growing up in a peer group where smoking is valued. There is now good evidence that genetic factors are important in the development of nicotine dependence. Taking a candidate gene approach, using a SNP association method to analyse a case control series, several cholinergic nicotinic receptor genes were identified as being associated with nicotine dependence [10]. Although the gene where variation was most strongly associated with nicotine dependence was *CHRNB3* (the β3 nicotinic receptor subunit gene), variation in *CHRNA5* (the α5 nicotinic receptor subunit gene) was felt to be the most biologically plausible result. This gene in the 15q25.1 locus was identified as a lung cancer susceptibility locus independent of smoking history by AMOS *et al.* [7] and HUNG *et al.* [8], and was shown to confer a twofold increased risk of nicotine dependence when the minor allele was homozygous. In a companion article, where the same cases and controls were used in a genome-wide association study, no individual SNPs were significantly associated with nicotine dependence after correcting for multiple comparisons [11].

The development of genomic techniques that can map the entire genome rapidly, accurately and cheaply has allowed significant progress to be made in the identification of genes that predispose to lung cancer or nicotine dependency. However, to date, the results have yet to be conclusively validated and the underlying biological mechanisms remain unclear. This type of research remains challenging from a technical and statistical perspective, and current data is limited to an ethnically European population.

Carcinogenesis

Stepwise carcinogenesis

In the classical multistep model of epithelial carcinogenesis, for a nonmalignant cell to be transformed into malignant cell, normal cell regulatory mechanisms must be overcome and this requires the accumulation of multiple genetic and epigenetic changes. These are generally thought to occur in a progressive sequential manner over a period of time and detection of early changes might allow intervention to prevent malignancy developing, such as with cervical cancer [12]. However, unlike other malignancies, such as bowel or cervical carcinoma, the stages that a nonmalignant pulmonary cell undergoes in order to become a lung cancer cell are relatively poorly understood. Indeed, the cell of origin or initiating cell type remains uncertain for different histological types of lung cancer, and the heterogeneity of "lung cancer" makes consideration of the process in each histological subtype separately more appropriate (fig. 1). More comprehensive understanding of the development of lung cancers is an important step towards prevention and early treatment, but may also identify novel potential therapeutic targets.

Squamous carcinoma. Lung carcinogenesis is best understood for squamous cell carcinoma (fig. 1a), since this is relatively common among the histological subtypes and is centrally located in the bronchial tree, making surveillance and sampling easier. Early histological changes of hyperplasia and squamous metaplasia are associated with allelic loss at several 3p sites and 9p21, and with telomerase dysregulation and $p16^{INK4a}$ methylation [12, 13]. At this stage, the 3p losses tend to be small but have been shown to increase in size as the lesions progress; 3p losses are common to all three major histological subtypes of lung cancer (squamous cell carcinoma, adenocarcinoma and small cell lung cancer (SCLC)) [15]. The lesions may progress to dysplasia and then to carcinoma *in situ* and invasive carcinoma. Progression is characterised by 8p changes, *FHIT* inactivation, and *TP53* inactivation [13]. However, it is clear that stepwise

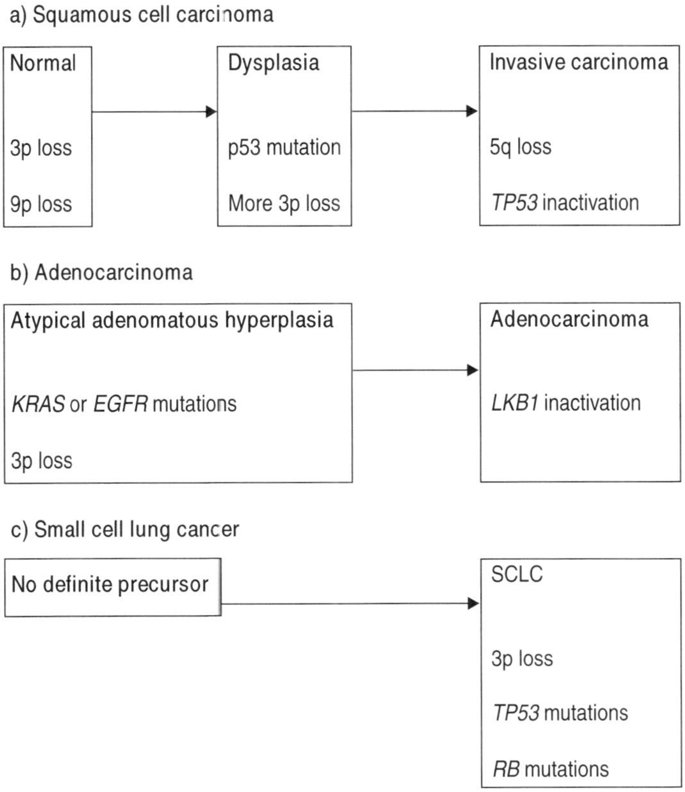

Fig. 1. – The multistep evolution of lung cancers [13, 14]. a) Squamous cell carcinoma; b) adenocarcinoma; and c) small cell lung cancer (SCLC). EGFR: epidermal growth factor receptor.

progression is not invariable and early lesions, including dysplasia, can regress [16]. Smoking induces a "field carcinogenesis" effect, with frequent areas of abnormality within the pulmonary epithelium of smokers with and without lung cancer [13, 15]. Differentiating lesions that are likely to progress from those likely to regress is currently not possible solely on the basis of histology [16].

Adenocarcinoma. Adenocarcinoma of the lung usually occurs in the periphery of the lung, making the development of the malignancy more difficult to study (fig. 1b). Atypical adenomatous hyperplasia (AAH) has been identified as a putative precursor, since these lesions often occur in the lungs of patients with adenocarcinoma and areas of AAH frequently have molecular changes, such as mutations in the *KRAS* oncogene, that are also found in adenocarcinoma [13]. The most compelling evidence identifying AAH as the precursor lesion of adenocarinoma comes from a conditional oncogenic *K-ras* mouse strain developed by JACKSON *et al.* [17]. In their mouse model [17], expression of oncogenic *K-ras* was inducible using recombinant adenovirus expressing Cre recombinase to remove a Stop element in the conditional allele, thus allowing gene transcription to be turned on. *K-ras* was selectively activated in the lungs of the mice by intranasal instillation of the adenovirus. The mice went on to develop AAH, then increasingly large adenomas and, finally, adenocarcinomas. However, *KRAS* mutations are only found in a subset of human lung adenocarcinomas, limiting the relevance of the model. Other mutations are also important in humans and the finding that epidermal growth factor receptor (EGFR) mutations are more common in adenocarcinomas from nonsmokers than smokers has led to the hypothesis that two separate pathways of carcinogenesis exist for adenocarcinoma, with *KRAS* mutations driving the process in smokers and *EGFR* mutations in nonsmokers [13]. A large genome-wide high-resolution analysis of 371 pulmonary adenocarcinoma resection specimens has identified *NKX2-1* as a potential lineage-survival oncogene, which may have an important role in carcinogenesis [18]. Interestingly, this gene encodes thyroid transcription factor-1, which has been widely used as a marker for tumours (particularly adenocarcinomas) of lung origin.

SCLC. No precursor lesion has been identified for SCLC, although there is now evidence that it is derived from an epithelial rather than neuroendocrine precursor [19]. The bronchial epithelium of patients with SCLC has been shown to have a higher burden of genetic abnormality than that of NSCLC [13], and the falling incidence of SCLC in the developed world has been attributed to changes in cigarette filters resulting in lower carcinogen exposure in the central airways and deeper penetration of smoke into the lung [20]. These observations have led to the suggestion that SCLC may develop rapidly without undergoing major histological changes associated with rapid genetic alterations (fig. 1c). This theory is known as the parallel theory of cancer development [14]. The key genetic changes associated with SCLC are mutations in *TP53* and *RB*, both tumour suppressor genes [14]. Their importance is underlined by the development of a mouse model of SCLC that develops tumours in response to conditional knockout of *Trp53* and *Rb1* [21].

Cancer stem cells

A cancer is composed of a heterogeneous population of cells and has a distinct microenvironment, analogous to organs within the body. It is increasingly clear that growth and cell renewal within organs is hierarchically organised with pluripotent stem cells, giving rise to more differentiated cells that have diminished capacity to renew themselves and are increasingly lineage restricted. The archetype is the haematopoietic system. The cancer stem cell hypothesis extends the analogy of the malignancy as an organ and suggests that cancers have their own stem cell compartment composed of cancer stem cells (CSCs). Evidence for this comes from the observation that only a small population of apparently immature cells from within a malignancy have the ability to form cancer on transplantation into immunocompromised mice. The theory has been recently reviewed by VERMEULEN *et al.* [22]. If the hypothesis is correct, then the only cells capable of driving cancer growth and progression, including metastasis, are the CSCs. This would make them the key target for therapy. An appealing inference is that CSCs are derived from normal tissue stem cells and therefore stem cells represent the cell of origin of cancer. However, this does not have to be the case, as CSCs could be derived from committed progenitors or even differentiated cells that have multiple genetic mutations rendering them more "stem cell-like".

The lung is a complex organ that has many functions and, therefore, has multiple different epithelial cell types within it. These are organised into anatomically distinct regions, each with their own stem cell, or at least progenitor cell, niche. It has been proposed that the stem/progenitor cells within these separate niches are the cells of origin for different types of lung cancer, thus explaining the clinicopathologically distinct lung cancer subtypes [23]. There is supporting evidence for this hypothesis from murine cancer models. In their conditional *K-Ras* mouse, which develops pulmonary adenocarcinoma on oncogenic *K-Ras* induction by intranasal infection with recombinant adenoviral Cre, KIM *et al.* [24] have identified bronchioalveolar stem cells (BASCs) at the bronchioalveolar duct junction. These cells were isolated and grown in tissue culture, where they were observed to proliferate in response to *K-Ras* induction and the BASC population was expanded in adenocarcinoma precursors and tumours *in vivo*. Whilst they were able to demonstrate that naphthalene airway injury prior to infection stimulated BASC proliferation and synergistically increased the tumour burden, they did not demonstrate that oncogenesis was dependent on the BASC population.

Subsequent work has shown that blocking the phosphatidylinositol 3-kinase (PI3K) signalling pathway reduces BASC expansion and reduces tumour growth, whereas enhancing PI3K signalling increases both parameters [25]. However, the link between the BASC population as the cell of origin and pulmonary adenocarcinoma still has to be conclusively demonstrated.

A recent important publication has identified a putative CSC population in each of the four main lung cancer subtypes [26]. In this study [26], the investigators used CD133, known to be a marker of cancer cells with stem cell properties in certain solid organ malignancies. They were able to isolate CD133+ cells from primary tumour tissue and, from a subset of the samples, these cells could be grown indefinitely *in vitro* in a selective medium. When the cells were injected into immunocompromised mice at low doses, tumours formed that were histologically similar to the original human tumours. CD133- cells were not able to form tumours, even when injected at high doses. This provides very strong evidence that the CD133+ cells identified from each type of lung cancer represent a CSC population and will allow CSCs to be isolated for further study. The CD133+ cells were also found to be relatively resistant to conventional chemotherapeutic agents *in vitro*.

Understanding CSCs offers an opportunity to improve treatment of lung cancer and possibly increase our understanding of pulmonary carcinogenesis. It is an exciting field where great progress is being made, but much remains to be done.

Disease progression and treatment response

Prognostication

A major problem in the treatment of lung cancer, as in many cancers, is selecting the most appropriate treatment modality and intensity for individual patients. Advances in genomics and proteomics has resulted in increased interest in methods of classification and prognostication and the concept of individualised treatment, where treatment is tailored to patients based on detailed analysis of both tumour and host factors at a molecular and genetic level.

Gene expression profiling has been shown to be able to reproduce histological classification of lung cancers and define new subtypes within both squamous carcinomas and adenocarcinomas [27–29]. These subtypes appear to have prognostic significance but, whilst one study identified four subgroups of adenocarcinoma [27], the other found only three [28]. Gene expression profiles can be used to predict outcome in lung cancer but there appears to be limited overlap between the genes and gene signatures found to be most significant by different groups [29–31]. This approach is limited by several factors. Genome-wide expression analysis is dependent on the quality of the RNA used, and a small difference in quality can result in large differences in apparent expression. To date, studies have only used surgical resection specimens, as it is relatively easy to extract high quality RNA from these specimens, thus restricting the findings to early stage NSCLC. Currently, gene expression profiling is limited to research use by the cost and technical expertise required for collection, processing and interpretation of results. These studies also offer little in the way of detailed biological information without further validation at the protein level and through mechanistic studies, as noted by WEIR *et al.* [18]. Indeed, whilst the metagene model [31] appears to be a potentially useful tool, it is entirely statistical in its construction and offers few novel insights into lung cancer biology.

SNPs may occur in protein-coding regions of a gene and give rise to a different amino acid sequence; these are known as nonsynonymous SNPs. If the SNP does not alter the protein sequence, it is synonymous. The Genetic Lung Cancer Predisposition Study cohort has been used to examine the effect of germline nonsynonymous SNPs in DNA repair enzymes on lung cancer outcome. 15 SNPs were identified where variation was significantly associated with overall survival in the cohort [32]. The SNPs were principally in genes of the base excision repair and nucleotide excision repair pathways where variation may lead to worse survival by promoting cancer progression through increased genetic instability or by modifying the response to treatment. This study was limited by a sample size of 700 patients, which is small when performing multiple comparisons in a complex analysis. However, it does provide an insight into how a patient's genotype might influence treatment response and outcome in addition to tumour characteristics.

MicroRNAs. MicroRNAs (miRNAs) are small (21–25 nucleotides long) noncoding RNAs that appear to have an important function in post-transcriptional regulation of gene expression. They act by binding to complimentary mRNA, thereby repressing translation, making miRNAs potential tumour suppressor genes or oncogenes.

Research into the expression profile of miRNAs in lung cancer has been conducted in a similar manner to the gene expression profiling studies that have attempted to improve prognostication. A study conducted in Taiwan identified a five-miRNA expression profile that was able to predict outcome in NSCLC independently of stage or histology [33]. The study was limited by requiring surgical tissue samples, in the same way as the prognostication studies, and it is not clear how miRNA expression profile relates to mRNA profiling, and whether they provide complimentary information or simply the same results. However, the study did make an attempt to investigate how the miRNAs identified might alter tumour biology, demonstrating that four of them appeared to increase the invasiveness of cells when overexpressed.

miRNA expression profiling may also have a role in identification of the primary site of malignancies that cannot be classified by conventional means. ROSENFELD *et al.* [34] reported good accuracy using a decision tree algorithm based on miRNA profile for identification of tumour samples. This has potentially important implications for the thoracic oncology team as this tool may be very useful; however, there is currently no evidence that better identification of primary tumour site in this group of poorly differentiated tumours, that are otherwise not classifiable, would lead to better outcomes.

A study that prospectively identified a candidate miRNA that regulates *EGFR* expression was able to demonstrate a biological effect, with the miRNA negatively regulating EGFR protein levels in a cell culture model [35]. Unfortunately, whilst loss of heterozygosity for the miRNA correlated with improved patient response to an EGFR tyrosine kinase inhibitor (TKI) and increased survival, miRNA loss of heterozygosity was not an independent predictor of outcome in multivariate analysis.

Growth factors and targeted therapies

The expression of growth factors is an essential element of the biology of all normal and malignant cells. Growth factors play a key role in regulating the proliferation, differentiation and death of cells. Tumour cells may be dependent on growth factors that are released either systemically or in a paracrine or autocrine fashion, both as signals for the tumour cells themselves to divide and grow, and also to stimulate the development of a new blood supply (neoangiogenesis). The growth factors may be peptide, steroid or other molecules.

Improvements in the understanding of cancer biology in general and lung cancer biology specifically have led to the development of new treatments designed to disrupt key processes within the tumour, such as growth factor signalling. These "targeted" therapies should have fewer side-effects than conventional treatment and have a major impact on the tumour.

EGFR inhibition. The EGFR family has been targeted for treatment in NSCLC. Overexpression has been demonstrated in 40–80% of NSCLC and is associated with clinically aggressive disease [36]. EGFR activation initiates downstream signalling through a variety of pathways including PI3K-Akt, Ras-Raf-mitogen-activated protein kinase (MAPK) and signal transducer and activator of transcription (STAT), which leads to regulation of cell proliferation, survival and migration. EGFR TKIs, such as gefitinib and erlotinib, target the ATP binding cleft of the tyrosine kinase domain of the receptor protein and prevent the recruitment of downstream effector proteins. Inhibition of EGFR by TKIs in NSCLC has been found to be beneficial in 10–20% of patients, with females, nonsmokers, people from South-East Asia and patients with adenocarcinoma being most likely to respond [37]. This observation has prompted further research in an attempt to determine the best biomarker to predict good clinical response to EGFR TKIs. Counterintuitively, EGFR protein detection by immunohistochemistry appears to have only a small predictive value for TKI response and is dependent on the antibody used and the cut-off value defining EGFR positivity [38]. In contrast, more accurate prediction of response is associated with activating mutations in the *EGFR* gene [37, 39]. Gene copy number amplification may also be an important predictor of response, although a precise role for this has yet to be defined [37]. *EGFR* mutations are more common in females, south-east Asians, nonsmokers and those with adenocarcinomas, thus explaining the pattern of response to inhibition and reinforcing the importance of *EGFR* mutation status as a predictor of response to TKIs [37]. The type of mutation present has a role in response, with exon 19 deletions conferring a higher response rate than exon 21 missense mutations [36]. Massarelli *et al.* [40] have recently provided evidence that, whilst *EGFR*-activating mutations are a good predictor of response, *KRAS* mutations may be an important predictor of failure to respond to EGFR TKIs irrespective of *EGFR* copy number increase. Most studies that define the genetic lesion in *EGFR* to predict drug response have been conducted in NSCLC refractory to chemotherapy using single-agent anti-EGFR treatment. In their analysis of the International Nifedipine Trial on Antiatherosclerotic Therapy (INTACT) study, Bell *et al.* [37] found that *EGFR* mutation-positive patients had an increased survival irrespective of gefitinib treatment and that the combination of gefitinib with chemotherapy had no impact on overall survival. They acknowledge the problem that analysis of EGFR status in diagnostic samples may not accurately reflect actual mutation status after chemotherapy, but current evidence does not support co-administration of gefitinib with chemotherapy. The median response to EGFR inhibition with gefitinib is 6–8 months, with relapse and subsequent resistance to treatment associated with a further *EGFR* mutation [36].

The feasibility of assessing genotype in patients prior to EGFR TKI treatment has been questioned, but evidence is accumulating that it is possible [39], and novel methods, such as the analysis of *EGFR* mutational status in tumour cells recovered from blood recently reported by MAHESWARAN *et al.* [41], may make this routine practice.

The role of EGFR inhibition in NSCLC demonstrates the complexity of apparently straight forward "targeted" treatments in lung cancer treatment, but also the potential role for tailored therapy. A more complete understanding of the biology of the EGFR pathway may allow treatment to overcome resistance. For instance, it has recently been demonstrated that insulin-like growth factor receptor 1 (IGF-R1) signalling can protect NSCLC cells from apoptosis induced by gefitinib and the use of gefitinib in conjunction with an inhibitor of IGF-R1 signalling increased apoptosis [42]. The IGF signalling axis has also been suggested as a target in SCLC [43] making inhibition of this pathway potentially very important.

SCLC. SCLC cells release a wide range of neuropeptide and polypeptide growth factors. These signals include angiotensin, insulin-like growth factor 1, serotonin, substance p and vasopressin together with gastrin-releasing peptide (the mammalian homologue of bombesin) [43, 44]. These peptide signals act as ligands for high affinity receptors on the tumour cell surface resulting in autocrine and paracrine signalling loops. Activation of the g-protein-coupled receptors results in an intracellular signal being transmitted and augmented such that the cell is stimulated to proliferate. Inhibition of neuropeptide paracrine signalling using substance p analogues has been shown to enhance the effects of chemotherapy [45]. This may lead to clinically useful applications however so far results with other growth factor inhibitors have been disappointing [43]. For example, c-kit is a transmembrane receptor for stem cell factor that is known to be involved in autocrine and paracrine growth stimulation in SCLC. Trials in SCLC patients using imatinib (a small-molecule TKI that blocks c-kit signalling) have been unsuccessful and, although the reason is not clear, it may be at least in part due to biological redundancy.

G-proteins and prenylation. G-proteins bind the nucleotide guanine and are important in the transduction of extracellular signals into intracellular responses. The RAS family of small G-proteins have been widely studied and several members, such as KRAS, are implicated in the oncogenic process in different tissues. Signal transduction in small G-proteins is achieved through their intrinsic GTPase activity and ability to bind both GDP and GTP. Binding of GTP places the protein in an active conformation, the protein dephosphorylates the GTP and the conformation changes to the biologically inactive GDP bound state. Oncogenic mutations in RAS family members that stabilise the GTP bound conformation leading to constitutive activation of the G-protein are well described and <20% of lung cancers (predominantly adenocarcinomas) have this type of *KRAS* mutation [13]. However, it is now clear that extensive post-translational modification of RAS family members that determines their subcellular location and precise function is also important in cancer. RAS GTPases undergo the attachment of a nonsterol isoprenoid (either farnesyl pyrophosphate or geranylgeranyl pyrophosphate), which targets the protein to the endoplasmic reticulum to undergo further post-translational modification before it is sent to the plasma membrane. This process is explained in more detail in a recent review [46]. Several drugs can interfere with the process of post-translational modification of RAS GTPases and have been shown, at least *in vitro*, to modify the growth and chemotherapy response of cancer cells.

KHANZADA *et al.* [47] showed that simvastatin could inhibit the growth of SCLC cell lines *in vitro* as well as in a xenograft model, and that this effect appeared to be a consequence of interference with RAS activation of the PI3K and mitogen-activating protein kinase kinase (MEK)/Erk pathways. This finding is important, as SCLC is not associated with RAS-activating mutations and demonstrates that mutant RAS is not necessary for RAS interference to be potentially beneficial. Statins are known to block the biosynthesis of isoprenoids and some promising results from clinical trials have been reported; a trial in SCLC is now underway.

Specific inhibitors of isoprenylation have also been developed and trialled in NSCLC. To date, results have been mixed and there are reports of dose-limiting toxicities, often exhibited as QT prolongation. However, there is evidence to suggest that combinations of drugs targeting different aspects of prenylation, or prenylation inhibitors with other chemotherapeutics may yield better results with less toxicity [46].

Angiogenesis inhibitors. The process of angiogenesis has long been recognised as fundamental in the growth and metastasis of cancers and, hence, tumour angiogenesis has been an attractive target for therapeutic intervention. Most angiogenesis would be expected to occur within the tumour in an otherwise healthy adult and so inhibition of angiogenesis would be expected to have limited side-effects but potentially significant anti-tumour effects.

Angiogenesis is a complex process that is not fully understood, however it is clear that vascular endothelial growth factor (VEGF) signalling through the receptor tyrosine kinase (RTK) VEGF receptor 2 is a key axis in both normal and tumour angiogenesis [48, 49]. VEGF is produced by tumour cells and is thought to act mainly in a paracrine manner on vascular endothelial cells, but VEGF can also be produced by cells other than the tumour cells, can bind to other receptors, such as neuropilins, and interference in other pathways, such as delta-like ligand 4 signalling through the Notch receptor, can also influence angiogenesis [49].

High VEGF levels in both serum and tumour samples are associated with poor outcome in NSCLC; VEGF inhibitors have had beneficial effects on human lung tumour xenografts [48]. These observations have led to the development of antiangiogenesis treatments for NSCLC, such as bevacizumab, a monoclonal antibody against VEGF, and several small molecule RTK inhibitors. These have been shown to have beneficial, although relatively modest, effects in NSCLC. Trials with bevacizumab (reviewed by GIACONNE [48]) have shown an increase in median survival of 2 months when combined with chemotherapy for NSCLC, coupled with an increased response rate. This contrasts with EGFR inhibitors, where co-administration with chemotherapy does not appear to increase survival [37]. It has been suggested that antiangiogenics may improve the access of chemotherapy to tumour cells by a process of vascular normalisation, where immature small new blood vessels in tumours are obliterated by the treatment, leaving more mature vessels intact and thus improving the effective blood flow to the tumour [49]. A recent study using a tissue microarray of NSCLC tumours and the associated tumour stroma showed that, in univariate analysis, high expression of VEGF in tumour tissue correlated with poor prognosis and in stromal tissue with good prognosis [50]. This finding demonstrates the complexity of angiogenesis, illustrating the difficulties in creating optimally targeted therapies. VEGF may play an anti-tumour role in cancer biology in certain situations and be pro-tumorigenic in others. Knowing when and where to target it may improve the efficacy of current treatments.

It is clear that targeting growth factors or indeed downstream signalling events within cancer cells has great promise as a therapeutic intervention and has already yielded important clinical benefits. The most successful treatments have targeted the best-understood processes, but even the most successful targeted therapies in lung cancer have yet to realise their theoretical potential when compared to the use of the same agents in other malignancies, for instance the use of VEGF inhibitors in renal cell carcinoma. This therapeutic shortfall is probably due to a combination of incomplete understanding of the targeted processes in lung cancer, lack of absolute specificity of the treatment and biological redundancy with other pathways taking over functions of the targeted pathway. A greater understanding of the signalling pathways involved and their complex inter-relationships in lung cancer is needed to fully realise the significant potential of targeted therapies.

Chemoresistance

The utility of conventional chemotherapy in lung cancer is limited by intrinsic resistance in NSCLC and acquired resistance in SCLC. Understanding the basic biological mechanisms of resistance to therapy might allow them to be circumvented improving patient outcomes.

Current understanding of chemoresistance mechanisms in general is classified by Agarwal and Kaye [51] into three broad categories: 1) pharmacokinetic factors relating to delivery of active drug to the tumour; 2) cell intrinsic factors, such as the presence of membrane drug efflux pumps; and 3) tumour–stroma interactions. Each type of resistance may contribute to the overall clinical resistance pattern different amounts in different types of cancer and different patients.

In lung cancer, the presence of drug efflux pumps has been described, but their prognostic significance remains uncertain and efforts to block their activity have failed to produce a survival benefit *in vivo* [52]. However, they do appear to be important *in vitro* and are noted to be expressed in high levels in stem cells [53]; thus, their precise role in chemoresistance remains a worthwhile research focus.

Other cell intrinsic mechanisms of chemoresistance reported to be important in lung cancer are the overexpression of DNA damage repair genes, such as excision repair cross-complementing 1 (*ERCC1*) [54], and overexpression of Bcl-2, an apoptosis inhibitor [55]. *ERCC1* performs an essential step of the nucleotide excision repair pathway, which, whilst being important in repairing tobacco-related DNA damage, is also involved in repairing damage caused by platinum chemotherapeutic drugs. High *ERCC1* levels in tumour tissue are associated with resistance to cisplatin in advanced NSCLC [56]. A phase III trial measuring *ERCC1* levels in tumour tissue to provide tailored chemotherapy (with or without cisplatin) has been performed [56]. Although there was a better response rate for tailored therapy compared to standardised chemotherapy (with cisplatin), this improved response rate did not translate into better survival, perhaps because of the universally poor survival in advanced NSCLC. The trial also had difficulties in specimen processing to extract RNA for *ERCC1* analysis, which led to a high dropout rate and a further round of patient recruitment. Simon *et al.* [54] approached the problem of obtaining good quality tissue for RNA analysis by collecting an extra biopsy solely for this purpose. They were able to measure *ERCC1* expression levels, as well as levels of ribonucleotide reductase subunit 1 (*RRM1*), the product of which determines gemcitabine efficacy. This demonstrates that it is possible to generate an individualised genetic profile for a tumour that could be used to tailor treatment using drugs to which the the tumour is sensitive. As basic research defines more markers of drug sensitivity, the accuracy and utility of such a profile should increase.

Tumour stroma interactions

Cancers within the body are not composed solely of malignant cells. Associated with the malignant cells is a connective tissue framework of matrix proteins and cells known as the stroma. This stroma creates a microenvironment for the tumour cells that can influence overall tumour responses and provides a context for cell–cell interactions. Key nonmalignant cell types in the tumour stroma are fibroblasts, which have been transformed by their reciprocal interaction with the tumour cells into cancer-associated fibroblasts, and immune cells. Tumour–stroma interactions have been recognised to influence growth, progression and chemoresistance of malignancies [57, 58].

In vitro experiments have shown that NSCLC cells can influence gene expression in pulmonary fibroblasts [59] and that fibroblasts can enhance NSCLC growth [60]. It has also been shown that *c-Met* expression in cancer-associated fibroblasts from resection specimens of NSCLC are an independent survival predictor [61].

In SCLC, there is also good evidence from laboratory investigations that stromal factors can influence chemotherapy response with both β-integrin-mediated adhesion to matrix proteins and fibroblast growth factor (FGF)-2 shown to protect SCLC cells from apoptosis [62, 63].

Taking this basic knowledge of tumour–stroma interactions forward, it may become possible to design treatments that render the tumour microenvironment hostile to the cancer, perhaps suppressing metastasis or further progression. The pathways that underlie the suppression of apoptosis in SCLC by both FGF-2 and β-integrin have been defined and represent potentially important targets for treatment. However, the exploitation of this knowledge for patient benefit currently remains elusive.

Immunology

There has been significant progress in the understanding of the interaction between the host immune system and cancer cells, which has led to optimism that manipulation of the immune response may lead to advances in cancer treatment. Two recent reviews summarise the field well [64, 65]. In order for a tumour to develop it must evade the normal host immune response. Tumour cells are antigenic but generally do not activate the immune system (they are nonimmunogenic). They evade immune activation by a variety of mechanisms, including the secretion of factors such as interleukin-6 and -10, which generate a local environment that leads to the suppression of T-cell function. For tumour antigens to activate the immune system effectively, they require presentation to naïve T-cells by antigen-presenting cells (such as dendritic cells) in the context of a local inflammatory response. However, a tumour generates little, if any, local inflammation, and this prevents a significant antitumour response. Even if an effective response occurs, the genetic instability of the cancer can lead to loss of the tumour antigen and escape from the immune response [64].

Attempts have been made to raise specific anti-tumour immune responses, particularly by vaccination with peptide antigens, in order to overcome tumour immune tolerance. The use of an adjuvant to stimulate the function of antigen presenting cells is often combined with the antigen to make the vaccine more effective [64]. An alternative strategy, using small molecule inhibitors to block immune evasion mechanisms also has promise [65].

In the lung cancer field, most data relates to the development of vaccines. A vaccine for SCLC has been developed using Bec2, a mouse antibody that mimics GD3 ganglioside expressed on the surface of SCLC. Despite promising early results, a recent phase III trial showed no benefit [66]. Cancer/testis antigens, such as the melanoma antigen-encoding

(MAGE) family of proteins, are attractive as antigens for the development of cancer vaccines as they are expressed by most cancers, but otherwise only in immunoprivileged sites within the body. Telomerase reverse transcriptase has an important role maintaining the cancer phenotype but is not expressed in normal tissue making it another potential cancer vaccine antigen. Both have been used to develop vaccines for NSCLC and have shown promise in early data; more definitive trials are awaited [67, 68].

Conclusions

Progress in the treatment of lung cancer has been slow, but advances, such as the use of targeted therapies, have been underpinned by improved understanding of the basic biology of lung cancer.

The development of genomic technologies has led to rapid accumulation of new knowledge about gene expression in lung cancer and identification of genes that may increase host susceptibility to cancer. Translating this knowledge into clinically useful interventions is the next major challenge facing both clinicians and scientists. The discovery of a genetic locus, 15q25, conferring increased susceptibility to lung cancer is the first step towards a polygenic susceptibility model that may allow targeted screening of high-risk patients, thus improving screening efficiency. That this locus contains genes for components of the nicotinic acetylcholine receptor is exciting, and further work investigating the mechanisms underlying the relationship between the risk allele and lung cancer might lead to important advances. Tantalisingly, the relationship between this locus and smoking dependency remains uncertain. Should these nicotinic receptor genes prove to have a role in nicotine dependence, then molecularly targeted treatment may improve smoking cessation rates.

The identification of stem cells in lung cancer specimens and the continuing development of the cancer stem cell field may lead directly to major clinical progress in treatment and avoidance of chemoresistance. Considerable further work needs to be done to understand the cell biology of CD133 positive lung cancer cells before benefit to patients is realised, but this work is feasible. However, the identification of the cells of origin of different histological types of lung cancer as stem cells remains controversial outside murine systems. Moving this stem cell research from animal models and into humans will be challenging.

Maximising the effectiveness of existing chemotherapeutic drugs by altering dose regimens and drug combinations in clinical trials continues to be important, but a better understanding of the basic mechanisms of drug resistance in cancer may hold greater hope for better treatment outcomes with these drugs. The development of techniques that allow individualised therapy to be formulated from standard biopsy techniques remains at an early stage but is now possible. Work on *ERCC1* and looking at *EGFR* mutation status shows that better identification of patients who would benefit from treatment is possible and this may lead to improved outcome. Despite several mechanisms of chemoresistance being identified in SCLC, no treatments based on this knowledge have yet been developed. As chemoresistance remains a key problem in limiting outcome in SCLC, translation of this knowledge into clinical benefit must be a priority.

The development of novel drugs, an area of great success in the last decade, relies on identification of novel targets, found and validated through basic scientific research. Drugs targeting prenylation of RAS family members are the "next generation" of targeted therapies and will undoubtedly find a place in the oncologist's armamentarium. They show promise in lung cancer and may succeed in fulfilling their potential as lung cancer treatments where perhaps EGFR inhibitors have been slightly disappointing.

Cancer immunology is a rapidly moving field where significant progress is occurring. Lung cancer vaccines that show promise in early trials continue to be developed and evaluated. Increasing sophistication in our understanding of how cancer evades the immune system and how this may be overcome, and the role of vaccines in relation to chemotherapy, makes this a particularly promising area.

Good progress in our understanding of the biology of lung cancer has occurred over the last decade. Unfortunately translation into improvements in the outcome of lung cancer treatment has not been rapid and this translational gap remains a major challenge to the clinical research community. Many fundamental questions in lung cancer biology remain unanswered, such as the identity of the cell of origin for different types of lung cancer, how chemoresistance develops and the best way to classify and prognosticate tumours. Addressing these questions and ensuring the answers translate into meaningful clinical interventions will make a difference to patient outcome.

Summary

Lung cancer is largely a smoking-induced tumour. Understanding of genetic predisposition to smoking dependency and lung cancer is increasing as powerful genomic technologies are developed. Whole genome microarray expression analysis has led to further subclassification of lung cancer, particularly adenocarcinoma, and the development of new prognostication methods.

Dissection of the genetic and morphological features of dysplastic and early malignant cells together with advances in our understanding of stem cell biology and the role of cancer stem cells may lead to the development of new strategies to detect and treat early lung cancers and prevent the development of chemoresistance.

As the cell biology of lung cancer becomes clearer, so new therapeutic targets become available. These therapeutic possibilities range from selection of the most appropriate chemotherapies, through inhibition of growth factors, angiogenesis and drug resistance to activation of the anti-tumour host immune response. The importance of tumour stroma interactions in determining cancer behaviour is also a new avenue that may bring improvements in treatment outcome through avoidance of chemoresistance to conventional drugs and through the development of new drugs to stromal targets.

The bewildering biological variety of superficially similar tumours underlines the future directions of the management of lung cancer. Interventions at all levels from prevention to chemotherapy for advanced disease will be increasingly influenced by genetic and cell biological analysis of individual patients and their tumours.

However, so far, this rapid progress has not translated to rapid clinical improvements. As this translational gap is bridged over time, significant improvements will result.

Keywords: Carcinogenesis, chemoresistance, genetics, growth factors, immunology, lung cancer.

Statement of interest

T. Eisen has received reimbursement for attending symposia from AstraZeneca and Roche; a speaker's fee from Roche; a fee for organising education from Boehringer Ingelheim; research funding from Bayer and Pfizer; and consulting fees from AstraZeneca, Roche, Bayer, Pfizer, Boehringer Ingelheim and Wyeth.

References

1. Lung Cancer and Smoking – UK. CancerStats 2004. http://info.cancerresearchuk.org/cancerstats/reports/ Date last updated: April 15, 2008. Date last accessed: April 20, 2009.
2. Verdecchia A, Francisci S, Brenner H, *et al.* Recent cancer survival in Europe: a 2000-02 period analysis of EUROCARE-4 data. *Lancet Oncol* 2007; 8: 784–796.
3. Lopez A, Collishaw N, Piha T. A descriptive model of the cigarette epidemic in developed countries. *Tobacco Control* 1994; 3: 242–247.
4. Doll R, Peto R, Boreham J, *et al.* Mortality in relation to smoking: 50 years' observations on male British doctors. *BMJ* 2004; 328: 1519.
5. Matakidou A, Eisen T, Houlston RS. Systematic review of the relationship between family history and lung cancer risk. *Br J Cancer* 2005; 93: 825–833.
6. Bailey-Wilson JE, Amos CI, Pinney SM, *et al.* A major lung cancer susceptibility locus maps to chromosome 6q23-25. *Am J Hum Genet* 2004; 75: 460–474.
7. Amos CI, Wu X, Broderick P, *et al.* Genome-wide association scan of tag SNPs identifies a susceptibility locus for lung cancer at 15q25.1. *Nat Genet* 2008; 40: 616–622.
8. Hung RJ, McKay JD, Gaborieau V, *et al.* A susceptibility locus for lung cancer maps to nicotinic acetylcholine receptor subunit genes on 15q25. *Nature* 2008; 452: 633–637.
9. Pharoah PD, Antoniou AC, Easton DF, *et al.* Polygenes, risk prediction, and targeted prevention of breast cancer. *N Engl J Med* 2008; 358: 2796–2803.
10. Saccone SF, Hinrichs AL, Saccone NL, *et al.* Cholinergic nicotinic receptor genes implicated in a nicotine dependence association study targeting 348 candidate genes with 3713 SNPs. *Hum Mol Genet* 2007; 16: 36–49.
11. Bierut LJ, Madden PA, Breslau N, *et al.* Novel genes identified in a high-density genome wide association study for nicotine dependence. *Hum Mol Genet* 2007; 16: 24–35.
12. Wistuba II, Mao L, Gazdar AF. Smoking molecular damage in bronchial epithelium. *Oncogene* 2002; 21: 7298–7306.
13. Wistuba II, Gazdar AF. Lung cancer preneoplasia. *Ann Rev Pathol* 2006; 1: 331–348.
14. Wistuba II, Gazdar AF, Minna JD. Molecular genetics of small cell lung carcinoma. *Semin Oncol* 2001; 28: Suppl. 4, 3–13.
15. Wistuba II, Behrens C, Virmani AK, *et al.* High resolution chromosome 3p allelotyping of human lung cancer and preneoplastic/preinvasive bronchial epithelium reveals multiple, discontinuous sites of 3p allele loss and three regions of frequent breakpoints. *Cancer Res* 2000; 60: 1949–1960.
16. Breuer RH, Pasic A, Smit EF, *et al.* The natural course of preneoplastic lesions in bronchial epithelium. *Clin Cancer Res* 2005; 11: 537–543.
17. Jackson EL, Willis N, Mercer K, *et al.* Analysis of lung tumor initiation and progression using conditional expression of oncogenic K-ras. *Genes Dev* 2001; 15: 3243–3248.
18. Weir BA, Woo MS, Getz G, *et al.* Characterizing the cancer genome in lung adenocarcinoma. *Nature* 2007; 450: 893–898.
19. Anbazhagan R, Tihan T, Bornman DM, *et al.* Classification of small cell lung cancer and pulmonary carcinoid by gene expression profiles. *Cancer Res* 1999; 59: 5119–5122.
20. Govindan R, Page N, Morgensztern D, *et al.* Changing epidemiology of small-cell lung cancer in the United States over the last 30 years: analysis of the surveillance, epidemiologic, and end results database. *J Clin Oncol* 2006; 24: 4539–4544.
21. Meuwissen R, Linn SC, Linnoila RI, *et al.* Induction of small cell lung cancer by somatic inactivation of both Trp53 and Rb1 in a conditional mouse model. *Cancer Cell* 2003; 4: 181–189.
22. Vermeulen L, Sprick MR, Kemper K, *et al.* Cancer stem cells – old concepts, new insights. *Cell Death Differ* 2008; 15: 947–958.
23. Giangreco A, Groot KR, Janes SM. Lung cancer and lung stem cells: strange bedfellows? *Am J Respir Crit Care Med* 2007; 175: 547–553.

24. Kim CF, Jackson EL, Woolfenden AE, *et al.* Identification of bronchioalveolar stem cells in normal lung and lung cancer. *Cell* 2005; 121: 823–835.
25. Yang Y, Iwanaga K, Raso MG, *et al.* Phosphatidylinositol 3-kinase mediates bronchioalveolar stem cell expansion in mouse models of oncogenic K-ras-induced lung cancer. *PLoS ONE* 2008; 3: e2220.
26. Eramo A, Lotti F, Sette G, *et al.* Identification and expansion of the tumorigenic lung cancer stem cell population. *Cell Death Differ* 2008; 15: 504–514.
27. Bhattacharjee A, Richards WG, Staunton J, *et al.* Classification of human lung carcinomas by mRNA expression profiling reveals distinct adenocarcinoma subclasses. *Proc Natl Acad Sci USA* 2001; 98: 13790–13795.
28. Garber ME, Troyanskaya OG, Schluens K, *et al.* Diversity of gene expression in adenocarcinoma of the lung. *Proc Natl Acad Sci USA* 2001; 98: 13784–13789.
29. Raponi M, Zhang Y, Yu J, *et al.* Gene expression signatures for predicting prognosis of squamous cell and adenocarcinomas of the lung. *Cancer Res* 2006; 66: 7466–7472.
30. Beer DG, Kardia SL, Huang CC, *et al.* Gene-expression profiles predict survival of patients with lung adenocarcinoma. *Nat Med* 2002; 8: 816–824.
31. Potti A, Mukherjee S, Petersen R, *et al.* A genomic strategy to refine prognosis in early-stage non-small-cell lung cancer. *N Engl J Med* 2006; 355: 570–580.
32. Matakidou A, el Galta R, Webb EL, *et al.* Genetic variation in the DNA repair genes is predictive of outcome in lung cancer. *Hum Mol Genet* 2007; 16: 2333–2340.
33. Yu SL, Chen HY, Chang GC, *et al.* MicroRNA signature predicts survival and relapse in lung cancer. *Cancer Cell* 2008; 13: 48–57.
34. Rosenfeld N, Aharonov R, Meiri E, *et al.* MicroRNAs accurately identify cancer tissue origin. *Nat Biotechnol* 2008; 26: 462–469.
35. Weiss GJ, Bemis LT, Nakajima E, *et al.* EGFR regulation by microRNA in lung cancer: correlation with clinical response and survival to gefitinib and EGFR expression in cell lines. *Ann Oncol* 2008; 19: 1053–1059.
36. Zhang X, Chang A. Somatic mutations of the epidermal growth factor receptor and non-small-cell lung cancer. *J Med Genet* 2007; 44: 166–172.
37. Bell DW, Lynch TJ, Haserlat SM, *et al.* Epidermal growth factor receptor mutations and gene amplification in non-small-cell lung cancer: molecular analysis of the IDEAL/INTACT gefitinib trials. *J Clin Oncol* 2005; 23: 8081–8092.
38. Hirsch FR, Dziadziuszko R, Thatcher N, *et al.* Epidermal growth factor receptor immunohisto-chemistry: comparison of antibodies and cutoff points to predict benefit from gefitinib in a phase 3 placebo-controlled study in advanced nonsmall-cell lung cancer. *Cancer* 2008; 112: 1114–1121.
39. Tamura K, Okamoto I, Kashii T, *et al.* Multicentre prospective phase II trial of gefitinib for advanced non-small cell lung cancer with epidermal growth factor receptor mutations: results of the West Japan Thoracic Oncology Group trial (WJTOG0403). *Br J Cancer* 2008; 98: 907–914.
40. Massarelli E, Varella-Garcia M, Tang X, *et al.* KRAS mutation is an important predictor of resistance to therapy with epidermal growth factor receptor tyrosine kinase inhibitors in non-small-cell lung cancer. *Clin Cancer Res* 2007; 13: 2890–2896.
41. Maheswaran S, Sequist LV, Nagrath S, *et al.* Detection of mutations in EGFR in circulating lung-cancer cells. *N Engl J Med* 2008; 359: 366–377.
42. Morgillo F, Kim WY, Kim ES, *et al.* Implication of the insulin-like growth factor-IR pathway in the resistance of non-small cell lung cancer cells to treatment with gefitinib. *Clin Cancer Res* 2007; 13: 2795–2803.
43. Fischer B, Marinov M, Arcaro A. Targeting receptor tyrosine kinase signalling in small cell lung cancer (SCLC): what have we learned so far? *Cancer Treat Rev* 2007; 33: 391–406.
44. Hodkinson PS, Mackinnon A, Sethi T. Targeting growth factors in lung cancer. *Chest* 2008; 133: 1209–1216.

45. Waters CM, MacKinnon AC, Cummings J, *et al.* Increased gastrin-releasing peptide (GRP) receptor expression in tumour cells confers sensitivity to [Arg6,D-Trp7,9,NmePhe8]-substance P (6–11)-induced growth inhibition. *Br J Cancer* 2003; 88: 1808–1816.
46. Konstantinopoulos PA, Karamouzis MV, Papavassiliou AG. Post-translational modifications and regulation of the RAS superfamily of GTPases as anticancer targets. *Nat Rev Drug Discov* 2007; 6: 541–555.
47. Khanzada UK, Pardo OE, Meier C, *et al.* Potent inhibition of small-cell lung cancer cell growth by simvastatin reveals selective functions of Ras isoforms in growth factor signalling. *Oncogene* 2006; 25: 877–887.
48. Giaccone G. The potential of antiangiogenic therapy in non-small cell lung cancer. *Clin Cancer Res* 2007; 13: 1961–1970.
49. Kerbel RS. Tumor angiogenesis. *N Engl J Med* 2008; 358: 2039–2049.
50. Donnem T, Al-Saad S, Al-Shibli K, *et al.* Inverse prognostic impact of angiogenic marker expression in tumor cells *versus* stromal cells in non small cell lung cancer. *Clin Cancer Res* 2007; 13: 6649–6657.
51. Agarwal R, Kaye SB. Ovarian cancer: strategies for overcoming resistance to chemotherapy. *Nat Rev* 2003; 3: 502–516.
52. Szakacs G, Paterson JK, Ludwig JA, *et al.* Targeting multidrug resistance in cancer. *Nat Rev Drug Discov* 2006; 5: 219–234.
53. Dean M, Fojo T, Bates S. Tumour stem cells and drug resistance. *Nat Rev* 2005; 5: 275–284.
54. Simon G, Sharma A, Li X, *et al.* Feasibility and efficacy of molecular analysis-directed individualized therapy in advanced non-small-cell lung cancer. *J Clin Oncol* 2007; 25: 2741–2746.
55. Rudin CM, Salgia R, Wang X, *et al.* Randomized phase II study of carboplatin and etoposide with or without the bcl-2 antisense oligonucleotide oblimersen for extensive-stage small-cell lung cancer: CALGB 30103. *J Clin Oncol* 2008; 26: 870–876.
56. Cobo M, Isla D, Massuti B, *et al.* Customizing cisplatin based on quantitative excision repair cross-complementing 1 mRNA expression: a phase III trial in non-small-cell lung cancer. *J Clin Oncol* 2007; 25: 2747–2754.
57. Bissell MJ, Radisky D. Putting tumours in context. *Nat Rev* 2001; 1: 46–54.
58. Kalluri R, Zeisberg M. Fibroblasts in cancer. *Nat Rev* 2006; 6: 392–401.
59. Fromigue O, Louis K, Dayem M, *et al.* Gene expression profiling of normal human pulmonary fibroblasts following coculture with non-small-cell lung cancer cells reveals alterations related to matrix degradation, angiogenesis, cell growth and survival. *Oncogene* 2003; 22: 8487–8497.
60. Zhu CQ, Popova SN, Brown ER, *et al.* Integrin α11 regulates IGF2 expression in fibroblasts to enhance tumorigenicity of human non-small-cell lung cancer cells. *Proc Natl Acad Sci USA* 2007; 104: 11754–11759.
61. Tokunou M, Niki T, Eguchi K, *et al.* c-MET expression in myofibroblasts: role in autocrine activation and prognostic significance in lung adenocarcinoma. *Am J Pathol* 2001; 158: 1451–1463.
62. Pardo OE, Wellbrock C, Khanzada UK, *et al.* FGF-2 protects small cell lung cancer cells from apoptosis through a complex involving PKCepsilon, B-Raf and S6K2. *EMBO J* 2006; 25: 3078–3088.
63. Sethi T, Rintoul RC, Moore SM, *et al.* Extracellular matrix proteins protect small cell lung cancer cells against apoptosis: a mechanism for small cell lung cancer growth and drug resistance *in vivo*. *Nat Med* 1999; 5: 662–668.
64. Gilboa E. The promise of cancer vaccines. *Nat Rev* 2004; 4: 401–411.
65. Muller AJ, Scherle PA. Targeting the mechanisms of tumoral immune tolerance with small-molecule inhibitors. *Nat Rev* 2006; 6: 613–625.
66. Giaccone G, Debruyne C, Felip E, *et al.* Phase III study of adjuvant vaccination with Bec2/bacille Calmette–Guerin in responding patients with limited-disease small-cell lung cancer (European Organisation for Research and Treatment of Cancer 08971-08971B; Silva Study). *J Clin Oncol* 2005; 23: 6854–6864.

67. Atanackovic D, Altorki NK, Cao Y, *et al.* Booster vaccination of cancer patients with MAGE-A3 protein reveals long-term immunological memory or tolerance depending on priming. *Proc Natl Acad Sci USA* 2008; 105: 1650–1655.
68. Bolonaki I, Kotsakis A, Papadimitraki E, *et al.* Vaccination of patients with advanced non-small-cell lung cancer with an optimized cryptic human telomerase reverse transcriptase peptide. *J Clin Oncol* 2007; 25: 2727–2734.

CHAPTER 7

Radiology of lung cancer

M.N. Taylor, P. Shaw

Dept of Radiology, University College Hospital, London, UK.

Correspondence: P. Shaw, Dept of Radiology, University College Hospital, 235 Euston Road, London NW1 2BU, UK. Fax: 44 02073809068; E-mail: penny.shaw@uclh.nhs.uk

There are 1.3 million new cases of lung cancer diagnosed annually, making it the most common cancer in the world [1]. In the UK, lung cancer rates in males have declined by >40% since the late 1970s, whilst in females they are currently stable, having risen until the late 1980s. Since the late 1990s, lung cancer has been superseded by breast cancer as the most commonly diagnosed cancer in the UK, but remains the leading cause of all deaths from cancer. In 2007, 34,509 people died of lung cancer in the UK, equating to someone dying of lung cancer almost every 15 min [2].

In England and Wales the latest figures show that 25% of all patients diagnosed with lung cancer are alive at 1 yr, and 7% at 5 yrs [3]. Whilst the 1-yr survival rates have risen significantly over the last 30 yrs, there has been little change in the 5-yr survival rates. In 2006, the median survival in England was just 5.3 months. Over two-thirds of patients with lung cancer are currently diagnosed at a late stage in the disease [4], highlighting the need for early detection.

The radiological presentation of lung cancer

Lung cancer presents in three main ways to the imaging department. Firstly, and most commonly, it can present as an abnormal chest radiograph in a patient referred with respiratory symptoms. Secondly, with the increasing use of cross-sectional imaging, lung cancer may also present incidentally, *e.g.* computed tomography (CT) coronary artery calcification scoring will include wide field of view images of the lungs, or CT imaging of the abdomen will include the lung bases. Thirdly, lung cancer may be detected radiologically by screening of high-risk populations using low dose CT.

Screening

In the 1970s and 1980s, large-scale screening programmes in the USA and Czechoslovakia, using chest radiographs and sputum analysis in high-risk populations, did not show any reduction in mortality from lung cancer. Since then, the interest has focused on low dose CT scanning of the chest. In the 1990s, a study by KANEKO *et al.* [5] detected 0.3% cancers on CT images, 73% of which were missed on chest radiographs. In 1999, the Early Lung Cancer Action Project in New York published data involving 1,000 volunteers. They found a malignant nodule prevalence rate of 2.7% for CT compared with 0.7% for chest radiography [6]. Three CT studies conducted in Japan found that 6.6% had an abnormality requiring further investigation, 0.47% of which had lung cancer [7–9]. Importantly, most of the tumours detected in these studies were stage

Eur Respir Mon, 2009, 44, 106–135. Printed in UK - all rights reserved. Copyright ERS Journals Ltd 2009; European Respiratory Monograph; ISSN 1025-448x.

1, and therefore potentially curable. In 2004, the US Preventive Services Task Force issued a statement citing that there was insufficient evidence to recommend for or against screening for lung cancer with either low-dose CT, chest radiography, sputum cytology, or a combination of these tests [9]. As of July 2006, the UK National Screening Committee's position is that screening for lung cancer in adult cigarette smokers using low-dose CT should not be offered, however, trials are ongoing. In the UK, 1,300 patients with COPD are currently being recruited into a 5-yr trial involving the combined use of low-dose CT and fluorescence bronchoscopy in those with abnormal sputum cytology [11]. In the USA, a screening programme using low dose CT and involving 50,000 people opened in 2002 and is due to close in 2009.

Imaging modalities

Chest radiography

Chest radiographs are often the first line of imaging, due to widespread availability, relatively low radiation dose (equivalent to a transatlantic flight), and low cost. Lung cancer may present as a simple mass lesion or with secondary features of post-obstructive lobar collapse, consolidation or air trapping. An unresolving pneumonia always requires further investigation as it may represent a post-obstructive phenomenon, or represent the tumour itself. In some cases, lung cancer may present as a mediastinal or hilar lymph node mass with little evidence of disease elsewhere. The S sign of Golden describes lobar collapse with a bulging contour caused by a primary central tumour, the combined outlines of which assume a reverse "S" shape. It is typically seen with right upper-lobe collapse (fig. 1). "Hidden areas" such as behind the heart, in the apices and below the hemidiaphragms should always be reviewed carefully (fig. 2). It is standard practice to proceed to CT if there is a suspicion of lung cancer on a chest radiograph.

Computed tomography

The use of a CT scan will evaluate a suspicious lesion, providing information on its position, size, composition, and relationship to other structures, as well as the presence or absence of disease elsewhere. CT of the liver and adrenal glands should be routinely included.

Spiral (helical) CT scanning was introduced in the late 1980s and quickly superseded single slice sequential scanning, having the advantage of a faster acquisition time, so images of the chest could be acquired in a single breath hold. The continuous and overlapping nature of the data acquisition improved multiplanar reformatting and nodule detection. However, the high heat loading of the tube required the dose to be reduced, thus limiting image quality. The introduction of multislice CT (or multidetector row CT) in the late 1990s overcame this problem by collecting data for more than one slice per tube rotation. Multislice CT allows faster scanning times, and improved image resolution. Because tube loading is not a restrictive factor, high quality thin slices (≤ 1 mm) can be obtained, improving nodule detection and reformatting in the coronal and sagittal planes. By 2005, 64 slice scanners were introduced, and more recently 256 and 320 slice scanners. The high spatial resolution of modern multislice CT scanning has meant that software algorithms for computer-aided detection (CAD) of pulmonary nodules have been developed, which have increasingly high sensitivity rates, albeit still moderate false positive rates [12]. Furthermore, nodule volumetry allows three-

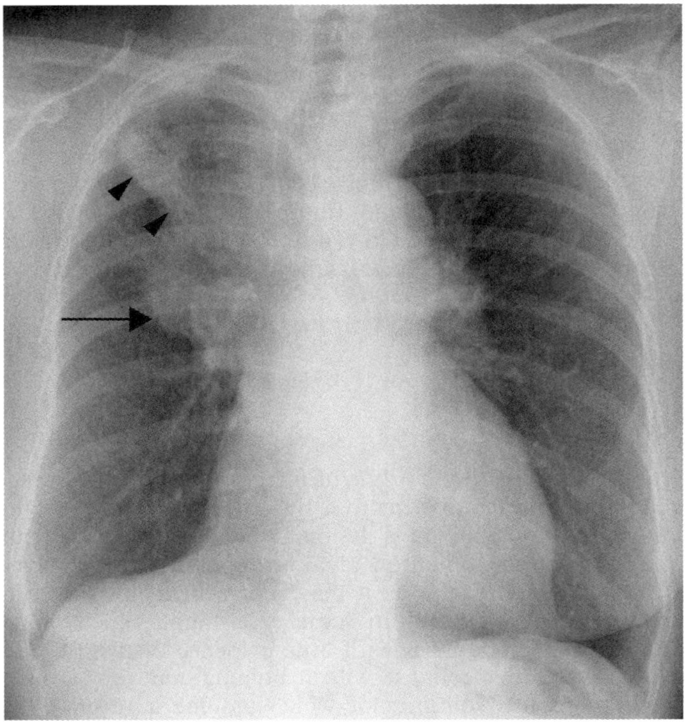

Fig. 1. – Chest radiograph showing S sign of Golden. There is partial right upper-lobe collapse (arrow heads), secondary to a central mass lesion (arrow).

dimensional (3D) measurements of nodules, allowing accurate monitoring of growth (fig. 3).

It is standard practice to acquire contiguous volume images of the chest at 36 s (the arterial phase) following the *i.v.* administration of 90 mL of iodinated contrast, followed by portal-venous phase images of the liver and adrenal glands. The *i.v.* contrast aids detection of mediastinal and hilar lymphadenopathy and is essential for liver metastases. Furthermore, indeterminate nodules may be assessed by sequential scanning at 1-min intervals, for up to 4 min, following contrast administration. Nodule enhancement of <15 Hounsfield Units (HU) is strongly predictive of benignity, with a sensitivity of 98% and specificity of 58% [13].

Positron emission tomography-computed tomography

Positron emission tomography (PET) scanning has secured its place in the assessment of lung cancer. It is used in the evaluation of indeterminate pulmonary nodules, and has a major role in the staging of lung cancer.

PET scanning involves the *i.v.* injection of the radiopharmaceutical, fluorine-18 fluorodeoxyglucose (FDG). The FDG component is a glucose analogue that is taken up by metabolically active cells, but which remains un-metabolised. The fluorine-18 component is a positron emitting radionuclide, which is annihilated in the cells by a negative electron, whereupon two photons are emitted simultaneously in opposite directions. It is these photons which are detected by a positron camera. Malignant cells metabolise increased

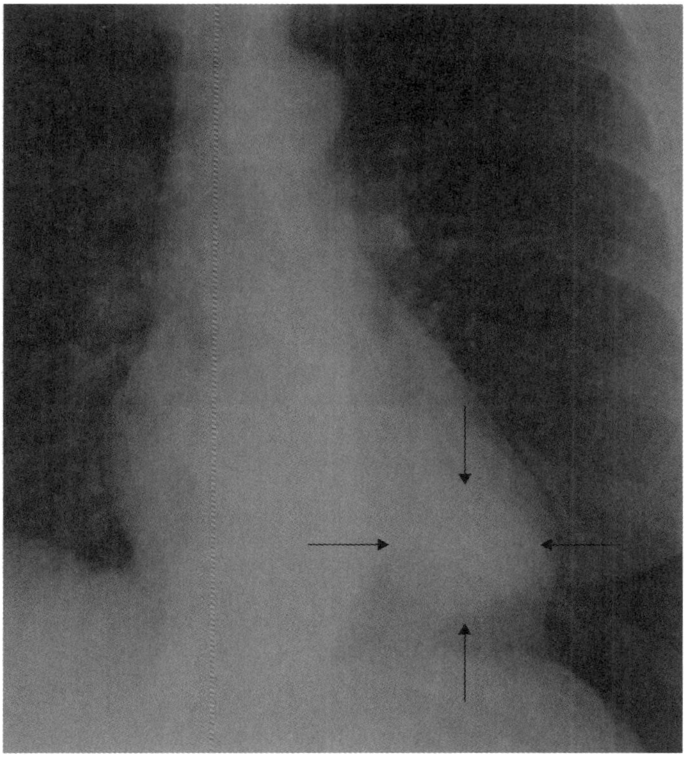

Fig. 2. – Chest radiograph showing a large retrocardiac mass (arrows).

amounts of glucose compared with normal cells, and it is this difference that allows the detection of neoplastic lesions. The uptake of FDG can be assessed both visually and quantitatively, the former simply by comparing uptake in the lesion with background uptake, and the latter using calculated standardised uptake values (SUV). An SUV <2.5 is in keeping with benignity. The uptake of FDG is directly proportional to the growth rate and aggressiveness of the tumour [14]. Patients with a negative PET scan who have subsequently been shown to have cancer have a significantly longer survival than those patients with a positive scan and cancer [15]. The sensitivity and specificity for the detection of malignant solid pulmonary nodules 1–3cm are ~94 and 83%, respectively [16], falling for nodules <1 cm in diameter. Bronchoalveolar cell carcinomas and carcinoid tumours have low rates of metabolism and are often PET negative. Infection or inflammatory conditions, such as sarcoidosis and rheumatoid, may yield false-positive results. A negative PET scan is associated with malignancy in <5% of patients for nodules 0.6–3 cm diameter [17].

PET scanning can identify mediastinal and hilar lymph node involvement by tumour, even when the nodes are not enlarged by CT criteria (*i.e.* <1 cm in short axis diameter). This is essential in the staging of disease. The negative predictive value of PET scanning for N3 disease is 96% [18], which is identical to mediastinoscopy. The most recent National Institute of Clinical Excellence (NICE; London, UK) guidelines on the diagnosis and treatment of lung cancer published in 2005 [19], stipulate that when an FDG-PET scan is negative for N2/3 disease, biopsy is not required even if the patient's nodes are enlarged by CT criteria (fig. 4). The same guidelines indicate which patients

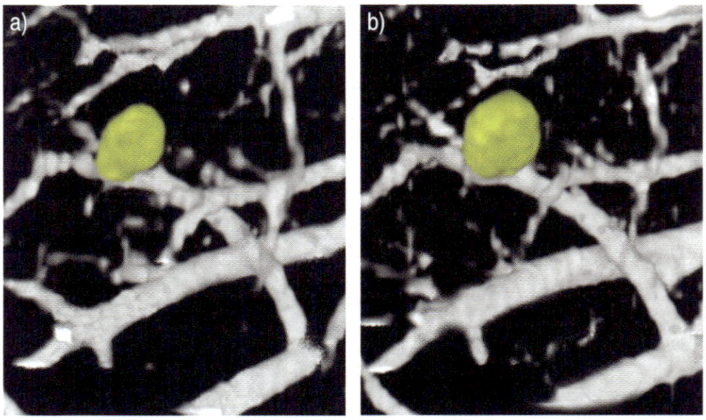

Fig. 3. – A computed tomography volumetric scan depicting three-dimensional images of an enlarging pulmonary nodule, b) was acquired 10 months after a). The nodule dimensions are: a) 129.65 mm^3 and b) 228.05 mm^3.

should have a PET scan: those who are staged as having resectable disease on CT; those that have limited (1–2 stations) N2/3 disease on CT of uncertain pathological significance but who are otherwise surgical candidates; and those who are candidates for radical radiotherapy. Extrathoracic spread is assessed at the time of the examination, as is the possibility of synchronous extrathoracic primary tumours. PET scanning can be used to guide the most appropriate site for tissue sampling.

By combining a positron camera and a CT scanner into a single gantry, dual modality images can be obtained sequentially in the same examination and superimposed into a co-registered set of PET-CT images. This provides both metabolic and anatomical information, and overcomes the problem of poor spatial resolution with PET alone.

Recently, novel tracers, such as fluorothymidine (FLT), have been investigated. Results of a multicenter Chinese clinical trial, published in 2008, showed that FLT is less sensitive than FDG in detecting lung cancer although it is more specific. However, by

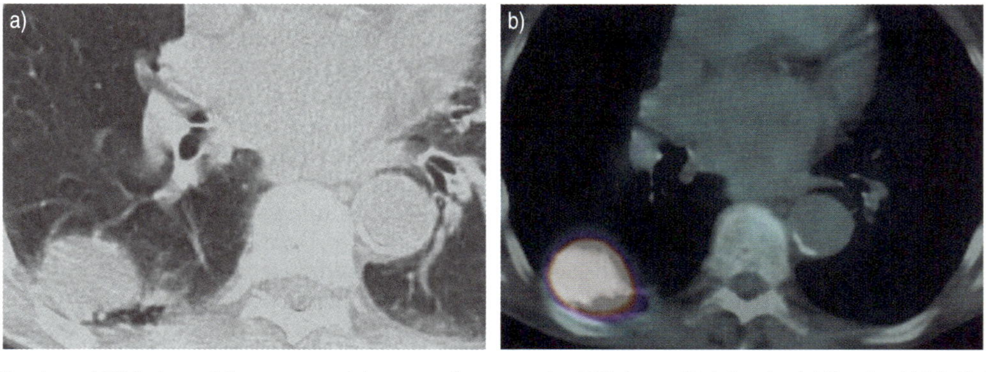

Fig. 4. – a) Right lower-lobe mass on axial computed tomography (CT) image. b) A fused axial fluorine-18 labelled fluorodeoxyglucose (FDG)-positron emission tomography and CT image. The mass has a high SUV in keeping with a tumour. No FDG uptake was seen elsewhere despite borderline nodes on CT. The patient underwent surgery.

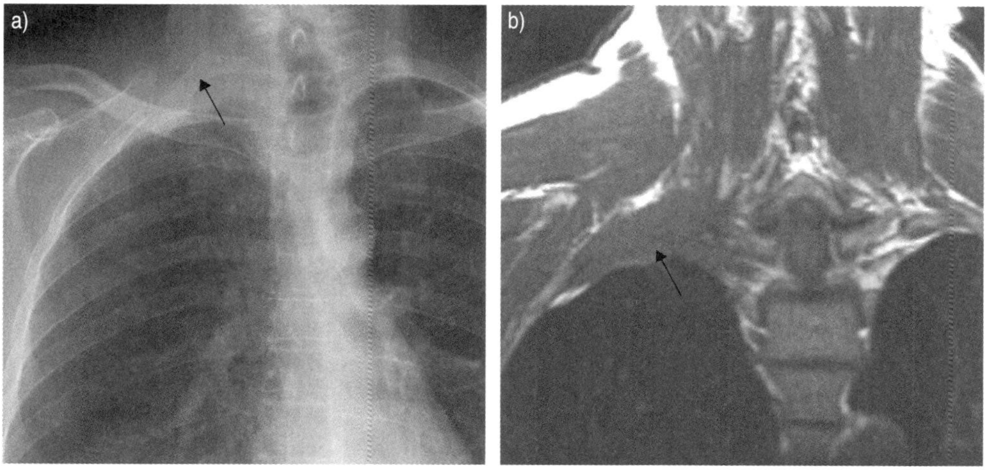

Fig. 5. – Superior sulcus (Pancoast) tumour. a) The chest radiograph demonstrates a right apical mass with destruction of the posterior portion of the second rib (arrow). b) Coronal T1 weighted magnetic resonance imaging in the same patient showing the mass infiltrating into the chest wall and posterior mediastinum (arrow).

combining both tracers the sensitivity and specificity of PET-CT rose to 100 and 89.7% respectively [20].

Magnetic resonance imaging

Magnetic resonance imaging (MRI) is not routinely used in the diagnosis and staging of lung cancer. Image acquisition is slower than with CT, more expensive, has poorer spatial resolution and provides little information on lung parenchyma. Being slow, respiratory motion artefact is a problem and may cause lymph node size to be over-estimated. T1 weighted MRI sequences allow visualisation of fat planes, whereas T2 weighted images are better at detecting tumour infiltration, which is usually of higher signal. The use of *i.v.* gadolinium further improves the diagnostic yield. MRI may be helpful when the use of *i.v.* contrast is contra-indicated in CT, and there is ambiguity over possible mediastinal invasion, or the presence of enlarged hilar nodes. Cardiac gating, which reduces cardiac pulsation artefact, allows accurate delineation of the heart and great vessels. This technique is also available with CT but rarely necessary due to fast scanning times. MRI retains a role in assessing superior sulcus tumours because of improved soft tissue contrast compared with CT, and multiplanar imaging capability, as well as the assessment of chest wall invasion, and spinal canal involvement (fig. 5)

Ultrasound

Ultrasound uses high frequency (>20 KHz) sound waves. Its short wavelength can be formed into a narrow beam which undergoes reflection at an interface between two different tissues, thus producing an image. Ultrasound is not used routinely to diagnose or stage lung cancer, although may be of use in the evaluation of chest wall invasion. Its main role is in aiding tissue sampling of lymph nodes, chest wall masses, subcutaneous soft tissue nodules, pleural deposits or effusions, and suspected liver metastases.

Imaging characteristics of different histological types of lung cancer

The imaging features of the most common histological types of lung cancer as categorised by the World Health Organization (WHO) [21] are summarised below.

Adenocarcinoma

There has been a sharp global rise in the incidence of adenocarcinoma of the lung in the last 50 yrs, perhaps as a result of low tar filtered cigarettes [22]. In the USA, adenocarcinoma of the lung is currently the most common histological subtype of lung cancer, representing ~50% of all lung cancers. Whilst a steep rise has also been reported in the UK and the rest of Europe [23], the rate of squamous cell carcinoma still exceeds that of adenocarcinoma. People who smoke low-tar filtered cigarettes tend to inhale deeply, and as a result, these tumours are often located peripherally within the lung. They are frequently found in scars and adjacent to pre-existing bullae. They are generally <4 cm in diameter and cavitation is seen in 4%. Air bronchograms or bronchiolograms are seen in 65% (fig. 6) and calcification in the periphery of the mass in 1%. Hilar and/or mediastinal lymph node involvement is seen in over 50% of cases at presentation. Adenocarcinomas may present either as a slow-growing localised area of ground glass opacity (GGO), or a faster growing solid mass. Atypical adenomatous hyperplasia, believed to be a possible precursor of adenocarcinoma, presents as a small (<2 cm), round, well-defined peripheral GGO without solid components [24, 25].

Bronchoalveolar cell carcinoma

Bronchoalveolar cell carcinoma (BACC) is a subtype of adenocarcinoma that accounts for ~5% of all bronchogenic carcinomas. It presents in both nodular and consolidative forms, and may be solitary or multifocal. The most common presentation is a solitary pulmonary nodule or mass, occurring in 41% [26]. Unresolving consolidation should always raise the possibility of BACC (fig. 7). A localised area of consolidation is the presentation in 22% of cases, and in 36% the disease is multicentric. The CT angiogram sign is seen in the consolidative form and describes enhancing branching pulmonary vessels in a homogeneous, low-attenuating, consolidation of lung

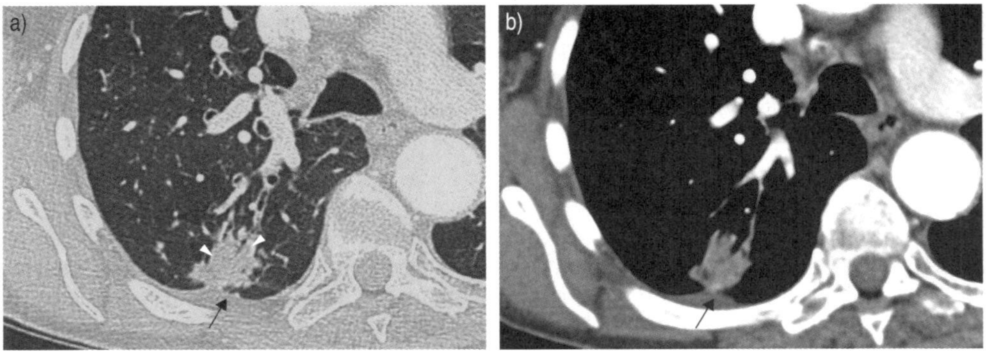

Fig. 6. – Adenocarcinoma. Axial computed tompography image on a) lung and b) mediastinal window settings. Note the peripheral air bronchograms (arrow heads) and the pleural tag (arrow).

parenchyma, relative to the chest wall musculature [27]. It has a low specificity and other malignant processes, such as lymphoma, as well as benign entities for example infective pneumonia and pulmonary oedema may also give this appearance. However, the consolidation seen in BACC tends to have a lower average HU than these other processes which have a similar HU to that of muscle. In their paper, IM *et al* [27] reported an average HU of 27.6 with BAC compared with 73.5 HU with consolidation due to other processes, and 74 HU for normal muscle. Air bronchiolograms, which have the appearance of bubble-like lucencies (and which are also termed pseudocavities), are seen in up to 55% of bronchoalveolar cell carcinomas. These occur as a result of airway distortion, which itself is caused by a desmoplastic reaction to the tumour. Hilar and mediastinal lymphadenopathy is uncommon.

Squamous cell carcinoma

People who smoke high-tar unfiltered cigarettes do not inhale as deeply and are more likely to develop centrally located squamous cell carcinomas [28]. In the UK and the rest of Europe, they are the most common type of lung cancer. They tend to grow to a larger size than adenocarcinomas, and cavitation is seen in 82% of them (fig. 8). Secondary segmental or lobar collapse is common. They are the least likely cell type to metastasise distally, the most likely to be radiologically occult, and the most common type to cause superior sulcus (Pancoast) tumours.

Adenosquamous carcinoma

Adenosquamous carcinoma represents ~2% of lung cancers. It has a propensity for metastases at the time of diagnosis and a poor prognosis. There is a spectrum of presentation, but most commonly a solitary peripheral nodule with an ill defined or spiculated margin is seen. Cavitation is seen in 13%. The mean diameter of peripheral tumours is 2.7 cm compared with 4.2 cm for centrally located tumours. Evidence of underlying pulmonary scarring or fibrosis is seen in 50% [29].

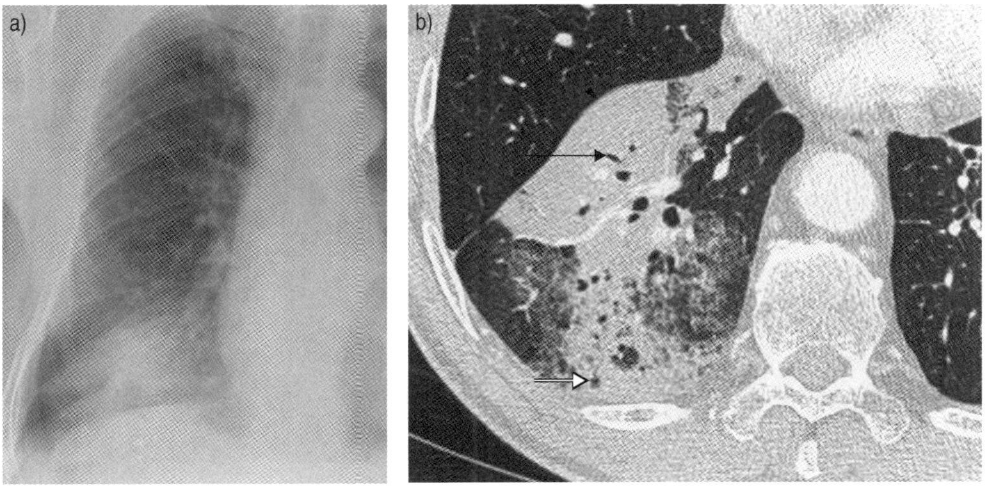

Fig. 7. – a) Chest radiograph of an unresolving right lower-lobe pneumonia. b) Axial computed tomographic image depicting dense and ground glass consolidation, subsequently confirmed as bronchoalveolar carcinoma. Note the bulging oblique fissure (arrow head), the air bronchograms (black arrow), and the pseudocavities (white arrow).

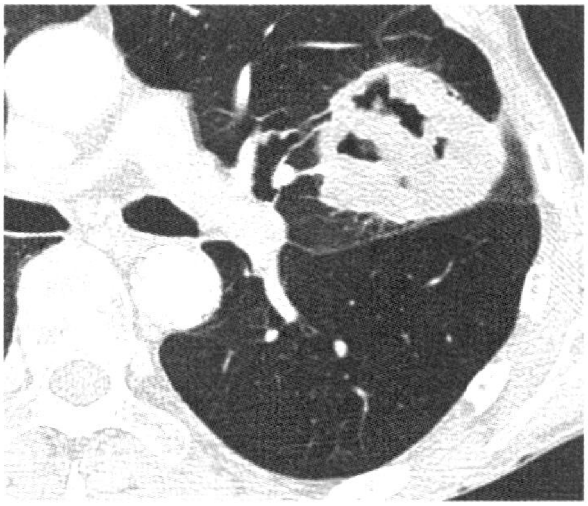

Fig. 8. – Axial computed tomographic image of an irregular thick-walled, spiculated, cavitating mass in the left upper-lobe, found to be a squamous cell carcinoma.

Small cell lung cancer

Small cell lung cancer (SCLC) accounts for 18% of lung cancers. These tumours represent the malignant end of the spectrum of neuroendocrine lung tumours. They are aggressive tumours, with a fast doubling time, and metastasise early (60–80% at the time of diagnosis). They usually present with large hilar and mediastinal lymph node masses (fig. 9). The primary tumour tends to be centrally located, and distinguishing this from adjacent lymph node metastases is often difficult. A separate parenchymal mass is identified in 41% of cases on CT. Cavitation is rare, and lobar collapse, obstructive pneumonitis, and superior vena cava obstruction are all recognised complications.

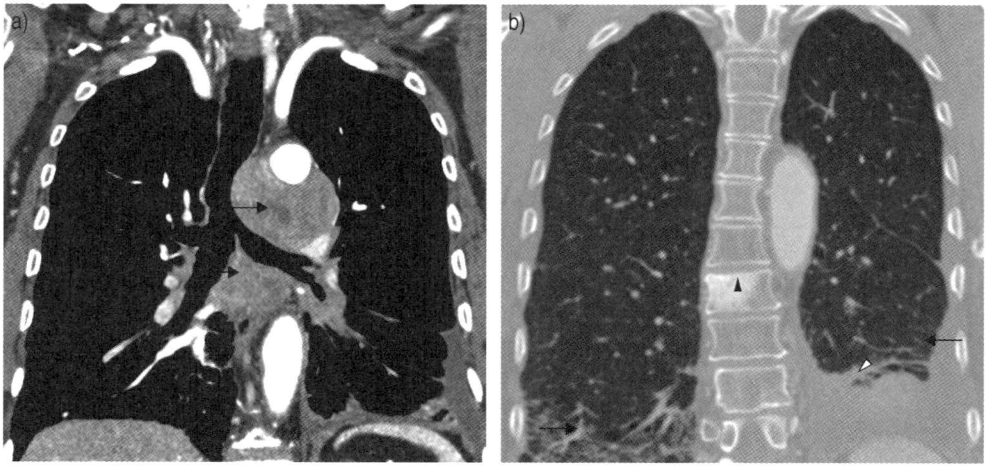

Fig. 9. – Coronal computed tomography reformats in a patient with small cell lung cancer. a) A large mediastinal tumour mass (arrows) compressing the trachea and origin of the left main bronchus. b) Additional findings were pulmonary fibrosis (arrows), atelectasis adjacent to a pleural effusion (white arrow head), and a sclerotic bony metastasis (black arrow head).

Large cell

Large cell carcinoma is the least common type of NSCLC and accounts for approximately 5% of lung cancers. Tumours tend to be peripherally located, grow rapidly and metastasise early. Tumours are >6 cm in size in 50% and contain large areas of necrosis. They include large cell neuroendocrine carcinoma as a subtype, which along with small cell cancers form the majority of malignant lung neuroendocrine tumours.

Carcinoid

Carcinoid tumours account for ~1–2% of lung cancers. Ninety per cent of these are typical carcinoids, which represent the most benign end of the spectrum of neuroendocrine tumours. These tumours tend to be slow-growing and metastasise infrequently. They more commonly arise centrally within the major airways, and are complicated by lobar collapse and post-obstructive pneumonitis. 10% are atypical tumours which are more aggressive, and arise from central and peripheral airways with equal frequency. Whereas typical carcinoids are usually <2.5 cm in size, atypical tumours tend to be >2.5 cm. The tumours tend to be well defined and calcification is seen in approximately one-third of them, being more frequently seen in central lesions.

The solitary pulmonary nodule

The finding of a solitary pulmonary nodule (SPN) is increasingly common with the use of multi-detector CT scanning. Differentiating benign from malignant nodules presents difficulties in management. The size, imaging characteristics (including the growth rate from previous imaging if available), as well as the clinical history are all helpful. Often a nodule is indeterminate, requiring either sampling or removal of the nodule, or follow-up imaging.

Definitions. The chest radiograph definition of a pulmonary nodule is a well or poorly defined rounded opacity measuring anything up to 3 cm in diameter [30]. At chest radiography, an SPN is seldom evident until it is at least 9 mm in diameter. The CT definition is as for a chest radiograph, but in addition further terminology applies: a micronodule is defined as measuring <3 mm in diameter; a ground glass nodule is defined as a hazy increase in attenuation in the lung; and a part-solid nodule is defined as consisting of both ground glass and solid components.

Differential diagnosis. The differential diagnosis of a solitary pulmonary nodule is wide and the more common causes are summarised in table 1. When interpreting a chest radiograph, it is important to be aware of pseudonodules such as rib fractures, skin lesions, and composite shadows, which together account for ~20% of suspected SPNs.

Benign nodules. Between 60–70% of solitary pulmonary nodules are benign. A number of factors are in keeping with benignity of a nodule: 1) Clinical history: no history of cigarette smoking, <35-yrs old and no history of pulmonary fibrosis or extrathoracic malignancy. 2) Serial imaging: no growth over at least 2 yrs. 3) Morphology of the nodule: benign nodules are usually homogenous with a smooth well defined margin. However, this cannot be taken as a reliable indicator of benignity. Homogeneity is seen in both benign (55%) and malignant (20%) nodules. The presence of fat within a nodule is a reliable indicator of a hamartoma (fig. 10). A characteristic pattern of calcification within a nodule: diffuse, central, and laminated (seen in granulomas) and popcorn-like

Table 1. – The differential diagnosis of a solitary pulmonary nodule

Infection	Inflammatory	Neoplastic	Vascular	Other
Granuloma (TB, fungal)	Sarcoid	Lung cancer	AVM	Intrapulmonary lymph node
Abscess	Wegener's	Metastasis	Contusion	Bronchogenic cyst
Rounded pneumonia	Rheumatoid	Carcinoid	Infarct	Mucoid impaction
Septic embolus	Amyloid	Hamartoma	Pulmonary artery aneurysm	Sequestration
Measles		1° pulmonary lymphoma	Haemangioma	Focal interstitial fibrosis

TB: tuberculosis; AVM: arteriovenous malformation; 1°: primary.

(seen in hamartomas), allows a near 100% diagnosis of a benign lesion. Calcification is also present in ~10% of malignant nodules, but this prevalence drops to only 2% in lesions <3 cm in diameter [31]. Approximately 50% of benign nodules are not calcified, and the reported incidence of calcification in hamartomas at CT is in the region of 30%. The presence of fat or calcification is often difficult to see on a chest radiograph. CT densitometry can be used to create a pixel map of a nodule, with HU values exceeding 200 in keeping with calcification and those between -50 and -100 in keeping with fat. Size is also an important factor, with 80% of benign lesions measuring <2 cm in diameter. Although the literature varies, there are reports suggesting that >90% of nodules that measure <2 cm in diameter are benign [32], but surgical series indicate a much lower figure.

Malignant nodules. Lung cancer presents as a SPN in 20–30% of cases. A history of smoking, asbestos exposure, pulmonary fibrosis, HIV, or head and neck cancer should increase suspicion. A spiculated or lobulated contour is suspicious for malignancy but 21% of malignant nodules have well-defined margins [33], and some benign nodules may appear slightly lobulated. Spiculation most often correlates pathologically with fibrosis

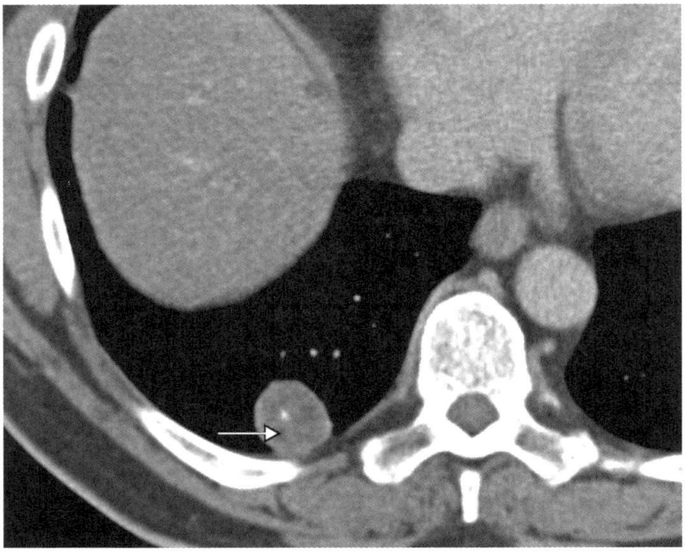

Fig. 10. – Well defined solitary pulmonary nodule which contains fat (arrow) and calcium, in keeping with a hamartoma.

secondary to a desmoplastic reaction, but may also represent localised lymphatic spread or infiltrative growth [34]. Although small size is more in keeping with a benign cause, it does not exclude malignancy: 15% of malignant nodules are <1 cm in diameter and ~42% are <2 cm in diameter [35]. However, the larger the nodule the more likely it is to be malignant. Calcification has already been discussed as being largely in keeping with benignity. However, calcification is seen in ~30% of carcinoid tumours (variable pattern), 6% of lung cancers (usually stippled or amorphous in appearance) and with metastases. Metastases from osteosarcomas or chondrosarcomas may demonstrate a benign diffuse pattern of calcification, whereas metastases from mucin-secreting tumours, such as ovary and colon, may give rise to a stippled pattern of calcification. Eccentric, punctate calcification may be seen as a result of engulfment of a pre-existing calcified granuloma by a lung cancer. The "solidity" of a nodule is an indeterminate feature, and ~34% of nonsolid (ground glass) nodules are malignant [36], usually in the form of a bronchoalveolar cell carcinoma or an invasive adenocarcinoma (fig. 11). Air bronchograms and air bronchiolograms within a nodule are more in keeping with malignancy, with one report suggesting an incidence of air bronchograms of 30% in malignant nodules compared with 6% in benign nodules [37]. Air bronchograms are suggestive of lymphoma, whereas air bronchiolograms, also termed pseudocavities, are suggestive of bronchoalveolar cell carcinoma. True cavitation in itself is not helpful in determining whether a nodule is benign or malignant, but the appearance of the cavity wall is. Smooth, thin walls (<4 mm) are in keeping with benignity, whereas irregular, thick walls (>16 mm) are in keeping with malignancy [35]. Whilst the location of the nodule cannot be used with any kind of certainty as to its aetiology, 70% of lung cancers originate in the upper lobes, and are one and a half times more common in the right lung.

The Fleischner guidelines. The Fleischner guidelines for the follow-up and management of small, noncalcified pulmonary nodules were drawn up in 2005 and are summarised in table 2 [38]. Prior to this, at a time when multidetector CT scanning was

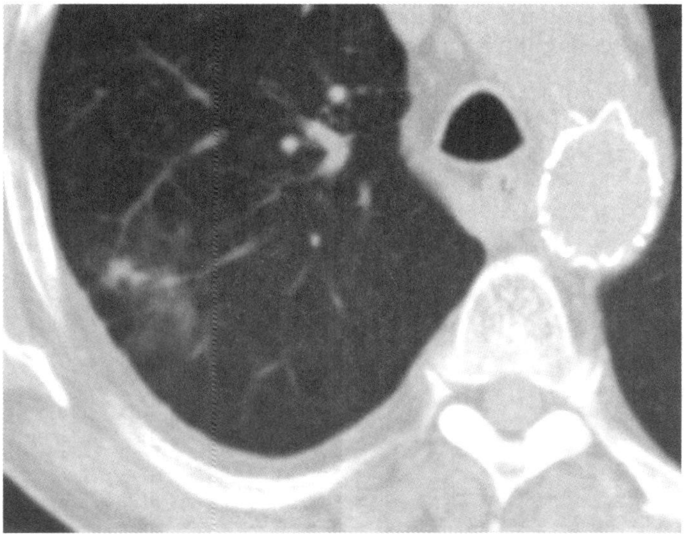

Fig. 11. – Axial computed tomography (CT) image of a ground glass nodular opacity discovered incidentally in a patient undergoing imaging of the aorta. A bronchoalveolar cell carcinoma was diagnosed following CT guided biopsy.

Table 2. – Fleischner recommendations for follow-up (FU) and management of nodules smaller than 8 mm detected incidentally at nonscreening computed tomography (CT)

Nodule size mm	Low-risk patient	High-risk patient
≤4	No FU	FU CT at 12 months and if unchanged no further FU
>4–6	FU CT at 12 months and if unchanged no further FU	FU CT at 6–12 months and at 18–24 months if no change
>6–8	FU CT at 6 to 12 months then at 18–24 months if no change	Initial FU CT at 3–6 months then at 9 months and then at 24 months if no change
>8	FU CT at 3, 9 and 24 months Dynamic contrast-enhanced CT PET and/or biopsy	Same as for low risk patient

PET: positron emission tomography.

not in wide use, the advice was that all indeterminate nodules should be followed up using serial CT for a minimum of 2 yrs.

Central tumours

Central tumours may present as a hilar mass or as post-obstructive collapse/consolidation. Distinguishing central tumours from proximal hilar and mediastinal lymph node masses, or from distal consolidation/collapse may prove difficult, as attenuation values are often similar. This differentiation is important in determining operability and for radiotherapy field planning. PET scans have been shown to be helpful in this regard (fig. 12). ONITSUKA *et al.* [39] found that with rapid sequence CT scanning there was preferential enhancement of the lung parenchyma between 40 s and 2 min following *i.v.* contrast, compared with minimal enhancement of the tumour. Ascertaining whether a central mass has arisen from the lung or from the mediastinum may be aided by assessing the interface between the mass and the lung. Spiculation or

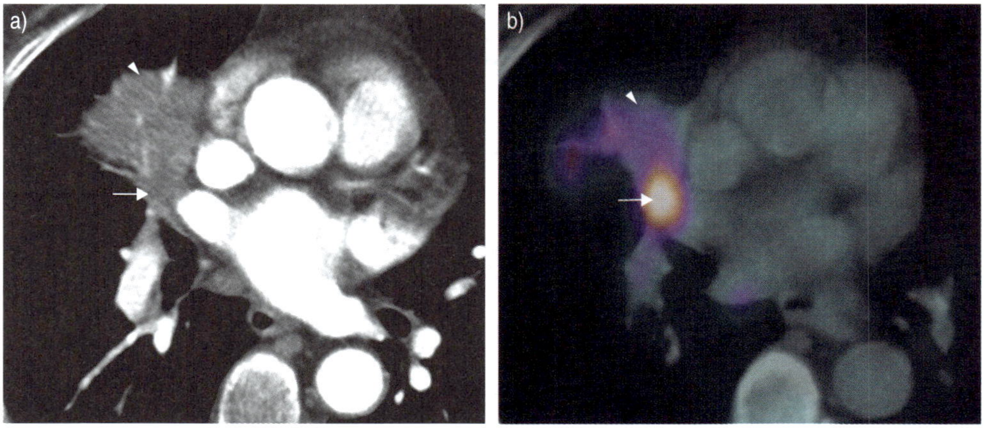

Fig. 12. – a) Axial computed tomographic (CT) image post *i.v.* contrast and b) fused axial fluorodeoxyglucose-positron emission tomographic and CT image. The latter allows differentiation of the involved hilar node (arrow), from distal collapse involving the right middle-lobe (arrow head).

irregularity at this interface usually indicates that the mass is of lung origin, whereas a smooth interface (with the exception of Hodgkin's lymphoma) usually indicates that the mass is mediastinal in origin.

Staging of lung cancer

Accurate staging is paramount in deciding whether a patient's tumour is potentially curable. It determines whether the tumour is resectable, and together with the clinical status, whether the patient is operable. If the tumour is nonresectable or the patient is unfit for surgery due to existing co-morbidity, staging will help guide medical management.

Staging of nonsmall cell lung cancer

Nonsmall cell lung cancer (NSCLC) includes squamous cell carcinoma, adenocarcinoma, and large cell carcinoma and is staged using the TNM system (T: primary tumour, N: regional lymph nodes, M: distant metastases). The current TNM staging system came into effect in 1997 [40]. It is being revised and is due for publication in 2009.

The International Association for the Study of Lung Cancer has recently published its proposals which include: subgroups within the T staging based on the size of the lesion (tumours >7 cm would move from T2 to T3); additional pulmonary nodules would be T3 in the same lobe, T4 in a different lobe but in the ipsilateral lung, and M1a in the contralateral lung; malignant pleural effusions would also be M1a. Furthermore, T2 N0 M0 would be upgraded from stage Ib to stage IIa; T2 N1 M0 cases would be downgraded from stage IIB to stage IIA, and T4 N0 M0 cases would be downgraded from stage IIIB to stage IIIA [41]. The new staging system is fully described in chapter 9 of this current *European Respiratory Monograph* (ERM).

A recent study by WEVER *et al.* [42], compared the TNM status of suspicious pulmonary nodules using integrated PET-CT, CT alone, PET alone and visually correlated PET-CT with the surgical TNM status. They found that integrated PET-CT was the most accurate imaging technique, correctly predicting tumour status in 86%, nodal status in 80% and metastatic status in 98%. The overall accuracy of determining TNM status was 70% for integrated PET-CT, 46% with CT alone, 30% with PET alone, and 54% with visually correlated PET-CT.

Tumour

Tumour status is based on its size, site and degree of local invasion. FDG-PET identifies 95% of T1 lesions [15]. The most important distinction is between T3 and T4 tumours as this distinguishes potential surgical from nonsurgical management. The sensitivity of CT for differentiating T3 from T4 tumours is low, and has been reported as 62% by WEBB *et al.* [43]. Some T4 tumours may be easily identifiable on CT, but diagnosing T3 or early T4 disease is often more difficult. Differentiating invasion, from tumour lying adjacent to the mediastinum, pleura, pericardium, chest wall, or diaphragm can prove challenging. The sensitivity and specificity for chest wall invasion using CT has been shown to be in the region of 38–87 and 40–90% respectively, with the only reliable finding being bony destruction [44] (fig. 13). The sensitivity for mediastinal invasion using CT has been reported to be as low as 40–44% [45]. Minimal mediastinal invasion limited to the fat, is considered resectable by many surgeons. Methods for assessing mediastinal or chest wall invasion have included the creation of artificial pneumothoraces to assess whether the pleura detaches from the structure in question. Results have been variable, with one study reporting 100 and 76% accuracy for mediastinal and chest wall involvement respectively, and another study reporting 100% sensitivity, and 80% specificity for both sites [46, 47]. Multisection expiratory dynamic CT has also been used, obtaining multiple images at 1 s intervals during a single expiration, and reviewing these in cine mode to assess movement of the tumour against the mediastinum or chest wall. In one study, the CT findings using this method correlated with pathological examination in all patients, but the numbers evaluated were small [48]. Although the study by GLAZER *et al* [49], which correlated CT scans considered indeterminate for mediastinal invasion with resectability at thoracotomy, predates the use of multidetector CT scanning, the findings probably remain valid. In their series of 80 CT scans, 36 out of 37 patients, with technically resectable disease, had one or more of the following features on a CT image: $\leq$3 cm contact of the mass with the mediastinum, $<$90° contact with the aorta, and/or a fat plane between the mass and mediastinal structures. Of these 36 masses, 28 were resectable with no evidence of mediastinal invasion, and eight were resectable with focal limited mediastinal invasion. A later study by HERMAN *et al.* [50] found that when $>$90° of contact was used as a positive CT finding, the sensitivity of CT for direct mediastinal invasion was only 40% but the specificity was 99%. The group also found that mediastinal structures with $>$180° of contact were involved by tumour. With the increasing use of multidetector CT and the capability for high quality multiplanar reformatting, the accuracy of CT in the assessment of T status is likely to have improved, but little exists in the literature at present to corroborate this.

MRI has also been used to assess both chest wall and mediastinal invasion. MRI has better soft tissue contrast than CT and fat planes are better delineated. The Radiologic Diagnostic Oncology Group found no significant difference in sensitivity and specificity between MRI (56 and 80%) and CT (63 and 84%) at distinguishing T3/4 tumours from T1/2 tumours [43]. However, with receiver operating characteristic (ROC) analysis, MRI was significantly more accurate than CT in diagnosing mediastinal invasion, but there was no difference in accuracy between the two modalities for bronchial involvement or chest wall invasion. MRI is of particular use in assessing myocardial invasion or tumour extending via the pulmonary veins into the left atrium [51]. MRI sensitivities and specificities of 90 and 86% have been reported for the detection of chest wall invasion

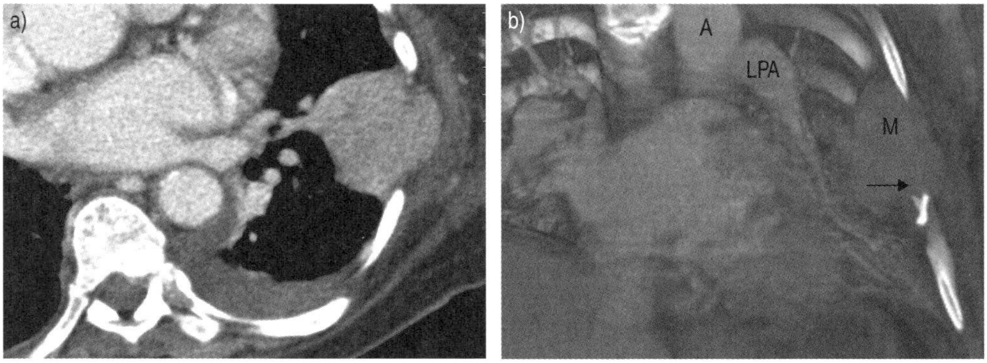

Fig. 13. – a) Axial computed tomography post *i.v.* contrast demonstrating a peripheral tumour mass clearly infiltrating through the chest wall. Note the associated left pleural effusion secondary to malignant infiltration of the pleura. b) A volume rendered image of the mass (M) clearly showing a destroyed rib (arrow). A: aorta; LPA: left pulmonary artery.

[52]. MRI remains the imaging modality recommended by NICE for the assessment of superior sulcus tumours, with a reported accuracy of 94% compared with 63% for CT [53]. MRI is particularly helpful at evaluating tumour extension through the intervertebral neural foramina, the spinal cord, the brachial plexus, and the subclavian artery. Thin section images using surface coils should be used.

The use of ultrasound, although not routinely performed, has recently been shown to have a sensitivity of 89% and specificity of 95% in assessing chest wall invasion, compared with 42 and 100% with CT [54]. The investigators assessed 90 patients with clinical suspicion of chest wall invasion, who underwent CT scanning, transthoracic ultrasound, and surgical exploration. Of the 26 patients that were confirmed to have chest wall invasion, ultrasound correctly identified 23, compared with CT which only identified 11. An earlier study, which reviewed 120 patients with tumour-chest wall contiguity on CT, found ultrasound to have a sensitivity of 100% and specificity of 98% compared with operative findings [55].

Malignant pleural infiltration renders a tumour unresectable. Benign pleural effusions occur with lung cancer and may be secondary to post-obstructive pneumonia. CT has been found to be indeterminate in 71% of patients with NSCLC and pleural abnormalities on CT. FDG-PET alone had a sensitivity and specificity of 100 and 71%, respectively, compared with 100 and 76% for combined CT and FDG-PET, respectively, in the detection of pleural malignancy in this patient group [56].

Regional lymph nodes

Nodal staging of the mediastinum is important, N2, unlike N3 disease, does not preclude surgery. N1 hilar nodes are resectable and although pre-operative detection is helpful, it does not generally influence whether to operate. Sarcoid-like reactions in lymph nodes occur in 1% of lung cancer patients [57] and may cause nodal enlargement, which is misinterpreted as metastatic spread.

Many studies were carried out in the 1990s comparing the accuracy of CT at staging nodal disease with the gold standard of mediastinoscopy or surgery. These studies found CT alone was not adequate as evidence of malignant nodal involvement, regardless of the size criteria, as 20% of nodes thought to be malignant on CT were benign [58]. The advent of PET scanning, which is now routine in most UK institutions, has revolutionised regional nodal staging. A recent meta-analysis by the American College of Chest Physicians found pooled sensitivity and specificity values for the identification of mediastinal lymph node metastases using CT to be 51 and 85% respectively. With PET scanning, pooled sensitivity and specificity values were 74 and 85% respectively [59]. These differences are supported by other published meta-analyses. These findings demonstrate that PET is better at staging mediastinal disease, but abnormal findings should be confirmed with tissue sampling (fig. 14). The limitation of PET scanning is poor image resolution (4–8 mm), which is overcome by the complementary use of CT. By using both the functional information afforded by PET and the anatomical information provided by CT, staging is improved. Central tumours can be differentiated from enlarged nodes and ipsilateral hilar nodes can be distinguished from mediastinal nodes (N1 *versus* N2). In patients with normal-sized mediastinal lymph nodes (*i.e.* <1 cm short axis diameter), PET has a sensitivity and specificity of 74 and of 96%, respectively, compared with 95 and 76, respectively, when the lymph nodes are enlarged [60]. The negative predictive value of PET scanning for N3 disease is equal to that of mediastinoscopy and current NICE guidelines stipulate that where FDG-PET is negative for N2/3 disease, despite the presence of enlarged lymph nodes on CT, confirmatory biopsy is not required. A recent study by AL-SARRAF *et al.* [61] sought to evaluate the incidence, pattern, and predictors of occult FDG-PET negative mediastinal lymph node involvement in patients with NSCLC who had undergone an integrated PET-CT scan. All 215 patients involved in the study underwent surgical resection and 16% were found to have occult N2 disease. They concluded that patients with centrally located tumours, right upper-lobe tumours and PET positive N1 nodes should have pre-operative cervical mediastinoscopy. Whilst PET scanning following induction therapy (chemotherapy, chemoradiation, radiotherapy), has a positive predictive value of 98% for detecting residual primary disease, it has been shown to be only 52% accurate at restaging mediastinal nodal status [62].

Single-photon emission CT (SPECT) using metastable technetium (^{99m}TC)-labelled tetrofosmin, when combined with CT has been shown to have a sensitivity of 94.7% and a specificity of 93.3% for the detection of mediastinal metastases in patients with NSCLC [63]. SPECT alone had a diagnostic accuracy of 85.3% compared with 73.5% for CT.

Historically MRI has been shown to have no advantage over CT in the evaluation of regional lymph node metastases, with reported sensitivities and specificities of 48 and 64% respectively, compared with 52 and 69% using CT [43] (the exception being when *i.v.* iodinated contrast is contraindicated *e.g.* in patients with renal failure or a history of contrast reaction). More recently, work has been undertaken using 3.0-T MRI. KIM *et al.* [64] assessed lymph node to tumour ratios (LTR's) of signal intensity and nodal morphology, such as eccentric cortical thickening and loss of the normal fatty hilum on T2-weighted (triple inversion black-blood fast spin-echo) images, and nodal short axis diameter on T1-weighted (3D fast field-echo) images. The group found that morphological details of lymph nodes on T2-weighted images were significant for the detection of mediastinal and hilar lymph node metastases, and had a sensitivity, specificity and accuracy values of 53, 91 and 86% respectively. A recently published study that assessed mediastinal lymph node metastases in 42 patients with NSCLC using diffusion weighted MRI reported a sensitivity, specificity, positive predictive value, negative predictive value and accuracy of 80, 97, 80, 97, and 95% respectively [65]. Short T1 inversion recovery (STIR) turbo spin echo (TSE) MRI has also been evaluated for this purpose with promising results. Further work is being undertaken looking at dynamic imaging with MRI.

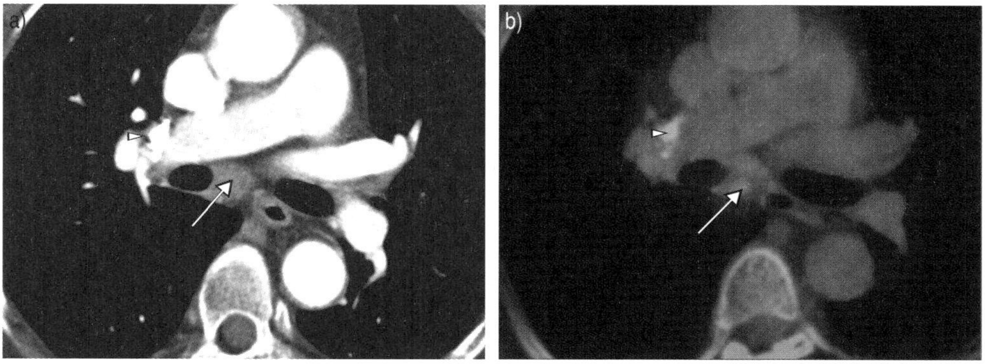

Fig. 14. – a) Axial computed tomography (CT) in a patient with a primary bronchogenic carcinoma. There is a subcarinal lymph node (arrow) and a calcified right hilar node (arrow head). b) Fused axial fluorodeoxyglucose-positron emission tomography (PET) and CT image showing significant increased uptake within the subcarinal node. Note the misregistration between mild uptake on PET and the right hilar-node on the CT.

Distant metastases

Using chest and abdominal CT scans in all patients, and CT brain and bone scans in symptomatic patients, QUINT *et al.* [66] found distant metastases in 21% of all NSCLC patients, most commonly brain (10%), bone (7%), liver (5%) and adrenal glands (3%). In the absence of clinical evidence of metastatic disease in patients with lung cancer, imaging using CT head, abdomen or bone scintigraphy, will detect occult metastases in $<$3% of patients [66]. The incidence of distant metastases in the absence of CT evidence of mediastinal involvement is $<$3% [68]. FDG-PET has been shown to improve the detection of extra-thoracic metastases in patients with NSCLC otherwise eligible for operation. In a study by WEDER *et al.* [69], extra-thoracic metastases were found in 14% of patients deemed to have stage IIIa disease or less by CT.

Brain

According to the current NICE guidelines, patients with clinical signs or symptoms of brain metastases should be imaged either with contrast-enhanced CT (fig. 15) or MRI, the latter being more sensitive. Whether to image the brain as part of routine staging in all patients has long been addressed and opinion varies. A metanalysis by SILVESTRI *et al.* [67] found that brain metastases were more frequent for adenocarcinoma and small cell than for squamous cell carcinoma. Furthermore, when the primary tumour is $>$3 cm in size, EARNEST *et al.* [70] found that 17% of patients had occult cerebral metastases as detected by gadolinium enhanced MRI. The high physiological uptake of FDG by the brain, precludes PET scanning for the exclusion of brain metastases. In a study of 100 patients by MAROM *et al.* [18], comparing whole body PET with thoracic and abdominal CT, bone scintigraphy, and brain CT or MRI, the sensitivity of PET for brain metastases was only 60%, compared with 100% using conventional imaging. SILVESTRI [71] recommended a routine search for metastatic disease in patients with known or suspected N2 disease being considered for surgery and this has been supported by others.

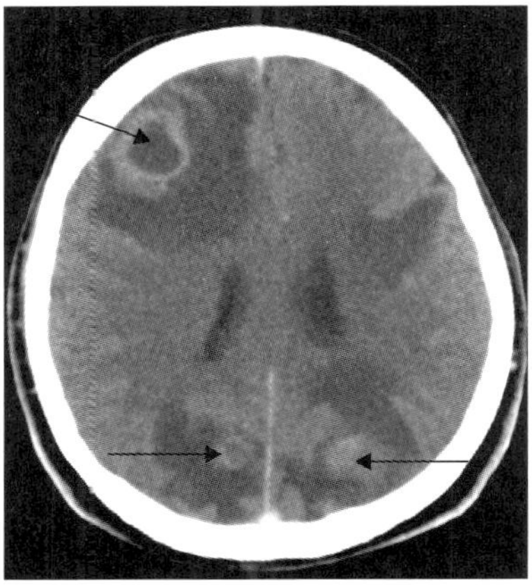

Fig. 15. – Axial computed tomography image of the brain post *i.v.* contrast. There are multiple ring-enhancing cerebral metastases with surrounding oedema.

Bone

The current NICE guidelines recommend that a radiograph should be performed in patients with localised signs or symptoms of bone metastases and if the results are negative or inconclusive, either a ^{99m}Tc methyl diphosphate (MDP) bone scan (fig. 16) or an MRI scan (fig. 17) should be offered. However, in one study, 75% of patients with bone metastases from NSCLC were asymptomatic [72]. Bone metastases are often picked up on PET imaging if this has been performed (fig. 18). In the study by MAROM *et al.* [18], the sensitivity, specificity, positive and negative predictive values of PET were 92, 99, 92, and 99%, respectively and those of bone scintigraphy were 50, 92, 50, and 92%, respectively. Whilst other studies have also shown F-18 FDG-PET to be more sensitive than ^{99m}Tc MDP bone scans for the detectionof bone metastases in patients with lung cancer, reported sensitivity values for bone scans are generally much higher than those reported by MAROM *et al.* [18].

Liver

Imaging of the liver is undertaken at the time of thoracic CT. In the study by MAROM *et al.* [18], the sensitivity, specificity, positive and negative predictive values of PET for the detection of liver metastases were 100% for all, whilst those of the CT scans were 100, 95, 55, and 100%, respectively.

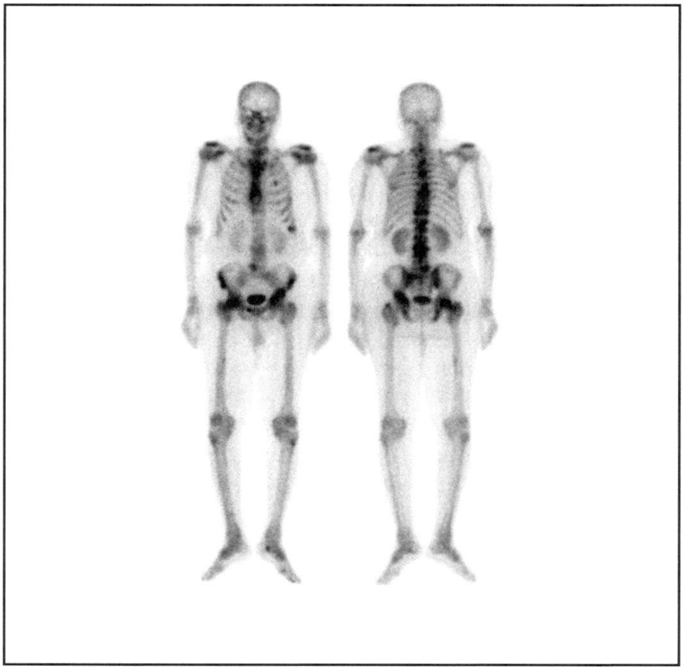

Fig. 16. – Bone scan image showing multiple areas of increased uptake in keeping with bone metastases.

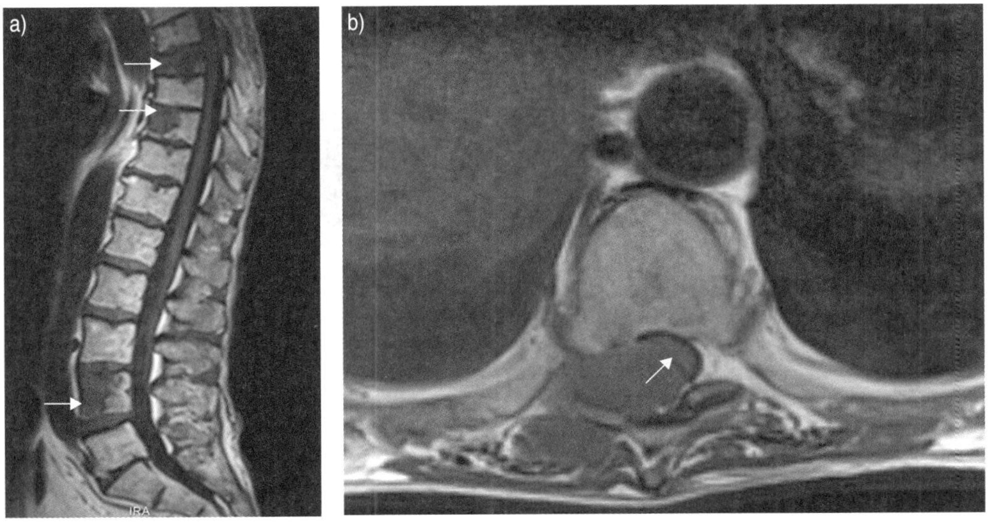

Fig. 17. – a) Sagittal T1 weighted magnetic resonance (MR) image demonstrating multiple low signal vertebral deposits in the lower thoracic and lumbar spine. b) Axial T1 weighted MR image in the same patient showing a large extradural mass extending through the right T7/8 neural exit foramen into the spinal canal, causing significant spinal cord compression (white arrow).

Adrenal glands

Up to 7% of patients with lung cancer have adrenal metastases [67] and staging CT should include the adrenal glands. It is known that up to 10% of the general population have benign adrenal adenomas and it is important to differentiate these from deposits. CT has a high specificity for the detection of adrenal metastases, but a low sensitivity. Benign adenomas tend to be <2 cm in diameter, of low attenuation (reflecting their fat content), well defined and involve only part of the gland. Malignant lesions tend to be > 5cm, heterogenous and irregular (fig. 19). If, on an unenhanced CT, an adrenal lesion has an attenuation value of $\leq$10 HU this is diagnostic of an adrenal adenoma. If the HU is >10, then a contrast scan should be performed with delayed images (10–15 min post *i.v.* contrast) to calculate the percentage of enhancement washout, a >60% washout is diagnostic of an adenoma [73, 74]. The use of chemical-shift MRI is recommended for lesions that are indeterminate on CTs. In the study by MAROM *et al.* [18], the sensitivity, specificity, positive and negative predictive values of PET for adrenal metastases detection were 100% for all whilst those for the CT scan were 100, 93, 46, and 100%, respectively.

Lung metastases and lymphangitis carcinomatosa

MAROM *et al.* [18] showed sensitivity, specificity, positive and negative predictive values of PET to be 94, 99, 94, and 99%, respectively, for the detection of lung metastases, and those of CT to be 78, 94, 74, and 95%, respectively. Lymphangitis carcinomatosa (malignant infiltration of the lymphatics and perilymphatic connective tissue) presents as smooth or nodular thickening of the interlobular septa with thickening of the peribronchovascular interstitium and preservation of the normal parenchymal architecture and it is usually asymmetrical (fig. 20).

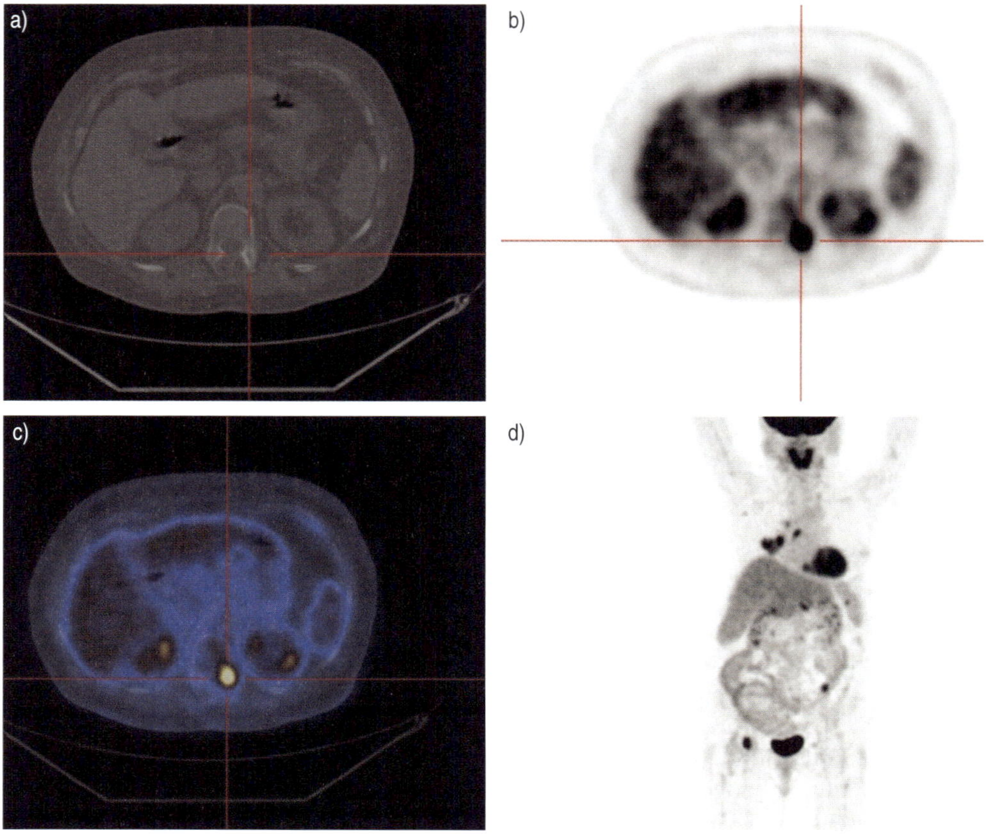

Fig. 18. – Vertebral metastatic deposit not evident on computed tomography (CT) but showing high fluorodeoxyglucose uptake on a positron emission tomography (PET) scan image. a) Axial CT on bone windows. b) Axial PET image. c) Fused axial CT-PET image. d) Coronal PET maximum intensity projection illustrating the primary lung cancer with nodal uptake in the mediastinum and further foci of uptake below the diaphragm. Note the normal high physiological uptake of tracer by the brain and left ventricle and excreted tracer within the bladder.

Staging of small cell lung cancer

The TNM system is not currently used to stage SCLC. Following recent review of TNM staging in 8,088 patients with small cell histology, Shephard *et al.* [75] found that survival did correlate with both T and N categorisation. They found that stage grouping differentiated survival (except between IA and IB) and concluded by recommending that the TNM staging system should also be used for SCLC. The current NICE guidelines advise that SCLC should be staged by a contrast-enhanced CT scan of the patient's chest, liver and adrenal glands and by selected imaging of any symptomatic area.

Synchronous primary lung tumours

Synchronous, primary, tumours occur secondary to field changes caused by the effect of carcinogens. Within the lung, differentiating synchronous, primary tumours from pulmonary metastases is difficult. The incidence is estimated at 0.5–2.3%.

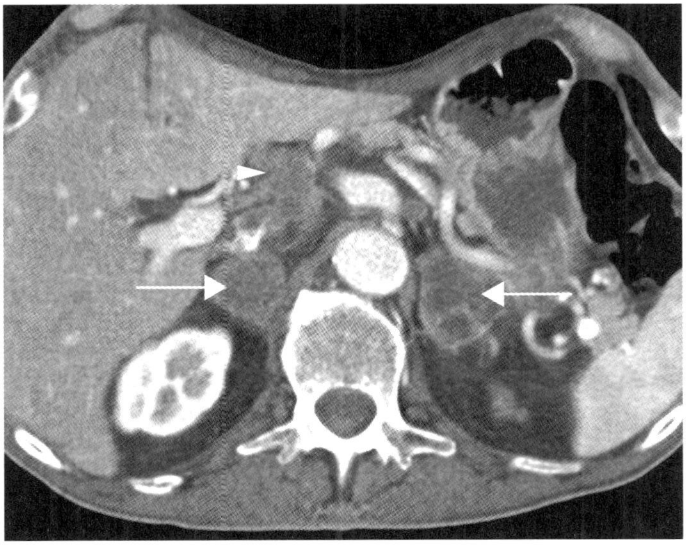

Fig. 19. – Axial computed tomography image through the upper abdomen post *i.v.* contrast depicting bilateral adrenal metastases (arrows). Note the necrotic porta hepatis and retroperitoneal nodes (arrow head).

Radiologically, suspicion is raised when a lesion is seen in the contralateral lung (as this is unusual at presentation), when spiculated margins are seen, and when there is a differential response to treatment. The current TNM staging system tends to upstage these tumours as they are not considered as separate entities. However, synchronous primary tumours carry a significantly better prognosis than stage IIIb and stage IV disease, which are the two categories into which multiple tumour nodules currently fall. The proposals for the new TNM staging system, which includes down staging of additional pulmonary nodules, will improve the situation.

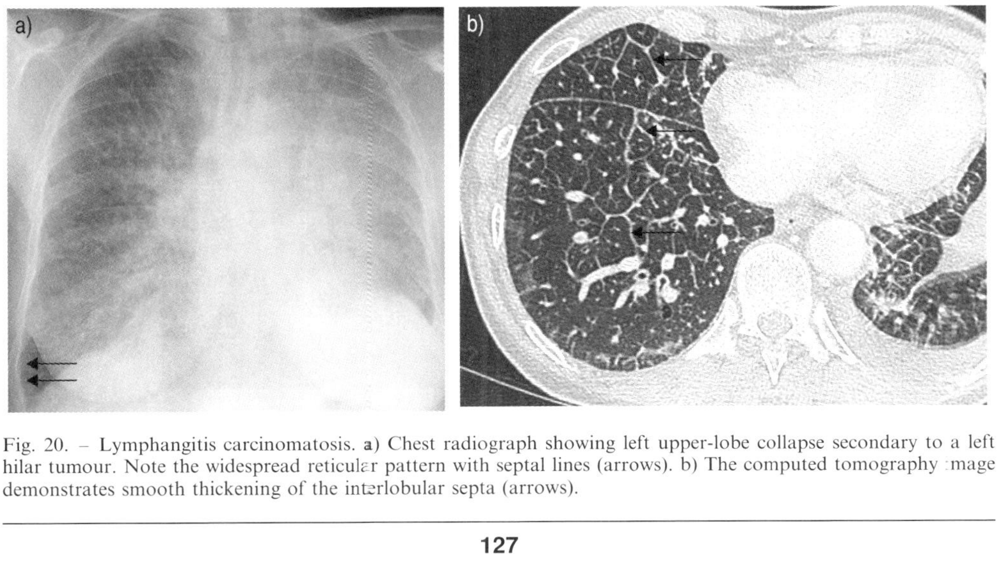

Fig. 20. – Lymphangitis carcinomatosis. a) Chest radiograph showing left upper-lobe collapse secondary to a left hilar tumour. Note the widespread reticular pattern with septal lines (arrows). b) The computed tomography image demonstrates smooth thickening of the interlobular septa (arrows).

Image guided biopsy of suspected lung cancer

Imaging will identify the site and appearance of the tumour, the quality of the surrounding lung parenchyma, and presence of possible metastatic disease. The radiologist can identify the optimum site for tissue sampling, the mode of access, and choice of imaging modality.

Indications for tissue sampling

The latest NICE guidelines on the diagnosis and treatment of lung cancer recommend the use of percutaneous transthoracic needle biopsies in patients with peripheral lung lesions. Where distant metastases are present, biopsies should be taken from the metastatic site to confirm tumour stage. Surgical biopsies should be reserved for patients where less invasive methods of tissue sampling are not feasible or have been unsuccessful. Patients who are staged as N0 or N1 and M0 (stages I and II) by CT and FDG-PET and who are surgical candidates do not need a biopsy prior to surgery to confirm nodal status. Where FDG-PET is positive for N2/3 disease, nodal sampling should be performed to confirm this (fig. 21). Where FDG-PET is negative for N2/3 disease, despite the presence of enlarged lymph nodes on CT (>1 cm in short axis diameter), biopsy is not required. However, if PET is not available in this latter situation, then sampling will be necessary in those patients who are potential candidates for either surgery or radical radiotherapy. Where there are definite distant metastases, and where there is a high probability that N2/3 disease is metastatic, histological or cytological confirmation may not be required.

Methods and sites of tissue sampling

Tissue may be obtained either by using fine needle aspiration (FNA) for cytology, or core biopsy for histology. There are many needles available. Those used for FNA are

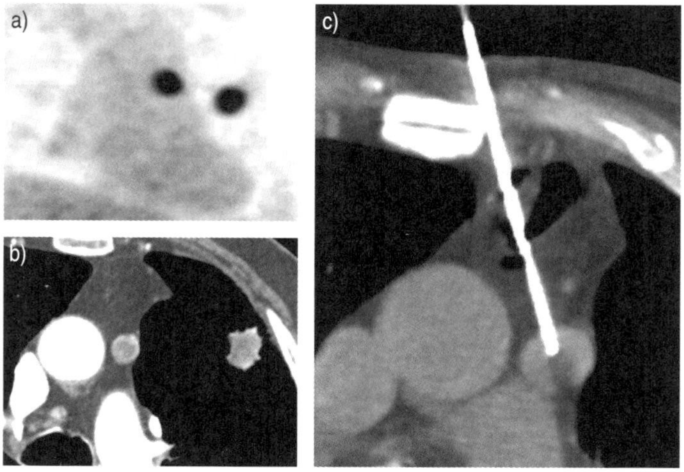

Fig. 21. – a) Positron emission tomography scan image showing a fluorodeoxyglucose avid nodule in the left lung, with similar uptake in an ipsilateral mediastinal lymph node. b) Axial computed tomography (CT) image post *i.v.* contrast confirming the nodule in the left upper lobe and a necrotic aorto-pulmonary node. c) CT guided biopsy of the mediastinal node. This confirmed nonsmall cell carcinoma (T1, N2).

generally 20–23 gauge in size, whereas core biopsy needles are generally 16–18 gauge. The common sites for tissue sampling in diagnosis and staging are illustrated in figure 22. Percutaneous sampling is performed by the radiologist using ultrasound or CT guidance. Common sites include the suspected primary lung lesion itself, nodal disease (supraclavicular, axillary, mediastinal, hilar or retroperitoneal), and metastatic disease (pleural, hepatic, adrenal, bone, and cutaneous deposits). A transbronchial approach using endoscopic ultrasound is preferable for central disease to sample suspected hilar or mediastinal nodal disease. Transoesophageal sampling is useful for suspicious subcarinal, or celiac axis lymph nodes (see chapter 8 in this ERM). If these methods are not feasible, then mediastinoscopy may be indicated.

Percutaneous transthoracic tissue sampling

There has been a shift in recent years from using FNA to sample pulmonary lesions, to using cutting needles which provide a core biopsy and more recently using a co-axial system to facilitate the latter. FNA involves using a fine needle attached to a syringe under suction and moving the needle gently in and out (within the lesion) to obtain cells. The core biopsy cutting needles use a spring-loaded mechanism that fires an inner notched stylet and an outer cutting cannula when a button is pushed. Newer needles have an inner stylet that is advanced prior to the firing of the cutting cannula. The needles are designed with both a 1 cm and a 2 cm "throw", the latter generally producing better cores. A co-axial system involves using a thin-walled introducer needle (usually 16 gauge), through which a smaller cutting needle (usually 18 gauge), or fine needle is introduced. This has the advantage that multiple cores can be obtained through a single pleural pass, thereby reducing the pneumothorax rate, and speeding up the procedure (fig. 23).

Percutaneous transthoracic tissue sampling of pulmonary and mediastinal lesions is performed using CT, which unlike ultrasound, allows visualisation of a lesion partially

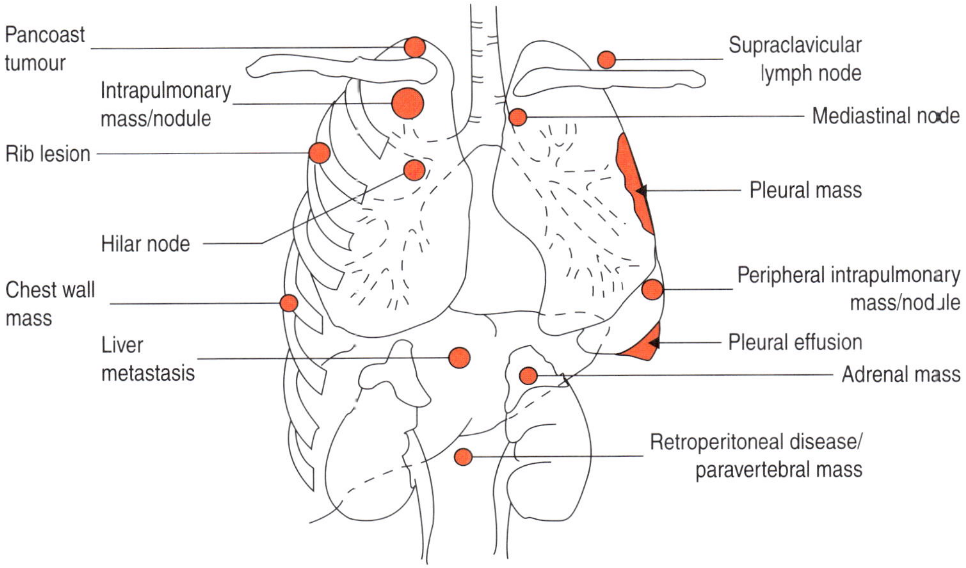

Fig. 22. – Common sites for tissue sampling.

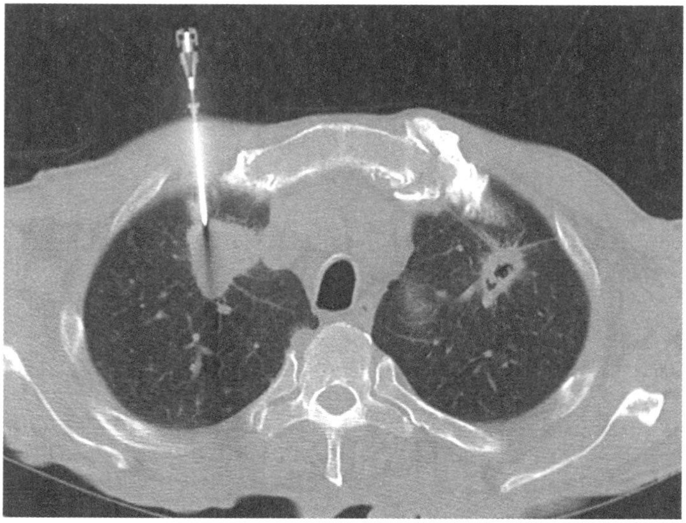

Fig. 23. – A computed tomography guided biopsy of a right upper-lobe mass using a co-axial system, in which a biopsy needle is passed through an introducer needle. This patient was found to have synchronous adenocarcinoma and squamous cell carcinomas in the right and left apices respectively.

or completely surrounded by air, and allows better visualisation of surrounding vascular structures. Chest wall lesions, pleural deposits (if accompanied by a pleural effusion), and cutaneous or soft tissue deposits related to bone metastases may be sampled under CT or ultrasound guidance.

The yield of both methods in malignant disease is very similar with a sensitivity of 90–95% [76]. The advantage of core biopsies lies in the diagnosis of benign disease [77], where this method has a sensitivity of 70% compared with 20–50% for FNA. Access to a cytologist during the procedure has been shown to increase the diagnostic yield of FNA. The procedure is limited with small lesions, which can move in and out of the biopsy plane depending on the phase of respiration. The main complications include pneumothoraces and haemorrhage (which may or may not manifest as haemoptysis). A rare complication is an air embolus. There is a popular misconception that the complication rate increases by using a larger cutting needle as opposed to a fine needle. A 2002 survey performed in the U.K., which reviewed data from 5,444 lung biopsies and FNAs, found no difference in the complication rate between the two methods [78]. This finding is supported by other studies. The pneumothorax rate for both procedures is in the range of 3–42% [79], and most are small enough that they do not require any intervention. Haemoptysis occurs in 4–5% of biopsies [78].

Relative contraindications include pulmonary fibrosis and emphysema, as a pneumothorax in these circumstances could be life-threatening. In these cases, it is important that the lesion is peripheral and lung parenchyma is not traversed. Each case is considered individually, following discussion at the lung cancer multidisciplinary meeting.

Percutaneous sampling of extrathoracic disease

The same methods described above can be used to sample extrathoracic disease. Supraclavicular and axillary lymphadenopathy are sampled under ultrasound, as are hepatic lesions, whereas adrenal lesions, retroperitoneal deposits, and paravertebral disease are usually biopsied under CT guidance. Ultrasound has the advantage of being fast, radiation-free and readily available, but does not always allow adequate visualisation of the target lesion or of surrounding structures to ensure a safe outcome. The deeper the lesion is to the skin, the poorer the resolution. It is important to note that 12–31% of patients presenting with lung cancer will have nonpalpable supraclavicular lymph node metastases detectable with ultrasound guided FNA or biopsy [80]. Ultrasound-guided sampling of this group of nodes may avoid more invasive tissue sampling and improve staging, avoiding unnecessary surgery.

Conclusion

Lung cancer is the most common cancer in the world and carries with it a poor prognisis. Most cancers are detected at a late stage in the disease, emphasising the need for early detection. Studies evaluating screening using low dose spiral CT are ongoing. Identification of lung cancer and accurate staging using a combination of CT and PET, and sometimes MRI and ultrasound is essential. Image-guided tissue sampling plays an important role in the staging and management of lung cancer. Recent advances include the introduction of multislice CT scanners, the routine use of FDG-PET and the co-registration of PET and CT images to facilitate interpretation.

Summary

Lung cancer is the most common cancer worldwide, and remains the leading cause of death from cancer in the UK. Despite its prevalence, screening is not currently recommended, although large scale trials using computed tomography (CT) are ongoing.
Chest radiographs remain the first line of imaging investigation usually. With the advent of multislice CT scans, image acquisition times and resolution have improved. Nodule detection has been ameliorated and high quality coronal and sagittal reformats can now be constructed. Positron emission tomography (PET) scanning has revolutionised staging and has a negative predictive value for N3 disease, which is equal to that of gold standard mediastinoscopy. In the UK, the National Institute of Clinical Excellence (London, UK) has recommended that when a PET scan is negative for N2/3 disease, then biopsy is not required even if the nodes are enlarged by CT criteria. Dual modality PET-CT images are increasingly performed, which overcome the poor spatial resolution of using PET alone. Magnetic resonance imaging is still recommended for the assessment of superior sulcus tumours, and research into its value for nodal staging is ongoing at present.
Lung cancer is divided into small cell lung cancer and nonsmall cell lung cancer (NSCLC). The imaging characteristics of the different tumours vary. At present the tumour, node, metastasis staging system only applies to NSCLC.
In addition to characterising and staging lung cancer, imaging is used to guide the best site for tissue sampling. This may involve computed tomography guided percutaneous transthoracic biopsies or ultrasound guided percutaneous nodal sampling. A co-axial system is increasingly used to perform radiologically guided biopsies.

Keywords: Computed tomography, lung cancer, magnetic resonance imaging, positron emission tomography, staging, tissue sampling.

Statement of interest
None declared.

References

1. Ferlay J, Autier P, Boniol M, *et al.* Estimates of the cancer incidence and mortality in Europe in 2006. *Ann Oncol* 2007; 18: 581–592.
2. Cancer Research UK. UK Lung. Cancer mortality statistics. http://info.cancerresearchukorg/cancerstats/types/lung/mortality/. Last updated: April 27, 2009. Date last accessed: May 16, 2009.
3. Coleman MP, *et al.* Trends and socioeconomic inequalities in cancer survival in England and Wales up to 2001. *Br J Cancer* 2004; 90: 1367–1373.
4. National Lung Cancer Audit Report 2006. UK, Information Centre for Health and Social Care (The IC) in conjunction with the Royal College of Physicians on behalf of The Healthcare Commission, 2006.
5. Kaneko M, Eguchi K, Ohmatsu H, *et al.* Peripheral lung cancer: screening and detection with low dose spiral CT *versus* radiography. *Radiology* 1996; 201: 798–802.
6. Henschke CI, McCauley DI, Yankelevitz DF, *et al.* Early Lung Cancer Action Project: overall design and findings from baseline screening. *Lancet* 1999; 354: 99–105.
7. Nawa T, Nakagawa T, Kusano S, *et al.* Lung cancer screening using low-dose spiral CT: results of baseline and 1-year follow up studies. *Chest* 2002; 122: 15–20.
8. Sone S, Li F, Yang ZG, *et al.* Results of three-year mass screening programme for lung cancer using mobile low-dose spiral computed tomography scanner. *Br J Cancer* 2001; 84: 25–32.
9. Sobue T, Moriyama N, Kaneko M, *et al.* Screening for lung cancer with low-dose helical computer tomography: anti-lung cancer association project. *J Clin Oncol* 2002; 20: 911–920.
10. Humphrey L, Teutsch S, Johnson M, *et al.* Lung cancer screening with sputum cytologic examination, chest radiography, and computed tomography: an update for the U.S. Preventative Services Task Force. *Ann Intern Med* 2004; 140: 740–753.
11. The Lung-SEARCH study UK. Phase 3 clinical trial. A randomised controlled trial of surveillance for the early detection of lung cancer in a high-risk group. UK Clinical Research Network. http://pfsearch.ukcrn.org.uk/StudyDetail.aspx?TopicID=1&studyID=2225
12. Wiemker, et al. Aspects of computer-aided detection (CAD) and volumetry of pulmonary nodules using multislice CT. *Br J Radiol* 2005; 78: S46–S56.
13. Swensen SJ, Viggiano RW, Midthun DE, *et al.* Lung nodule enhancement at CT: multicenter study. *Radiology* 2000; 214: 73–80.
14. Duhaylongsod FG, Lowe VJ, Patz EF Jr, *et al.* Lung tumor growth correlates with glucose metabolism measured by fluoride18 fluorodcoxyglucose positron emission tomography. *Ann Thorac Surg* 1995; 60: 1348–1352.
15. Marom EM, Sarvis S, Herndon JE II, *et al.* T1 lung cancers: sensitivity of diagnosis with fluorodeoxyglucose PET. *Radiology* 2002; 223: 453–459.
16. Gould MK, Maclean CC, Kuschner WG, *et al.* Accuracy of positron emission tomography for diagnosis of pulmonary nodules and mass lesions: a meta-analysis. *JAMA* 2001; 285: 914–924.
17. Gupta NC, Maloof J, Gunel E. Probability of malignancy in solitary pulmonary nodules using fluorine-18-FDG and PET. *J Nucl Med* 1996; 37: 943–948.
18. Marom E, McAdams HP, Erasmus JJ, *et al.* Staging non-small cell lung cancer with whole-body PET. *Radiology* 1999; 212: 803–809.
19. Lung cancer: The diagnosis and treatment of lung cancer, clinical guideline 24. London, National Institute for Clinical Excellence, 2005. http://www.nice.org.uk/CG024NICEguideline

20. Tian J, Yang X, Yu L, *et al.* A multicenter clinical trial on the diagnostic value of dual-tracer PET/CT in pulmonary lesions using 3′-deoxy-3′-18F-fluorothymidine and 18F-FDG. *J Nuc Med* 2008; 49: 186–194.
21. Brambilla E, Travis W, Colby T, *et al.* The new World Health Organization classification of lung tumours. *Eur Respir J* 2001; 18: 1059–1068.
22. Strauss G, Jemal A, McKenna M, *et al.* The epidemic of smoking-related adenocarcinoma of the lung: The role of the tobacco industry and filtered and low-tar cigarettes. 12th World Conference on Lung Cancer, Seoul, Korea, September 2–6. *J Thorac Oncol* 2007; 2: Suppl. 4, S305.
23. Janssen-Heijnen ML, Coebergh JW. The changing epidemiology of lung cancer in Europe. *Lung Cancer* 2003; 41: 245–258.
24. Park CM, Goo JM, Lee HJ, *et al.* CT Findings of atypical adenomatous hyperplasia in the lung. *Korean J Radiol* 2006; 7: 80–86.
25. Kawakami S, Sone S, Takashima S, *et al.* Atypical adenomatous hyperplasia of the lung: correlation between high-resolution CT findings and histopathologic features. *Eur Radiol* 2001; 11: 811–814.
26. Bonomo L, Storto ML, Ciccotosto C, *et al.* Bronchioloalveolar carcinoma of the lung. *Eur Radiol* 1998; 8: 996–1001.
27. Im JG, Han MC, Yu EJ, *et al.* Lobar bronchioloalveolar cell carcinoma: angiogram sign on CT scans. *Radiology* 1990; 176: 749–753.
28. Thun MJ, Lally CA, Flannery JT, *et al.* Cigarette smoking and changes in the histopathology of lung cancer. *J Natl Cancer Inst* 1997; 89: 1580–1586.
29. Kazerooni EA, Bhalla M, Shepard JA, *et al.* Adenosquamous carcinoma of the lung: radiologic appearance. *AJR Am J Roentgenol* 1994; 163: 301–306.
30. Hansell DM, Bankier AA, MacMahon H, *et al.* Fleischner Society: glossary of terms for thoracic imaging. *Radiology* 2008; 246: 697–722.
31. Grewal RG, Austin JH. CT demonstration of calcification in carcinoma of the lung. *J Comput Assist Tomogr* 1994; 18: 867–871.
32. Swensen SJ, Jett JR, Hartman TE, *et al.* CT screening for lung cancer: 5-year prospective experience. *Radiology* 2005; 235: 259–265.
33. Siegelman SS, Zerhouni EA, Leo FP, *et al.* CT of the solitary pulmonary nodule. *AJR Am J Roentgenol* 1980; 135: 1–13.
34. Zwirewich CV, Vedal S, Miller RR, *et al.* Solitary pulmonary nodule: high-resolution CT and radiologic-pathologic correlation. *Radiology* 1991; 179: 469–476.
35. Erasmus JJ, Connolly JE, McAdams HP, *et al.* Solitary pulmonary nodules: Part I. Morphologic evaluation for differentiation of benign and malignant lesions. *Radiographics* 2000; 20: 43–58.
36. Henschke CI, Yankelevitz DF, Mirtcheva R, *et al.* CT screening for lung cancer: frequency and significance of part solid and non-solid nodules. *AJR Am J Roentgenol* 2002; 178: 1053–1057.
37. Kui M, Templeton PA, White CS, *et al.* Evaluation of the air bronchogram sign on CT in solitary pulmonary lesions. *J Comput Assist Tomogr* 1996; 20: 983–986.
38. MacMahon H, Austin J, Gamsu G, *et al.* Guidelines for management of small pulmonary nodules detected on CT scans: A statement from the Fleischner Society. *Radiology* 2005; 237: 395–400.
39. Onitsuka H, Tsukuda M, Araki A, *et al.* Differentiation of central lung tumor from postobstructive lobar collapse by rapid sequence computed tomography. *J Thorac Imaging* 1991; 6: 28–31.
40. Mountain CF. Revisions in the International System for Staging Lung Cancer. *Chest* 1997; 111: 1710–1717.
41. Goldstraw P, Crowley J, Chansky K, *et al.* The IASLC Lung Cancer Staging Project: Proposals for the Revision of the TNM Stage Groupings in the Forthcoming (Seventh) Edition of the TNM Classification of Malignant Tumours. *J Thorac Oncol* 2007; 2: 706–714.
42. Wever W, Ceyssens S, Mortelmans L, *et al.* Additional value of PET-CT in the staging of lung cancer: comparison with CT alone, PET alone and visual correlation of PET and CT. *Eur Radiol* 2007; 17: 23–32.

43. Webb WR, Glatsonis C, Zerhouni EA, *et al.* CT and MR imaging in staging non-small cell bronchogenic carcinoma: report of the Radiologic Diagnostic Oncology Group. *Radiology* 1991; 178: 705–713.
44. Quint LE, Francis IR. Radiologic staging of lung cancer. *J Thorac Imaging* 1999; 14: 235–246.
45. Rankin S. Advances in radiological staging of non-small cell lung cancer (NSCLC). *Cancer Imaging* 2004; 4: S22–S24.
46. Yokoi K, Mori K, Miyazawa N, *et al.* Tumor invasion of the chest wall and mediastinum in lung cancer: evaluation with pneumothorax CT. *Radiology* 1991; 181: 147–152.
47. Watanabe A, Shimokata K, Saka H, *et al.* Chest CT combined with artificial pneumothorax: value in determining origin and extent of tumor. *AJR Am J Roentgenol* 1991; 156: 707–710.
48. Murata K, Takahashi M, Mori M, *et al.* Chest wall and mediastinal invasion by lung cancer: evaluation with multisection expiratory dynamic CT. *Radiology* 1994; 191: 251–255.
49. Glazer HS, Kaiser LR, Anderson DJ, *et al.* Indeterminate mediastinal invasion in bronchogenic carcinoma: CT evaluation. *Radiology* 1989; 173: 37–42.
50. Herman SJ, Winton TL, Weisbrod GL, *et al.* Mediastinal invasion by bronchogenic carcinoma: CT signs. *Radiology* 1994; 190: 841–846.
51. McLoud TC, Swenson SJ. Lung carcinoma. *Clin Chest Med* 1999; 20: 697–713.
52. Padovani B, Mouroux J, Seksik L, *et al.* Chest wall invasion by bronchogenic carcinoma: evaluation with MR imaging. *Radiology* 1993; 187: 33–38.
53. Heelan RT, Demas BE, Caravelli JF, *et al.* Superior sulcus tumours: CT and MRI imaging. *Radiology* 1989; 170: 637–641.
54. Bandi V, Lunn W, Ernst A, *et al.* Ultrasound *vs* CT in Detecting Chest Wall Invasion by Tumor. *Chest* 2008; 133: 881–886.
55. Suzuki N, Saitoh T, Kitamura S. Tumor invasion of the chest wall in lung cancer: diagnosis with US. *Radiology* 1993; 187: 39–42.
56. Schaffler G, Wolf G, Schoellnast H, *et al.* Non–small cell lung cancer: evaluation of pleural abnormalities on CT scans with ^{18}F FDG PET[1]. *Radiology* 2004; 231: 858–865.
57. Tomimaru Y, Higashiyama M, Okami J, *et al.* Surgical results of lung cancer with sarcoid reaction in regional lymph nodes. *Jpn J Clin Oncol* 2007; 37: 90–95.
58. McLoud T. A System for the Clinical Staging of Lung Cancer—A Commentary. *AJR Am J Roentgenol* 2006; 187: 269–270.
59. Silvestri G, Gould M, Margolis M, *et al.* American College of Chest Physicians- noninvasive staging of non-small cell lung cancer ACCP evidenced-based clinical practice guidelines (2nd Edition). *Chest* 2007; 132: 178S–201.
60. Dietlein M, Weber K, Gandjour A, *et al.* Cost-effectiveness of FDG-PET for the management of potentially operable non–small cell lung cancer: priority for a PET-based strategy after nodal-negative CT results. *Eur J Nucl Med* 2000; 27: 1598–1609.
61. Al-Sarraf N, Aziz R, Gately K, *et al.* Pattern and predictors of occult mediastinal lymph node involvement in non-small cell lung cancer patients with negative mediastinal uptake on positron emission tomography. *Eur J Cardiothorac Surg* 2008; 33: 104–109.
62. Akhurst T, Downey RJ, Ginsberg MS, *et al.* An initial experience with FDG-PET in the imaging of residual disease after induction therapy for lung cancer. *Ann Thorac Surg* 2002; 73: 259–64.
63. Shiun SC, Sun SS, Hsu NY, *et al.* Detecting mediastinal lymph node metastases in non–small cell lung cancer using a combination of technetium-99m tetrofosmin chest single photon emission computed tomography and chest computed tomography. *Cancer Invest* 2002; 20: 311–317.
64. Kim HY, Yi C, Lee KS, *et al.* Nodal metastasis in non–small cell lung cancer: accuracy of 3.0-T MR imaging. *Radiology* 2007; 246: 596–604.
65. Hasegawa I, Boiselle P, Kuwabara K, *et al.* Mediastinal lymph nodes in patients with non-small cell lung cancer. Preliminary experience with diffusion-weighted MR imaging. *J Thorac Imaging* 2008; 23: 157–161.
66. Quint LE, Tummala S, Brisson LJ, *et al.* Distribution of distant metastases from newly diagnosed non-small cell lung cancer. *Ann Thorac Surg* 1996; 62: 246–250.

67. Silvestri GA, Littenberg B, Colice GL. The clinical evaluation for detecting metastatic lung cancer. A meta-analysis. *Am J Respir Crit Care Med* 1995; 152: 225–230.
68. Grant D, Edwards D, Goldstraw P. Computed tomography of the brain, chest, and abdomen in the preoperative assessment of non-small cell lung cancer. *Thorax* 1988; 43: 883–886.
69. Weder W, Schmid RA, Bruchhaus H, *et al.* Detection of extrathoracic metastases by positron emission tomography in lung cancer. *Ann Thorac Surg* 1998; 66: 886–893.
70. Earnest FT, Ryu JH, Miller GM, *et al.* Suspected non–small cell lung cancer: incidence of occult brain and skeletal metastases and effectiveness of imaging for detection: pilot study. *Radiology* 1999; 211: 137–145.
71. Silvestri GA. Invited commentary. *Ann Thorac Surg* 2001; 71: 433–434.
72. Lau CL, Harpole DH Jr, Patz E. Staging techniques for lung cancer. *Chest Surg Clin N Am* 2000; 10: 781–801.
73. Mayo-Smith W. CT Characterization of adrenal masses. *Radiology* 2003; 226: 289–290.
74. Caoili EM, Korobkin M, Francis IR, *et al.* Adrenal masses: characterization with combined unenhanced and delayed enhanced CT. *Radiology* 2002; 222: 629–633.
75. Shepherd F, Crowley J, Van Houtte P, *et al.* The International Association for the Study of Lung Cancer Lung Cancer Staging Project: Proposals regarding the clinical staging of small cell lung cancer in the forthcoming (seventh) edition of the tumor, node, metastasis classification for lung cancer. *J Thorac Oncol* 2007; 2: 1067–1077.
76. Klein JS, Salomon G, Stewart EA. Transthoracic needle biopsy with a coaxially placed 20-gauge automated cutting needle: results in 122 patients. *Radiology* 1996; 198: 715–720.
77. Grief J, Marmor S, Schwarz Y, Man A, Staroselsky AN. Percutaneous core needle biopsy *versus* fine needle aspiration in diagnosing benign lung lesions. *Acta Cytol* 1999; 43: 756–760.
78. Richardson CM, Pointon KS, Manhire AR, *et al.* Percutaneous lung biopsies. A survey of UK practice based on 5444 biopsies. *Br J Radiol* 2002; 75: 731–735.
79. Lacasse Y, Wong E, Guyatt G, *et al.* Transthoracic needle aspiration biopsy for the diagnosis of localised pulmonary lesions: a meta-analysis. *Thorax* 1999; 54: 884–893.
80. Fultz PJ, Feins RH, Strang JG, *et al.* Detection and diagnosis of nonpalpable supraclavicular lymph nodes in lung cancer at CT and US. *Radiology* 2002; 222: 245–251.

CHAPTER 8

Diagnostic endoscopic investigations in lung cancer

N. Navani, S.M. Janes

Centre for Respiratory Research, University College London, London, UK.

Correspondence: N. Navani, Centre for Respiratory Research, University College London, Rayne Building, 5 University Street, London WC1E 6JJ, UK. Fax: 44 2073809476; E-mail: n.navani@ucl.ac.uk

Distinguishing nonsmall cell lung cancer (NSCLC) from small cell lung cancer (SCLC) is of paramount importance, since the treatment and prognosis of the cancers are often significantly different. SCLC is well known to exhibit massive lymphadenopathy, direct mediastinal invasion and paraneoplastic syndromes [1]. However, there is considerable clinical overlap between NSCLC and SCLC such that clinical differentiation is often not possible and pathological diagnosis is essential. A small number of patients who are unfit for any oncological or surgical treatment and are candidates for best supportive care only may not benefit from pathological diagnosis. In these patients, a clinical diagnosis of lung cancer may have to suffice on the basis of imaging alone. The remaining majority of patients undergo various investigations to determine the histological subtype. An initial diagnosis should be pursued from the most distal site of suspected disease in order to provide staging as well as diagnostic information.

Cytology or histology may be provided for pathological analysis, depending on the source and technique employed to generate the sample. Either histology or cytology can discriminate NSCLC from SCLC. Although histology may generally be preferred, cytological samples are also reliable, particularly for NSCLC. Meta-analysis of data from sputum, bronchoscopy and transthoracic needle aspiration compared cytology to histology samples for patients with NSCLC and SCLC [2]. The probability of diagnosing NSCLC in error on the basis of cytology was 0.02 (range 0.01–0.07); however, the converse is less robust. A diagnosis of SCLC had a probability of actually being a NSCLC of 0.09 (range 0–0.33). Therefore, if a diagnosis of SCLC is made on a cytological sample, but the clinical and radiological findings are discordant with the cytological diagnosis, then a histological biopsy should be obtained where possible [2].

In order to achieve a tissue diagnosis of lung cancer, patients may undergo sputum cytology analysis, bronchoscopy, transbronchial needle aspiration (with or without endobronchial ultrasound guidance), endoscopic ultrasound fine needle aspiration, or surgical procedures; these are discussed below. Radiologically guided transthoracic sampling is discussed in chapter 7 in this *European Respiratory Monograph*.

Sputum cytology

Sputum cytology is a noninvasive method of diagnosing lung cancer by detecting exfoliated malignant cells (fig. 1). Sensitivity is higher for central squamous cell and small cell carcinomas, bloody sputum, tumours >2.4 cm in size and in patients with low forced expiratory volume in 1 s values [3]. Yield may be maximised by collecting at least

Eur Respir Mon, 2009, 44, 136–149. Printed in UK - all rights reserved. Copyright ERS Journals Ltd 2009; European Respiratory Monograph; ISSN 1025-448x.

three samples [4]. A meta-analysis of 29,245 patients who underwent sputum cytology analysis demonstrated a pooled sensitivity of 66% and specificity of 99% [2]. The indication for sputum analysis varied considerably and the pooled prevalence of disease was only 15%. One study specifically evaluated sputum cytology in patients with suspected lung cancer and found a sensitivity of 87% and specificity of 90% [5]. However, much of the published data came from centres that have established protocols in sputum analysis. It is likely that sensitivity in routine practice is lower.

Abnormal cells may arise from anywhere in the aero-digestive tract or from pre-invasive lesions, such that a false-positive rate for sputum cytology of ~9% is observed when the disease prevalence is 15% [2]. Furthermore, discordant results have occurred between sputum cytology and histological findings at bronchoscopy. Therefore, sputum analysis as a sole test is reserved for patients who are unable or unwilling to undergo further diagnostic procedures.

Bronchoscopy

Fibreoptic bronchoscopy was first performed in the 1960s in Japan and is now a standard investigation worldwide for the diagnosis and staging of lung cancer. Advances in microtechnology have resulted in fibreoptic bronchoscopes evolving into video-bronchoscopes, which are increasingly used in clinical practice (fig. 2a). The procedure is most commonly performed under conscious sedation with topical anaesthesia in the outpatient setting.

Yield from bronchoscopy is primarily determined by the location of the tumour. Bronchoscopy has a higher sensitivity for the diagnosis of central tumours compared to peripheral tumours and is the primary investigation of choice for centrally located lung cancer. Central lesions (up to a segmental bronchus) may present at bronchoscopy with an exophytic endobronchial mass, tumour infiltration of the bronchial wall or extrinsic

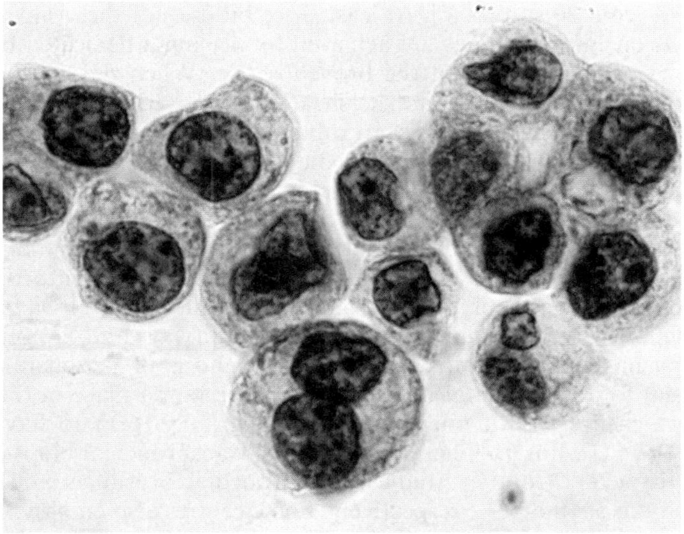

Fig. 1. – Sputum showing adenocarcinoma/alveolar cell carcinoma. A cluster of glandular cells with eccentric nuclei, mild anisonucleosis, prominent nucleoli, irregular nuclear margins and well-defined nonphagocytic cytoplasm. (Papanicoulaou stain; magnification ×1,000, using oil immersion).

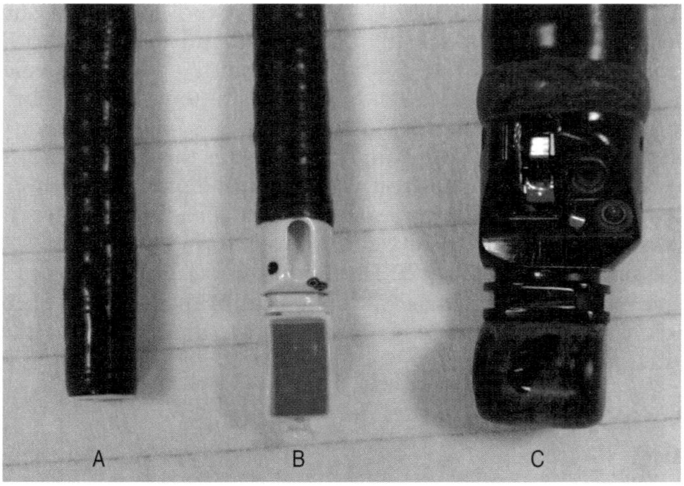

Fig. 2. – A) Standard videobronchoscope. B) Endobronchial ultrasound, which allows real-time ultrasound-guided transbronchial needle aspiration. C) Endoscopic ultrasound, which allows real-time ultrasound guided fine-needle aspiration and biopsy.

compression by a peribronchial mass. Diagnostic yield is highest when the tumour is visible. Meta-analysis of 4,507 patients with central disease from 35 studies has demonstrated a pooled sensitivity of 88% [2].

At bronchoscopy, a combination of biopsy, brush, wash and bronchoalveolar lavage (BAL) is performed. Biopsy of a visible endobronchial lesion is performed by introducing forceps into the working channel of a bronchoscope and carrying out the biopsy under direct vision. Yield for this technique in isolation is reported as 74%, with a range of 50–92% from 20 studies [6]. At least three biopsies of the visible lesion should be performed. Bronchial brushings are achieved by placing a dedicated brush within a sheath into the working channel of the bronchoscope. When the site for sampling is located, the brush is extended beyond the sheath and moved to and fro on the target area. Samples for cytological analysis are obtained and smeared directly onto glass slides. When the lesion is visible, a diagnosis may be obtained by bronchial brushings in ~60% of cases (range 23–92%) [6]. Bronchial washings occasionally add to the diagnostic yield of biopsy and brushings in central tumours. Saline is instilled into the bronchial tree and a sample is collected for cytological (and microbiological) analysis. BAL is performed by obtaining a "wedge" of the bronchoscope into the most distal airway. 120–180 mL of saline is then introduced into the distal airway. The saline is returned by suction, allowing evaluation of the distal airways and alveoli.

Bronchoscopy has a more limited role in the diagnosis of peripheral lung lesions, which arise distal to the segmental bronchus. It may retain a place in the diagnosis of lung lesions, which are shown on computed tomography (CT) to have a bronchus extending into them [7]. For peripheral lung lesions, transbronchial biopsies provide the highest sensitivity (57% from 21 studies) [2]. Bronchial brushings and BAL have a pooled sensitivity of 54 and 43%, respectively. Some centres also employ fluoroscopy to direct bronchoscopic procedures, which may improve the diagnostic yield of peripheral lesions [8]. Transbronchial biopsy of lung parenchyma (with or without screening) is useful in the diagnosis of lymphangitis carcinomatosis.

Autofluorescence bronchoscopy

The advent of autofluorescence bronchoscopy (AFB), which uses blue light rather than the standard white light bronchoscopy (WLB), allows identification of pre-invasive lesions that may be missed by usual techniques. Observations in the lung have shown that dysplasia, carcinoma *in situ* (CIS), and microinvasive carcinomas exhibit weaker green fluorescence than normal tissues when illuminated by blue light. Normal endobronchial mucosa therefore appears green while the abnormal areas appear purplish (using the D-Light AF system; Stortz, Tuttlingen, Germany). Several systems are in clinical use. These include light-induced fluorescence endoscopy (LIFE; Xillix Technologies, Vancouver, Canada), as well as integrated AFB and white light bronchoscopes (D-Light AF system and the SAFE 1000 System; Pentax, Tokyo, Japan). The systems appear to be broadly equivalent clinically [9, 10]. Much of the reported data on AFB surrounds the use of the LIFE system and demonstrates the superiority of AFB over WLB for the detection of pre-invasive lesions. A multi-centre randomised study using the D-Light AF device recruited 1,173 participants who were current smokers, >40 yrs of age with at least 20 pack-yrs of smoking and had either symptoms concerning for lung carcinoma (new cough, haemoptysis, or new dyspnoea) or radiological suspicion for carcinoma [11]. Participants were randomised to WLB only, or to WLB plus AFB examination. Only 3.9% of patients had high-grade dysplasia or CIS. Despite the low incidence of detected disease, combined AFB and WLB improved detection of dysplastic lesions by a factor of 2.1 over WLB. However, there was no statistical difference between WLB and combined WLB and AFB in the rate of detection of CIS. The authors concluded that the study confirmed the hypothesis that AFB and WLB are superior to WLB alone for the detection of pre-invasive disease. However, the study did demonstrate a low positive predictive value (PPV) of 25.1% and a low specificity of 58.4% [11]. Similarly low PPVs have been confirmed in other studies.

One explanation for the low specificity of abnormal AF is that inflammation, metaplasia and low-grade dysplasia may display abnormal AF and may be difficult to distinguish from high-grade lesions. Furthermore, the natural history of high-grade lesions remains unclear. One study of 22 patients by George *et al.* [12] followed pre-invasive lesions with AFB every 4–12 months with CT scan annually. The risk of developing lung cancer in patients with a high-grade lesion was 33% at 1 yr and 54% at 2 yrs [12]. Interestingly, some of the high-grade pre-invasive lesions regressed. Therefore, the best management of high grade pre-invasive lesions remains unresolved and the role of AFB in the early detection of lung cancer requires clarification. Currently AFB may be indicated following the detection of moderate dysplasia, severe dysplasia, CIS, or invasive carcinoma graces in sputum cytology [13], particularly in the context of normal WLB.

Bronchoscopy as a staging tool

In addition to providing pathological information, bronchoscopy also allows assessment of the location and extent of the endobronchial lesion (which may impact significantly on treatment). Careful assessment of the vocal cords is mandatory, as the presence of vocal cord palsy may provide evidence of mediastinal invasion (and inoperability) in a patient with the appropriate radiological features. Bronchoscopy also allows for accurate assessment of the location of an endobronchial tumour within the bronchial tree. NSCLCs involving the carina are staged as T4 disease and are not considered as candidates for surgery. If a tumour is measured to be within 2 cm distal of the carina, it is currently staged as a T3 lesion. If the NSCLC is in a main bronchus and >2 cm from the carina, it is deemed a T2 lesion.

Transbronchial needle aspiration

Blind transbronchial needle aspiration (TBNA) is a safe but underutilised procedure for mediastinal lymph node staging and was first described in 1978 [14]. It is planned with the aid of CT (and positron emission tomography (PET) if available) to identify the lymph node to be sampled and to note its relationship to bronchial landmarks. During standard bronchoscopy, a TBNA needle is introduced into the working channel of the bronchoscope. The needle punctures the bronchial wall allowing the mediastinal lymph node to be aspirated. This is most commonly performed in the subcarinal lymph node station, but lower paratracheal and hilar lymph nodes can also be sampled. The procedure may be carried out with an 18, 19 or 22 gauge needle.

A meta-analysis of patients undergoing TBNA showed a pooled sensitivity as low as 39% for the technique when the prevalence of mediastinal metastases was 34% [15]. Several modifiable factors have been shown to optimise the diagnostic yield of blind TBNA. First, at least five and up to seven passes in the same area may maximise diagnostic tissue [16]. Secondly, the presence of a cytologist within the endoscopy suite to evaluate aspirates as they are produced, may significantly improve accuracy [17]. Rapid on-site evaluation of samples allows an immediate diagnosis of malignancy or can confirm the adequacy of a specimen by identifying lymphocytes. Thirdly, the use of CT fluoroscopy allows imaging of MLN during TBNA and may improve yield [18]. Finally, since blind TBNA is highly operator dependent, focused education and experience in the technique are invaluable in improving results [19]. The highest yield is seen in lymph nodes >1 cm in the right paratracheal and subcarinal locations [20], and it is this patient group that may benefit most from TBNA.

Assessment of the endobronchial tree is performed at the same sitting as TBNA. In addition, it is a relatively inexpensive and well-tolerated outpatient procedure that can be performed under conscious sedation. A positive result from TBNA may prevent further invasive tests, particularly when combined with PET [21]. However, its generally low diagnostic yield and negative predictive value mean that TBNA has been slow to be embraced by respiratory physicians. Further invasive sampling always remains necessary in the event of a negative or nondiagnostic sample.

Endobronchial ultrasound

Endobronchial ultrasound-guided transbronchial needle aspiration (EBUS-TBNA) is an important new and minimally invasive technique for the diagnosis and staging of NSCLC. A catheter with a radial ultrasound mini-probe at the tip was the first to be developed. The catheter is placed in the biopsy channel of the bronchoscope. When the lymph node to be sampled has been identified using the radial ultrasound scanner, the catheter was withdrawn and replaced with a conventional TBNA needle. The lymph node is then aspirated blindly. Conflicting evidence exists as to whether EBUS-TBNA using the mini-probe is superior to conventional blind TBNA. More recently, an integrated curvilinear ultrasound bronchoscope has been developed (fig. 2b) and allows TBNA under real-time ultrasound guidance. This progress in technology allows the pulmonologist and thoracic surgeon for the first time to sample the mediastinum in a minimally invasive manner under direct vision and with high sensitivity [22].

The integrated scope has a convex ultrasound transducer at the distal end with a 7.5 MHz frequency and allows visualisation of parabronchial structures up to a depth of 5 cm. The outer diameter of the insertion tube is 6.2 mm and that of the tip is 6.9 mm. The distal end of the scope can be adjusted 160° upwards and 90° downward and the endoscope has a biopsy channel of 2 mm. The fibreoptic lens is oblique forward-viewing at 30° and the ultrasound image is in parallel to the scope, with a scanning angle of 50°. After intubation with the EBUS scope, a saline-filled balloon is inflated to maintain contact with the airway wall. Vascular structures are located using power Doppler imaging. Once the target lymph node is identified on the ultrasonography monitor, a dedicated 22 gauge needle is inserted into the working channel. The needle can then be observed to pierce and enter the lymph node under direct ultrasound vision. Suction is applied and the needle is moved to and fro within the lesion. Using this technique, mediastinal lymph nodes as small as 5 mm may be sampled. The procedure is carried out in the ambulatory setting, under conscious sedation or general anaesthesia. Lymph nodes that may represent N3 (contralateral mediastinal or hilar) metastases are sampled first, followed by N2 nodes and finally ipsilateral hilar nodes, so that any contamination will not result in false over-staging. A diagnostic plateau may be reached after three passes per lymph node [23].

EBUS-TBNA affords access to the upper and lower paratracheal nodes, the subcarinal lymph node station and the hilar lymph nodes (fig. 3). Cytological samples are produced, although occasionally histological cores may be obtained. Currently, one single centre trial has compared blind TBNA to EBUS-TBNA and demonstrated that the ultrasound-guided technique has a higher sensitivity for detecting malignant mediastinal nodes [24]. In addition, a growing body of cohort series have illustrated that EBUS-TBNA is a safe and efficacious procedure for the detection of mediastinal metastases. In the largest cohort of 502 patients, the sensitivity of EBUS-TBNA for diagnosing mediastinal disease was 94% in the context of a disease prevalence of 98% [26]. A meta-analysis of the first 918 patients from expert centres revealed a pooled sensitivity of 90%, when the disease prevalence was 68% (table 1) [27].

Importantly, the false negative rate of EBUS-TBNA is currently 20% and therefore negative or benign aspirates should be followed by further invasive mediastinal staging [27]. No complications of the technique have been reported, and the leaning curve may be a short as 10 cases [29]. EBUS-TBNA has several advantages over standard mediastinoscopy. It is less invasive, can be performed without general anaesthetic, enables visualisation of the endobronchial tree and allows access to hilar as well as mediastinal nodes. In the first study to compare EBUS-TBNA with mediastinoscopy, Ernst *et al.* [30] performed both procedures on 66 patients. In this study [30], the diagnostic yield from EBUS-TBNA was 91% compared to 78% from mediastinoscopy. The technique may even be able to detect metastatic disease in mediastinal lymph nodes <1 cm in short axis that are negative on PET scanning [31]. EBUS-TBNA is therefore a safe and efficacious procedure for the diagnosis of mediastinal metastases of NSCLC. However, the relatively low negative predictive value, as well as the lack of randomised controlled trials and healthcare cost data, mean that the precise role of EBUS-TBNA in the diagnostic and staging algorithm for NSCLC requires clarification. Currently, it is most commonly employed as an alternative to mediastinoscopy, with the caveat that negative results are followed by surgical sampling.

In addition to the mediastinal staging of NSCLC, EBUS-TBNA may have an important role in the diagnosis of para-tracheal and para-bronchial lesions. These primary lesions lie extrinsic to the bronchial wall and are not visible at standard bronchoscopy. Two retrospective studies totalling 95 patients have suggested that EBUS-TBNA has a high sensitivity for the diagnosis of these lung lesions, reducing the need for transthoracic or surgical biopsy [32, 33].

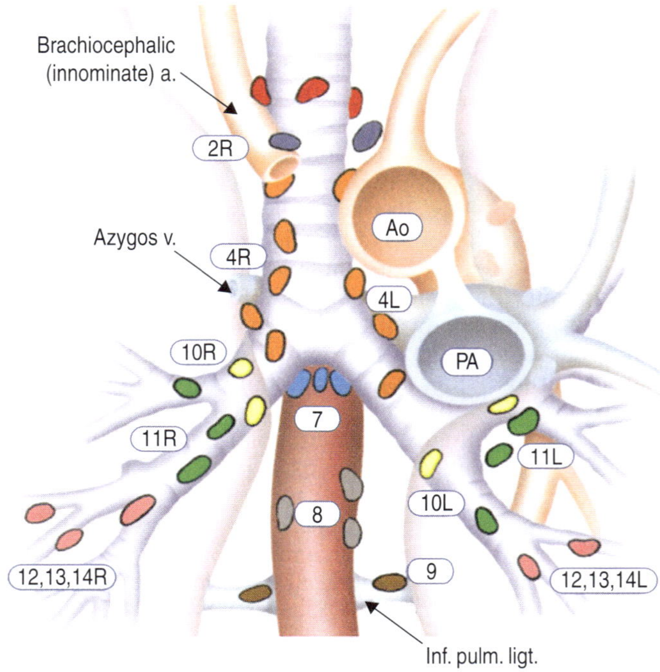

Fig. 3. – Lymph node stations (depicted numerically) that are accessed by endobronchial ultrasound-guided transbronchial needle aspiration and endoscopic ultrasound-guided fine-needle aspiration. Ao: aorta; PA: pulmonary artery; R: right; L: left; a.: artery; v.: vein; inft. pulm. ligt.: inferior pulmonary ligament. Reproduced from [24], with permission from the publisher.

A further important application of linear EBUS-TBNA may be the re-staging of mediastinal disease following neo-adjuvant treatment. Repeat surgical evaluation of the mediastinum is often complicated by adhesions and is performed by few thoracic surgeons. EBUS-TBNA however, may be repeated in the same patient without

Table 1. – Sensitivity, specificity and false negative rates for diagnostic endoscopic investigations in lung cancer

Investigation	Sensitivity	Specificity	False negative rate	Disease prevalence	Comments
Sputum cytology	66	99	6	15	Reserved for patients unable or unwilling to undergo more invasive tests
Bronchoscopy (for central tumours)	88	100	12	100	Standard procedure for the diagnosis of central tumours
TBNA (for mediastinal disease)	78	99	28	75	Highly operator dependent
EBUS-TBNA (for mediastinal disease)	90	100	20	68	Access to para-bronchial mediastinal and hilar lesions
EUS-FNA (for mediastinal disease)	84	99.5	19	61	Access to left-sided and posterior mediastinal lesions

Data are presented as %. TBNA: transbronchial needle aspiration; EBUS-TBNA: endobronchial ultrasound-guided TBNA; EUS-FNA: endoscopic ultrasound-guided fine-needle aspiration. Data are taken from [2] and [27]. Table adapted from [28], with permission from the publisher.

difficulty. Herth *et al.* [34] evaluated 126 consecutive patients with stage IIIA (N2) disease who had undergone induction chemotherapy. EBUS-TBNA had a sensitivity of 76% for detecting residual mediastinal metastases and is therefore a promising tool for mediastinal re-staging, although corroborating data from other centres is required.

Although real-time linear EBUS-TBNA using an integrated scope has largely superseded the radial mini-probe technique for the diagnosis of mediastinal lymph nodes and para-bronchial lesions, the mini-probe may retain a role in the diagnosis of peripheral lung lesions and in the assessment of airway invasion. A mini-probe placed in a distal airway may identify peripheral pulmonary lesions. In one study of 50 patients with peripheral pulmonary lesions inaccessible to standard bronchoscopy, a histological diagnosis was made in 31 patients and was effective in diagnosing lesions >2 cm in diameter [35]. This technique of guiding transbronchial biopsies with the EBUS mini-probe may be particularly useful in patients with peripheral lesions in whom percutaneous transthoracic biopsy is hazardous due to poor respiratory reserve and does not incur the radiation exposure required with fluoroscopy. The radial view provided by the mini-probe may also be employed to assess the depth of invasion of centrally located early stage lung cancer and therefore accurately select those patients who may benefit most from photodynamic therapy [36].

Endoscopic ultrasound

EUS-FNA is an important investigation for the mediastinal staging of NSCLC. The procedure is commonly performed by gastroenterologists and has been increasingly utilised for sampling the mediastinum in the last 10 yrs. A modified endoscope with an ultrasound scanner at its distal end is placed in the oesophagus under conscious sedation. Radial echo-endoscopes provide cross-sectional imaging and may be used in the assessment of mediastinal invasion of primary tumours. One study demonstrated a sensitivity of 88%, but over-staging occurred in 30% of patients limiting its clinical use [37]. Radial echo-endoscopes do not allow tissue samples to be obtained and have been largely replaced by an integrated linear ultrasound probe that allows sampling of the mediastinum under direct vision (fig. 2c). Aspiration with a 22-gauge, adjustable-length needle is performed through the wall of the oesophagus. Due to the anatomical location of the oesophagus, EUS-FNA provides minimally invasive access to left paratracheal, aorto-pulmonary window, subcarinal and para-oesophageal lymph nodes (fig. 3). In addition, EUS-FNA allows aspiration of the celiac axis nodes, left lobe of the liver and left adrenal gland providing crucial further diagnostic and staging information.

Cytology samples are obtained by EUS-FNA with a 22-gauge needle. However, in lymph nodes >2 cm in their short axis, core samples for histopathological analysis may be obtained, using a 19-gauge Trucut needle (Wilson-Cook, Winston-Salem, NC, USA). The availability of rapid on-site evaluation of samples may improve diagnostic yield from the procedure. This involves a cytologist being present in the endoscopy suite and by using rapid staining techniques (*e.g.* modified May–Grunwald–Giemsa stain), the cytologist is able to make an immediate assessment of the sample with high accuracy, eliminating inconclusive or inadequate samples [38]. This arrangement has also been shown to be cost-effective [39]. Diagnostic yield is maximised by performing 3–5 passes.

Studies have demonstrated that EUS-FNA is a safe and efficacious procedure for the mediastinal staging of NSCLC. A meta-analysis of 16 studies, totalling 1,003 patients demonstrated a pooled sensitivity of 84% (range 45–100%) and specificity of 99.5% when the prevalence of mediastinal disease was 61% [28]. The false negative rate from the pooled data was 19% (table 1). In an important study, SINGH *et al.* [40] employed EUS-FNA as a first test after CT scan in 93 patients. By sampling the mediastinum and extra-thoracic sites, they were able to provide a tissue diagnosis and stage in a single test in 70% of cases. Metastases to coeliac axis nodes were diagnosed in 11% of cases, half of which were in nodes <1 cm in short axis and therefore not suspected on CT scan. The study highlights the improved accuracy of EUS-FNA over CT and PET scanning for the detection of metastases from lung cancer as well as the poor prognosis of coeliac axis nodal involvement [40].

To date, EUS-FNA has been examined in two randomised studies, suggesting that EUS-FNA may reduce the need for mediastinoscopy in the staging of NSCLC [41], and that it may also reduce the number of futile thoracotomies if employed routinely [42]. However, data from these studies on healthcare costs are unavailable. In cohort studies, the high diagnostic accuracy of EUS-FNA has been demonstrated in mediastinal nodes <1 cm as well as PET-positive mediastinal nodes. A study based in the Netherlands evaluated PET-positive mediastinal lesions in 81 patients with proven or suspected lung cancer [43]. A total of 50 patients in this trial had a positive diagnosis of metastatic disease by EUS-FNA. EUS-FNA of PET-positive nodes was a cost-effective strategy, reducing surgical staging procedures by >50% and saving 40% of staging costs. The unreliability of negative EUS-FNA samples, however, means that surgical staging techniques still have an important role.

EUS-FNA therefore represents an important advance in the mediastinal staging of NSCLC. The technique offers a minimally invasive and potentially cost-effective alternative to mediastinoscopy when sampling of left-sided or posterior mediastinal lymph nodes is required. In addition it may diagnose previously unsuspected extra-thoracic disease. Despite these advantages, EUS-FNA has been slow to be incorporated into local diagnostic and staging algorithms. As with other minimally invasive techniques for mediastinal lymph node sampling, negative results must be verified by surgical techniques.

Combining EBUS/EUS

Endobronchial and endoscopic ultrasound provide complimentary access to the mediastinum. Combining EBUS and EUS at the same sitting allows minimally invasive sampling of the entire mediastinum except for the para-aortic nodes which lie anterior and lateral to the ascending aorta and aortic arch. Early results suggest that the combination procedure may be performed safely and have a combined accuracy of approaching 100% [25, 44]. Expertise and availability of the necessary equipment is not universally available and some centres employ the EBUS scope in the oesophagus, having already undertaken EBUS-TBNA. The combination of EBUS and EUS does however, enable more complete access to the mediastinum than standard mediastinoscopy and in the future may be considered the gold standard for mediastinal staging. Results from a European randomised trial comparing combined EBUS/EUS *versus* mediastinoscopy in the mediastinal staging of NSCLC are awaited.

Surgical procedures

Mediastinoscopy is the current gold standard technique for pre-operative mediastinal lymph node (MLN) staging in NSCLC. Performed under general anaesthesia, an incision is made above the suprasternal notch and the mediastinoscope is inserted along the trachea, allowing visualisation and biopsy of MLNs. The procedure is increasingly performed as a day-case with low morbidity (2%); mortality is rare. Mediastinoscopy affords access to paratracheal nodes, pre-tracheal nodes and anterior subcarinal nodes. However, lymph nodes in the aorto-pulmonary window, anterior mediastinal nodes, posterior subcarinal nodes and inferior mediastinal nodes are not accessible by this technique. The technique allows the surgeon to determine extra-capsular spread (and inoperability) at the time of the operation. Large biopsy samples also allow micro-metastases to be detected, even in normal sized lymph nodes. However, a meta-analysis of 6,505 patients demonstrated a pooled sensitivity of 78% (range 40–97%), and a false negative rate of 11% when the overall prevalence of disease was 39% [27]. This inaccuracy (for the gold standard technique) is in part explained by the limited access of mediastinoscopy to the mediastinum.

Invasive mediastinal sampling (by mediastinoscopy or needle aspiration technique) is currently indicated for the evaluation of any PET positive mediastinal lymph nodes, nodes that are >16 mm in short axis on staging CT scan, central tumours, PET positive hilar disease and in the scenario of low fluorodeoxyglucose uptake of the primary tumour [45]. Surgical mediastinal staging is not currently justified in patients with clinical stage 1 NSCLC with negative CT and PET scan of the mediastinum, on the basis that the prevalence of mediastinal disease in this group of patients is very low. However, mediastinoscopy does appear to be underutilised in clinical practice and when it is carried out, is not uniformly performed to the highest standards. Best practice at mediastinoscopy would require that five nodal stations (upper and lower left and right paratracheal and subcarinal areas) are routinely sampled. SMULDERS *et al.* [46] demonstrated that systematic mediastinal lymph node sampling was performed in only 50% of cases and estimated that 18% of thoracotomies that were subsequently proven futile could have been avoided if gold standard techniques had been observed [46]. Of 39 cases with unexpected N2 disease at thoracotomy, 16 were retrospectively noted to be accessible to mediastinoscopy [46].

The advent of videomediastinoscopy has improved the standard procedure allowing better visualisation and in addition to usual mediastinal lymph node stations, sampling of posterior subcarina lymph nodes. Video-assisted mediastinal lymphadectomy (VAMLA) may also be performed using this technique allowing complete lymph node dissection without the need for thoracotomy. VAMLA offers a standardised approach to surgical MLN sampling and may be superior to standard cervical mediastinoscopy with an accuracy of 88% and negative predictive value of 83% in a recent cohort of 234 patients [47]. Surgical expertise in this technique however is far from universal and further data is required.

Primary NSCLCs of the left upper lobe have a predilection for metastasis to mediastinal lymph nodes in the aorto-pulmonary window (station 5) and para-aortic lymph nodes (station 6), often skipping left hilar (N1) nodes. Although EUS-FNA is able to sample station 5 nodes, the para-aortic area is generally inaccessible to minimally invasive techniques. Few studies have evaluated the best approach for the staging of patients with left upper lobe tumours. A retrospective study of 112 patients with suspected metastases in lymph node stations 5 or 6 suggested that EUS-FNA had an accuracy of 66%, whereas the preferred staging procedure was left video-assisted thorascopic surgery (VATS), with an accuracy of 100% in this group of patients [48]. Nodes in the aorto-pulmonary window (APW), to which left upper lobe cancers commonly spread, can also be accessed by anterior mediastinotomy, also known as the Chamberlain procedure. An incision is made under general anaesthetic in the second or third intercostal space just to the left of the sternum; overnight stay is usually required. Few studies have addressed the accuracy of this procedure, although it is employed as the definitive staging technique for nodes in the APW. Extended cervical mediastinoscopy is also performed in some centres for the staging of left upper lobe tumours. In one series, this was found to have a sensitivity of 69% and false negative rate of 11% in 100 patients with a prevalence of mediastinal disease of 29% [49].

VATS is performed under general anaesthetic and can directly access one side of the mediastinum, with the right side being technically easier. Few prospective data are available, although the procedure appears to have an acceptable safety and accuracy profile and may be regarded as an adjunct procedure to standard techniques. It may be best suited to the diagnosis of parenchymal lesions inaccessible by other means, assessment of mediastinal invasion (T4 disease) and sampling of APW nodes. In addition, VATS has a key role in the diagnosis and therapeutics of a malignant pleural effusion. The procedure allows the surgeon visual access to the pleural space and biopsy of the pleura, and drainage of the pleural space and pleurodesis is also commonly performed, allowing a tissue diagnosis to be made as well as achieving effective palliation in a single procedure.

Future techniques in diagnostic endoscopy

Progress in technology is resulting in promising advances in diagnostic endoscopy. Medical thoracoscopy is currently performed in many centres for pleural effusions and is analogous to a VATS procedure, but does not require general anaesthesia. Recently an autoclavable semi-rigid thorascope has been introduced into clinical practice. Initial experience with this thorascope in 56 patients has demonstrated a diagnostic yield of over 90% and also allowed talc poudrage [50].

Electromagnetic navigation for peripheral pulmonary lesions is useful for lesions that are not accessible to standard bronchoscopy and is performed under general anaesthesia. Following detailed review of the CT scan, the patient is placed within an electromagnetic field and a sensor probe within a steerable catheter is introduced *via* a bronchoscope. During registration, the probe is touched onto pre-defined anatomical landmarks and data from the CT scan of the thorax are then merged with electromagnetic information using specific computer software. The precise three-dimensional location of the sensor probe can therefore be established and guided precisely towards the target lesion. Once the target lesion has been identified, the sensor probe is withdrawn, leaving the catheter in place. Biopsy forceps or brush may then be inserted into the catheter, which acts as an extended working channel of the bronchoscope. The procedure has been assessed in several series demonstrating diagnostic yields of up to 74% for peripheral lesions and 100% for mediastinal lymph nodes [51]. The addition of a radial EBUS probe to confirm the lesion location may further improve the yield of peripheral lesions to 88% [52].

Confocal laser fluorescent microscopy (alveoloscopy) is at the development stage but is an exciting new technique that allows microscopic tissue views *in vivo* for the first time. When combined with autofluorescence, real-time noninvasive imaging, known as "optical biopsy", is possible and may improve yield from conventional biopsy samples. A probe that emits and detects light is inserted into the working channel of the bronchoscopy. The probe is ≤ 1 mm in diameter and therefore may be advanced beyond distal airways. Thin section images of the microscopic autofluorescence structure may be obtained. A French group reported 29 patients who underwent confocal laser fluorescent microscopy. Alterations of the autofluorescence microstructure were seen in 19 out of 22 pre-invasive lesions, all CIS and two (out of two) invasive lesions [53]. The specificity of this technique remains to be defined and image quality can be hindered by endobronchial secretions.

Summary

A tissue diagnosis of lung cancer is crucial to differentiate nonsmall cell lung cancer (NSCLC) from small cell lung cancer. In patients with intra-thoracic disease, bronchoscopy remains a standard, routinely performed procedure that can provide important diagnostic as well as staging information. Surgical biopsy and mediastinoscopy are still considered to be gold standard investigations. However, rapid advances in technology have allowed the bronchoscopist's role to be expanded considerably. Autofluorescence bronchoscopy aids in the diagnosis of pre-invasive lesions and early lung cancers, while endobronchial and endoscopic ultrasound have become established for the mediastinal staging of NSCLC. In the current epidemic of lung cancer, these techniques are at the forefront of establishing a diagnosis and disease stage and are central to the multidisciplinary management of lung cancer.

Keywords: Autofluorescence bronchoscopy, bronchoscopy, endobronchial ultrasound, endoscopic ultrasound, mediastinoscopy, sputum cytology.

Statement of interest
None declared.

References

1. Foster BB. Neuroendocrine carcinomas of the lung: clinical, radiologic and pathologic correlation. *Radiology* 1989; 170: 441–445.
2. Rivera MP, Mehta AC. Initial diagnosis of lung cancer: ACCP evidence-based clinical practice guidelines (2nd edition). *Chest* 2007; 132: 131–148.
3. Risse EK, Van't Hof MA, Vooijs GP. Relationship between patient charcteristics and the sputum cytologic diagnosis of lung cancer. *Acta Cytol* 1987; 31: 159–165.
4. Bocking A, Biesterfield S, Chatelain R, *et al.* Diagnosis of bronchial carcinoma on sectinos of paraffin-embedded sputum: sensitivity and specificity of an alternative to routine cytology. *Acta Cytol* 1992; 36: 37–47.
5. Jay SJ, Wehr K, Nicholson DP, *et al.* Diagnostic sensitivity and specificity of pulmonary cytology: comparison of techniques used in conjunction with flexible fiber optic bronchoscopy. *Acta Cytol* 1980; 24: 302–312.
6. Schreiber G, McCrory DC. Performance characteristics of different modalities for diagnosis of suspected lung cancer: summary of published evidence. *Chest* 2003; 123: 115S–128S.
7. Gaeta M, Pandolfo I, Volta S, *et al.* Bronchus sign on CT in peripheral carcinoma of the lung: value in predicting results of transbronchial biopsy. *Am J Roentgenol* 1991; 157: 1181–1185.
8. Cox ID, Bagg LR, Russell NJ, *et al.* Relationship of radiologic position to the diagnostic yield of fibreoptic bronchoscopy in bronchial carcinoma. *Chest* 1984; 85: 519–522.
9. Herth FJ, Ernst A, Becker HD. Autofluorescence bronchoscopy – a comparison of two systems (LIFE and D-Light). *Respiration* 2003; 70: 395–398.
10. Philippe P, Benoit M, Verdebout JM, *et al.* Flourescence bronchoscopy in high risk patients: a comparison of LIFE and Pentax systems. *J Bronchol* 2001; 8: 251–254.
11. Haussinger K, Becker H, Stanzel F, *et al.* Autofluorescence bronchoscopy with white light bronchoscopy compared with white light bronchoscopy alone for the detection of precancerous lesions: a European randomised controlled multicentre trial. *Thorax* 2005; 60: 496–503.

12. George PJ, Banerjee AK, Read CA, *et al.* Surveillance for the detection of early lung cancer in patients with bronchial dysplasia. *Thorax* 2007; 62: 43–50.
13. Kennedy TC, McWilliams A, Edell E, *et al.* Bronchial intraepithelial neoplasia/early central airways: lung cancer ACCP evidence-based clinical practice guidelines (2nd Edition). *Chest* 2007; 132: 221S–233S.
14. Wang KP, Terry P, Marsh B. Bronchoscopic needle aspiration biopsy of paratracheal tumors. *Am Rev Respir Dis* 1978; 118: 17–21.
15. Holty JE, Kuschner WG, Gould MK. Accuracy of transbronchial needle aspiration for mediastinal staging of non-small cell lung cancer: a meta-analysis. *Thorax* 2005; 60: 949–955.
16. Chin R, McCain TW, Lucia MA, *et al.* Transbronchial needle aspiration in diagnosing and staging lung cancer: how many aspirates are needed? *Am J Respir Crit Care Med* 2002; 166: 377–381.
17. Diacon AH, Schuurmans MM, Theron J, *et al.* Transbronchial needle aspirates: how many passes per target site? *Eur Respir J* 2007; 29: 112–116.
18. Garpestad E, Goldberg S, Herth F, *et al.* CT fluoroscopy guidance for transbronchial needle aspiration: an experience in 35 patients. *Chest* 2001; 119: 329–332.
19. Hsu LH, Liu CC, Ko JS. Education and experience improve the performance of transbronchial needle aspiration: a learning curve at a cancer center. *Chest* 2004; 125: 532–540.
20. Harrow EM, Abi-Saleh W, Blum J, *et al.* The utility of transbronchial needle aspiration in the staging of bronchogenic carcinoma. *Am J Respir Crit Care Med* 2000; 161: 601–607.
21. Bernasconi M, Chhajed PN, Gambazzi F, *et al.* Combined transbronchial needle aspiration and positron emission tomography for mediastinal staging of NSCLC. *Eur Resp J* 2006; 27: 889–894.
22. Krasnik M, Vilmann P, Larsen SS, *et al.* Preliminary experience with a new method of endoscopic transbronchial real time ultrasound guided biopsy for diagnosis of mediastinal and hilar lesions. *Thorax* 2003; 58: 1083–1086.
23. Lee HS, Lee GK, Lee HS, *et al.* Real-time endobronchial ultrasound-guided transbronchial needle aspiration in mediastinal staging of non-small cell lung cancer: how many aspirations per target lymph node station? *Chest* 2008; 134: 368–374.
24. Mountain CF, Dresler CM. Regional lymph node classification for lung cancer staging. *Chest* 1997; 111: 1718–1723.
25. Wallace MB, Pascual JM, Raimondo M, *et al.* Minimally invasive endoscopic staging of suspected lung cancer. *JAMA* 2008; 299: 540–546.
26. Herth FJ, Eberhardt R, Vilmann P, *et al.* Real-time endobronchial ultrasound guided transbronchial needle aspiration for sampling mediastinal lymph nodes. *Thorax* 2006; 61: 795–798.
27. Detterbeck FC, Jantz MA, Wallace MB, *et al.* Invasive mediastinal staging of lung cancer: ACCP evidence-based clinical practice guidelines (2nd edition). *Chest* 2007; 132: 202–220.
28. Navani N, Spiro SG, Janes SM, *Advances in mediastinal staging of non-small cell lung cancer. Nature Rev Clin Oncol* 2009; 6: 278–286.
29. Groth SS, Whitson BA, D'Cunha J, *et al.* Endobronchial ultrasound-guided fine-needle aspiration of mediastinal lymph nodes: A single institution's early learning curve. *Ann Thorac Surg* 2008; 86: 1104–1110.
30. Ernst A, Anantham D, Eberhardt R, *et al.* Diagnosis of mediastinal adenopathy-real-time endobronchial ultrasound guided needle aspiration *versus* mediastinoscopy. *J Thorac Oncol* 2008; 3: 577–582.
31. Herth FJ, Eberhardt R, Krasnik M, *et al.* Endobronchial ultrasound-guided transbronchial needle aspiration of lymph nodes in the radiologically and positron emission tomography-normal mediastinum in patients with lung cancer. *Chest* 2008; 133: 887–891.
32. Tournoy KG, Rintoul RC, van Meerbeeck JP, *et al.* EBUS-TBNA for the diagnosis of central parenchymal lung lesions not visible at routine bronchoscopy. *Lung Cancer* 2009; 63: 45–49.
33. Nakajima T, Yasufuku K, Fujiwara T, *et al.* Endobronchial ultrasound-guided transbronchial needle aspiration for the diagnosis of intrapulmonary lesions. *J Thorac Oncol* 2008; 3: 985–988.

34. Herth FJ, Annema JT, Eberhardt R, *et al.* Endobronchial ultrasound with transbronchial needle aspiration for restaging the mediastinum in lung cancer. *J Clin Onc* 2008; 26: 3346–3350.
35. Dooms CA, Verbeken E, Becker H, *et al.* Endobronchial ultrasonography in bronchoscopic occult pulmonary lesions. *J Thorac Onc* 2007; 2: 121–124.
36. Miyazu Y, Miyazawa T, Kurimoto N, *et al.* Endobronchial ultrasonography in the assessment of centrally located early-stage lung cancer before photodynamic therapy. *Am J Respir Crit Care Med* 2002; 165: 832–837.
37. Varadarajulu S, Schmulewitz N, Wildi SM, *et al.* Accuracy of EUS in staging of T4 lung cancer. *Gastrointest Endosc* 2004; 59: 345–348.
38. Tournoy KG, Praet MM, Van Maele G, *et al.* Esophageal endoscopic ultrasound with fine-needle aspiration with an on-site cytopathologist: high accuracy for the diagnosis of mediastinal lymphadenopathy. *Chest* 2005; 128: 3004–3009.
39. Pellisé Urquiza M, Fernández-Esparrach G, Solé M, *et al.* Endoscopic ultrasound-guided fine needle aspiration: predictive factors of accurate diagnosis and cost-minimization analysis of on-site pathologist. *Gastroenterol Hepatol* 2007; 30: 319–324.
40. Singh P, Camazine B, Jadhav Y, *et al.* Endoscopic ultrasound as a first test for diagnosis and staging of lung cancer: a prospective study. *Am J Respir Crit Care Med* 2007; 175: 345–354.
41. Tournoy KG, De Ryck F, Vanwalleghem LR, *et al.* Endoscopic ultrasound reduces surgical mediastinal staging in lung cancer: a randomized trial. *Am J Respir Crit Care Med* 2008; 177: 531–535.
42. Larsen SS, Vilmann P, Krasnik M, *et al.* Endoscopic ultrasound guided biopsy performed routinely in lung cancer staging spares futile thoracotomies: preliminary results from a randomised clinical trial. *Lung Cancer* 2005; 49: 377–385.
43. Kramer H, van Putten JW, Post WJ, *et al.* Oesophageal endoscopic ultrasound with fine needle aspiration improves and simplifies the staging of lung cancer. *Thorax* 2004; 59: 596–601.
44. Vilmann P, Krasnik M, Larsen SS, *et al.* Transesophageal endoscopic ultrasound-guided fine-needle aspiration (EUS-FNA) and endobronchial ultrasound-guided transbronchial needle aspiration (EBUS-TBNA) biopsy: a combined approach in the evaluation of mediastinal lesions. *Endoscopy* 2005; 37: 833–839.
45. De Leyn P, Lardinois D, Van Schil PE, *et al.* ESTS guidelines for preoperative lymph node staging for non-small cell lung cancer. *Eur J Cardiothorac Surg* 2007; 32: 1–8.
46. Smulders SA, Smeenk FW, Janssen-Heijnen ML, *et al.* Surgical mediastinal staging in daily practice. *Lung Cancer* 2005; 47: 243–251.
47. Leschber G, Sperling D, Klemm W, *et al.* Does video-mediastinoscopy improve the results of conventional mediastinoscopy? *Eur J Cardiothorac Surg* 2008; 33: 289–293.
48. Cerfolio RJ, Bryant AS, Eloubeidi MA. Accessing the aortopulmonary window (#5) and the paraaortic (#6) lymph nodes in patients with non-small cell lung cancer. *Ann Thorac Surg* 2007; 84: 940–945.
49. Ginsberg RJ, Rice TW, Goldberg M, *et al.* Extended cervical mediastinoscopy. A single staging procedure for bronchogenic carcinoma of the left upper lobe. *J Thorac Cardiovasc Surg* 1987; 94: 673–678.
50. Munavvar M, Khan MA, Edwards J, *et al.* The autoclavable semirigid thoracoscope: the way forward in pleural disease? *Eur Respir J* 2007; 29: 571–574.
51. Gildea TR, Mazzone PJ, Karnak D, *et al.* Electromagnetic navigation diagnostic bronchoscopy: a prospective study. *Am J Respir Crit Care Med* 2006; 174: 982–989.
52. Eberhardt R, Anantham D, Ernst A, *et al.* Multimodality bronchoscopic diagnosis of peripheral lung lesions: a randomized controlled trial. *Am J Respir Crit Care Med* 2007; 176: 36–41.
53. Thiberville L, Moreno-Swirc S, Vercauteren T, *et al.* *In vivo* imaging of the bronchial wall microstructure using fibered confocal fluorescence microscopy. *Am J Respir Crit Care Med* 2007; 175: 22–31.

CHAPTER 9

Staging of lung cancer

J-P. Sculier

Correspondence: J-P. Sculier, Dept of Critical Care and Thoracic Oncology, Institut Jules Bordet, Université Libre Bruxelles (ULB), 1, rue Héger-Bordet, B-1000 Brussels, Belgium.

Staging has a key role in the rational clinical management of lung cancer patients [1], whatever the histological subtype, small cell lung cancer (SCLC) or nonsmall cell lung cancer (NSCLC). A system classifying lung cancer based on the status of primary tumour (T), regional lymph nodes (N), and metastatic involvement (M) was originally proposed in 1946 by DENOIX [2]. It was designed and mainly used by surgeons [3], because at that time, the only effective treatment was surgical and staging was oriented for this particular therapeutic modality. In 1953, the Union Internationale Contre le Cancer (UICC) created a committee for the anatomical classification of tumours based on TNM. The concept of stage grouping of patients with similar prognoses came later. The practical advantage of such a definition is relevant to patient care and the TNM staging system has thus been internationally accepted. The stage is called "clinical" when staging is performed prior to treatment; it is called "pathological" when it is performed after surgery, taking into account the data obtained by the anatomopathological examination of the resected specimen.

In 1968, the UICC published the first edition of its manual, *The TNM Classification of Malignant Tumours*. In 1973, the American Joint Committee on Cancer (AJCC) described its own classification, based on the TNM system. Tumours were grouped into one of three stages: stages I and II were for operable disease and III for inoperable tumours. A study performed on a large series of patients with bronchogenic carcinoma confirmed the role of stage in the prognosis and the AJCC classification was adopted by Japan in 1973 and by the UICC in 1978 [4].

The TNM classification for lung cancer was revised for the first time in 1986 [5]. This revision, as with the following ones, was carried out on the basis of outcome data analysis demonstrating different prognoses for each new stage. A new definition of the T, N and M classification was adopted by the various national TNM committees and by the UICC in 1986 and became the International Staging System (ISS). The main changes were in T3 and T4 categories for tumour status, in N2 and N3 categories for regional nodal spread and in M1 category for distant metastatic involvement. Stage III, which represents locally advanced disease, was subdivided into IIIA and IIIB on the basis of potential complete surgical resection (A) and not (B), and stage IV has been added to include patients with distant metastatic disease (M1). This classification was modified for the second time in 1997.

The 1997 international staging system

In the description of ISS revised in 1997 [6], descriptors of the TNM components (table 1) remain the same as in 1986 except for two points: 1) satellite tumour nodule(s) in the primary tumour lobe of the lung represent(s) T4 disease, and 2) separate

Eur Respir Mon, 2009, 44, 150–168. Printed in UK - all rights reserved. Copyright ERS Journals Ltd 2009; European Respiratory Monograph; ISSN 1025-448x.

metastatic tumour nodule(s) in the ipsilateral nonprimary-tumour lobe(s) of the lung are designated M1 disease.

Stage grouping (table 2) is a classification of patients according to TNM descriptors into categories on the basis of treatment options and prognosis. Stage I includes patients with no evidence of lymph node involvement or distant metastasis and those who are candidates for definitive surgical treatment. It is subdivided into categories A and B. Stage IA represents patients with T1N0M0, who have the best outcome, and stage IB patients with T2N0M0, who are also expected to survive >5 yrs after treatment, but with a statistically significant difference from the first group. Stage II usually consists of resectable lesions completely within the lung with ipsilateral intrapulmonary, hilar or peribronchial nodes (T1–2, N1, M0). This stage is categorised in IIA (T1N1M0) and IIB (T2N0M0) on basis of prognostic criteria. Moreover, in the 1997 classification, T3N0M0 disease has been shifted from stage IIIA to IIB because the survival of these patients was nearly the same as those of the T2N1M0 ones. Stage III represents locally advanced disease and had been subdivided in a previous revision into stage IIIA and IIIB according to possible surgical resectability. Stage IIIA designates T3N1M0 and T1–3N2M0 disease; T3N0M0 is no longer in this category. Stage IIIB remains unchanged from the 1986 ISS classification, with T4N0–2M0 and T1–4N3M0 diseases. Stage IV consists of distant disease, with poorer prognosis: any T, any N and M1.

Table 1. – TNM system description according to the 1997 Union Internationale Contre le Cancer classification

Primary tumour (T factor)	
TX	Primary tumour cannot be assessed, or tumour proven by the presence of malignant cells in sputum or bronchial washings but not visualised by imaging or bronchoscopy
T0	No evidence of primary tumour
Tis	Carcinoma *in situ*
T1	Tumour <3 cm in greatest dimension, surrounded by lung or visceral pleura, without bronchoscopic evidence of invasion more proximal than the lobar bronchus (*i.e.* not in the main bronchus)[#]
T2	Tumour with any of the following features of size or extent: >3 cm in greatest dimension, involves main bronchus, >2 cm distal to the carina, invades the visceral pleura, associated with atelectasis or obstructive pneumonitis that extends to the hilar region but does not involve the entire lung
T3	Tumour of any size that directly invades any of the following: chest wall (including superior sulcus tumours), diaphragm, mediastinal pleura, parietal pericardium; or tumour in the main bronchus <2 cm distal to the carina, but without involvement of the carina; or associated atelectasis or obstructive pneumonitis of the entire lung
T4	Tumour of any size that invades any of the following: mediastinum, heart, great vessels, trachea, oesophagus, vertebral body, carina; or tumour with a malignant pleural or pericardial effusion[¶]; or tumour with satellite tumour nodule(s) within the ipsilateral primary-tumour lobe of the lung
Regional lymph nodes (N factor)	
NX	Regional lymph nodes cannot be assessed
N0	No regional lymph node metastasis
N1	Metastasis to ipsilateral peribronchial and/or ipsilateral hilar lymph nodes, and intrapulmonary nodes involved by direct extension of the primary tumour
N2	Metastasis to ipsilateral mediastinal and/or subcarinal lymph node(s)
N3	Metastasis to contralateral mediastinal, contralateral hilar, ipsilateral or contralateral scalene, or supraclavicular lymph node(s)
Distant metastasis (M factor)	
MX	Presence of distant metastasis cannot be assessed
M0	No distant metastasis
M1	Distant metastasis present (separate metastatic tumour nodule(s) in the ipsilateral nonprimary-tumour lobe(s) of the lung also are classified M1)

[#]: uncommon superficial tumour of any size with its invasive component limited to the bronchial wall, which may extend proximal to the main bronchus, is also classified T1. [¶]: most pleural effusions associated with lung cancer are due to tumour. However, there are a few patients in whom multiple pathological examinations of pleural fluid show no tumour. In these cases, the fluid is nonbloody and is not an exudate. When these elements and clinical judgement dictate that the effusion is not related to the tumour, the effusion should be excluded as a staging element.

Table 2. – Stage grouping according to 1986 and 1997 international staging system

Staging classification 1986	
Stage I	T1 N0 M0
	T2 N0 M0
Stage II	T1 N1 M0
	T2 N1 M0
Stage IIIA	T3 N0–1 M0
	T1–3 N2 M0
Stage IIIB	Any T N3 M0
	T4 any N M0
Stage IV	Any T any N M1
Staging classification 1997	
Stage IA	T1 N0 M0
Stage IB	T2 N0 M0
Stage IIA	T1 N1 M0
Stage IIB	T2 N1 M0
	T3 N0 M0
Stage IIIA	T3 N1 M0
	T1–3 N2 M0
Stage IIIB	Any T N3 M0
	T4 any N M0
Stage IV	Any T any N M1

In conclusion, the 1997 ISS includes revised descriptors for T4 and M1 and divides stages I and II into A and B categories and modifies stage IIIA with the shift of T3N0M0 to stage IIB.

Problems with the 1997 international staging system

Many criticisms [7, 8] can be levelled at the 1997 ISS, still the current system used at the time the present chapter was being written. It is derived from a single-institution database analysis, constructed between 1975 and 1988, without internal and external validity. Indeed, prior to adoption, the results were not validated in other independent series. patients' work-up often did not use modern imaging techniques, such as computed tomography, magnetic resonance imaging and positron emission tomography (PET) scan. Finally, and more to the point, it is not based on a patient population treated with modern therapeutic modalities, including chemotherapy, and does not take into consideration the data obtained with multimodal therapeutic modalities. Today, the treatment of NSCLC is no longer primarily surgical with adjuvant therapy decided after surgical resection. It is the object of a multidisciplinary approach based on the clinical staging as defined prior to any treatment administration. The pathological staging is in fact a post-therapeutic staging and has to be considered at the same level as a response to chemotherapy or to radiotherapy. As the initial therapeutic approach of NSCLC is becoming more often nonsurgical for stage III disease and possibly also in the future for earlier stages, it seems appropriate to have a TNM staging system that is adapted to decisions taken on the basis of clinical data. The main publications providing data suggesting that the 1997 ISS needs to be improved will now be reviewed.

Surgical series of completely resected NSCLCs

The 1997 ISS has been assessed in various surgical series from different countries. Although most of the revisions made were supported by analyses, some proposals or observations were performed for subsequent revisions, such as moving T3N1M0 to stage IIB and T3N2M0 to stage IIIB [9]; the grouping of stages IB and IIA [10–12]; and the absence of different prognosis for clinical staging, but pathological staging between stages IB and IIA [13], or between pIIIA and pIIIB [12] without much corroborative evidence. It should also be pointed out that prognosis is predicted more accurately by the pathological stage than the clinical stage in the main series [6, 11, 13–15].

Tumour size

Multiple publications have examined the role of the tumour size in the prognosis and the importance to take into account that parameter in the T definition. In 1999, the Spanish Bronchogenic Carcinoma Cooperative Group proposed the definition of four different prognostic groups: size 0–2 cm, 2.1–4 cm, 4.1–7 cm and >7 cm [16]. A tumour with a diameter >7 cm had, in their series of 2,361 cases, a prognosis similar to that of stage T3 or stage IIB. The analysis of the data of National Cancer Centre of Tokyo (545 cases with a size >3 cm) [17], of the study performed in Valencia (637 patients with stage IB) [18] and of an Italian group (548 resected stage I cases) [19] suggested a cut-off point of 5 cm for prognosis. American authors from Boston (9,191 stage I tumours) [20] and from Bethesda (665 cases) [21], as well as the data provided by the California Cancer Registry (19,702 stage I cases) [22], proposed the choice of a 4 cm cut-off point.

In stage IA (T1N0 with T defined as <3 cm), many studies have shown that the smaller tumours have a significantly better survival prognosis, proposing a split into two substages. The cut-off proposed was either 1.5 cm [23, 24] or 2 cm [16, 19–21, 25]. The analysis of the SEER (Surveillance, Epidemiology and End Results) registry (84,152 cases) [26] suggested cut-offs in tumour size at 15, 25, 35 and 45 mm.

Other T descriptors

Only a few studies have been performed concerning the other T descriptors that are not based on the tumour size.

For T2 tumours, descriptors include visceral pleural invasion, hilar atelectasis, obstructive pneumonitis and main bronchus involvement ≥2 cm from the carina. In the SEER registry analysis (10,545 stage IB NSCLC), the prognostic significance of descriptors are mainly dependent on tumour size [27]. Concerning visceral pleural invasion, Japanese authors have proposed a classification based on outcome assessment [28] taking into account the tumour size: if it is >3 cm with visceral pleural invasion, the tumour should be upgraded to T3 status.

For T3 tumours, descriptors include direct invasion of the chest wall, diaphragm, mediastinal pleura and parietal pericardium, and tumour in the main bronchus <2 cm from the carina but not involving it. In a French series of 261 resected T3 NSCLCs, bronchial pT3 tumours tended to have a better prognosis and chest wall pT3 tumours a worse one [29]. The nodal status can have a strong influence on the prognosis. The analysis of the SEER registry (5,254 NSCLC T1N1M0, T2N1M0 or T3N0M0) has shown that patients with T3N0 tumours have a survival pattern that resembles those with T1N1 ones and T3N0 diseases should thus be considered as stage II [30].

For T4 tumours, the descriptors include direct invasion of the mediastinum, heart, great vessels, trachea, carina, oesophagus, vertebral body or the presence of a malignant pleural or pericardial effusion or of satellite tumour nodules within the ipsilateral primary tumour lobe. In a surgical series of resected T4 tumours, pleural disease appears to be associated with a worse prognosis [31].

Pulmonary nodules

Pulmonary nodules are designated as T4 if they are within the same lobe as the primary tumour (often called satellite nodules) and as M1 if they are in another lobe. A literature review [32] supported the staging proposed by MOUNTAIN [5, 6], as did the database analysis by the National Cancer Centre of Tokyo [33]. Nevertheless, more recent data obtained in the USA [34], Japan [35] and Canada [36] have shown that tumours that are T4 by satellite nodule have a better prognosis than T4 by invasion, and that this prognosis is closer to the prognosis of T3 tumours.

N descriptors

N descriptors might be improved by taking into account some of the following considerations. Lymph node status has a different prognosis according to the extent of the metastatic involvement. In resected N2 tumours, when N2 is not detected preoperatively (so called minimal N2), prognosis is better than if N2 involvement has been diagnosed before surgery (clinical N2) [37]. Extranodal extension of regional lymph nodes is, conversely, an independent poor prognostic factor [38].

Lymph node metastases can skip the intrapulmonary nodes directly to the mediastinum (N2 disease without N1 involvement). The patients with N2 skip metastasis have a better prognosis than those with N1 and N2 diseases. Skip metastases are thus a unique group of pN2 disease [39]. Finally, prognosis may be related to the lymph node stations involved, which depend on the lobe of the primary tumour [40].

Clinical stage III

As suggested by some studies performed before the 1997 edition of classification, the available classification needs to be improved in stage III disease, for which the treatment has become multimodal and is mainly based on the clinical TNM, which requires a more operational staging system [41, 42].

In a large prospective Radiation Therapy Oncology Group series of >600 patients treated by hyperfractionated radiation therapy [43], stage IIIA (1986 ISS classification) had a better survival prognosis than stage IIIB and, in stage IIIA, tumours with chest wall invasion (T3) had a significantly worse survival than those without it. This observation led the authors to propose a subdivision of stage IIIA into two subsets according to presence or absence of clinically documented chest wall invasion. This proposal was in apparent contradiction with the 1997 ISS classification, where T3N0 diseases have been moved into stage II; however, this change was based on surgical and not on radiotherapy data.

In a prospective Cancer and Leukemia Group B series of 112 patients treated by chest irradiation either with or without induction chemotherapy [44], patients with stage IIIA disease had superior survival to those with stage IIIB and, in univariate analysis, the T status but not the N status was a prognostic factor for survival. The prognostic value of subsets of tumours according to T and N has not been investigated, probably because of the small number of patients.

In a cohort of 428 patients with clinical stage III initially inoperable NSCLC treated by the same induction chemotherapy regimen, the European Lung Cancer Working Party has investigated the prognostic value of clinical T and N subgroupings in order to validate the 1986 ISS classification [45]. Patients with stage IIIA had a significantly better survival than those with stage IIIB (median survival 47 *versus* 36 weeks; $p=0.01$). A recursive partitioning and amalgamation (RECPAM) analysis showed that patients with T1–2 N3 and T4 N0–2 stages had a prognosis closer to those with stage IIIA disease. That result had allowed the definition of two new sub-groups: stage IIIα (T3–4 N0–1; any T1–3N2; T1–T2 N3) and IIIβ (T3–T4 N3), with a highly significant difference in survival between them (median survival 45 *versus* 29 weeks; $p<0.0001$). This observation was confirmed by a validation study performed in a consecutive series of 328 patients [46].

An Australian study, performed on 243 patients treated by radiotherapy [47], failed to identify T and N status as a prognostic factor in univariate and multivariate analyses.

In a Japanese surgical series including 152 stage III NSCLC [48], no difference in survival between patients with T3 and T4 diseases was observed. The authors classified the patients into different groups on the basis of the TNM descriptors and were able to obtain survival differences. They reclassified T4 tracheal invasion and T4 pulmonary metastasis with T3 and T3 bronchial invasion to T2. With those changes, they observed significant survival differences between T3 and T4 tumours and between stage IIIA and IIIB.

The International Association for the Study of Lung Cancer international staging project

The studies just described clearly show that improvement of the current clinical TNM classification is necessary. Indeed, the ISS, even in its 1997 revision, is not necessarily totally appropriate for an optimal management of lung cancer, when modern methods of staging and treatment are taken into consideration. For that reason, P. Goldstraw, Thoracic Surgeon at Royal Brompton Hospital, London, UK, took the initiative to organise, since 1999, international multidisciplinary meetings of physicians and scientists who had databases and wished to collaborate for changing the TNM classification with an adequate statistical methodology. Those meetings led to the development of a staging project within the International Association for the Study of Lung Cancer (IASLC), which is the international multidisciplinary scientific society most dedicated to that purpose. The IASLC agreed with the creation of the IASLC Staging Project Committee, chaired by GOLDSTRAW *et al.* [49]. The committee was structured in subcommittees for T descriptors (Rami-Porta), N descriptors (Rusch), M descriptors (Postmus), prognostic factors (Sculier), SCLC (Shepherd), nodal chart (Tsuchiya), and validation and methodology (Groome).

Methodology

The proposal of modifications of the lung cancer classification for the seventh edition that will be published in 2009, required data analysed in 2006. For evident follow-up reasons (a minimal 5-yr period required for all included patients), only a retrospective study was possible. The IASLC staging project has been able to collect data on 100,869 patients [49] from 45 different sources and 20 countries: registries, clinical trials, surgical series, and hospital series. Cancers were diagnosed between 1990 and 2000. Data about stage and survival follow-up were sufficient in 81,495 cases, including 13,032 SCLC and 68,463 NSCLC. Treatment was surgery in 41%, radiotherapy in 11%, chemotherapy in 23% and combined modalities for the remaining patients.

The databases and the statistical analysis were managed by Cancer Research and Biostatistics, conducted by J. Crowley in Seattle, WA, USA. The committee and subcommittees have had multiple meetings and electronic mailing has mainly helped communication between members. The subcommittee "Methodology and Validation" has supervised all the analyses performed for ensuring homogeneity [50]. For each proposal, one-third of the cases of the databases of the IASLC staging project was used for internal validation. External validation was performed by using the data of the SEER registry, through an authorisation of the American authorities [50].

The overall results and those of each subcommittee have been the topic of separate articles, published in the *Journal of Thoracic Oncology*, which is the official journal of the IASLC. These articles are freely accessible on line.

Results of the retrospective study

The TNM classification was studied in the group of patients with NSCLC in the databases of the IASLC staging project.

T descriptors. Metastatic cases (M1) were excluded. For analysis purposes, there were enough data for 18,018 patients for clinical T and 15,234 for pathological T, whatever the N status [51].

Tumour size appeared to be a strong prognostic factor with different thresholds defining different prognoses (table 3): 2 cm, 3 cm, 5 cm and 7 cm. Tumours with a size >7 cm had a prognosis similar to T3. It has thus been proposed to divide T1 into two categories, T1a and T1b, according to a size either smaller or greater than 2 cm and T2 into T2a and T2b according to a size either smaller or greater than 5 cm while those >7 cm become T3.

Tumours classified as T4 and M1 by the presence of an ipsilateral lung nodule (either in the same lobe or in another lobe to the primary tumour, respectively) were shown to have a better prognosis, similar to T3 if in the same lobe or to T4 if in another lobe of the same lung. Finally, tumours designated T4 by pleural involvement had a worse prognosis than the other T4 tumours with respective 5-yr survivals of 2% and 14% ($p<0.0001$).

N descriptors. In the case of N descriptors, not enough sufficiently detailed data describing N existed to be able to propose new changes, because of the use of different nodal charts: the one of Naruke in a Japanese series and the American Thoracic

Table 3. – International Association for the Study of Lung Cancer staging project: role of tumour size in the prognosis of the T descriptor

T	N0			All N		
	Patients n	5-yr survival	p-value	Patients n	5-yr survival	p-value
Pathological stages						
pT1 ≤2 cm	1959	76		2389	71	
pT2 >2–3 cm	1800	70	<0.0001	2484	62	<0.0001
pT2 >3–5 cm	3175	58	<0.0001	5242	49	<0.0001
pT2 >5–7 cm	936	49	<0.0001	1615	40	<0.0001
pT2 >7 cm	426	35	<0.0001	788	28	<0.0001
pT3	711	38	0.2739	1224	31	0.1597
Clinical stages						
cT1 ≤2 cm	423	53		518	48	
cT2 >2–3 cm	445	47	0.0932	543	43	0.1400
cT2 >3–5 cm	1345	43	0.1032	1793	39	0.0388
cT2 >5–7 cm	411	36	0.0010	572	32	0.0001
cT2 >7 cm	173	26	0.0076	258	24	0.0182
cT3	486	29	0.6111	677	27	0.6482

Data are presented as %, unless otherwise indicated.

Table 4. – International Association for the Study of Lung Cancer staging project: data supporting the introduction of new M substages

	Patients n	1-yr survival	Comparison	p-value
T4M0 all N	1106	53		
Pleural extent	771	45	With T4	<0.0001
Contralateral lung nodule	369	46	With pleural extent	0.3816
Distant metastases	4350	22	With contralateral lung nodule	<0.0001
			With pleural extent	<0.0001

Data are presented as %, unless otherwise indicated.

Society's one in the others [52]. It has been impossible to obtain an accurate correspondence between both charts and a proposal for a universal chart will be made for the future. Nevertheless, exploratory analyses suggest that the use of nodal zones, as follows, might be helpful: superior (areas 1 to 4), aorto-pulmonary (5 and 6), subcarinal (7), inferior (8 and 9), hilar (10 and 11), and peripheral (12 and 13). The involvement of multiple zones appears to give poor prognosis.

M descriptors. In the case of pleural involvement, prognosis is significantly worse than if the tumour is T4M0 for another reason, but better than if the tumour is M1 by distant metastases, except in the case of contralateral lung nodules (table 4) [53]. It has thus been proposed to classify pleural extent as M1 and to subdivide M1 into substages M1a for pleural extent or contralateral lung nodules and M1b for distant metastases.

Regrouping by stages. In addition to the changes already proposed, statistical analyses by RECPAM suggest reclassification of T2aN1 in stage IIA (instead of IIB), T2bN0 in stage IIA (instead of IB) et T4N0 and T4N1 in stage IIIA (instead of IIIB) [54]. All the proposed changes are summarised in table 5.

As shown in table 6 for clinical stages (the results are similar for pathological stages), the new system predicts the prognosis better than that of the sixth edition. It should be remembered that those data were validated in the internal validation group of the IASLC staging databases and in the SEER registry used for external validation [50].

Proposed classification

All the analyses performed have led to the proposal [54] of a new classification by TNM (table 7) and by stage (table 8) that, in 2010, will become the official UICC classification.

Node chart

NARUKE *et al.* [55], from the National Cancer Hospital in Tokyo, Japan, first proposed a nodal map for lung cancer drainage and assigned specific numbers to node stations and differentiated the bronchopulmonary and hilar lymph nodes from the mediastinal lymph nodes [55]. This map was modified by the American Thoracic Society and subsequently accepted by the AJCC and by UICC, with the last version being published in 1997 by MOUNTAIN and DRESLER [56]. There is considerable discordance in the designation of nodal stations between Japanese and occidental surgeons [57], and this high variability makes it very difficult to make comparisons between published data.

Table 5. – International Association for the Study of Lung Cancer staging project: changes (in bold) proposed for TNM regrouping by stages

Descriptor T/M (6th edition)	T/M change proposed	N0	N1	N2	N3
T1 (≤2 cm)	T1a	IA	IIA	IIIA	IIIB
T1 (>2–3 cm)	T1b	IA	IIA	IIIA	IIIB
T2 (≥3–5 cm)	T2a	IB	**IIA**	IIIA	IIIB
T2 (>5–7 cm)	T2b	**IIA**	IIB	IIIA	IIIB
T2 (≥7 cm)	T3	**IIB**	**IIIA**	IIIA	IIIB
T3 by invasion		IIB	IIIA	IIIA	IIIB
T4 (nodule same lobe)		**IIB**	**IIIA**	IIIA	IIIB
T4 by extension	T4	**IIIA**	**IIIA**	IIIB	IIIB
M1 (ipsilateral other lobe nodule)		**IIIA**	**IIIA**	**IIIB**	**IIIB**
T4 (pleural involvement)	M1a	**IV**	**IV**	**IV**	**IV**
M1 (contralateral lung nodule)		IV	IV	IV	IV
M1 (distant metastasis)	M1b	IV	IV	IV	IV

The IASLC staging project has worked to a map that might be accepted by all surgeons for international validation; this map should be available shortly.

SCLC and neuroendocrine tumours

Two main systems can be used to define the extent of disease: the ISS with TNM according to the last version published in 1997 by the UICC [6] or the two-stage system developed by the Veterans Administration Lung Cancer Study Group (either limited or extensive disease) [58]. In the latter system, patients with limited disease (LD) have involvement restricted to the ipsilateral hemithorax, which can be included within a single radiation port. In the definition of LD, the IASLC also includes the presence of contralateral hilar and/or ipsilateral and/or contralateral supraclavicular nodes and/or pericardial and/or ipsilateral pleural effusion, regardless of the cytology [59].

The classification proposed by the IASLC staging project has been assessed in the cases of SCLC available in its databases [60]. A total of 8,088 patients were eligible for the analysis; as shown in table 9, the classification appeared to adequately discriminate for predicting prognosis (except in stage IIA whose case number was small). These results have been confirmed with the SEER registry. Taking into consideration those results, it has been proposed to use the TNM system to describe stage in SCLC, as it is the rule in NSCLC.

Table 6. – International Association for the Study of Lung Cancer (IASLC) staging project: prediction of prognosis (Cox models) by the classification of the sixth Union Internationale Contre le Cancer edition and by the system proposed by the IASLC (clinical stage)

Comparison	Hazard ratio		p-value	
	6th edition	IASLC	6th edition	IASLC
IB *versus* IA	1.31	1.19	<0.0001	0.0035
IIA *versus* IB	1.35	1.23	0.1978	0.0020
IIB *versus* IIA	1.20	1.46	0.4344	<0.0001
IIIA *versus* IIB	1.30	1.27	<0.0001	<0.0001
IIIB *versus* IIIA	1.47	1.54	<0.0001	<0.0001
IV *versus* IIIB	1.71	1.64	<0.0001	<0.0001
R^2	25.86	26.77		

Table 7. – International Association for the Study of Lung Cancer staging project: TNM classification

cTNM clinical classification	
Primary tumour (T-factor)	
TX	Primary tumour cannot be assessed, or tumour proven by the presence of malignant cells in sputum or bronchial washings but not visualised by imaging or bronchoscopy
T0	No evidence of primary tumour
Tis	Carcinoma *in situ*
T1	Tumour <3 cm in greatest dimension, surrounded by lung or visceral pleura, without bronchoscopic evidence of invasion more proximal than the lobar bronchus (*i.e.* not in the main bronchus)[#]
T1a	Tumour <2 cm in greatest dimension
T1b	Tumour >2 cm but not >3 cm in greatest dimension
T2	Tumour >3 cm but not >7 cm; or tumour with *any* of the following features[¶] Involves main bronchus, ≥2 cm distal to the carina Invades visceral pleura Associated with atelectasis or obstructive pneumonitis that extends to the hilar region but does not involve the entire lung
T2a	Tumour >3 cm but not >5 cm in greatest dimension
T2b	Tumour >5 cm but not >7 cm in greatest dimension
T3	Tumour more than 7 cm or one that directly invades any of the following: chest wall (including superior sulcus tumours), diaphragm, phrenic nerve, mediastinal pleura, parietal pericardium; *or* tumour in the main bronchus less than 2 cm distal to the carina1 but without involvement of the carina; *or* associated atelectasis or obstructive pneumonitis of the entire lung or separate tumour nodule(s) in the same lobe
T4	Tumour of any size that invades any of the following: mediastinum, heart, great vessels, trachea, recurrent laryngeal nerve, oesophagus, vertebral body, carina; separate tumour nodule(s) in a different ipsilateral lobe
Regional lymph nodes (N-factor)	
NX	Regional lymph nodes cannot be assessed
N0	No regional lymph node metastasis
N1	Metastasis in ipsilateral peribronchial and/or ipsilateral hilar lymph nodes and intrapulmonary nodes, including involvement by direct extension
N2	Metastasis in ipsilateral mediastinal and/or subcarinal lymph node(s)
N3	Metastasis in contralateral mediastinal, contralateral hilar, ipsilateral or contralateral scalene, or supraclavicular lymph node(s)
Distant metastasis (M-factor)	
MX	Distant metastasis cannot be assessed
M0	No distant metastasis
M1	Distant metastasis
M1a	Separate tumour nodule(s) in a contralateral lobe; tumour with pleural nodules or malignant pleural (or pericardial) effusion[+]
M1b	Distant metastasis
pTNM pathological classification	
The pT, pN, and pM categories correspond to the T, N, and M categories	
pN0	Histological examination of hilar and mediastinal lymphadenectomy specimen(s) will ordinarily include 6 or more lymph nodes. If the lymph nodes are negative, but the number ordinarily examined is not met, classify as pN0
G histopathological grading	
GX	Grade of differentiation cannot be assessed
G1	Well differentiated
G2	Moderately differentiated
G3	Poorly differentiated
G4	Undifferentiated

[#]: the uncommon superficial spreading tumour of any size with its invasive component limited to the bronchial wall, which may extend proximal to the main bronchus, is also classified as T1. [¶]: T2 tumours with these features are classified T2a if ≤5 cm. [+]: most pleural (and pericardial) effusions with lung cancer are due to tumour. In a few patients, however, multiple cytopathological examinations of pleural (pericardial) fluid are negative for tumour, and the fluid is nonbloody and is not an exudate. Where these elements and clinical judgment dictate that the effusion is not related to the tumour, the effusion should be excluded as a staging element and the patient should be classified as T1, T2, T3 or T4.

Table 8. – International Association for the Study of Lung Cancer staging project: stage grouping

Occult carcinoma	TX N0 M0
Stage 0	Tis N0 M0
Stage IA	T1a, b N0 M0
Stage IB	T2a N0 M0
Stage IIA	T1a, b N1 M0
	T2a N1 M0
	T2b N0 M0
Stage IIB	T2b N1 M0
	T3 N0 M0
Stage IIIA	T1, T2 N2 M0
	T3 N1, N2 M0
	T4 N0, N1 M0
Stage IIIB	T4 N2 M0
	Any T N3 M0
Stage IV	Any T Any N M1

Prognostic implications

In addition to stage, information about potential prognostic variables, such as age, sex, histological type and performance status (PS), was available in the databases of the IASLC staging project. 12,428 eligible patients with NSCLC and 6609 with SCLC were available for multivariate analyses by Cox models and RECPAM, allowing the largest prognostic factor analysis ever made for lung cancer to be performed [61]. For SCLC, stage was defined as limited or extensive according to the data provided by the local database holders, as information on the descriptors were too limited to reclassify disease according to TNM. The main results are shown in tables 10 and 11. Stage, PS, sex and age were all independent prognostic factors. For NSCLC, squamous cell carcinoma was associated with a better prognosis.

RECPAM analysis identified four groups of patients with significant prognostic difference for NSCLC, as follows: group 1 with stages IA–IIA (any age, any PS); group 2 with stages IIB/IIIA and PS 0–1 (any age); group 3 with stages IIB/IIIA and PS 2 (any age) or with stages IIIB/IV and PS 0 (any age) or with stages IIIB/IV, age <81 yrs and PS 1; and group 4 with stages IIB/IIIA and PS 3–4 (any age) or with stages IIIB/IV and PS 2–4 (any age) or with stages IIIB/IV, PS 1 and age >80 yrs. Median survival times for groups 1–4 were 53, 16, 8 and 3 months, respectively (fig. 1). The same type of analysis performed in SCLC also identified four groups, as follows: group 1 with LD, PS 0 and age <60 yrs or with LD, PS 1–2 and age <65 yrs; group 2 with LD, PS 1–2 and age ≥65 yrs or females with extensive disease (ED), PS 0 and age <65 yrs; group 3 with females with ED, PS 0 and age ≥65 yrs or males with ED and PS 0 or with both sexes

Table 9. – International Association for the Study of Lung Cancer staging project: application of the proposed classification to the databases cases with small cell lung cancer

Stage	Patients n	1-yr survival	5-yr survival	p-value[#]
IA	211	77	38	
IB	325	67	21	0.0003
IIA	55	85	38	0.0075
IIB	270	70	18	0.0118
IIIA	1170	59	13	0.0003
IIIB	1399	50	9	<0.0001
IV	4530	22	1	<0.0001

Data are presented as %, unless otherwise indicated. #: comparison with the earlier stage.

Table 10. – Multivariate analysis of prognostic factors for survival in nonsmall cell lung cancer performed in the International Association for the Study of Lung Cancer staging project databases, using general characteristic variables

Variable	Subjects	HR (95% CI)	p-value[#]
Clinical TNM stage			
Stage II	1531 (12)	1.80 (1.65–1.97)	<0.001
Stage IIIA	2048 (16)	2.71 (2.49–2.95)	<0.001
Stage IIIB/IV	7280 (59)	5.34 (4.95–5.76)	<0.001
Age (continuous)	12426	1.01 (1.00–1.01)	<0.001
Squamous cell type	5304 (43)	0.93 (0.89–0.97)	<0.001
Male	9764 (79)	1.17 (1.11–1.23)	<0.001
PS 1 (*versus* 0)	6294 (51)	1.38 (1.32–1.44)	<0.001
PS 2 (*versus* 0)	1423 (11)	2.09 (1.95–2.23)	<0.001
PS 3–4 (*versus* 0)	579 (5)	3.48 (3.17–3.83)	<0.001

Data are presented as n (%), unless otherwise indicated. HR: hazard ratio; CI: confidence interval PS: performance status. [#]: p-value from Wald Chi-squared test in Cox regression.

and ED, PS 1 and age <70 yrs; and group 4 with LD and PS 3–4 or with ED, PS 1 and ≥70 yrs or with ED and PS 2–4. Median survival times for groups 1–4 were 17, 12, 10 and 6 months, respectively (fig. 2).

Exploratory statistical analyses have suggested that in advanced disease, some routine biological data could have a prognostic role, *e.g.* calcium, albumin, sodium, white blood cells and haemoglobin [61]. In addition to those results, it should be added the meta-analysis performed on the published data in the literature [62] concerning the prognostic role of the maximum standardised uptake value (SUV_{max}) obtained by PET.

All the prognostic factors identified by the IASLC staging project are summarised in table 12, with a grading as follows. ++++ and +++: factors present in any model; ++: factors significant in recursive partitioning and amalgamation and Cox models; +: factors significant in Cox models (or in a meta-analysis for SUV_{max}); +§: biological factors significant in Cox models not taking into consideration other biological variables.

With regard to the role of molecular or biological markers in lung cancer, >5,000 articles have been published, of varying methodological quality. The best evidence available in the literature at present on this subject has come from the meta-analyses summarised in table 13. The estimate of the prognostic value of the variables reported in these studies is limited by their use of univariate analyses. The independent role of the prognostic factors identified needs to be confirmed in prospective studies using methodology, such as that recently proposed by Zhu *et al.* [81] and the international recommendations for marker evaluation [82].

Table 11. – Multivariate analysis of prognostic factors for survival in small cell lung cancer, using general characteristic variables

Variable	Subjects	HR (95% CI)	p-value[#]
Age yrs	6609	1.01 (1.01–1.02)	<0.001
Extensive stage (*versus* limited)	3739 (57)	2.13 (2.02–2.25)	<0.001
Male	4368 (66)	1.25 (1.19–1.32)	<0.001
PS 1	3161 (48)	1.36 (1.28–1.44)	<0.001
PS 2	1060 (16)	1.93 (1.78–2.09)	<0.001
PS 3–4	349 (5)	3.45 (3.05–3.89)	<0.001

Data are presented as n (%), unless otherwise indicated. HR: hazard ratio; CI: confidence interval; PS: performance status. [#]: p-value from Wald Chi-squared test in Cox regression.

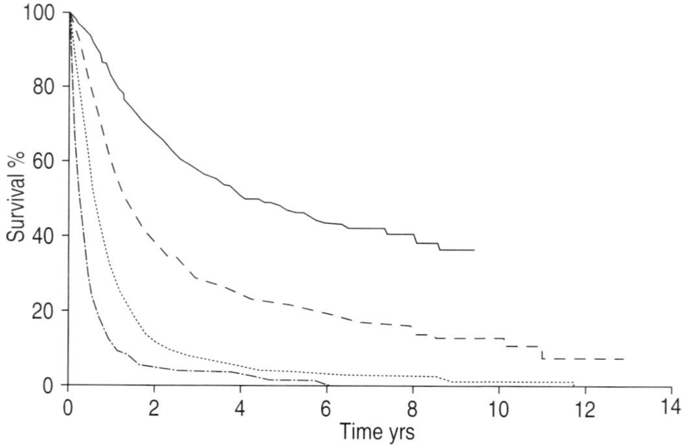

Fig. 1. – Survival obtained for the four amalgamated groups of different prognosis for nonsmall cell lung cancer (validation set of 4,227 patients). ——: IA/IB/IIA, any age, any performance status (PS); 351 deaths, n=639, median survival 53 months. – – – –: IIB/IIIA, any age, PS 0–1; 790 deaths, n=1,037, median survival 16 months. ······: IIB/IIIA, any age, PS 2; IIIB/IV, any age, PS 0; IIIB/IV, age <81 yrs, PS 1; 1,758 deaths, n=1,932, median survival 8 months. – · – · –: IIB/IIIA, any age, PS 3–4; IIIB/IV, any age, PS 2–4; IIIB/IV, age ≥81 yrs, PS 1; 557 deaths, n=619, median survival 3 months.

Conclusions, limitations and perspectives

The stage of lung cancer has a key prognostic and operational role in the management of the patient. Over ~40 yrs, successive improvements in the staging system have been performed. In the last version by the ISS, and as proposed by the IASLC staging project for the forthcoming seventh edition of the TNM classification (due to be published in

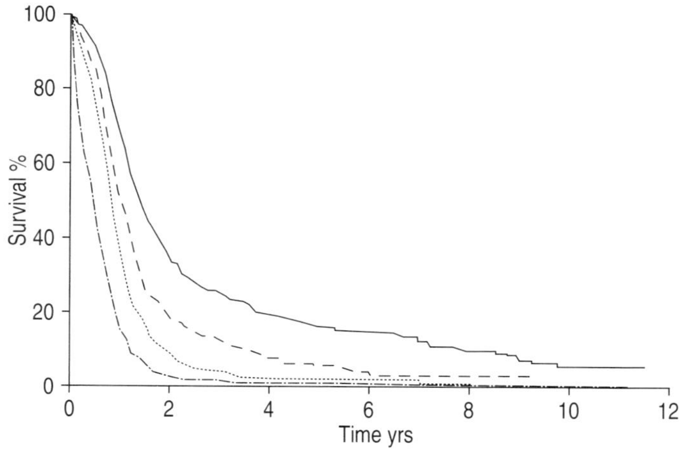

Fig. 2. – Survival obtained for the four amalgamated groups of different prognosis in small cell lung cancer (validation set of 2,250 patients). ——: limited disease (LD), performance status (PS) 0; LD, PS 1–2, age <65 yrs; 577 deaths, n=696, median survival 17 months. – – – –: LD, PS 1–2, age ≥65 yrs; extensive disease (ED), PS 0, female, age <65 yrs; 277 deaths, n=307, median survival 12 months. ······: ED, PS 0, female, age ≥65 yrs; ED, PS 0, male; ED, PS 1, age <70 yrs; 727 deaths, n=765, median survival 10 months. – · – · –: LD, PS 3–4; ED, PS 1, age ≥70 yrs; ED, PS 2–4; 459 deaths, n=482, median survival 6 months.

Table 12. – Summary of the prognostic factors with grading[#]

Variable	NSCLC	SCLC
Clinical extent of disease[¶]	++++	++++
Performance status[+]	+++ (≥IIB only)	+++
Age	++ (≥IIIB only)	++
Sex male	+	++
Squamous cell type	+ (IIIA only)	N/A
PET SUVmax	+	N/A
Calcium	+[§]	
Albumin	+[§]	+
Sodium	+§[§]	+§
White blood cells	+[§]	
Haemoglobin	+§[§]	

NSCLC: nonsmall cell lung cancer; SCLC: small cell lung cancer; PET: positron emission tomography; SUVmax: maximum standardised uptake value; N/A: not applicable or not available. #: grading is as follows. ++++ and +++: factors present in any model; ++: factors significant in recursive partitioning and amalgamation and Cox models; +: factors significant in Cox models (or in a meta-analysis for SUVmax); +§: biological factors significant in Cox models not taking into consideration other biological variables. ¶: extent of disease by TNM stage for NSCLC and with limited/extensive disease for SCLC. +: performance status by Zubrod scale. §: advanced stage IIIB/IV for NSCLC.

2009), the major modifications have taken into account tumour size, pleural involvement and pulmonary nodules, and have used a more adequate methodology (*i.e.* large database, multiple sources of original cases, more contemporary cases with adequate follow-up, modern statistical methods, and internal and external validations). It should be noted that the translation of pre-existing databases using the 1997 system into the new TNM classification will require precise information about the descriptors that have been modified (tumour size, lung nodules and pleural extent), and that the use of management algorithms based on the past staging system will have to be carried out very carefully when patients are staged using the new system.

Table 13. – Meta-analyses published on the prognostic value of biological or genetic markers for survival in lung cancer

Biological variable	Prognostic factor	First author [ref.]
Bcl-2	Good	Martin [63]
TTF1	Poor	Berghmans [64]
Cox2	Poor	Mascaux [65]
EGFR	Poor	Nakamura [66] Meert [67]
Ras	Poor	Mascaux [68] Huncharek [69]
Ki-67	Poor	Martin [70]
HER2	Poor	Meert [71] Nakamura [72]
VEGF	Poor	Delmotte [73]
Microvascular density	Poor	Meert [74] Trivella [75]
p53	Poor	Steels [76] Mitsudomi [77] Huncharek [78]
Aneuploidy	Poor	Choma [79]
Surviving	Poor	Fan [80]

TTF: thyroid transcription factor; Cox: cyclooxygenase; EGFR: epidermal growth factor receptor; VEGF: vascular endothelial growth factor.

Nevertheless, because of the retrospective approach taken, some limitations exist in the proposal due to the impossibility to obtain with accuracy the characteristics of the T, N and M descriptors, and as a result of the heterogeneity of the data collected from the various local database sources. For these reasons, the IASLC wants to perform an international prospective multicentric study with an established list of data in order to define even more accurately the TNM descriptors and their prognostic value.

Summary

The stage of lung cancer has a key role in the management of the patient. The system classifying lung cancer based on the status of primary tumour (T), regional lymph nodes (N) and metastatic involvement (M) was originally proposed in 1946, and has been the subject of many modifications to improve its prognostic and operational roles.
In the present chapter, the 1997 classification is described, as well as the various problems reported in the literature concerning its application.
In order to improve the staging system, an international initiative, International Association for the Study of Lung Cancer staging project, was undertaken to make a huge databases and to propose a revision of the 1997 system. The proposal, which will be used as official staging classification in 2009, is presented and discussed, as well as the role of stage in prognosis. Indeed, stage is so far the main prognostic factor in lung cancer.
In the future, proposals for further TNM revisions should be based on a prospective international multicentric databases where the details of the T, N and M descriptors should be available.

Keywords: Lung cancer, nonsmall cell lung cancer, prognosis, small cell lung cancer, staging, TNM.

Statement of interest
None declared.

References

1. Miller JD, Gorenstein LA, Patterson GA. Staging: the key to rational management of lung cancer. *Ann Thorac Surg* 1992; 53: 170–178.
2. Denoix PF. Enquête permanente dans les centres anti-cancéreux. *Bull Inst Natl Hyg* 1946; 1: 70–75.
3. Patel AM, Dunn WF, Trastek VF. Staging systems of lung cancer. *Mayo Clin Proc* 1993; 68: 475–482.
4. Mountain CF, Carr DT, Anderson WAD. A system for the clinical staging of lung cancer. *Am J Roentgenol* 1974; 120: 130–138.
5. Mountain CF. A new international staging system for lung cancer. *Chest* 1986; 89: Suppl. 4, 225S–233S.
6. Mountain CF. Revisions in the International System for Staging Lung Cancer. *Chest* 1997; 111: 1710–1717.
7. Leong SS, Lima CM, Sherman CA, *et al.* The 1997 International Staging System for non-small cell lung cancer: have all the issues been addressed? *Chest* 1999; 115: 242–248.

8. Sculier JP. Doit-on améliorer la classification TNM de 1997? *Rev Mal Respir* 1999; 16: Suppl. 3, S111–S112.
9. Inoue K, Sato M, Fujimura S, *et al.* Prognostic assessment of 1310 patients with non-small-cell lung cancer who underwent complete resection from 1980 to 1993. *J Thorac Cardiovasc Surg* 1998; 116: 407–411.
10. van Rens MT, de la Riviere AB, Elbers HR, *et al.* Prognostic assessment of 2,361 patients who underwent pulmonary resection for non-small cell lung cancer, stage I, II, and IIIA. *Chest* 2000; 117: 374–379.
11. Goya T, Asamura H, Yoshimura H, *et al.* Prognosis of 6644 resected non-small cell lung cancers in Japan: a Japanese lung cancer registry study. *Lung Cancer* 2005; 50: 227–234.
12. Duque JK, Lopez-Encuentra A, Porta RR. Survival of 2,991 patients with surgical lung cancer: the denominator effect in survival. *Chest* 2005; 128: 2274–2281.
13. Naruke T, Tsuchiya R, Kondo H, *et al.* Prognosis and survival after resection for bronchogenic carcinoma based on the 1997 TNM-staging classification: the Japanese experience. *Ann Thorac Surg* 2001; 71: 1759–1764.
14. Lopez-Encuentra A, Garcia-Lujan R, Rivas JJ, *et al.* Comparison between clinical and pathologic staging in 2,994 cases of lung cancer. *Ann Thorac Surg* 2005; 79: 974–979.
15. D'Cunha J, Herndon JE, Herzan DL, *et al.* Poor correspondence between clinical and pathologic staging in stage 1 non-small cell lung cancer: results from CALGB 9761, a prospective trial. *Lung Cancer* 2005; 48: 241–246.
16. Bronchogenic Carcinoma Cooperative Group of the Spanish Society of Pneumology and Thoracic Surgery (GCCB-S). Clinical tumour size and prognosis in lung cancer. *Eur Respir J* 1999; 14: 812–816.
17. Carbone E, Asamura H, Takei H, *et al.* T2 tumors larger than five centimeters in diameter can be upgraded to T3 in non-small cell lung cancer. *J Thorac Cardiovasc Surg* 2001; 122: 907–912.
18. Padilla J, Calvo V, Penalver JC, *et al.* Survival and risk model for stage IB non-small cell lung cancer. *Lung Cancer* 2002; 36: 43–48.
19. Christian C, Erica S, Morandi U. The prognostic impact of tumor size in resected stage I non-small cell lung cancer: evidence for a two thresholds tumor diameters classification. *Lung Cancer* 2006; 54: 185–191.
20. Mery CM, Pappas AN, Burt BM, *et al.* Diameter of non-small cell lung cancer correlates with long-term survival: implications for T stage. *Chest* 2005; 128: 3255–3260.
21. Mulligan CR, Meram AD, Proctor CD, *et al.* Lung cancer staging: a case for a new T definition. *Ann Thorac Surg* 2006; 82: 22022–22026.
22. Ou SH, Zell JA, Ziogas A, *et al.* Prognostic factors for survival of stage I nonsmall cell lung cancer patients: a population-based analysis of 19,702 stage I patients in the California Cancer Registry from 1989 to 2003. *Cancer* 2007; 110: 1532–1541.
23. Gajra A, Newman N, Gamble GP, *et al.* Impact of tumor size on survival in stage IA non-small cell lung cancer: a case for subdividing stage IA disease. *Lung Cancer* 2003; 42: 51–57.
24. Wisnivesky JP, Yankelevitz D, Henschke CI. The effect of tumor size on curability of stage I non-small cell lung cancers. *Chest* 2004; 126: 761–765.
25. Flieder DB, Port JL, Korst RJ, *et al.* Tumor size is a determinant of stage distribution in t[illegible] non-small cell lung cancer. *Chest* 2005; 128: 2304–2308.
26. Wisnivesky JP, Yankelevitz D, Henschke CI. Stage of lung cancer in relation to its size: part 2. Evidence. *Chest* 2005; 127: 1136–1139.
27. Ou SH, Zell JA, Ziogas A, *et al.* Prognostic significance of the non-size-based AJCC T2 descriptors: visceral pleura invasion, hilar atelectasis, or obstructive pneumonitis in stage IB non-small cell lung cancer is dependent on tumor size. *Chest* 2008; 133: 662–669.
28. Shimizu K, Yoshida J, Nagai K, *et al.* Visceral pleural invasion classification in non-small cell lung cancer: a proposal on the basis of outcome assessment. *J Thorac Cardiovasc Surg* 2004; 127: 1574–1578.

29. Riquet M, Lang-Lazdunski L, Le PB, *et al.* Characteristics and prognosis of resected T3 non-small cell lung cancer. *Ann Thorac Surg* 2002; 73: 253–258.
30. Wisnivesky JP, Henschke C, McGinn T, *et al.* Prognosis of stage II non-small cell lung cancer according to tumor and nodal status at diagnosis. *Lung Cancer* 2005; 49: 181–186.
31. Osaki T, Sugio K, Hanagiri T, *et al.* Survival and prognostic factors of surgically resected T4 non-small cell lung cancer. *Ann Thorac Surg* 2003; 75: 1745–1751.
32. Urschel JD, Urschel DM, Anderson TM, *et al.* Prognostic implications of pulmonary satellite nodules: are the 1997 staging revisions appropriate? *Lung Cancer* 1998; 21: 83–87.
33. Okumura T, Asamura H, Suzuki K, *et al.* Intrapulmonary metastasis of non-small cell lung cancer: a prognostic assessment. *J Thorac Cardiovasc Surg* 2001; 122: 24–28.
34. Bryant AS, Pereira SJ, Miller DL, *et al.* Satellite pulmonary nodule in the same lobe (T4N0) should not be staged as IIIB non-small cell lung cancer. *Ann Thorac Surg* 2006; 82: 1808–1813.
35. Nagai K, Sohara Y, Tsuchiya R, *et al.* Prognosis of resected non-small cell lung cancer patients with intrapulmonary metastases. *J Thorac Oncol* 2007; 2: 282–286.
36. Rao J, Sayeed RA, Tomaszek S, *et al.* Prognostic factors in resected satellite-nodule T4 non-small cell lung cancer. *Ann Thorac Surg* 2007; 84: 934–938.
37. André F, Grunenwald D, Pignon JP, *et al.* Survival of patients with resected N2 non-small-cell lung cancer: evidence for a subclassification and implications. *J Clin Oncol* 2000; 18: 2981–2989.
38. Lee YC, Wu CT, Kuo SW, *et al.* Significance of extranodal extension of regional lymph nodes in surgically resected non-small cell lung cancer. *Chest* 2007; 131: 993–999.
39. Riquet M, Assouad J, Bagan P, *et al.* Skip mediastinal lymph node metastasis and lung cancer: a particular N2 subgroup with a better prognosis. *Ann Thorac Surg* 2005; 79: 225–233.
40. Okada M, Sakamoto T, Yuki T, *et al.* Border between N1 and N2 stations in lung carcinoma: lessons from lymph node metastatic patterns of lower lobe tumors. *J Thorac Cardiovasc Surg* 2005; 129: 825–830.
41. Green MR, Lilenbaum RC. Stage IIIA category of non-small-cell lung cancer: a new proposal. *J Natl Cancer Inst* 1994; 86: 586–588.
42. Grunenwald D, Le Chevalier T. Re: Stage IIIA category of non-small-cell lung cancer: a new proposal. *J Natl Cancer Inst* 1997; 89: 88–89.
43. Curran WJ Jr, Cox JD, Azarnia N, *et al.* Comparison of the Radiation Therapy Oncology Group and American Joint Committee on Cancer staging systems among patients with non-small cell lung cancer receiving hyperfractionated radiation therapy. A report of the Radiation Therapy Oncology Group protocol 83-11. *Cancer* 1991; 68: 509–516.
44. Kreisman H, Lisbona A, Olson L, *et al.* Effect of radiologic stage III substage on nonsurgical therapy of non- small cell lung cancer. *Cancer* 1993; 72: 1588–1596.
45. Sculier JP, Paesmans M, Ninane V, *et al.* Evaluation of the TN sub-staging in patients with initially unresectable stage III non-small cell lung cancer treated by induction chemotherapy. The European Lung Cancer Working Party. *Lung Cancer* 1998; 22: 201–213.
46. Berghmans T, Lafitte JJ, Thiriaux J, *et al.* Survival is better predicted with a new classification of stage III unresectable non-small cell lung carcinoma treated by chemotherapy and radiotherapy. *Lung Cancer* 2004; 45: 339–348.
47. Ball D, Smith J, Wirth A, *et al.* Failure of T stage to predict survival in patients with non-small-cell lung cancer treated by radiotherapy with or without concomitant chemotherapy. *Int J Radiat Oncol Biol Phys* 2002; 54: 1007–1013.
48. Kameyama K, Huang CL, Liu D, *et al.* Problems related to TNM staging: patients with stage III non-small cell lung cancer. *J Thorac Cardiovasc Surg* 2002; 124: 503–510.
49. Goldstraw P, Crowley J, on behalf of the IASLC International Staging Project. The International Association for the Study of Lung Cancer international staging project on lung cancer. *J Thorac Oncol* 2006; 1: 281–286.
50. Groome PA, Bolejack V, Crowley JJ, *et al.* The IASLC Lung Cancer Staging Project: validation of the proposals for revision of the T, N, and M descriptors and consequent stage groupings in the

forthcoming (seventh) edition of the TNM classification of malignant tumours. *J Thorac Oncol* 2007; 2: 694–705.

51. Rami-Porta R, Ball D, Crowley J, *et al.* The IASLC Lung Cancer Staging Project: proposals for the revision of the T descriptors in the forthcoming (seventh) edition of the TNM classification for lung cancer. *J Thorac Oncol* 2007; 2: 593–602.
52. Rusch VW, Crowley J, Giroux DJ, *et al.* The IASLC Lung Cancer Staging Project: proposals for the revision of the N descriptors in the forthcoming seventh edition of the TNM classification for lung cancer. *J Thorac Oncol* 2007; 2: 603–612.
53. Postmus PE, Brambilla E, Chansky K, *et al.* The IASLC Lung Cancer Staging Project: proposals for revision of the M descriptors in the forthcoming (seventh) edition of the TNM classification of lung cancer. *J Thorac Oncol* 2007; 2: 686–693.
54. Goldstraw P, Crowley J, Chansky K, *et al.* The IASLC Lung Cancer Staging Project: proposals for the revision of the TNM stage groupings in the forthcoming (seventh) edition of the TNM Classification of malignant tumours. *J Thorac Oncol* 2007; 2: 706–714.
55. Naruke T, Suemasu K, Ishikawa S. Lymph node mapping and curability at various levels of metastasis in resected lung cancer. *J Thorac Cardiovasc Surg* 1978; 76: 832–839.
56. Mountain CF, Dresler CM. Regional lymph node classification for lung cancer staging. *Chest* 1997; 111: 1718–1723.
57. Watanabe S, Ladas G, Goldstraw P. Inter-observer variability in systematic nodal dissection: comparison of European and Japanese nodal designation. *Ann Thorac Surg* 2002; 73: 245–248.
58. Zelen M. Keynote address on biostatistics and data retrieval. *Cancer Chemother Rep 3* 1973; 4: 31–42.
59. Stahel R, Aisner J, Ginsberg R, *et al.* Staging and prognostic factors in small cell lung carcinoma. Consensus report. *In*: Hansen HH, Kristjansen PE, eds. Management of small cell lung cancer. Elsevier, Amsterdam, 1989; pp. 1–8.
60. Shepherd FA, Crowley J, Van HP, *et al.* The International Association for the Study of Lung Cancer lung cancer staging project: proposals regarding the clinical staging of small cell lung cancer in the forthcoming (seventh) edition of the tumor, node, metastasis classification for lung cancer. *J Thorac Oncol* 2007; 2: 1067–1077.
61. Sculier JP, Chansky K, Crowley JJ, *et al.* The impact of additional prognostic factors on survival and their relationship with the anatomical extent of disease expressed by the 6th Edition of the TNM Classification of Malignant Tumors and the proposals for the 7th Edition. *J Thorac Oncol* 2008; 3: 457–466.
62. Berghmans T, Dusart M, Paesmans M, *et al.* Primary tumor standardized uptake value (SUVmax) measured on fluorodeoxyglucose positron emission tomography (FDG-PET) is of prognostic value for survival in non-small cell lung cancer (NSCLC): a systematic review and meta-analysis (MA) by the European Lung Cancer Working Party for the IASLC Lung Cancer Staging Project. *J Thorac Oncol* 2008; 3: 6–12.
63. Martin B, Paesmans M, Berghmans T, *et al.* Role of Bcl-2 as a prognostic factor for survival in lung cancer: a systematic review of the literature with meta-analysis. *Br J Cancer* 2003; 89: 55–64.
64. Berghmans T, Paesmans M, Mascaux C, *et al.* Thyroid transcription factor 1 – a new prognostic factor in lung cancer: a meta-analysis. *Ann Oncol* 2006; 17: 1673–1676.
65. Mascaux C, Martin B, Paesmans M, *et al.* Has Cox-2 a prognostic role in non-small-cell lung cancer? A systematic review of the literature with meta-analysis of the survival results. *Br J Cancer* 2006; 95: 139–145.
66. Nakamura H, Kawasaki N, Taguchi M, *et al.* Survival impact of epidermal growth factor receptor overexpression in patients with non-small cell lung cancer: a meta-analysis. *Thorax* 2006; 61: 140–145.
67. Meert AP, Martin B, Delmotte P, *et al.* The role of EGF-R expression on patient survival in lung cancer: a systematic review with meta-analysis. *Eur Respir J* 2002; 20: 975–981.
68. Mascaux C, Iannino N, Martin B, *et al.* The role of RAS oncogene in survival of patients with lung cancer: a systematic review of the literature with meta-analysis. *Br J Cancer* 2005; 92: 131–139.

69. Huncharek M, Muscat J, Geschwind JF. K-ras oncogene mutation as a prognostic marker in non-small cell lung cancer: a combined analysis of 881 cases. *Carcinogenesis* 1999; 20: 1507–1510.
70. Martin B, Paesmans M, Mascaux C, *et al.* Ki-67 expression and patients survival in lung cancer: systematic review of the literature with meta-analysis. *Br J Cancer* 2004; 91: 2018–2025.
71. Meert AP, Martin B, Paesmans M, *et al.* The role of HER-2/neu expression on the survival of patients with lung cancer: a systematic review of the literature. *Br J Cancer* 2003; 89: 959–965.
72. Nakamura H, Kawasaki N, Taguchi M, *et al.* Association of HER-2 overexpression with prognosis in nonsmall cell lung carcinoma: a metaanalysis. *Cancer* 2005; 103: 1865–1873.
73. Delmotte P, Martin B, Paesmans M, *et al.* [VEGF and survival of patients with lung cancer: a systematic literature review and meta-analysis]. *Rev Mal Respir* 2002; 19: 577–584.
74. Meert AP, Paesmans M, Martin B, *et al.* The role of microvessel density on the survival of patients with lung cancer: a systematic review of the literature with meta-analysis. *Br J Cancer* 2002; 87: 694–701.
75. Trivella M, Pezzella F, Pastorino U, *et al.* Microvessel density as a prognostic factor in non-small-cell lung carcinoma: a meta-analysis of individual patient data. *Lancet Oncol* 2007; 8: 488–499.
76. Steels E, Paesmans M, Berghmans T, *et al.* Role of p53 as a prognostic factor for survival in lung cancer: a systematic review of the literature with a meta-analysis. *Eur Respir J* 2001; 18: 705–719.
77. Mitsudomi T, Hamajima N, Ogawa M, *et al.* Prognostic significance of p53 alterations in patients with non-small cell lung cancer: a meta-analysis. *Clin Cancer Res* 2000; 6: 4055–4063.
78. Huncharek M, Kupelnick B, Geschwind JF, *et al.* Prognostic significance of p53 mutations in non-small cell lung cancer: a meta-analysis of 829 cases from eight published studies. *Cancer Lett* 2000; 153: 219–226.
79. Choma D, Daures JP, Quantin X, *et al.* Aneuploidy and prognosis of non-small-cell lung cancer: a meta-analysis of published data. *Br J Cancer* 2001; 85: 14–22.
80. Fan J, Wang L, Jiang GN, *et al.* The role of survivin on overall survival of non-small cell lung cancer, a meta-analysis of published literatures. *Lung Cancer* 2008; 61: 91–96.
81. Zhu CQ, Shih W, Ling CH, *et al.* Immunohistochemical markers of prognosis in non-small cell lung cancer: a review and proposal for a multiphase approach to marker evaluation. *J Clin Pathol* 2006; 59: 790–800.
82. McShane LM, Altman DG, Sauerbrei W, *et al.* Reporting recommendations for tumor marker prognostic studies. *J Clin Oncol* 2005; 23: 9067–9072.

CHAPTER 10

Functional evaluation for treatment

C.F.N. Koegelenberg, D. Plekker, C.T. Bolliger

Division of Pulmonology, Dept of Medicine, University of Stellenbosch and Tygerberg Academic Hospital, Cape Town, South Africa.

Correspondence: C.F.N. Koegelenberg, Dept of Medicine, Faculty of Health Sciences, University of Stellenbosch and Tygerberg Academic Hospital, P.O. Box 19063, Tygerberg, 7505, Cape Town, South Africa. E-mail: coeniefn@sun.ac.za

Only 15–25% of all lung cancers are operable, and despite advances in chemo- and radiotherapy, pulmonary resection represents the only curative intervention [1, 2]. The pre-operative assessment of patients with bronchogenic carcinoma comprises three entities: 1) tumour type, 2) tumour stage, and 3) cardiopulmonary reserves (fig. 1) [3]. Depending on the extent, pulmonary resections lead to permanent loss of pulmonary function. A previously healthy person tolerates a pneumonectomy remarkably well. However, 90% of lung cancer patients, are current or past smokers and frequently have varying degrees of concomitant chronic obstructive pulmonary disease (COPD) and/or ischaemic heart disease [1, 2]. Lung cancer patients who undergo resection are therefore at particular risk of developing post-operative complications and dying. Moreover, patients are at risk of ending up with permanent respiratory disability. BECHARD [4] suggested that the term "operability" be used to denote the ability of the patient to endure the physical stress of the operation itself and that "resectability" should refer to the amount of lung tissue that can be resected without rendering the patient a respiratory cripple. The term resectability is, however, more often used to indicate the anatomical resectability of a tumour. Most authorities therefore simply use the term operability to denote both the short- and long-term ability of a patient to endure pulmonary resection [1–3].

In the present chapter, we will review the current evidence base for various parameters of functional operability and post-operative complications, discuss the assessment of regional lung function and the calculation of predicted post-operative lung function, and conclude with a practical algorithm for the functional assessment prior to pulmonary resection.

Parameters of functional operability

The chief parameters for the functional evaluation are summarised in table 1 and discussed below. It remains imperative that all pulmonary function tests and other functional parameters are measured when patients are at their personal best. Patients may require an intensive course of bronchodilator therapy and a short course of oral steroids.

General clinical assessment

Advanced age. Advanced age, often defined as >70 yrs, has been shown to predict complications following lung resection [5, 6]. Co-morbidities associated with increased

Eur Respir Mon, 2009, 44, 169–186. Printed in UK - all rights reserved. Copyright ERS Journals Ltd 2009; European Respiratory Monograph; ISSN 1025-448x.

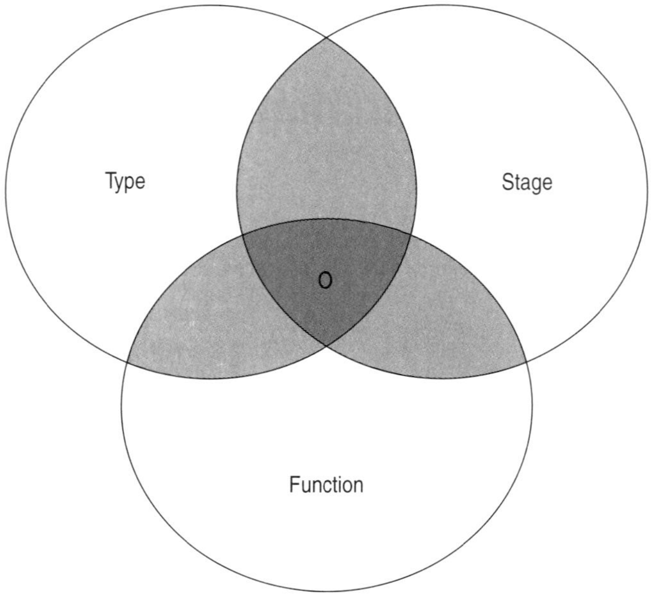

Fig. 1. – The three entities that determine the management of a patient with lung cancer: tumour type, tumour extent (stage) and functional class. Only 15–25% of all patients are operable (O) at the time of diagnosis. The tumour type can be either nonsmall cell lung cancer (NSCLC) or small cell lung cancer (SCLC). Tumour stage refers to either the TNM staging for NSCLC or limited *versus* extensive disease in the case of SCLC. The cardiopulmonary reserve (functional class) is assessed by means of various parameters (see text).

age, rather than ageing itself, are likely to be responsible for this observation [7]. In fact, CONTI *et al.* [8] found that patients >70 yrs of age with a good performance status (Karnofsky score: 70 points) and intact cardiopulmonary reserves had a long-term survival comparable with younger surgical patients. Elderly patients therefore should not be excluded from surgery solely on the basis of their age [1].

Cigarette smoking. The fact that smoking is a risk factor for post-operative pulmonary complications has been known for >60 yrs [9]. Cigarette smoking increases this risk irrespective of the presence of chronic pulmonary disease [7]. The relative risk may be as

Table 1. – Important parameters of functional operability

General clinical assessment	Age Smoking status Chronic obstructive lung disease General health and nutritional state
Spirometry	FEV_1 $FEV_{1,ppo}$
Diffusion capacity	$D_{L,CO}$ $D_{L,CO,ppo}$
Exercise capacity	$V'_{O_2,max}$ $V'_{O_2,max,ppo}$
Cardiac risk assessment	See table 2
Extent of resection	Estimation of post-operative lung function

FEV_1: forced expiratory volume in 1 s; ppo: predicted post-operative value; $D_{L,CO}$, diffusing capacity of the lung for carbon monoxide; $V'_{O_2,max}$: maximal oxygen uptake.

high as 4.3 [9], and only decreases significantly after 8 weeks of cessation [8]. Postponing pulmonary resection for 8 weeks purely for the sake of smoking cessation is impractical, especially in lung cancer patients who should undergo resection with the shortest possible delay, and the impact of <8 weeks of smoking on post-operative complications is controversial. At least two studies have shown that quitting <8 weeks prior to surgery may paradoxically increase the risk for complications [10, 11].

COPD. COPD is the most frequently identified risk factor for pulmonary complications amongst patients undergoing any form of surgery [12]. Patients with overt COPD have a relative risk of 4.7 of developing post-operative complications following thoracic surgery [7]. Moreover, both the presence of abnormalities on physical examination (*e.g.* prolonged expiration and wheezes), and the degree of obstruction (as measured by means of spirometry) correlate with these events. It is therefore paramount to institute optimal medical management of COPD prior to pulmonary resection. There is currently no prospective evidence to estimate the risk of post-operative complications in patients with restrictive ventilatory impairment [12]. Well-controlled asthma is not associated with post-operative complications, neither is a short course of oral corticosteroids [12].

General health and nutritional status. The American Society of Anesthesiologists' (ASA) classification has been shown to predict post-operative complications. Patients with an ASA class of III (patient with a systemic disease that is not incapacitating) or higher have an odds ratio of 2.6 for post-operative pulmonary complications when compared to patients with ASA class I and II [12]. Partial and total dependence have been shown to be major risk factors [13]. Patients who are dependent are therefore unlikely to be candidates for major pulmonary resection.

Metabolic disturbances contribute to post-operative complications. Malnutrition (albumin <30 $g \cdot L^{-1}$, odds ratio 2.5) reduces ventilatory drive to hypoxia and hypercapnia, contributes to respiratory muscle dysfunction, alters lung elasticity and impairs immunity. Nutritional intervention prior to surgery does not attenuate the risk. A blood urea >30 $mg \cdot dL^{-1}$ (10.7 $mmol \cdot L^{-1}$) carries an odds ratio of 2.3 for post-operative complications [12, 13].

Other risk factors. Notwithstanding the assumption that obesity is a risk factor for post-operative complications, multiple prospective studies have found no significant increase in complications [12]. The same is true for alcohol abuse.

Spirometry

Background. Various parameters of pulmonary mechanics have been recommended. As early as 1955, GAENSLER *et al.* [14] recommended the use of the vital capacity (VC), and suggested a cut-off of >2 L before pulmonary resection, without mentioning the extent. Although other authors have also reported the use of the VC, either in absolute values or in percentage of predicted, it has been abandoned over time. Other parameters, such as peak flow, maximal midexpiratory flow and the maximal voluntary ventilation could also not be validated as pre-operative parameters [15]. In fact, only measurements of the forced expiratory volume in 1 s (FEV1) have stood the test of time.

FEV1. Early recommendations of FEV1 values for safe resections were >2 L for pneumonectomy [16, 17] and >1.5 L for lobectomy [17, 18]. These absolute cut-off values that are currently still endorsed by the British Thoracic Society (BTS) [19], were based on data from >2,000 patients in three large series in the 1970s [20]. Unfortunately none of these series reported percentages of predicted. The use of absolute values has never been universally accepted, as they do not take sex, height, weight and age into consideration, nor do they consider the actual functional contribution of the tissue to be removed [15, 20].

Three authors suggested cut-offs for FEV_1 in percentage predicted: MITTMAN [21] suggested >70%, whereas NAGASAKI *et al.* [5] and, more recently, PATE *et al.* [22] suggested >40%. None of the three studies mentioned the extent of resection possible with these values.

Predicted post-operative FEV_1. In recent years, interest has shifted to the so-called predicted post-operative (ppo) function. The techniques used for this estimation are discussed later in the present chapter, as they are not only used to measure $FEV_{1,ppo}$, but also the post-operative diffusing capacity of the lung for carbon monoxide ($D_{L,CO,ppo}$) and maximal oxygen consumption on exercise testing ($V'_{O_2,max,ppo}$). OLSEN *et al.* [23] suggested a $FEV_{1,ppo}$ threshold of 800 mL as a lower limit for pulmonary resection. PATE *et al.* [22] suggested lowering the limit to 700 mL. These values, as is the case with pre-operative FEV_1, inherently discriminated against short individuals, females and elderly people. It therefore became apparent that establishing the threshold for spirometry expressed as a percentage ppo (%ppo) would be ideal.

Numerous prospective studies have validated a $\%FEV_{1,ppo}$ of <40% as a prohibitive threshold for pulmonary resection. MARKOS *et al.* [24], WAHI *et al.* [25] and BOLLIGER *et al.* [26] all found mortality rates of ~50% in patients with a $\%FEV_{1,ppo}$ of <40%. NAKAHARA *et al.* [27] found an even higher mortality (60%) in patients with a $\%FEV_{1,ppo}$ of <30%.

Diffusion capacity

$D_{L,CO}$. The $D_{L,CO}$ is a proxy measurement of alveolar oxygen exchange [28]. As early as 1963, CANDER [29] suggested that a value of <50% of predicted precluded pulmonary resections. FERGUSON *et al.* [30] first demonstrated $D_{L,CO}$ to be an independent predictor of post-operative mortality. They identified a $D_{L,CO}$ of <60% of predicted as a cut-off value for major pulmonary resection. Similar findings were reported by MARKOS *et al.* [31].

The predicted post-operative $D_{L,CO}$. The predicted post-operative $D_{L,CO}$ ($D_{L,CO,ppo}$), rather than the actual value, is increasingly being used as a further refinement, particularly in patients with impaired pulmonary reserves [28]. A $D_{L,CO,ppo}$ value of <40% identifies high-risk patients [32]. The $D_{L,CO,ppo}$ values derived from various methods (discussed below) have been shown to overestimate immediate post-operative values, but there is a significant correlation between actual values 1 month after resection and $D_{L,CO,ppo}$ values [28]. Despite being included in current guidelines, the European Thoracic Surgery Database recently suggested that in only one-quarter of patients were actual $D_{L,CO}$ values measured prior to pulmonary resection [33].

Exercise testing

Background. Exercise testing differs conceptually from the other indices discussed thus far in that it provides an ideal overall parameter for the assessment of cardiopulmonary reserves, as it evaluates the fitness of a patient [1]. It is increasingly being used to assess the aerobic reserves of pulmonary resection candidates. Patients with marginal aerobic reserves more often have major difficulties coping with the multiple pathophysiological changes associated with major surgery. Formal cardiopulmonary exercise testing (CPET) is well validated, but requires a significant degree of expertise and is not universally available. Several cheaper surrogates that require less technology have been suggested, including stair climbing and walking tests.

Formal CPET. Currently, maximal or symptom-limited exercise tests with a cycle or treadmill are recommended. They are performed in a controlled environment and have the advantage of good reproducibility, Furthermore, various parameters, including cardiac ischaemia, are assessed in real-time. Although in 1952, TAYLOR *et al.* [34] had already showed that $V'_{O_2,max}$ measured during CPET was an objective parameter of cardiopulmonary reserves, it was not before 1982 that the assessment of $V'_{O_2,max}$ gained interest after a report by EUGENE *et al.* [35]. In a small series of only 19 patients, they were able show that a $V'_{O_2,max}$ <1,000 mL was associated with a 75% peri-operative mortality.

Subsequent studies better defined cut-off $V'_{O_2,max}$ values [26, 36–40]. A value of >20 mL·kg^{-1}·min^{-1} or >75% of predicted [36] qualifies for resection up to pneumonectomy, whereas a value <10 mL·kg^{-1}·min^{-1} (or <40% of predicted) is generally prohibitive for any resection, as it caries a high risk for mortality. Another frequently cited cut-off for safe resection of at least one lobe is a $V'_{O_2,max}$ of ≥15 mL·kg^{-1}·min^{-1} [37–39]. With regards to $V'_{O_2,max,ppo}$, prospective evidence indicates that values of <10 mL·kg^{-1}·min^{-1} are associated with a high risk of post-operative complications and death [26].

Low-technology (minimal achievement) exercise tests. In the absence of sophisticated exercise equipment, low-technology (minimal achievement) exercise tests are sometimes utilised to estimate the post-operative risk. Stair climbing is by far the most used and best validated of these tests, although it is still not universally accepted, mostly because of a lack of standardisation [40].

The major advantages of stair climbing lie in its availability, simplicity, brevity and in the familiarity of subjects with this form of exercise. It has even been reported that stair climbing yields greater values of V'_{O_2} values than cycle ergometry [41, 42]. BRUNELLI *et al.* [43] published the largest prospective study (n=160) to evaluate the capability of stair climbing to predict cardiopulmonary complications following pulmonary resection for lung cancer. Patients who experienced no complications on average climbed to a height of 20.6 m, whereas those with complications could only master a mean height of 14.96 m ($p<0.001$). The authors concluded that stair climbing was safe, and that height achieved was the best predictor of serious cardiopulmonary complications (irrespective of the extent of resection). Several smaller studies yielded comparable results.

In a recent study performed by KOEGELENBERG *et al.* [40] on pulmonary resection candidates, the average speed of ascent over a 20 m standardised climb was compared to $V'_{O_2,max}$ values measured by means of cycle ergometry. A significant linear correlation was demonstrated ($R^2=0.67$), and the authors were able to identify potential cut-off values with relation to pulmonary resection. A speed of elevation of 15 m·min^{-1} correlated with a $V'_{O_2,max}$ of 20 mL·kg^{-1}·min^{-1} (potential cut-off for pneumonectomy), whereas a speed of 12 m·min^{-1} correlated with a $V'_{O_2,max}$ of 15 mL·kg^{-1}·min^{-1} (potential cut-off for lobectomy).

Walking tests have been suggested by some authorities [28]. Both 6- and 12-min walking distances have been shown to correlate with $V'_{O_2,max}$ in patients with COPD. The shuttle walk test has been reported to be even more reproducible and more highly correlated with $V'_{O_2,max}$ measured by formal CPET [44, 45]. SINGH *et al.* [46] suggested that 25 shuttles on a shuttle walk test indicate a $V'_{O_2,max}$ of 10 mL·kg^{-1}·min^{-1}, and this cut-off value was even suggested in the functional algorithm proposed by the BTS [19]. Unfortunately, numerous prospective studies failed to validate either the 6- and 12-min walking distances or the shuttle walk test [47, 48]. Therefore, the use of these tests can currently not be advocated.

Cardiac risk assessment

Principles. In comparison to the abundant literature on pulmonary function evaluation prior to pulmonary resection, less has been published on the evaluation of cardiac risk specific to lung cancer surgery. Yet cardiac complications are second only to pulmonary complications as a cause of peri-operative morbidity and mortality after pulmonary resection. In 1961, MITTMAN [21] had already showed that an abnormal ECG was associated with an increased risk of suffering an intraoperative or post-operative cardiac event. Many authors subsequently reported similar findings. GOLDMAN *et al.* [49] published the multifactorial cardiac risk index in 1977, which has since been validated by many reports. In 1999, LEE *et al.* [50] revised Goldman's criteria for cardiac risk index and developed six independent predictors/variables (see table 2) that correlated with post-operative cardiac complications. Patients with more than two variables have a post-operative cardiac complication rate of >10% and are considered to be high risk. The revised Goldman's criteria are currently used by many authorities. Pulmonary resection remains high risk surgery (*i.e.* one variable positive), and any patient with more than one variable positive needs urgent review and potential intervention by a cardiologist.

Interventions. Coronary angioplasty and stenting may be performed prior to pulmonary resection, although there is little evidence that it influences cardiac risk [2]. Previously it was suggested that, if necessary, patients undergo coronary artery bypass surgery prior to lung cancer surgery, although this approach may delay curative resection of bronchogenic carcinoma. Furthermore, when conventional coronary artery bypass surgery is combined with lung cancer surgery, there is an increased risk of morbidity and mortality [51, 52]. DYSZKIEWICZ *et al.* [53] investigated combining minimally invasive ("off-pump") direct coronary artery bypass with lung cancer resection. Complications were comparable with lung resection alone and there were no post-operative myocardial infarctions or episodes of myocardial ischaemia.

Table 2. – Revised Goldman Cardiac Risk Index: six independent predictors of major cardiac complications

1. High-risk type of surgery
2. History of ischaemic heart disease
   a. History of myocardial infarction (within 6 months)
   b. Positive exercise test
   c. Current complaint of ischaemic chest pain
   d. Use of nitrate therapy
   e. Pathological Q waves on ECG

(Not included: prior coronary revascularisation procedure unless one of the other criteria for ischaemic heart disease is present)

3. History of cardiac failure
4. History of cerebrovascular disease
5. Diabetes mellitus requiring treatment with insulin
6. Pre-operative serum creatinine >2.0 mg·dL^{-1} (177 μmol·L)$^{-1}$

The number of positive variables correlates with the risk for major post-operative cardiac complication: with no risk factors, the risk is 0.4%; with one risk factor the risk is 0.9%; with two risk factors it is 7%; and with ≥3, the risk is 11.0%. Reproduced from [50] with permission from the publisher.

Other parameters

Extent of resection. There is a clear correlation between the extent of resection and post-operative morbidity and mortality. The mortality after pneumonectomy is usually twice that after lobectomy: A lobectomy, for example, caries a 30-day mortality of up to 2–3% and a pneumonectomy up to 4–6% [1, 2]. The estimation of the amount of lung tissue that can safely be removed is therefore very important in the pre-operative evaluation, and the development of split-function studies has made it possible to calculate the relative function of the tissue to be removed to the total function of both lungs, and thereby to predict post-operative function (see later in the present chapter).

Static lung volumes and related indices. Static lung volumes and related indices measured by body plethysmography have been suggested to appreciate the extent of overinflation as a potential risk factor [15]. Published recommendations for the residual volume and airway resistance varied greatly, and the use of these parameters has been abandoned over time.

Blood gas measurements. The predictive value of arterial blood gas measurements remains uncertain. There is no general agreement regarding a value of the arterial oxygen tension that would indicate a definite increased risk for pulmonary resections. A raised carbon dioxide tension of >6 kPa (45 mmHg) has an increased risk of post-operative complications [5, 22], but is not considered sufficient (as a single parameter) to preclude pulmonary resection.

Pulmonary haemodynamics. Early investigators found that following major lung resection, exercise capacity was decreased due to a reduced maximal cardiac output [15]. It was postulated that the reduction of the pulmonary vascular bed led to pulmonary artery hypertension and subsequently to right ventricular failure. Pre-operative right ventricular and pulmonary vascular reserve with the use of temporary unilateral occlusion of the pulmonary artery was therefore assessed by numerous investigators. With this technique, the pulmonary artery pressure and the arterial oxygen tension (P_{a,O_2}) at rest and during exercise were measured while the pulmonary artery of the lung to be resected was occluded by a balloon tipped catheter [15]. Many investigators showed that an increased pulmonary artery pressure and a fall in the P_{a,O_2} on temporary unilateral occlusion of the pulmonary artery were associated with increased operative risk. This technique has, however, largely been abandoned due to its invasiveness, high failure rate, complications and the conflicting results published by various investigators.

The assessment of regional lung function

The assessment of regional lung function forms an essential part of the pre-operative evaluation of pulmonary resection candidates with impaired lung function. Physicians involved in the pre-operative evaluation of such patients need to be able to utilise the various means of estimating the relative contribution of the pulmonary parenchyma earmarked for resection. As discussed earlier, patients with impaired pulmonary functions (FEV1 and/or $D_{L,CO}$ of <80% of predicted) warrant more extensive evaluation of their pulmonary reserves, which should include CPET. A decision regarding operability is subsequently based not only on the pre-operative percentage of predicted for spiromeric values (most importantly FEV1, $D_{L,CO}$ and $V'_{O_2,max}$), but more importantly on the ppo of these parameters. The ppo value for these parameters (be it a spirometric volume, diffusion capacity or oxygen uptake) is equal to the pre-operative values × (1-fractional contribution of tissue earmarked for resection) [1–3]. There are four validated ways of estimating the relative functional contribution or split function: anatomic calculation, split radionucleotide perfusion scanning, quantitative computer tomography scanning and dynamic perfusion magnetic resonance imaging (MRI) [54].

Techniques available to estimate regional lung function and calculate ppo values

Anatomical calculations. Anatomical calculations of the ppo values are the simplest and oldest method of predicting regional lung function. They were initially introduced in the 1930s; numerous refinements were then described up to 1970. Following the introduction of scintigraphy, anatomical calculations were abandoned for some years, but again revived in the 1990s, and subsequently firmly re-established as reasonable predictors of post-resectional pulmonary function [54].

Anatomical calculations are usually based on the number of segments to be resected, thereby estimating ppo function as the fraction of the segments remaining [55, 56], or similarly the number of subsegments [57]. Further distinctions between occluded and patent segments or subsegments are often made, whereby the loss of occluded segments is disregarded. The current validated formulae are summarised in table 3. In clinical practicality, the $FEV_{1,ppo}$ is most frequently estimated by means of the segmental formula, *i.e.* pre-operative FEV_1 × [(19-patent segments removed)/19]. For a right lower lobectomy, for example, $FEV_{1,ppo}$ would be equal to the pre-operative FEV_1 × (14/19), provided that the segments are all endoscopically patent. If a patient with an actual pre-operative FEV_1 of 2.40 L (63.2% of a predicted 3.80 L) undergoes this procedure, then the $FEV_{1,ppo}$ will be 2.40 × 14/19=1.77 l (46.6% of a predicted 3.80 L). The $D_{L,CO,ppo}$ and $V'_{O_2,max,ppo}$ are calculated in a similar way.

Prospective data comparing post-operative estimations based on the various anatomical calculations with actual post-operative lung function are limited. BOLLIGER *et al.* [58] found similar and equally significant correlations when they studied these calculations in pulmonary resection candidates. They were able to show a correlation coefficient (r) of 0.88 when comparing anatomical estimates to actual lung functions 6 months post-operatively for FEV_1, 0.85 for forced vital capacity (FVC), 0.84 for $D_{L,CO}$ and 0.75 for $V'_{O_2,max}$. They also showed that anatomical calculations were less accurate at predicting ppo function following pneumonectomy than lobectomy. Stratifying patients according to obstructive airflow limitation did not alter the correlations.

Radionucleotide perfusion scanning. Radiospirometry (with xenon-133) for the analysis of regional ventilation described >50 yrs ago, was in general use up to the

Table 3. – Anatomical calculations: validated formulae

1. Number of segments:
   ppo function=pre-operative function × (1-*y*/19), where y is the number of segments to be removed, and 19 the total number of segments.
2. Number of functional segments:
   ppo function=pre-operative function (1-*y*/*z*), where *y* is the number of functional segments to be removed, and *z* the total number of functional segments.
3. Number of subsegments:
   ppo function=pre-operative function × (1-(b-n)/(42-n)), where n is the number of obstructed and b the total number of subsegments in the resected lobe; it is assumed that b=6, 4, 12 in the right upper, middle and lower lobes, respectively, and 10 each in the left upper and lower lobes.

1970s. Several studies validated the use of this modality, and the functional loss as predicted by radiospirometry was considered accurate as long as the resection involved more than three segments. OLSEN *et al.* [59] published a landmark study in 1974, which showed that split perfusion scans using intravenous technetium-99 macroaggregates accurately predicted functional loss 3 months post-pneumonectomy. Numerous authors confirmed the feasibility of estimating ventilatory function by perfusion scanning. Radionucleotide perfusion scanning ultimately replaced radiospirometry, given its general availability, ease of performance and superior reproducibility [54].

Technetium-99m-macroaggregated albumin remains the radiopharmaceutical of choice with regards to pulmonary perfusion [54]. It is trapped in the pulmonary capillary bed, and emits gamma rays proportional to local perfusion. Patients should be scanned in the sitting position and in four projections (anterior, posterior, left posterior oblique and right posterior oblique) with 5×10^5 counts per image each on a one-head gamma camera (single photon emission computed tomography (SPECT) scan) [60]. Figure 2 contains examples of images from a SPECT scan. Quantification is performed by means of a system-integrated region-ratio programme in the anterior and posterior projections for right–left lung quantification (geometric mean), in the left posterior oblique projection for left lung and the right posterior oblique projection for right lung lobar quantification [58].

In a prospective study by BOLLIGER *et al.* [58], radionucleotide perfusion scanning outperformed anatomical calculations and quantitative computed tomography (CT) scanning with regards to the range of functional parameters. Estimates of post-operative function based on perfusion scans consistently exhibited the highest correlations with post-operatively measured values for FEV1 (r=0.92), FVC (r=0.90), $D_{L,CO}$ (r=0.85) and $V'_{O_2,max}$ (r=0.85). Other investigators found similar correlations [61].

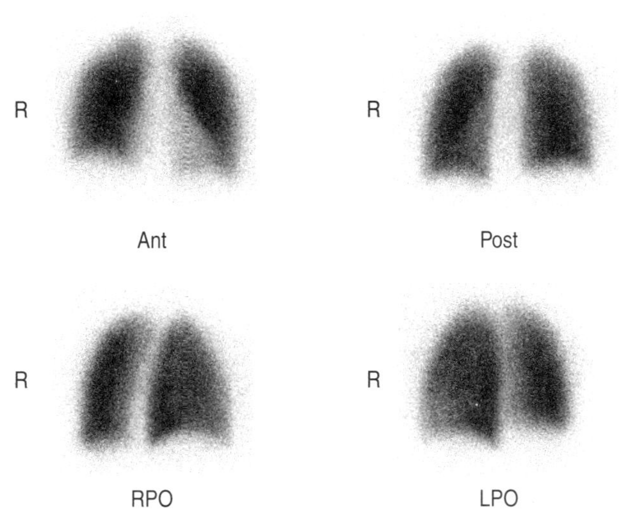

Fig. 2. – Radionucleotide perfusion scan. An example of a radionucleotide perfusion scan performed on a patient with normal pulmonary perfusion (technetium-99m single photon emission computed tomography). Quantification is performed by means of a system-integrated region-ratio programme in the anterior (Ant) and posterior (Post) projections for right–left lung quantification (geometric mean), in the right posterior oblique (RPO) projection for right lung lobar quantification and in the left posterior oblique (LPO) projection for the left lung. R: right. (Scans kindly provided by A. Ellmann, Medical Imaging and Clinical Oncology, University of Stellenbosch and Tygerberg Academic Hospital, Cape Town, South Africa.)

Pulmonary quantitative CT scanning. Pulmonary quantitative CT scanning has become an extremely popular modality, given its simplicity, the universal availability of CT scans and the fact that most lung cancer patients invariably have chest CT scans. WU *et al.* [62] pioneered the technique in the early 1990s and later refined it following technological advances in the field of CT [63]. Quantitative CT scans should be performed at full inspiration and viewed with a standard-spatial-frequency reconstruction algorithm. Semi-automated analyses of the parenchymal views are then performed by means of commercially available software in order to identify the "total functional lung volume" (TFLV). The lung parenchyma is outlined from the outer mediastinum and inner chest wall by means of a cursor. Three quantitative segments are then generated (three different colours) by applying thresholds of more than -500 Hounsfield units (HU), -500 to -910 HU and less than -910 HU, respectively (fig. 3). The TFLV is then automatically calculated as a volume (the product of colour segments areas and section thickness). The volume of the tumour-bearing lobe(s) or lung is measured in a similar way and designated the "regional functional lung volume" (RFLV). The CT-ppo FEV_1 values are then calculated as follows: $FEV_{1,ppo}$=pre-operative $FEV_1 \times (1-(RFLV/TFLV))$ [62, 63]. Similar calculations are performed for FVC_{ppo}.

Predictions by CT correlate well with actual post-operative measurements. In their landmark study, WU *et al.* [62] found that, irrespective of the extent of resection, $FEV_{1,ppo}$ and FVC_{ppo} showed statistically significant correlations with post-operative measured values (r=0.93 and 0.86, respectively) [62]. BOLLIGER *et al.* [58], WU *et al.* [63] and OHNO *et al.* [64] subsequently found comparable correlations. Furthermore, BOLLIGER *et al.* [58] and WU *et al.* [63] also concluded that quantitative CT was more accurate at predicting functional loss after lobectomy (r=0.90) than pneumonectomy (r=0.88). Only BOLLIGER *et al.* [58] reported prospective data on the ability of quantitative CT scans to predict post-operative $D_{L,CO}$ and $V'_{O_2,max}$. They showed that

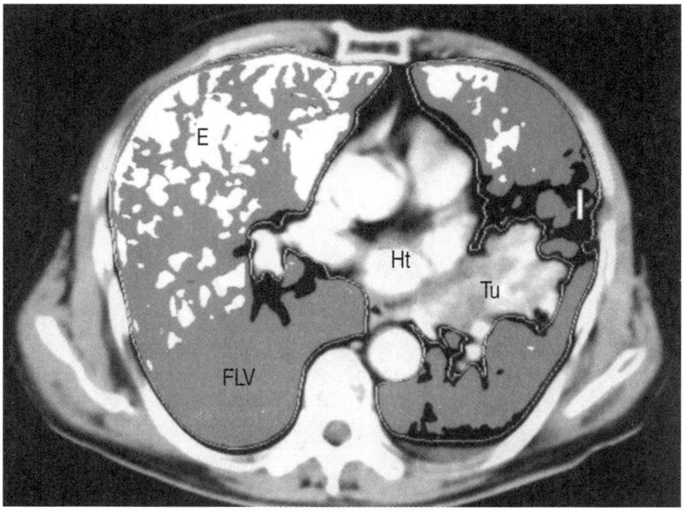

Fig. 3. – Pulmonary quantitative computed tomography (CT) scan. Quantitative CT map shows functional lung volume of representative slice. Lung parenchyma was first outlined from mediastinum and chest wall by default range of -200 and -1,024 HU (white line contours). Tumour (Tu) was also excluded. After applying dual threshold, three segments in lung parenchyma were generated. The white area below -910 HU denoted emphysema (E), black area above -500 HU denoted infiltration and atelectasis, and grey area between -500 and -910 HU denoted functional lung volume (FLV). Ht: heart. Reproduced from [63], with permission from the publisher.

the CT-derived $D_{L,CO,ppo}$ correlated well, whereas $V'_{O_2,max,ppo}$ correlated less well than perfusion scan-derived estimates (r=0.77 *versus* 0.85).

Dynamic contrast-enhanced perfusion MRI. Although dynamic perfusion MRI is well established in the evaluation of regional pulmonary perfusion in healthy volunteers, its potential role in predicting post-operative lung function was only recently appreciated following a landmark study by OHNO *et al.* [65]. Dynamic perfusion MRI studies are performed on a 1.5-T scanner using a phased array coil. The studies are acquired with a three-dimensional radiofrequency-spoiled gradient-echo sequence (fig. 4). A bolus of 3–5 mL of gadopentetate dimeglumine is administered with an automatic infusion system prior to the scan. Analysing and interpreting the data acquired by means of dynamic contrast-enhanced perfusion MRI requires some degree of expertise, as well as appropriate computer software. Regional pulmonary blood volume is calculated from the MRI signal intensity–time course curve. The $FEV_{1,ppo}$ (perfusion MRI) value=$FEV_1 \times$(1-(percentage of perfusion resected lobe or lung/100)) [64, 65].

The study by OHNO *et al.* [65] is arguably the largest prospective study in the field of ppo lung functions. OHNO *et al.* [65] compared dynamic perfusion MRIs ability to predict post-operative FEV_1 with that of CT and SPECT. They found the ability of perfusion MRI (r=0.87) and quantitative CT (r=0.88) to predict actual post-operative FEV_1 superior to that of SPECT (r=0.83). It is noteworthy that the investigators did not assess the ppo of other parameters (most notably $D_{L,CO}$ and $V'_{O_2,max}$).

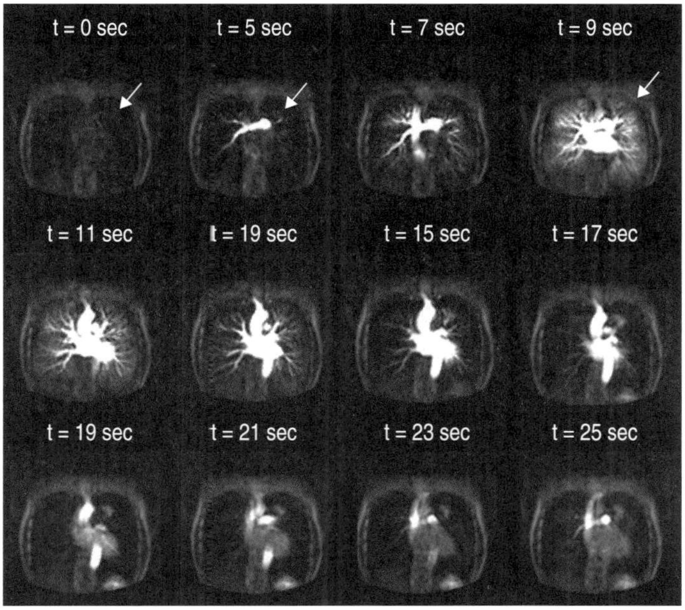

Fig. 4. – Dynamic perfusion magnetic resonance imaging (MRI). A dynamic perfusion MRI of a 63-yr-old male subject with adenocarcinoma in upper lobe of left lung. The images show heterogeneous but well-enhanced pulmonary parenchyma at 5 and 13 s in portions of lungs not affected by lung cancer (arrows). Lung cancer also is enhanced after 13 s. Reproduced from [64], with permission from the publisher.

Practical approach to the assessment of regional lung function prior to pulmonary resection

Patients with an FEV1 and/or a *D*L,CO of <80% of the predicted warrant a formal exercise test and, if their exercise capacity is impaired ($V'O_{2,max}$ <20 mL·kg^{-1}·min^{-1} or 75% of predicted), calculations of the ppo values of FEV1, *D*L,CO and $V'O_{2,max}$ are needed. Some authorities even advocate the performance of split studies prior to formal exercise tests, but the cost effectiveness of this approach has been questioned, as exercise tests are cheap and noninvasive [1–3].

Estimations of ppo lung function based on anatomical calculations are by far the simplest way of predicting post-resectional lung function. Although these calculations are less accurate than other techniques, they remain useful screening tools as they err on the side of safety. Anatomical estimations have been shown in prospective studies to overestimate functional loss [54], as there may be minimal loss after removal of destroyed and collapsed lung parenchyma [54]. A reasonable approach, therefore, would be to perform anatomical calculations in each pulmonary resection candidate requiring assessment of predicted post-operative lung function, and to reserve the more complex techniques for the borderline or apparent inoperable cases.

Until recently, radionucleotide perfusion scanning was considered the gold standard for the assessment of regional lung function. Recent advances in radiology with regards to quantitative CT scanning and dynamic contrast-enhanced perfusion MRI have certainly challenged this notion [54]. Variations in study protocols, local expertise and equipment complicate the direct comparison between different modalities. Furthermore, some studies only evaluated the ability of the modalities to predict post-operative FEV1. Both *D*L,CO,ppo and $V'O_{2,max,ppo}$ predict post-operative complications [1–3], and radionucleotide perfusion scanning may be superior to quantitative CT scanning at predicting the post-operative values of these parameters [52, 58].

In summary, anatomical calculations of ppo values should be performed on all patients who require pre-operative estimation of post-operative lung function. Patients who require further evaluation will require either radionucleotide perfusion scanning, quantitative CT scanning or dynamic contrast-enhanced perfusion MRI. All three techniques perform comparatively well at predicting post-operative FEV1. Cost, local expertise and availability, as well as the need to predict $V'O_{2,max,ppo}$, should dictate the choice between these modalities. Staging CT scans are invariably performed pre-operatively on practically all lung cancer patients. Quantitative CT scanning is therefore arguably the investigation of choice with regards to the prediction of post-operative function in lung cancer patients, as it is well validated [52, 58, 63], generally available and relatively cheap. A degree of expertise and the appropriate software are, however, required.

Algorithm for the functional assessment prior to pulmonary resection

All pulmonary resection candidates should undergo a pre-operative clinical evaluation, focussing on respiratory, cardiovascular and other clinical parameters discussed above. A resting ECG should be performed on all candidates. Airflow limitation should be optimised prior to further evaluation and cardiac disease identified and managed either medically or surgically. The initial pulmonary function evaluation should include at least an FEV1, FVC and *D*L,CO. Values >80% of predicted for FEV1 and *D*L,CO are associated with an uncomplicated surgical course for resection up to a pneumonectomy, whereas an FEV_1 of <40% of predicted generally precludes major lung resection.

It is highly desirable to follow a structured algorithm for the further pre-operative assessment. One of the most widely used algorithms initially proposed by and subsequently validated by BOLLIGER *et al.* [15, 60] is based on the principle of successive steps from simple to more complex investigations (fig. 5). The aim of this (and other) algorithms is to include rather than to exclude as many patients as possible. Patients with a relatively poor FEV_1 can, for example, compensate with a relative preserved $V'_{O_2,max}$. It remains of paramount importance to estimate the relative contribution of the tissue earmarked for resection (which can range from a pneumonectomy, to a lobectomy, right down to a segmentectomy) by means of the methods discussed in patients who do not have an FEV_1 and $D_{L,CO}$ >80% of predicted or at least a $V'_{O_2,max}$ >20 $mL \cdot kg^{-1} \cdot min^{-1}$ or >75% of predicted.

Once a candidate is deemed operable, it remains imperative to appreciate that the "resection up to calculated extent" (fig. 5) refers to the extent that was used in estimation of the ppo values (*i.e.* the tissue earmarked for resection), which once again may vary from a pneumonectomy right down to a segmentectomy. It is also important to bear in mind that this algorithm only serves as a guide, and that common sense still needs to prevail (*e.g.* subjecting a patient with an FEV_1 and a $D_{L,CO}$ <30% of predicted to a formal exercise test is unlikely to alter their "high-risk" status).

An alternative algorithm, an unvalidated consensus product, has been proposed in the recent second edition of the American College of Chest Physicians evidence-based practice guidelines for the diagnosis and management of lung cancer [66].

Patients considered high risk for any resection by any algorithm are generally inoperable. However, exceptions can be made on an individual basis, provided that the patient and surgeon are aware of the significant risk of post-operative morbidity and more importantly, mortality. This has been confirmed in a very recent study by the Cancer and Leukemia Group B, which retrospectively applied the algorithm previously validated by BOLLIGER *et al.* [67] to a subset of their patients and found it to be somewhat too conservative, as a sizable number of patients considered at high risk by the algorithm underwent resection without increased complications. Furthermore, advances in surgical techniques (*e.g.* minimal invasive procedures), as well as limited resection combined with lung volume reduction surgery [68], has to an extent challenged the current thresholds. It remains to be determined whether the formal assessment of regional lung function alters the risk stratification of patients who undergo tumour resection in conjunction with lung volume reduction surgery, although upper lobe predominance of the emphysematous changes have been associated with a more favourable outcome [69].

Conclusions

Pulmonary resection remains the only curative intervention for bronchogenic carcinoma, but is considered to be a high-risk surgical procedure. All pulmonary resection candidates should undergo a structured stepwise pre-operative evaluation, starting with a full cardiac and general risk assessment. The initial pulmonary function evaluation should include at least an FEV_1, FVC (to determine and treat airflow obstruction), and $D_{L,CO}$. Patients with impaired pulmonary functions warrant formal cardiopulmonary exercise testing, and if impaired, assessment of their regional lung functions in order to calculate ppo lung functions. This should be done by means of anatomical calculations, with either radionucleotide perfusion scanning or quantitative CT scanning reserved for indeterminate cases.

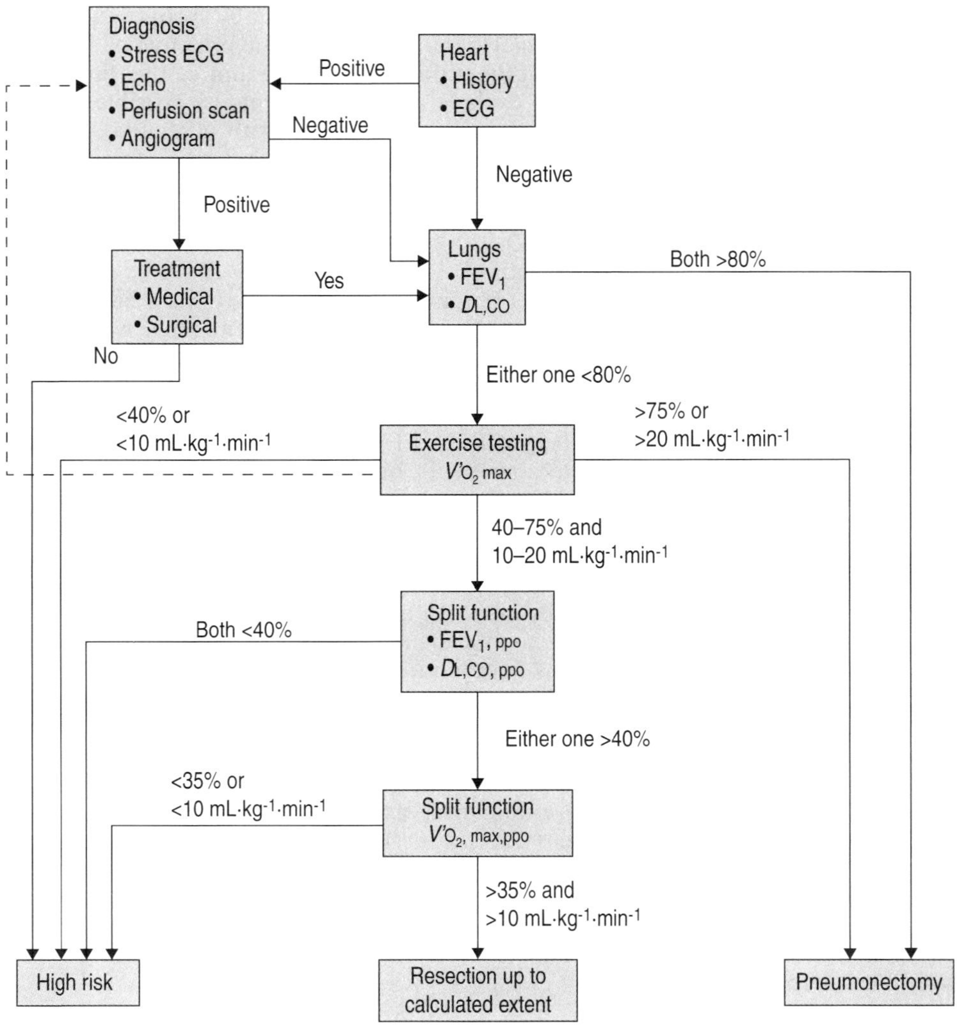

Fig. 5. – Algorithm for the assessment of cardiorespiratory reserve and operability of lung resection candidates. Patients undergo successive steps from top to bottom until they either qualify for varying extents of resection or are deemed inoperable. Split lung function testing allows a more accurate estimate of predicted post-operative (ppo) function (see text for details). This is usually calculated by means of anatomical calculations, computed tomography scan or using split perfusion scanning. A safety loop for patients with possible cardiac disease detected on exercise testing (signs or symptoms of myocardial ischaemia) is shown by the dashed line in the upper left hand corner. Note that all percentages refer to % of predicted. Care must be taken to understand that ppo calculations by implication take the calculated extent of resection into account, and that this may vary from a pneumonectomy to a lobectomy right down to a segmentectomy. FEV1: forced expiratory volume in 1 s; $D_{L,CO}$: carbon monoxide diffusing capacity; $V'_{O_2,max}$: maximal oxygen consumption. Adapted from [15].

Summary

Pulmonary resection remains the only curative intervention for bronchogenic carcinoma, but is considered to be a high-risk surgical procedure. Furthermore, pulmonary resection candidates often suffer from concomitant chronic obstructive lung disease or ischaemic heart disease. Pulmonary resection candidates therefore should undergo a structured pre-operative evaluation while they are at their personal best. The clinical assessment should focus on respiratory, cardiovascular and other general clinical parameters, including the smoking status. A resting ECG should be performed on all candidates. Serious cardiovascular pathology should be diagnosed and corrected prior to continuing with the stepwise approach.

The initial pulmonary function evaluation should at least include forced expiratory volume in 1 s (FEV1), forced vital capacity and diffusing capacity of the lung for carbon monoxide ($D_{L,CO}$). Values > 80% of predicted for FEV1 and $D_{L,CO}$ are associated with an uncomplicated surgical course for resection up to a pneumonectomy. Patients with impaired pulmonary functions warrant formal cardiopulmonary exercise testing. A maximal oxygen uptake ($V'_{O_2,max}$) value of >20 mL·kg^{-1}·min^{-1} or >75% predicted qualifies for resection up to pneumonectomy, whereas a value <10 mL·kg^{-1}·min^{-1} (or <40% predicted) is generally prohibitive for any resection. The cut-off value for a lobectomy is 15 mL·kg^{-1}·min^{-1}.

Intermediate cases ($V'_{O_2,max}$ 10–20 mL·kg^{-1}·min^{-1} or 40–75%) require some form of assessment of their regional lung functions in order to predict post-operative values. This should be done by means of anatomical calculations, with either radionucleotide perfusion scanning or quantitative computed tomography scanning reserved for borderline or indeterminate cases. Patients with predicted post-operative FEV1 and $D_{L,CO}$ >40% or $V'_{O_2,max}$ >10 mL·kg^{-1}·min^{-1} may still have a resection up to a calculated extent.

Lung volume reduction surgery may be combined with lung cancer surgery in selected individuals, who may otherwise have been deemed inoperable.

Keywords: Maximal oxygen uptake, operability, pre-operative functional evaluation, regional lung function, spirometry.

Statement of interest

None declared.

References

1. Bolliger CT. Evaluation of operability before lung resection. *Curr Opin Pulm Med* 2003; 9: 321–326.
2. Bolliger CT, Koegelenberg CF, Kendal R. Preoperative assessment for lung cancer surgery. *Curr Opin Pulm Med* 2005; 11: 301–306.
3. Bolliger CT. Pre-operative assessment of the lung caner patient. *S Afr Med J* 2001; 91: 120–123.
4. Bechard DE. Pulmonary function testing. *In*: LoCicero J III, ed. Diagnostic Procedures for Thoracic Diseases. Chest Surgery Clinics. WB Suanders Co, Philadelphia, 1992; pp. 565–586.
5. Nagasaki F, Flehinger BJ, Martini N. Complications of surgery in the treatment of carcinoma of the lung. *Chest* 1982; 82: 25–29.

6. Didolkar MS, Moore RH, Takita H. Evaluation of the risk in pulmonary resection for bronchogenic carcinoma. *Am J Surg* 1974; 127: 700–703.
7. Smetana GW. Preoperative pulmonary evaluation. *N Eng J Med* 1999; 340: 937–943.
8. Conti B, Brega Massone PP, Lequaglie C, *et al.* Major surgery in lung cancer in elderly patients? Risk factors analysis and long-term results. *Minerva Chir* 2002; 57: 317–321.
9. Morton HJV. Tobacco smoking and pulmonary complications after surgery. *Lancet* 1944; 1: 368–370.
10. Warner DO, Offord KP, Warner MA, *et al.* Role of preoperative cessation of smoking and other factors in postoperative pulmonary complications: a blinded prospective study of coronary artery bypass patients. *Mayo Clin Proc* 1989; 64: 609–616.
11. Bluman LG, Mosca L, Newman N, *et al.* Preoperative smoking habits and postoperative pulmonary complications. *Chest* 1998; 113: 883–889.
12. Smetana GW, Lawrence VA, Cornell JE. Preoperative pulmonary risk stratification for noncardiothoracic surgery: systemic review for the American College of Physicians. *Ann Intern Med* 2006; 144: 581–595.
13. Arozullah AM, Khuri SF, Henderson WG, *et al.* Development and validation of a multifactorial risk index for predicting postoperative pneumonia after major noncardiac surgery. *Ann Intern Med* 2001; 135: 845–857.
14. Gaensler EA, Cugell DW, Lindgren I, *et al.* The role of pulmonary insufficiency in mortality and invalidism following surgery for pulmonary tuberculosis. *J Thorac Cardiovasc Surg* 1955; 29: 163–187.
15. Bolliger CT, Perruchoud AP. Functional evaluation of the lung resection candidate. *Eur Respir J* 1998; 11: 198–212.
16. Peters RM, Clausen JL, Tisi GM. Extending resectability for carcinoma of the lung in patients with impaired pulmonary function. *Ann Thorac Surg* 1978; 26: 250–260.
17. Boushy SF, Billig DM, North LB, *et al.* Clinical course related to preoperative and postoperative pulmonary function in patients with bronchogenic carcinoma. *Chest* 1971; 59: 383–391.
18. Perruchoud A, Meili U, Kopp C, *et al.* Preoperative evaluation of pulmonary function in patients with bronchogenic carcinoma [Präoperative Abklärung der Lungenfunktion bei Patienten mit Bronchialkarzinom]. *Schweiz Med Wschr* 1979; 109: 832–835.
19. British Thoracic Society; Society of Cardiothoracic Surgeons of Great Britain and Ireland Working Party. BTS Guidelines: guidelines on the selection of patients with lung cancer for surgery. *Thorax* 2001; 56: 89–108.
20. Brunelli A, Rocco G. Spirometry: predicting risk and outcome. *Thorac Surg Clin* 2008; 18: 1–8.
21. Mittman C. Assessment of operative risk in thoracic surgery. *Am Rev Respir Dis* 1961; 84: 197–207.
22. Pate P, Tenholder MF, Griffin JP, *et al.* Preoperative assessment of the high risk patient for lung resection. *Ann Thorac Surg* 1996; 61: 1494–1500.
23. Olsen GN, Block AJ, Tobias JA. Prediction of postpneumonectomy pulmonary function using quantitative macroaggregate lung scanning. *Chest* 1974; 66: 13–16.
24. Markos J, Mullan BP, Hillman DR, *et al.* Preoperative assessment as a predictor of mortality and morbidity after lung resection. *Am Rev Respir Dis* 1989; 139: 902–910.
25. Wahi R, McMurtry MJ, DeCaro LF, *et al.* Determinants of perioperative morbidity and mortality after pneumonectomy. *Ann Thorac Surg* 1989; 48: 33–37.
26. Bolliger CT, Wyser C, Roser H, *et al.* Lung scanning and exercise testing for the prediction of postoperative performance in lung resection candidates: at increased risk for complications. *Chest* 1995; 108: 341–348.
27. Nakahara H, Ohno K, Hashimoto J, *et al.* Prediction of postoperative respiratory failure in patients undergoing lung resection for lung cancer. *Ann Thorac Surg* 1988; 46: 549–552.
28. Ferguson MK, Lehman AG, Bolliger CT, *et al.* The role of diffusing capacity and exercise tests. *Thorac Surg Clin* 2008; 18: 9–17.

29. Cander L. Physiologic assessment and management of preoperative patient with pulmonary emphysema. *Am J Cardiol* 1963; 12: 324–326.
30. Ferguson MK, Little L, Rizzo L, *et al.* Diffusing capacity predicts morbidity and mortality after pulmonary resection. *J Thorac Cardiovasc Surg* 1988; 96: 894–900.
31. Markos J, Mullan BP, Hillman DR, *et al.* Preoperative assessment as a predictor of mortality and morbidity after lung resection. *Am Rev Respir Dis* 1989; 139: 902–910.
32. Ferguson MK, Reeder LB, Mick R. Optimizing selection of patients for major lung resection. *J Thorac Cardiovasc Surg* 1995; 109: 275–281.
33. Berrisford R, Brunelli A, Rocco G, *et al.* The European Thoracic Surgery Database project: modelling the risk of in-hospital death following lung resection. *Eur J Cardiothorac Surg* 2005; 28: 306–311.
34. Taylor HL, Buskirk E, Henschel A. Maximal oxygen intake as an objective measurement of cardiorespiratory performance. *J Appl Physiol* 1955; 8: 73–80.
35. Eugene J, Brown SE, Light RW, *et al.* Maximum oxygen consumption: a physiologic guide to pulmonary resection. *Surg Forum* 1982; 33: 260–262.
36. Bolliger CT, Jordan P, Solèr M, *et al.* Exercise capacity as a predictor of postoperative complications in lung resection candidates. *Am J Respir Crit Care Med* 1995; 151: 1472–1480.
37. Wang JS, Abboud RT, Evans KG, *et al.* Role of CO diffusion capacity during exercise in the preoperative evaluation for lung resection. *Am J Respir Crit Care Med* 2000; 162: 1435–1444.
38. Morice RC, Peters EJ, Ryan MB, *et al.* Exercise testing in the evaluation of patients at high risk for complications from lung resection. *Chest* 1992; 101: 356–361.
39. Smith TP, Kinasewitz GT, Tucker WY, *et al.* Exercise capacity as a predictor of post-thoracotomy morbidity. *Am Rev Respir Dis* 1984; 129: 730–734.
40. Koegelenberg CF, Diacon AH, Irani S, *et al.* Stair climbing in the functional assessment of lung resection candidates. *Respiration* 2008; 75: 374–379.
41. Holden DA, Rice TW, Stelmach K, *et al.* Exercise testing, 6-min walk, and stair climb in the evaluation of patients at high risk for pulmonary resection. *Chest* 1992; 102: 1774–1779.
42. Pollock M, Roa J, Benditt J, *et al.* Estimation of ventilatory reserve by stair climbing. A study in patients with chronic airflow obstruction. *Chest* 1993; 104: 1378–1383.
43. Brunelli A, Al Refai M, Monteverde M, *et al.* Stair climbing test predicts cardiopulmonary complications after lung resection. *Chest* 2002; 121: 1106–1110.
44. Bernstein ML, Despars JA, Sing NP, *et al.* Reanalysis of the 12-minute walk in patients with chronic obstructive lung disease. *Chest* 1994; 105: 163–167.
45. Swinburn CR, Wakefield JM, Jones PW. Performance, ventilation and oxygen consumption in three different types of exercise test in patients with chronic obstructive lung disease. *Thorax* 1985; 40: 581–586.
46. Singh SJ, Morgan MD, Hardman AE, *et al.* Comparison of oxygen uptake during a conventional treadmill test and the shuttle walking test in chronic airflow limitation. *Eur Respir J* 1994; 7: 2016–2020.
47. Win T, Jackson A, Groves AM, *et al.* Relationship of shuttle walk test and lung cancer surgical outcome. *Eur J Cardiothorac Surg* 2004; 26: 1216–1219.
48. Win T, Jackson A, Groves AM, *et al.* Comparison of shuttle walk with measured peak oxygen consumption in patients with operable lung cancer. *Thorax* 2006; 61: 57–60.
49. Goldman L, Caldera DL, Nussbaum SR, *et al.* Multifactorial index of cardiac risk in noncardiac surgical procedures. *N Engl J Med* 1977; 297: 845–850.
50. Lee TH, Marcantonio ER, Mangione CM, *et al.* Derivation and prospective validation of a simple index for prediction of cardiac risk of major noncardiac surgery. *Circulation* 1999; 100: 1043–1049.
51. Johnson JA, Landreneau RJ, Boley TM, *et al.* Should pulmonary lesions be resected at the time of open heart surgery? *Am Surg* 1996; 62: 300–303.
52. Miller DL, Orszulak TA, Pairolero PC. Combined operation for lung cancer and cardiac disease. *Ann Thorac Surg* 1994; 58: 989–993.

53. Dyszkiewicz W, Jemielity MM, Piwkowski CT, *et al.* Simultaneous lung resection for cancer and myocardial revascularization without cardiopulmonary bypass (off-pump coronary artery bypass grafting). *Ann Thorac Surg* 2004; 77: 1023–1027.
54. Koegelenberg CF, Bolliger CT. Assessing regional lung function. *Thorac Surg Clin* 2008; 18: 19–29.
55. Pierce RJ, Copland JM, Sharpe K, *et al.* Preoperative risk evaluation for lung cancer resection: Predicted postoperative product as a predictor of surgical mortality. *Am J Respir Crit Care Med* 1994; 150: 947–955.
56. Beccaria M, Corsico A, Fulgonie P, *et al.* Lung cancer resection. The prediction of postsurgical outcomes should include long-term functional results. *Chest* 2001; 120: 37–42.
57. Nakahara K, Monden Y, Ohno K, *et al.* A method for predicting postoperative lung function and its relation to postoperative complications in patients with lung cancer. *Ann Thorac Surg* 1985; 39: 260–265.
58. Bolliger CT, Guckel C, Engel H, *et al.* Prediction of functional reserves after lung resection: comparison between quantitative computed tomography, scintigraphy, and anatomy. *Respiration* 2002; 69: 482–489.
59. Olsen GN, Block AJ, Tobias JA. Prediction of postpneumonectomy pulmonary function using quantitative macroaggregate lung scanning. *Chest* 1974; 66: 13–16.
60. Wyser C, Stulz P, Soler M, *et al.* Prospective evaluation of an algorithm for the functional assessment of lung resection candidates. *Am J Respir Crit Care Med* 1999; 159: 1450–1456.
61. Beccaria M, Corsico A, Fulgonie P, *et al.* Lung cancer resection. The prediction of postsurgical outcomes should include long-term functional results. *Chest* 2001; 120: 37–42.
62. Wu MT, Chang JM, Chiang AA, *et al.* Use of quantitative CT to predict postoperative lung function in patients with lung cancer. *Radiology* 1994; 191: 257–262.
63. Wu MT, Pan HB, Chiang AA, *et al.* Prediction of postoperative lung function in patients with lung cancer: comparison of quantitative CT with perfusion scintigraphy. *Am J Roentgenol* 2002; 178: 667–672.
64. Ohno Y, Koyama H, Nogami M, *et al.* Postoperative lung function in lung cancer patients: comparative analysis of predictive capability of MRI, CT, and SPECT. *Am J Roentgenol* 2007; 189: 400–408.
65. Ohno Y, Hatabu H, Higashino T, *et al.* Dynamic perfusion MRI *versus* perfusion scintigraphy: prediction of postoperative lung function in patients with lung cancer. *Am J Roentgenol* 2004; 182: 73–78.
66. Colice GL, Shafazand S, Griffin JP, *et al.* Physiologic evaluation of the patient with lung cancer being considered for resectional surgery: ACCP evidenced-based clinical practice guidelines (2nd edition). *Chest* 2007; 132: 161S–177S.
67. Loewen GM, Watson D, Kohman L, *et al.* Preoperative exercise $V O_2$ measurement for lung resection candidates: results of Cancer and Leukemia Group B Protocol 9238. *J Thorac Oncol* 2007; 2: 619–625.
68. Choong CK, Meyers BF, Battafarano RJ, *et al.* Lung cancer resection combined with lung volume reduction in patients with severe emphysema. *J Thorac Cardiovasc Surg* 2004; 127: 1323–1331.
69. National Emphysema Treatment Trial Research Group. A randomized trial comparing lung-volume reduction surgery with medical therapy for severe emphysema. *N Engl J Med* 2003; 348: 2059–2073.

CHAPTER 11

The surgical treatment of lung cancer

E. Potton*, S.M. Janes#, S.G. Spiro¶,+

*University College London Hospitals, #Centre for Respiratory Research, University College London, ¶Division of Cancer Medicine, University College London Hospitals, and +Royal Brompton Hospital, London, UK.

Correspondence: S.G. Spiro, 66 Grange Gardens, Pinner, Middlesex, HA55QF, UK. E-mail: stephenspiro@btinternet.com

The best chance to cure lung cancer is by surgery; however, the number of patients going to pulmonary resection has not increased dramatically over the years. Clinicians are getting better at selecting those fit enough to do well and still have a reasonable respiratory reserve post-operatively. Also, staging has become more refined, with positron emission tomography (PET) scanning and better techniques for assessing the mediastinum. In general, surgery is offered to patients with nonsmall cell lung cancers (NSCLC), apart from the occasional small cell tumour confined to the lung (stage IA or IB). These occasional patients, who, after extensive and careful staging, are considered resectable, have a reasonable long-term survival, not too different from equivalent stage NSCLC.

It is now increasingly common for surgery to be combined with other modalities, such as neoadjuvant or adjuvant chemotherapy. This is described in detail in chapter 13 of this *European Respiratory Monograph* (*ERM*). Post-operative radiotherapy has not proven to be of clear benefit and may even be deleterious to long-term survival [1] (see chapter 12 of this *ERM*). Trials are also in progress examining the role of combining surgery with concurrent chemoradiation in patients with locally advanced (N2) disease. In these trials, disease is confined to one or two mediastinal lymph node stations (K.S. Albain, Loyola University Chicago Stritch School of Medicine, Maywood, IL, USA, and J.P. Van Meerbeeck, Dept of Respiratory Medicine and Thoracic Oncology, University Hospital, Ghent, Belgium; personal communication).

Stage at diagnosis is still the single most important factor in determining resectability and long-term survival. There was some controversy over the maximum size of a resectable tumour, which in the literature has ranged up to 7 cm in diameter. This is reviewed in chapter 9 of this *ERM*, which addresses the topic of staging. For example, Patz *et al.* [2] reviewed a large series of IA lung cancers collected over 19 yrs and showed that there was no effect of tumour size on survival for tumours of <3 cm diameter. They examined survival for different streams of tumour sizes within stage I patients and showed no difference in 5-yr survival for smaller tumours (<2 cm) than those 2–3 cm at resection. This may reflect tumour biology, *i.e.* there is more to survival prediction than just size of the primary lesion, which does not take biological aggression into account. However, most agree that tumour size at presentation correlates reasonably well with survival and is an important prognostic factor. The "tumour, node, metastasis" (TNM) staging classification remains based around this. In fact, in the new International Association for the Study of Lung Cancer (IASLC) classification described in chapter 9, the new staging system for the "T" denominator is based on tumour size and, because of the strong association of size and prognosis, T1 becomes

Eur Respir Mon, 2009, 44, 187–206. Printed in UK - all rights reserved. Copyright ERS Journals Ltd 2009; European Respiratory Monograph; ISSN 1025-448x.

T1a (<2 cm) and T1b (>2 cm), with T2 becoming T2a (<5 cm) and T2b (>5 cm). T3 is >7 cm, showing, from the 15,000 pathologically staged patients in the classification, that tumour size is very important.

Accurate staging is vital, but can be viewed as a "negative advance", as better staging identifies smaller deposits of disease and thus more patients will be turned down for resection because of discovering what previously would have been occult disease. PET scanning and mediastinal endoscopic ultrasound (EUS) are two such techniques that have led to upstaging of previously resectable cases.

The use of computed tomography (CT) is routine for all newly diagnosed patients and should precede bronchoscopy, as CT may allow both diagnosis and staging to be performed by a single investigative biopsy. The sensitivity and specificity of CT have been described in chapter 7, and it is clear that defining probable metastatic disease by lymph node size is both unreliable and misleading with this modality. PET has taken staging to new levels of accuracy and will identify tumour masses down to 7 mm in diameter. PET has saved thoracotomy in up to 30% of otherwise clinically resectable patients [3] and, in general, changes the clinical stage in up to 40% of newly diagnosed cases. It may also give a clue for the biology of the tumour, as initial studies showed that those primary tumours with high standardised uptake values (SUVs), indicating high biological activity, may respond better to treatment with radiotherapy and/or chemotherapy than those with lower SUVs [4]. However, the high SUV tumours relapsed earlier with poorer overall survival. Newer studies have confirmed these findings and, clearly, PET does provide a glimpse of tumour activity that intuitively seems likely to represent biological activity and rate of cell turnover. This has also been shown to affect the 5-yr survival after surgery, with better outcomes for those with low SUV tumours, although different studies have used different thresholds for making this comparison (table 1) [5].

Less aggressive tumours, such as bronchoalveolar cell cancers, carcinoid tumours and adenoid cystic carcinomas, have much lower SUV uptakes, and the SUV may be less of a predictive marker here.

Number of patients undergoing surgical resection for lung cancer

A much greater number of patients with NSCLC undergo surgical intervention than with small cell lung cancer. The numbers vary between countries, depending on the stage cut-off accepted in different units, the quality of staging, the incidence of significant

Table 1. – Positron emission tomography, standardised uptake value (SUV) and prognosis for survival post-surgery for lung cancer

First author [ref.]	Patients n	SUV threshold	Stage	Upper 5-yr survival threshold %	Lower 5-yr survival threshold
VANSTEENKISTE [4]	125	>7.0	I and II	83	43% (2 yrs)
GOODGAME [6]	136	>5.5	I		3 × recurrence rate
	136	>5.5		54	39%
HANIN [7]	96	>7.8	I		Worse
			II		No difference
OHTSUKA [8]	100	>3.3	I adenocarcinoma		Worse
CERFOLIO [9]	315	>median	IB and II		Worse at 4 yrs
			IB	92	51%
			II	64	47%

Data taken from [5].

comorbidities and the experience and availability of thoracic surgeons (for example, in the USA, much lung cancer surgery is still carried out by general surgeons). Other factors leading to a decision to operate may depend on whether clinically detected mediastinal nodal involvement in any station renders the subject inoperable, or whether intracapsular disease or single station disease is acceptable, albeit with a lower chance of cure than for lesser stage disease. There also is a wide variation of resection rates between regions within some countries. The reasons for these variations are not clear. High rates of resection, however, may not imply that the resection rate of NSCLC is a surrogate marker for survival, as quality of staging and cut-off decisions will vary. In a Swedish study, there was considerable variation of resection rates between counties, ranging from 10 to 30% [10]. Accessibility to referral centres may play a part in the rate of resection within each county.

The overall resection rate in this Swedish population study was 17.5% [10]. All patients were logged with a *pre mortem* histological diagnosis of NSCLC and then data was prospectively collected about their treatment and survival. The Lung Cancer Register was used in seven counties across Sweden but only represented 21% of the whole population. Diagnosis, staging and management were guided by uniform treatment guidelines and local multidisciplinary meetings (these were developed throughout the regions during the study period 1995–2003). The study spanned the introduction of the amended staging system for lung cancer [11] and the introduction of PET. In a sub-analysis it was noted that, in the later time period, patients presenting with stage I disease were more likely to undergo a surgical resection. However, there were wide variations in practice, despite uniform guidelines.

Another study, from the Netherlands [12], documented a similar rate of surgical resection to that in Sweden. The data was from one surgical centre serving a population of 2.2 million between 1984 and 1992, with 7,899 histologically confirmed diagnoses of lung cancer. 24% of these patients underwent surgery.

In 713,043 patients from the Surveillance Epidemiology and End Results (SEER) database in the USA, the resection rate was 27% for NSCLC between 1967 and 1976 [13]. The 5-yr survival of these patients was between 55 and 63%. This study was conducted prior to the 1997 re-classification of the staging system and it is possible that, with more accurate staging, a lower proportion of these patients would have been suitable for surgical resection.

Studies and audits in the UK have documented a much lower rate of surgical resection (10%) in lung cancer patients [14–17], but it is not clear why resection rates are so low. LAROCHE *et al.* [16] measured the improvement in resection rates after introduction of a two-stop investigation service at one cardiothoracic centre in the UK. At the end of the study period, resection rates were 25% with a futile thoracotomy rate of 11%. This was attributed to shorter time to diagnosis (<4 weeks), higher percentage of histological confirmation and prompt surgical review of every patient.

One study looked at why there may be low resection rates within parts of the UK by comparing rates between Varese in Italy and Hull in the UK [17]. There was a similar incidence of lung cancer, but the rate of resection was significantly lower in Hull (7%) than in Varese (25%). The patient group in Hull was older, had a higher proportion of smokers and a poorer performance status compared with the Varese population. The authors hypothesised that part of the reason for the lower resection rate in the Hull population was due to its demographics.

It is not easy to compare studies from different countries because the denominators are different. For example, UK data include some patients with just a clinical diagnosis of lung cancer, *i.e.* without histological confirmation. The other European and American studies quoted only included patients with a histological diagnosis (therefore the proportions that undergo resection are higher).

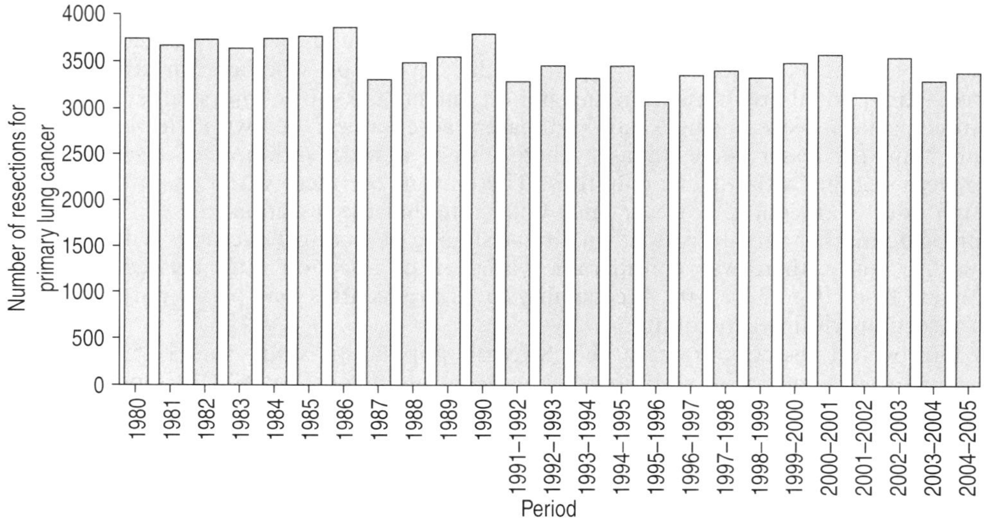

Fig. 1. – The number of patients undergoing a lung resection for primary lung cancer over time in Great Britain and Ireland. n=87,367 over whole period shown. From the Society for Cardiothoracic Surgery in Great Britain and Ireland, reproduced from [14] with permission from the publisher.

There has been a downward trend in the number of patients undergoing resections within the UK, as demonstrated in figure 1, and this may reflect improvements in staging techniques.

Another study from the SEER database looked at trends for resection in subjects with NSCLC over the age of 66 yrs [18]. The study reviewed patients selected for surgery between 1992 and 2002 and the hypothesis was that resection rates would increase. Although the SEER database seems partial, comprising 14–25% of incident tumours in the USA, 24,030 patients went to thoracotomy. Of these, 25% were aged 66–70 yrs, 32% were aged 71–75 yrs, 26% were aged 76–80 yrs, 12.6% were aged 81–85 yrs and 3.8% were over 86 yrs of age. The results showed a 14% drop in resection rates over the 10 yrs, with a reduction in the odds for a resection falling by 5% per annum. It was not apparent why this fall had occurred; possibilities included too many inexperienced surgeons in the USA, and no effect for advancing age or increased comorbidity was found. Since approximately 70% of those presenting with stage I disease would expect to be cured by surgery, this was a worrying trend.

Early detection of lung cancer and better clinical staging

Low-dose CT screening of populations at varying degrees of risk for lung cancer has identified a wide-ranging incidence of noncalcified lung nodules, up to 51% on prevalence screens, with up to 2.7% of noncalcified lung nodules proven to be malignant [19–22]. Whether CT will prove to be a useful method of screening will not be clear until the results of randomised controlled trials are reported, as most studies to date have not been randomised and are hypothesis generating. Compared with the chest radiograph, CT will identify up to four times as many cancers [22], but cure rate will not be known for several years. The topic is discussed in detail in chapter 4.

Clinical staging has become more accurate with PET, which has reduced the number of futile thoracotomies in patients clinically judged suitable for thoracotomy [3]. As PET has a predictive false positive rate of up to 25%, positive lesions require a confirmatory biopsy, particularly if it is the only contraindication to resection. A negative PET scan, however, has a predictive value close to 98% and no biopsy is needed (see chapters 7 and 8). This has led to the increasing use of endobronchial ultrasound (EBUS) to stage disease in the mediastinum, in order to facilitate accurate pre-operative staging in patients without requiring mediastinoscopy. Use of EBUS and EUS for the aspiration and biopsy of mediastinal lymph nodes is becoming increasingly adopted for staging, and it has a much greater access to the mediastinal nodes than cervical mediastinoscopy. It will prevent mediastinoscopy in many cases, and its value is discussed in chapter 8. It may be best used for staging prior to a PET scan as, if EBUS/EUS is positive, PET becomes unnecessary in those cases [23]. Currently, EBUS/EUS is only routinely used in a few specialist centres, but it inevitably will become a potential gold standard for clinical and pathological staging. PET, EBUS and EUS have not been available for long enough to reflect long-term surgical survival data. Very few of the >100,000 patients in the IASLC 2009 staging classification had undergone PET (see chapter 9). Virtually none would have had EUS/transbronchial needle aspiration. It will, therefore, be some years before the place of these techniques in selection for surgery becomes clear.

Surgical results for lung cancer

Stage I (T1N0 and T2N0) and stage II (T1N1, T2N1 and T3N0) NSCLC, in the 1997 staging system, are regarded as resectable [24]. The aim of an operative procedure is to cure and minimise the chance of recurrence, while preserving optimal functional capacity. Lobectomy and pneumonectomy are the main surgical procedures, but segmentectomy, wedge resection and video-assisted thoracoscopic surgery (VATS) lobectomy are also performed. Sleeve lobectomy is performed if tumours occlude the right upper lobe orifice, making a conventional upper lobectomy impossible. It allows the intermediate bronchus to be transected below the right upper lobe orifice, and the middle and lower lobe airways anastomosed to the right main bronchus, *i.e.* preventing a more major resection. This procedure is performed in less than 5% of cases and would be preferable to pneumonectomy. Comparing outcome of sleeve resection with pneumonectomy showed better 5-yr results for sleeve resection (39%, *versus* 27% following pneumonectomy) [25]. However, the two groups were not fully comparable as those undergoing pneumonectomy tended to have worse stage tumours. Physiologically there is an advantage for sleeve resection as more lung function is preserved.

Mortality and morbidity

The current, immediate post-operative mortality for pulmonary resections are quoted at between 1 and 8% [24]. ALLEN *et al.* [26] reported overall mortality following lobectomy as 1%, and as 2–3% for more advanced cases requiring more extensive resections. Older patients aged ≥70 yrs and those of ≥80 yrs fared no worse, due to careful case selection. This study sets a benchmark for surgical mortality and morbidity following pulmonary resection. Earlier studies reported a mortality of 3.8% from 2,220 resections, with a 6.2% mortality for pneumonectomy and 2.9% mortality for lobectomy [27]. The improvement will reflect the better case selection, intra-operative techniques and post-operative management that have developed over the last 20 yrs. Also, the pneumonectomy rate was around 25% in the 1970s and 1980s, compared with 4% in recent reports. Other studies have reported an operative mortality of 3% for lobectomy and 11.8% for pneumonectomy [28], and a rate of 3.2% for pneumonectomy in Japan with an overall mortality of 1.3% [29]. These studies did not report a consistent cause of death, the most common being multisystem organ failure. The post-operative complication rate was 38% in the recent study of ALLEN *et al.* [26]. The commonest problems were atrial arrhythmias, prolonged air leaks and excessive tube drainage. The frequencies of these complications, which prolong hospital admission, have not changed much in the last two decades. Pulmonary embolism remains a post-operative problem. Prolonged post-operative pain is another.

Post-operative complications are more prevalent in smokers, and those with nodal disease, right sided resections, bilobectomies and squamous cell cancers. The main identifiable causes of death are pneumonia, septic shock and acute respiratory distress syndrome. In order to prevent these early and potentially fatal complications, early extubation, use of thoracic epidurals and regular suctioning can be helpful.

Of the major complications, bronchial anastomotic complications occur at around 6%. Tumour invasion of the stump may predispose patients to this complication. If this problem occurs early in the post-operative course, surgical intervention is advocated. Stump dehiscence can be a result of residual tumour at the anastomosis or devascularisation at lymph node dissection. The tumour margins examined after the initial operation will give an indication of whether the tumour was completely resected. However, if it is a late complication it is usually managed with pleural drainage and an open window thoracostomy.

Quality of life studies after surgery are few, but it is higher after a lobectomy than after a pneumonectomy [30]. Much of this is due to less physiological damage and deficit to the individual. Morbidity is often quoted at similar rates for these resections, but this is likely to be due to the selection of patients to undergo each type of surgery.

Lymph node sampling and lymph node dissection

Mediastinal lymph node dissection at pulmonary resection rather than sampling remains a controversial area within NSCLC surgery. Because the prognosis of lung cancer is related to whether lymph node metastasis has occurred, accurate lymph node assessment is crucial both to give patients an accurate prognosis and to offer them an appropriate resection and the possibility for adjuvant therapy. A large randomised trial of complete mediastinal lymphadenectomy *versus* nodal sampling only, in 1,111 patients with clinical stage I lung cancer, is in progress [31]. This has already shown that there were a handful of patients (20 in the lymph node dissection arm) who were upstaged when N2 positive nodes were found at operation. There is controversy about whether there is an increase in post-operative morbidity and a higher complication rate with dissection [26], but this ongoing trial did not report a higher complication rate in the lymph node dissection arm [31]. Complications anticipated, such as recurrent laryngeal nerve injury, bronchial devascularisation and increase in chylothorax or bleeding, did not occur [26], and there was no difference in incidence in the two arms.

The relationship to improved survival and extent of lymph node sampling in stage I disease was shown in a study by GAJRA *et al.* [32]. They analysed 442 patients who underwent surgical resection and some form of mediastinal node sampling. Sampling was random, systematic or complete, as defined by sampling at levels 4, 7 and 10 for right-sided lesions, and levels 5 or 6 and 7 for left-sided tumours (fig. 2).

Patients who underwent random sampling had a 5-yr disease-free survival of 51%, compared with 80% for both systematic and complete dissections. This confirms the similar findings in earlier studies [34]. While there is support for radical nodal dissection (as opposed to sampling), with an improved outcome for N2 disease, a randomised trial addressing this issue found that, for pN0 disease, lymphadenectomy had little effect on

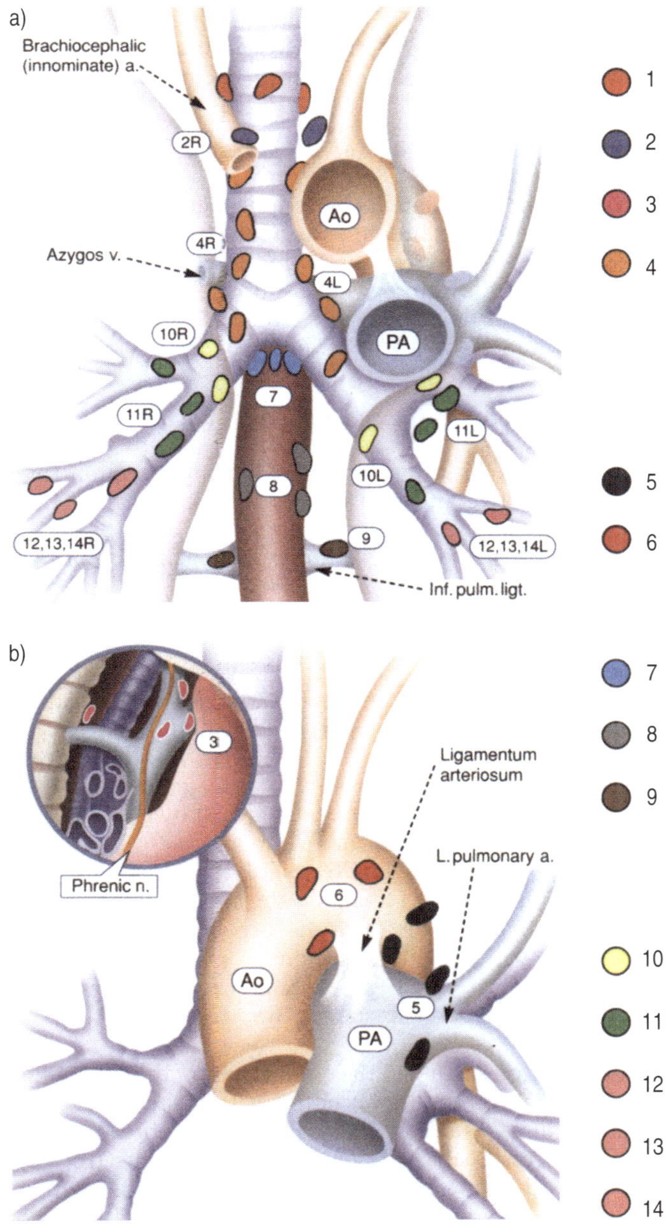

Fig. 2. – Regional lymph node stations for lung cancer staging. Reproduced from [33] with permission from the publisher. Superior mediastinal nodes: 1) highest mediastinal; 2) upper paratracheal; 3) pre-vascular and retrotracheal; 4) lower paratracheal (including azygos nodes). N_2=single digit, ipsilateral; N_3=single digit, contralateral or supraclavicular. Aortic nodes: 5) subaortic (A-P window); 6) para-aortic (ascending aorta or phrenic). Inferior mediastinal nodes: 7) subcarinal; 8) para-oesophageal (below carina); 9) pulmonary ligament. N_1 nodes: 10) hilar; 11) interlobar; 12) lobar; 13) segmental; 14) subsegmental.

survival but did prolong survival for pN1 and pN2 disease [35]. However, a more recent retrospective study in patients with stage II and IIIa disease showed that systematic nodal sampling seemed as effective as complete mediastinal dissection [36]. Subset analysis did show that complete mediastinal dissection identified significantly more levels of N2 disease and was associated with improved survival.

Pre-operative assessment and decisions about surgical intervention

The pre-operative assessment of patients undergoing surgery for lung cancer has been discussed in chapter 10. The pre-operative assessment inevitably has an impact on the surgical procedure that the patient can undergo. It is a balance of achieving clear margins and sampling the mediastinum with ensuring that the patient has functional capacity after their operation. Lung function, exercise testing and ventilation–perfusion scans are used in this assessment as discussed in chapter 10.

Survival of patients undergoing resection for lung cancer

There are many large series showing survival following resection for NSCLC in the literature. They are retrospective and the stage of disease will have been based on the 1997 classification. The 2009 IASLC modification was based on multicentre international data collected from patients who underwent resection between 1990 and 2000 [37]. Even this huge series of more than 64,000 cases of NSCLC will have produced its guidelines without full benefit from PET and routine mediastinal exploration pre-operatively.

Most large studies [38–41] report the overall 5-yr survival of patients following surgery to range from 36 to 52%, depending on pathological disease stage. While clinical stage is the main determinate of outcome, pathological stage after resection provides better information. The numbers remaining in the same stage post-operatively is always fewer but with a better outcome, as the clinical stage underestimates disease due to inability to identify small volumes of tumour. This is shown in the survival curves in figure 3 and in tables 2 and 3.

PFANNSCHMIDT *et al.* [38] published a series of 2,083 patients who had surgery between 1996 and 2005 in one centre. Patients were staged clinically by the use of chest CT, ultrasound, bone scintigram and fibreoptic bronchoscopy. Mediastinoscopy was not routinely performed. Further investigations were employed to exclude extra-pulmonary disease but the authors did not specify what these were or whether PET scans were employed at any stage. The staging was based on the 1997 revised TNM classification.

GOYA *et al.* [40] retrospectively studied the clinical and pathological stage and survival of patients with lung cancer from multiple centres within Japan. They selected patients who had a resection for lung cancer in 1994. They followed the 1997 staging system. There were a few differences in survival compared with results from other studies. In particular, clinically staged IA lung cancer had a worse survival rate than pathologically staged IA lung cancer. This may be because lymph node dissection is regularly performed in Japan and, therefore, there may be a large number of cases that are upstaged to IB using the pathological staging system post-operatively. They noted that pathological staging IA and IIB have a similar prognosis.

The study by NARUKE *et al.* [41] included 3,043 patients resected between 1961 and 1995 and encompassed many improvements in the staging systems. In the clinical stage there were significant prognostic differences for 5-yr survival between stage IA and IB, stage IIB and IIIA, and stage IIIA and IIIB. There were no differences between stage IB

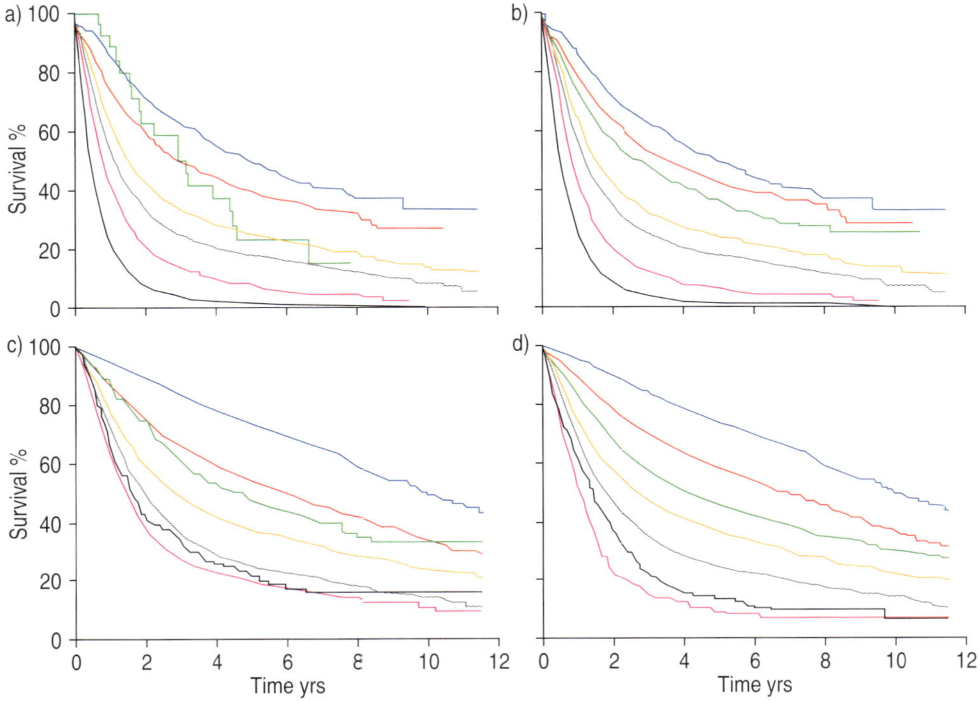

Fig. 3. – Overall survival according to a and b) clinical and c and d) pathological staging using the a and c) sixth and b and d) seventh edition of the TNM classification of malignant tumours. Reproduced from [37] with permission from the publisher. Blue: stage IA; red: stage IB; green: stage IIA; yellow: stage IIB; grey: stage IIIA; pink: stage IIIB; black: stage IV. See table 2 for additional data.

Table 2. – Survival data for curves shown in figure 3

Stage	6th edition				7th edition			
	Deaths n	Total n	MST months	5-yr survival %	Deaths n	Total n	MST months	5-yr survival %
Clinical								
IA	443	831	60	50	443	831	60	50
IB	1133	1842	37	40	750	1284	43	43
IIA	19	25	38	24	318	483	34	36
IIB	1571	2151	18	25	1652	2248	18	25
IIIA	2397	3005	14	18	2528	3175	14	19
IIIB	1088	1224	10	8	676	758	10	7
IV	2343	2458	6	2	2627	2757	6	2
Pathological								
IA	1168	3666	119	73	1168	3666	119	73
IB	2231	4426	70	54	1450	3100	81	58
IIA	306	562	54	48	1485	2579	49	46
IIB	1951	2982	33	38	1502	2252	31	36
IIIA	2348	3091	23	25	2896	3792	22	24
IIIB	838	1042	16	19	263	297	13	9
IV	146	183	18	21	224	266	17	13

Reproduced from [37] with permission from the publisher. MST: median survival time.

Table 3. – 5-yr survival rates for post-surgical nonsmall cell lung cancer by clinical (C) and pathological post-operative (P) stage according to the 1997 TNM staging system, as reported in studies with ≥2,000 patients

	PFANNSCHMIDT [38][#]		GOYA [40][¶]		NARUKE [41][+]	
	C stage	P stage	C stage	P stage	C stage	P stage
IA		68.5	72.0	79.5	70.8	79
IB		66.6	49.9	60.1	44.0	59.7
IIA		55.3	48.7	59.9	41.1	56.9
IIB		49.0	40.6	42.2	38.8 (T2N1M0) 32.6 (T3N0M0)	45
IIIA		35.8	35.9	29.8	22.3 (T1-2 N2M0) 22.9 (T3 N1-2 M0)	23.6
IIIB		35.4	28.0	19.3	11.7 (any T, N3M0) 24.3 (T4, any N, M0)	16.5
IV		Not defined	20.8	20.0		5.1

Data are presented as percentages. #: n=2,083; ¶: n=6,644; +: n=3,043.

and IIA, stage IIA and IIB, and stage IIIB and IV. In the post-operative staging there were significant differences in 5-yr survival rates between each stage except IB and IIA. The sixth international classification by MOUNTAIN [11] in 1997 showed a similar lack of survival difference for stage IB and IIA, which have now separated in the new IASLC classification. The clinical and pathological stage survival curves for the old and new classifications are summarised in figure 3 and table 2, illustrating the effect of the much larger dataset in the latest classification (see also chapter 9, table 6).

Stage I and II disease. About 25% of newly diagnosed lung cancers will be clinically stage I and stand a high chance of cure with surgery. At resection, about 20% of cases will have mediastinal lymph node involvement, and this is highest in adenocarcinomas. The usual procedure is lobectomy, for which the mortality should be no greater than 1% and complications rare, the commonest being a cardiac arrhythmia (14% of complications) [26]. Overall long-term survival is 67–83% for stage IA and 57–75% for IB. In Japanese studies, 5-yr survival tends to be better due to their high incidence of stage IA adenocarcinomas: 90% survival for IA and 75% for IB [42]. In general, lobectomy is well tolerated physiologically, with post-operative forced expiratory volume in 1 s (FEV1) of 86%, forced vital capacity of 81% and a shuttle walk test of 83% of pre-operative values. The same applies to elderly patients.

For all resections the same principles should apply: the tumour and its draining lymph nodes should be resected completely whenever possible; there should be an *en bloc* dissection of adjacent structures to the tumour if there is local invasion; and a complete ipsilateral lymph node dissection or extensive sampling should be performed. This is important even in stage IA disease, as lymph node involvement is quite common. If the primary tumour is <1 cm diameter, which is unusual, there is much less likelihood of nodal disease. However, tumours between 1 and 2 cm can have nodes in up to 20% of cases and this is commoner for adenocarcinomas. Those tumours larger than 2 cm can have nodal disease in up to 40% of cases, making mediastinal dissection imperative. The evidence that mediastinal node dissection is better for cure than random sampling of suspicious nodes has been summarised earlier.

Limited resection for early stage disease. With CT screening and more intensive investigation of patients with chronic obstructive pulmonary disease, stage I tumours are being identified more frequently. This population will have significant comorbidity and is ageing, which has led to an increase in tissue-sparing surgery: wedge resection, segmentectomy and VATS lobectomy. However, as a cancer operation, wedge resection produces inferior survival to lobectomy [43], but segmentectomy is superior to wedge for long-term survival [44]. Physiological performance is better following a segmentectomy compared with lobectomy and the long-term survival data is similar.

Although there are no randomised trials of lobectomy *via* VATS compared with thoracotomy and lobectomy, the segment resected and the width of the resection margin will influence the rates of recurrence [45]. For similar extents of lymph node involvement and dissection, there is no survival disadvantage for a VATS lobectomy [46]. However, performing a segmentectomy by VATS is difficult and not done routinely, although this may be dependent both on the previous experience of the surgeon and the segment to be excised. In 180 patients undergoing VATS lobectomy, the mortality was 0.6% and 14 (9.2%) patients underwent a conversion thoracotomy [46]. The median length of stay was 4 days. The data for patients older than 80 yrs were identical. All patients underwent mediastinal lymph node dissection. There was also less post-operative pain than in other series of patients who underwent an open lobectomy. If adjuvant chemotherapy is contemplated, it should be noted that patients recover faster from VATS lobectomy than from routine thoracotomy and more will agree to chemotherapy [47].

The place of sublobar resection for lung cancer has been the subject of a recent comprehensive review [48]. Sublobar resections remain a controversial area in surgery. There has only been one randomised, controlled trial of lobectomy *versus* segmentectomy or wedge resection and that was concluded in 1988 and published in 1995 [43]. The study was for T1N0 disease and staging included CT scans. Mediastinoscopy was not performed, and patients only entered the trial during surgery if frozen sections of lymph nodes were negative. 247 patients were eligible for assessment and the results showed that with limited resection there were 75% more recurrences, a 30% (nonsignificant) increase in the death rate, and no long-term survival advantage. They concluded that lobectomy remained the procedure of choice. However, of the 122 patients undergoing a limited resection, 40 had a wedge procedure only.

A recent meta-analysis has confirmed the results of the randomised trial, showing no differences in survival in stage I disease between the two resection procedures, but with a small benefit for the lobectomy group [49]. However, the advent of CT screening for lung cancer, especially in Japan, has increased the detection of very small cancers (<2 cm) and ground-glass opacities, for which lobectomy may appear excessive, by four-fold. In these very small tumours, the 5-yr survival rates seem the same for segmentectomy and for lobectomy. However, it is worse for wedge resection, where in one study the recurrence rate was significantly higher after wedge resection (38.5%) compared with segmentectomy (16.7%) and lobectomy (14.7%) [50]. With wedge resection, the resection margin is often narrower than with segmentectomy, with recurrence highest if this margin was <1 cm. In an uncontrolled trial of segmentectomy *versus* wedge, the procedure chosen at the surgeon's discretion, the results were inferior for wedge, with a significantly worse 5-yr survival than segmentectomy (48 *versus* 71%) and a higher local recurrence rate [51]. Tumour size seems critical, and Rami-Porta and Tsuboi [48], in their review, point out that the best results are for tumours <2 cm in diameter. Age is another important factor for sublobar resection, as lobectomy seems to have a better survival for those aged <70 yrs; however, the benefit of lobectomy disappears in those aged ≥71 yrs. Bronchoalveolar carcinomas (BACs) may be a special case for sublobar resection, as pure BAC with no features of invasion or lymph node involvement does particularly well. Small BACs are classically detected on CT screening and most series reviewed in the article by Rami-Porta and Tsuboi [48] are from Japan, where they are detected as ground-glass opacities, usually <2 cm diameter. If the tumour is removed by sublobar resection, attention must be paid to its histology intra-operatively by frozen section, as if it contains elements of adenocarcinoma, commoner if the ground-glass lesion is partially solid, a lobectomy should be performed, as the mixed BAC or pure adenocarcinoma does less well following a minor resection. Both lobectomy and sublobar resection for BAC is associated with a 5-yr survival rate of 100% if the tumour is <2 cm diameter.

In stage II disease with N1 involvement, surgery is often more extensive, needing either a pneumonectomy or a sleeve resection. Once the intrapulmonary or hilar nodes are involved, the 5-yr survival decreases considerably. About 20% of these patients will need a pneumonectomy. For upper lobe tumours where lymph nodes involve the main bronchus or adjacent pulmonary artery, sleeve resection can be performed to save lung function. For right lower lobe tumours with nodal disease at the origin of the lower lobe bronchus, or in the territory of the middle lobe airway, a right middle and lower lobectomy is required. The dissection of the mediastinum will reveal occult disease in up to 20% of cases, although with PET and EBUS/EUS, this figure may drop in the future.

The rate of relapse for stage I disease is the lowest for all resected lung cancers. Most relapses are distant, with only a 10% chance of local recurrence. Brain relapse can occur as a common distal site, especially for upper lobe lesions, right lung commoner than left, and adenocarcinoma or large cell tumours more likely than squamous cell.

For stage II, relapse is much commoner and again is usually distant; survival is considerably worse than for stage IA and IB disease (fig. 3 and table 2).

Stage III disease. Approximately 30% of NSCLC presents with stage III disease. This is a very heterogeneous stage classification. 10% of patients will be stage IIIA and some of these will be considered resectable (T3N1 and T1-3N2). There is a huge difference between these two groups, as a chest wall tumour with hilar nodal involvement is likely to fare better and may be resectable compared with a primary tumour (any T) with clinical mediastinal nodal involvement. The 20% in stage IIIB (T4N0-2, T1-4N3) are inoperable. Some may receive neoadjuvant chemotherapy or chemoradiotherapy in an attempt to downstage and become resectable, but this is quite uncommonly truly successful. The 5-yr survival for IIIB cases is only 3–7%.

In stage IIIA, N2 disease can vary considerably. A single mediastinal node found at pathology after apparently curative resection carries a 5-yr survival of about 40%. A single node found to be positive at thoracotomy, despite normal staging tests, will have a survival rate of 25–40%, with nodal disease confined to within the node capsule. Extracapsular spread in a single node still has a 5-yr survival of about 11%, but multilevel disease or clinical mediastinal disease detected pre-operatively has only a 7% survival rate [52].

The role of surgery in clinical N2 has still to be clarified. There have been several studies attempting to downstage this presentation by both chemotherapy alone and by combination chemoradiotherapy. Downstaging to the extent of clearing disease from lymph nodes at restaging mediastinoscopy (a difficult procedure, particularly after chemoradiotherapy) does influence the prospect of long-term survival. However, studies of neoadjuvant therapy and then randomising responders to surgery or radical radiotherapy have not shown a survival advantage for surgery [52]. Two studies, one from the USA (K.S. Albain; personal communication) and one from Europe (J.P. Van Meerbeeck; personal communication), have only been reported as abstracts and are negative for surgery. There are a number of factors that also affect survival after resection for lung cancer. These include age, sex and histological type of lung cancer. Post-operatively, females have a higher 5-yr survival rate. This is demonstrated consistently in trials [38–40, 53].

Most studies have demonstrated that patients with adenocarcinoma had a higher 5-yr survival (~56%) compared with squamous cell (48%) and large cell lung cancer [39–41].

This is not repeated in all studies The series studied by PFANNSCHMIDT *et al.* [38] showed that post-operative 5-yr survival was higher for squamous cell lung cancer.

Pancoast tumours. These apical or superior sulcus tumours are relatively uncommon but are important, as they are frequently missed despite early symptoms and tend to cause local problems of pain and neurological damage, rather than spreading widely to cause death. Even after successful resection, local recurrence remains relatively common. By the time these tumours come to resection, chest and/or shoulder pain is almost invariable and root pain in the C8 or T1 dermatome is common with sensory and motor changes; Horner's syndrome is less frequent. Most large surgical units will operate on fewer than 10 such tumours per annum and, therefore, controlled trials of novel therapies are rare and most of the literature is of a series of cases, or sequential therapies over a period of time, making direct comparisons difficult. Surgical approaches vary, with either a posterolateral thoracotomy or a combined transcervical and transthoracic approach [54]. In most series the commonest resection is by lobectomy and most cases are IIB, with occasional patients having a worse clinical stage. For possible cure, the resection must be complete and, with modern staging, including magnetic resonance imaging (MRI) of the neck and PET, most resections are carefully chosen, yielding a high complete resection rate. In the series of 67 cases reported by ALIFANO *et al.* [54], the peri-operative mortality was 8.9% (six cases) and the complete resection rate was 82% without routine MRI or PET. The overall 5-yr survival rate was 36% and this was poorest in those with incomplete resection and/or significant comorbid illness. There was no survival disadvantage for worsening stage, but these numbers were small. Also, 53 patients received post-operative treatment, mainly radiotherapy, but the additional effect of this was not evaluated in the study. Furthermore, local recurrence, usually treated with further radiotherapy and/or chemotherapy, was relatively ineffective. In general, most cures arise from resection T4N0 disease and the presence of hilar and, in particular, mediastinal node involvement is associated with a much poorer prognosis.

If the tumour seems confined to the lung apex but has penetrated adjacent structures, *i.e.* is T4, these subjects do relatively poorly with surgery alone and there are now several reports on pre-operative chemoradiation followed, where possible, by curative surgery and, often, further chemoradiation therapy. The latest such study gathered 32 cases of T4 superior sulcus or central T4 tumours over a period of 6 yrs [55]. All were staged with CT, MRI and PET, with mediastinoscopy where indicated. They received two courses of cisplatin-etoposide chemotherapy and concomitant radiotherapy at 45 Gy. In all, two patients progressed, 15 had stable disease and there were 14 partial responses. 27 (84%) patients underwent thoracotomy and in 25 a complete resection was achieved. 11 patients required a pneumonectomy. Their median length of follow-up is only 26.5 months and the projected 5-yr survival is 74% in intention to treat and 77% in those having a complete resection. Those with Pancoast tumours fared better to date than the central T4 lesions, with a projected 5-yr survival of 85% compared with 60% for central disease. This compares well with other nonrandomised series of chemoradio-therapeutic induction for superior sulcus tumours. For example, the biggest series from the South West Oncology Group, of 110 patients, had 80% go to surgery with an operative mortality of 2.3% and a 46% overall 5-yr survival [56]. It seems, therefore, that the current treatment approach to superior sulcus tumours, because most will have penetrated the chest wall and associated vertebral bodies (T4), is trimodality treatment. Whether this is an advance in the treatment of the tumour, or oncologists are tackling more advanced disease than T3, is not clear, as there are no comparative trials. One of the reasons why results are better than those first described by surgeons in the 1960s and 1970s is likely to be better selection of operable subjects due to better staging today.

Another issue for these tumours is the high rate of relapse in the brain, a feature of both adenocarcinomas and upper lobe tumours. Prophylactic cranial irradiation in these cases that have curative pulmonary procedures does reduce the incidence of brain relapse, but does not improve overall survival.

Chest wall tumours. Many tumours are approximate to the chest wall but do not penetrate the parietal pleura. The depth of the chest wall invasion probably does not affect survival, although it will influence the extent of the resection necessary. In a recent Japanese study of 97 patients who were staged using CT and isotope bone scans collected between 1985 and 1997, 50% were squamous cell tumours and 89% were resected by lobectomy [57]. More than half had T3N0 disease and in 40 only resection up to and including the pleura was required, while subpleural soft tissue (10 cases) and rib resection (26 cases) was needed. The survival was similar in all three groups at 30–38% at 5 yrs. Once N2 disease was present at resection, survival at 5 yrs was 6%. Some patients received pre-operative induction therapy and others post-operative treatment, but this was haphazard and difficult to analyse. Another Japanese study used careful staging with CT and MRI to determine the extent of chest wall invasion in 132 patients who had cancers resected that involved the chest wall, to see if staging could predict invasion and whether an *en bloc* dissection of the chest wall would become necessary [58]. In fact, if there was no chest pain and the CT failed to show soft tissue or rib invasion, an *en bloc* resection was not needed. However, there was no survival disadvantage for those requiring chest wall resection and the N stage dominated 5-yr outcome.

Small cell lung cancer

For small cell lung cancer (SCLC) a clinical trial in the 1970s did show that the median survival time of patients with SCLC who underwent surgery was shorter than for those who received radiotherapy alone and concluded that there was no place for surgery in this cell type [59]. However, this probably reflects the rudimentary staging at this time, with just the chest radiograph, and much disease was missed as 30% of the surgical arm patients had too advanced disease to undergo a resection. Subsequent trials have demonstrated that early SCLC (stage I disease) has a much better survival rate after modern staging [60]. A recent series from the Royal Brompton Hospital (London, UK) reported a 52% 5-yr survival in a small number of highly selected cases [61]. However, although of interest, these small selective studies are hard to interpret in relation to "usual practice". The authors' resection rate for small cell tumours, in a busy referral centre, was 2% of that for NSCLC. In 26 yrs 52 patients underwent surgery. Although staging was thorough and "modern", changing with developments in staging, there was no difference in survival according to clinical or pathological stage. There were only nine cases of stage IIIA. This is odd and makes the selection criteria for surgery somewhat opaque, especially as the 2009 staging classification shows a clear stage progression based on TNM (see chapter 9, fig. 2). Nevertheless, the outcome for the occasional patient with SCLC who can be resected is, on average, better than the survival following routine treatment, although there are no randomised trials to prove this.

Surgery for node-positive disease has been evaluated by the Lung Cancer Study Group, who randomised patients with node-positive disease to surgery after chemotherapy or to just chemotherapy alone [62]. There was no difference in the 2-yr survival rates, suggesting no role for resection in patients with nodal spread. Thus, the role for surgery remains very limited. A small primary tumour found to be stage IA and small cell on needle biopsy may be a carcinoid tumour at resection, and therefore an open mind needs to be kept and patients judged on individual merits.

Surgical intervention in the elderly

While overall the mortality and morbidity for lung cancer surgery is falling, age remains a major risk factor. The overall incidence of pulmonary resection has declined, especially in the elderly, perhaps due to age bias, the known higher risk for the surgeon, comorbidity and even lack of availability of specialised thoracic surgeons [18]. The main factors that influence outcome in the elderly are post-operative FEV1, history of cardiac disease and the extent of the planned resection. Assessment by the Charlston index is also a useful predictor of outcome [63]. The majority of elderly patients operated on tend have stage I disease. The mortality for patients aged >70 yrs with resection was 2.3–9% overall, with a rise to 22% for pneumonectomy, and a morbidity of up to 83% [64]. More recent data suggest that these values have improved and nearly halved, except for those aged >74 yrs, where the risk remains four times higher than for younger subjects [65, 66].

The post-operative mortality and morbidity are, to a large extent, determined by the size of resection. While sublobar resections have a similar mortality and morbidity to a lobectomy, they can be performed in patients with less cardiopulmonary reserve, and the survival benefit of lobectomy seems less obvious in patients aged >71 yrs.

The effects on quality of life following surgery in the elderly are no different than for younger patients. The post-operative quality of life, despite a higher incidence of post-operative complications, is well maintained [67]. In the very elderly, where series are small, resection seems safe, with no peri-operative mortality in one series of 41 patients [68], and an acceptable 5-yr survival of 57–34% depending on stage. Nevertheless, elderly patients are turned down for surgery in greater proportions than their younger counterparts.

In another study looking at the effects of age on survival, patients having a potentially curative procedure were divided into three groups: <65 yrs (n=1,315), <75 yrs (n=587) and ≥75 yrs (n=119) [69]. There was no significant difference in mortality between the age groups but performance status was closely linked to survival in those aged >65 yrs. BROKX *et al.* [70] looked at a country-wide database to identify patients aged >80 yrs who had undergone thoracic surgery for NSCLC. They also commented that the numbers were few compared with other age groups (6% of patients aged >80 yrs who were diagnosed with NSCLC underwent surgery whereas 23% of those aged 70–79 yrs and 30% of those aged <70 yrs underwent surgery). The mortality for those aged >80 yrs was, again, similar to their younger counterparts. There was no comorbidity data.

The SEER data from more than 300,000 lung cancer patients in the USA identified 145 patients aged >80 yrs and 33% aged 70–79 yrs [71]. Those aged >80 yrs were much less likely to receive any form of curative treatment but, for those who did, the results were comparable to younger subjects.

Finally, VATS in the elderly, with good selection for lobotomy by this technique, showed little effect due to age [72]. Data for stage II and IIIa patients are very scanty and clearly most are turned down on risk factors, comorbidity and extent of planned resection.

Conclusions

There have been many advances and changes in the treatment of lung cancer. In particular, the improvements in staging technology and in the actual classification are likely to have a big impact on selection for surgery and for induction and adjuvant therapy in the future. Surgery in the elderly is perfectly feasible depending on careful selection. Sublobar resection in those aged <70 yrs seems sensible, as those with poor physiology now achieve the chance for curative resection. Pre-operative assessment and post-operative care has improved greatly in the last 20 yrs, reflecting the improving morbidity and mortality around resection. Most, if not all surgery, is in NSCLC, although each case of SCLC should be assessed on its merits.

Summary

Surgery remains the best option for cure in nonsmall cell lung cancer (NSCLC) and for the occasional small cell tumour. About 10–15% of NSCLC cases go to pulmonary resection, although the resection rate varies across different countries and within countries. Staging is paramount with regard to case selection for resection, and the introduction of positron emission tomography scanning and endoscopic mediastinal lymph node sampling will further refine this. The new International Association for the Study of Lung Cancer staging classification, based on a very large number of cases, has further defined prognosis by stage, and will influence selection of patients for surgery. The mortality of resection is falling and in large centres is now about 1% for lobectomy and 3–4% for pneumonectomy. Sublobar resections are becoming increasingly common as more patients are found to have stage I disease following computed tomography screening or more intensive investigation for chronic obstructive pulmonary disease. Segmentectomy appears as successful as lobectomy of patients below 71 yrs of age, with better preservation of lung function. However the non-anatomic wedge resection carries a worse long-term survival than both segmentectomy and lobectomy. Following careful case selection, older patients fare no worse than their younger counterparts. While patients presenting with stage I and II disease are suitable for curative surgery, stage IIA remains a complex constellation of presentations. Those with N1 disease can do relatively well, but for presentations such as superior sulcus tumours and chest wall tumours, if there is nodal involvement and the stage is worse than T3N0, the prognosis is much worse. The evidence for surgery after chemoradiation induction for locally advanced stage IIIA or IIIB has not yet been made, and chemoradiotherapy alone may be the treatment of choice. Trial results are awaited. In addition to age (half of lung cancer patients present aged $\geq$70 yrs), comorbidity remains a major reason for inoperability. For small cell lung cancer, there are only small series of patients who have undergone resection. Each case should be reviewed on its merits and if at a truly early stage after the best possible staging, resection must be considered.

Keywords: Lobectomy, mortality, pneumonectomy, sublobar resection, surgery, survival.

Statement of interest
None declared.

References

1. Dautzenberg B, Arriagada R, Chammard AB, *et al.* A controlled study of postoperative radiotherapy for patients with completely resected nonsmall cell lung carcinoma. *Cancer* 1999; 86: 265–273.
2. Patz EF Jr, Rossi S, Harpole DH Jr, *et al.* Correlation of tumor size and survival in patients with stage IA non-small cell lung cancer. *Chest* 2000; 117: 1568–1571.

3. van Tinteren H, Hoekstra OS, Smit EF, *et al.* Effectiveness of positron emission tomography in the preoperative assessment of patients with suspected non-small-cell lung cancer: the PLUS multicentre randomised trial. *Lancet* 2002; 359: 1388–1393.
4. Vansteenkiste JF, Stroobants SG, Dupont PJ, *et al.* Prognostic importance of the standardized uptake value on 18F-fluoro-2-deoxy-glucose-positron emission tomography scan in non-small-cell lung cancer: an analysis of 125 cases. Leuven Lung Cancer Group. *J Clin Oncol*, 17: 3201–3206.
5. Erasmus JJ, Rohren E, Swisher SG. Prognosis and re-evaluation of lung cancer by positron emission tomography imaging. *Proc Am Thorac Soc* 2009; 6: 171–179.
6. Goodgame B, Pillot GA, Yang Z, *et al.* Prognostic value of preoperative positron emission tomography in resected stage I non-small cell lung cancer. *J Thorac Oncol* 2008; 3: 130–134.
7. Hanin FX, Lonneux M, Cornet J, *et al.* Prognostic value of FDG uptake in early stage non-small cell lung cancer. *Eur J Cardiothorac Surg* 2008; 33: 819–823.
8. Ohtsuka T, Nomori H, Ebihara A, *et al.* FDG-PET imaging for lymph node staging and pathologic tumor response after neoadjuvant treatment of non-small cell lung cancer. *Ann Thorac Cardiovasc Surg* 2006; 12: 89–94.
9. Cerfolio RJ, Bryant AS, Ohja B, *et al.* The maximum standardized uptake values on positron emission tomography of a non-small cell lung cancer predict stage, recurrence, and survival. *J Thorac Cardiovasc Surg* 2005; 130: 151–159.
10. Myrdal G, Lamberg K, Lambe M, *et al.* Regional differences in treatment and outcome in non-small cell lung cancer: a population-based study (Sweden). *Lung Cancer* 2009; 63: 16–22.
11. Mountain CF. Revisions in the International System for Staging Lung Cancer. *Chest* 1997, 111: 1710–1717.
12. Damhuis RA, Schütte PR. Resection rates and postoperative mortality in 7,899 patients with lung cancer. *Eur Respir J* 1996; 9: 7–10.
13. Fry WA, Phillips JL, Menck HR. Ten-year survey of lung cancer treatment and survival in hospitals in the United States: a national cancer data base report. *Cancer* 1999; 86: 1867–1876.
14. Page R, Keogh B, Kinsman R. The Society for Cardiothoracic Surgery in Great Britain and Ireland. First National Thoracic Surgery Activity and Outcomes Report 2008. Available from http://www.scts.org/documents/PDF/ThoracicSurgeryReport2008.pdf
15. Peake MD, Stanley R, Chanarin N. The National Lung Cancer Audit Programme (LUCADA) – Highlights from the First Annual Report. *Clin Oncol (R Coll Radiol)* 2007; 19: Suppl. 3, S42.
16. Laroche C, Wells F, Coulden R, *et al.* Improving surgical resection rate in lung cancer. *Thorax* 1998; 53: 445–449.
17. Imperatori A, Harrison RN, Leitch DN, *et al.* Lung cancer in Teesside (UK) and Varese (Italy): a comparison of management and survival. *Thorax* 2006; 61: 232–239.
18. Farjah F, Wood DE, Yanez D 3rd, *et al.* Temporal trends in the management of potentially resectable lung cancer. *Ann Thorac Surg* 2008; 85: 1850–1855.
19. Stephenson SM, Mech KF, Sardi A. Lung cancer screening with low-dose spiral computed tomography. *Am Surg* 2005; 71: 1015–1017.
20. MacRedmond R, McVey G, Lee M, *et al.* Screening for lung cancer using low dose CT scanning: results of 2 year follow up. *Thorax* 2006; 61: 54–56.
21. Swensen SJ, Jett JR, Hartman TE, *et al.* CT screening for lung cancer: five-year prospective experience. *Radiology* 2005; 235: 259–265.
22. Henschke CI, McCauley DI, Yankelevitz DF, *et al.* Early Lung Cancer Action Project: overall design and findings from baseline screening. *Lancet* 1999; 354: 99–105.
23. Navani N, Spiro SG, Janes SM. Mediastinal staging of NSCLC with endoscopic and endobronchial ultrasound. *Nat Rev Clin Oncol* 2009; 6: 278–286.
24. British Thoracic Society, Society of Cardiothoracic Surgeons of Great Britain and Ireland Working Party. BTS guidelines: guidelines on the selection of patients with lung cancer for surgery. *Thorax* 2001; 56: 89–108.

25. Ludwig C, Stoelben E, Olschewski M, *et al.* Comparison of morbidity, 30-day mortality, and long-term survival after pneumonectomy and sleeve lobectomy for non-small cell lung carcinoma. *Ann Thorac Surg* 2005; 79: 968–973.
26. Allen MS, Darling GE, Pechet TT, *et al.* Morbidity and mortality of major pulmonary resections in patients with early-stage lung cancer: initial results of the randomized, prospective ACOSOG Z0030 trial. *Ann Thorac Surg* 2006; 81: 1013–1019.
27. Ginsberg RJ, Hill LD, Eagan RT, *et al.* Modern thirty-day operative mortality for surgical resections in lung cancer. *J Thorac Cardiovasc Surg* 1983; 86: 654–658.
28. Silvestri GA, Handy J, Lackland D, *et al.* Specialists achieve better outcomes than generalists for lung cancer surgery. *Chest* 1998; 114: 675–680.
29. Wada H, Nakamura T, Nakamoto K, *et al.* Thirty-day operative mortality for thoracotomy in lung cancer. *J Thorac Cardiovasc Surg* 1998; 115: 70–73.
30. Balduyck B, Hendriks J, Lauwers P, *et al.* Quality of life after lung cancer surgery: a prospective pilot study comparing bronchial sleeve lobectomy with pneumonectomy. *J Thorac Oncol* 2008; 3: 604–608.
31. Su X, Wang X, Long H, *et al.* Mediastinal lymph node dissection affects survival in patients with stage I non-small cell lung cancer. *Thorac Cardiovasc Surg* 2008; 56: 226–230.
32. Gajra A, Newman N, Gamble GP, *et al.* Effect of number of lymph nodes sampled on outcome in patients with stage I non-small-cell lung cancer. *J Clin Oncol* 2003; 21: 1029–1034.
33. Mountain CF, Dresler CM. Regional lymph node classification for lung cancer staging. *Chest* 1997; 111: 1718–1723.
34. Martini N, Bains MS, Burt ME, *et al.* Incidence of local recurrence and second primary tumors in resected stage I lung cancer. *J Thorac Cardiovasc Surg* 1995; 109: 120–129.
35. Izbicki JR, Passlick B, Pantel K, *et al.* Effectiveness of radical systematic mediastinal lymphadenectomy in patients with resectable non-small cell lung cancer: results of a prospective randomized trial. *Ann Surg* 1998; 227: 138–144.
36. Keller SM, Adak S, Wagner H, *et al.* Mediastinal lymph node dissection improves survival in patients with stages II and IIIa non-small cell lung cancer. Eastern Cooperative Oncology Group. *Ann Thorac Surg* 2000; 70: 358–365.
37. Goldstraw P, Crowley J, Chansky K, *et al.* The IASLC Lung Cancer Staging Project: proposals for the revision of the TNM stage groupings in the forthcoming (seventh) edition of the TNM classification of malignant tumours. *J Thorac Oncol* 2007; 2: 706–714.
38. Pfannschmidt J, Muley T, Bülzebruck H, *et al.* Prognostic assessment after surgical resection for non-small cell lung cancer: experiences in 2083 patients. *Lung Cancer* 2007; 55: 371–377.
39. Duque JK, López-Encuentra A, Porta RR, *et al.* Survival of 2,991 patients with surgical lung cancer: the denominator effect in survival. *Chest* 2005; 128: 2274–2281.
40. Goya T, Asamura H, Yoshimura H, *et al.* Prognosis of 6644 resected non-small cell lung cancers in Japan: a Japanese lung cancer registry study. *Lung Cancer* 2005; 50: 227–234.
41. Naruke T, Tsuchiya R, Kondo H, *et al.* Prognosis and survival after resection for bronchogenic carcinoma based on the 1997 TNM-staging classification: the Japanese experience. *Ann Thorac Surg* 2001; 71: 1759–1764.
42. Okada M, Nishio W, Sakamoto T, *et al.* Evolution of surgical outcomes for nonsmall cell lung cancer: time trends in 1465 consecutive patients undergoing complete resection. *Ann Thorac Surg* 2004; 77: 1926–1930.
43. Ginsberg RJ, Rubinstein LV. Randomized trial of lobectomy *versus* limited resection for T1 N0 non-small cell lung cancer. Lung Cancer Study Group. *Ann Thorac Surg* 1995; 60: 615–622.
44. Schuchert MJ, Pettiford BL, Keeley S, *et al.* Anatomic segmentectomy in the treatment of stage I non-small cell lung cancer. *Ann Thorac Surg* 2007; 84: 926–932.
45. Sienel W, Stremmel C, Kirschbaum A, *et al.* Frequency of local recurrence following segmentectomy of stage IA non-small cell lung cancer is influenced by segment localisation and width of resection margins – implications for patient selection for segmentectomy. *Eur J Cardiothorac Surg* 2007; 31: 522–527.

46. Shaw JP, Dembitzer FR, Wisnivesky JP, *et al.* Video-assisted thoracoscopic lobectomy: state of the art and future directions. *Ann Thorac Surg* 2008; 85: S705–S709.
47. Demmy TL, Nwogu C. Is video-assisted thoracic surgery lobectomy better? Quality of life considerations. *Ann Thorac Surg* 2008; 85: S719–S728.
48. Rami-Porta R, Tsuboi M. Sublobar resection for lung cancer. *Eur Respir J* 2009; 33: 426–435.
49. Nakamura H, Kazuyuki S, Kawasaki N, *et al.* History of limited resection for non-small cell lung cancer. *Ann Thorac Cardiovasc Surg* 2005; 11: 356–362.
50. Miller DL, Rowland CM, Deschamps C, *et al.* Surgical treatment of non-small cell lung cancer 1 cm or less in diameter. *Ann Thorac Surg* 2002; 73: 1545–1550.
51. Sienel W, Dango S, Kirschbaum A, *et al.* Sublobar resections in stage IA non-small cell lung cancer: segmentectomies result in significantly better cancer-related survival than wedge resections. *Eur J Cardiothorac Surg* 2008; 33: 728–734.
52. Betticher DC, Hsu Schmitz SF, Tötsch M, *et al.* Mediastinal lymph node clearance after docetaxel-cisplatin neoadjuvant chemotherapy is prognostic of survival in patients with stage IIIA pN2 non-small-cell lung cancer: a multicenter phase II trial. *J Clin Oncol* 2003; 21: 1752–1759.
53. Båtevik R, Grong K, Segadal L, *et al.* The female gender has a positive effect on survival independent of background life expectancy following surgical resection of primary non-small lung cancer: a study of absolute and relative survival over 15 years. *Lung Cancer* 2005; 47: 173–181.
54. Alifano M, D'Aiuto M, Magdeleinat P, *et al.* Surgical treatment of superior sulcus tumors: results and prognostic factors. *Chest* 2003; 124: 996–1003.
55. De Leyn P, Vansteenkiste J, Lievens Y, *et al.* Survival after trimodality treatment for superior sulcus and central T4 non-small cell lung cancer. *J Thorac Oncol* 2009; 4: 62–68.
56. Rusch VW, Giroux DJ, Kraut MJ, *et al.* Induction chemoradiation and surgical resection for superior sulcus non-small-cell lung carcinomas: long-term results of Southwest Oncology Group Trial 9416 (Intergroup Trial 0160). *J Clin Oncol* 2007; 25: 313–318.
57. Matsuoka H, Nishio W, Okada M, *et al.* Resection of chest wall invasion in patients with non-small cell lung cancer. *Eur J Cardiothorac Surg* 2004; 26: 1200–1204.
58. Kawaguchi K, Mori S, Usami N, *et al.* Preoperative evaluation of the depth of chest wall invasion and the extent of combined resections in lung cancer patients. *Lung Cancer* 2009; 64: 41–44.
59. Fox W, Scadding JG. Medical Research Council comparative trial of surgery and radiotherapy for primary treatment of small-celled or oat-celled carcinoma of bronchus. Ten-year follow-up. *Lancet* 1973; 2: 63–65.
60. Shields TW, Higgins GA Jr, Matthews MJ, *et al.* Surgical resection in the management of small cell carcinoma of the lung. *J Thorac Cardiovasc Surg* 1982; 84: 481–488.
61. Lim E, Belcher E, Yap YK, *et al.* The role of surgery in the treatment of limited disease small cell lung cancer: time to reevaluate. *J Thorac Oncol* 2008; 3: 1267–1271.
62. Lad T, Piantadosi S, Thomas P, *et al.* A prospective randomized trial to determine the benefit of surgical resection of residual disease following response of small cell lung cancer to combination chemotherapy. *Chest* 1994; 106: Suppl. 6, 320S–323S.
63. Wang CY, Lin YS, Tzao C, *et al.* Comparison of the Charlson comorbidity index and Kaplan-Feinstein index in patients with stage I lung cancer after surgical resection. *Eur J Cardiothorac Surg* 2007; 32: 877–881.
64. Birim O, Zuydendorp HM, Maat AP, *et al.* Lung resection for non-small-cell lung cancer in patients older than 70: mortality, morbidity, and late survival compared with the general population. *Ann Thorac Surg* 2003; 76: 1796–1801.
65. Mery CM, Pappas AN, Bueno R, *et al.* Similar long-term survival of elderly patients with non-small cell lung cancer treated with lobectomy or wedge resection within the Surveillance, Epidemiology and End Results database. *Chest* 2005; 128: 237–245.
66. Aelony Y. Lung resection in the elderly. *Chest* 2006; 129: 496–497.
67. Ferguson MK, Parma CM, Celauro AD, *et al.* Quality of life and mood in older patients after major lung resection. *Ann Thorac Surg* 2009; 87: 1007–1012.

68. Brock MV, Kim MP, Hooker CM, *et al.* Pulmonary resection in octogenarians with stage I nonsmall cell lung cancer: a 22-year experience. *Ann Thorac Surg* 2004; 77: 271–277.
69. Schneider T, Pfannschmidt J, Muley T, *et al.* A retrospective analysis of short and long-term survival after curative pulmonary resection for lung cancer in elderly patients. *Lung Cancer* 2008; 62: 221–227.
70. Brokx HA, Visser O, Postmus PE, *et al.* Surgical treatment for octogenarians with lung cancer: results from a population-based series of 124 patients. *J Thorac Oncol* 2007; 2: 1013–1017.
71. Owonikoko TK, Ragin CC, Belani CP, *et al.* Lung cancer in elderly patients: an analysis of the Surveillance, Epidemiology and End Results database. *J Clin Oncol* 2007; 25: 5570–5577.
72. Cattaneo SM, Park BJ, Wilton AS, *et al.* Use of video-assisted thoracic surgery for lobectomy in the elderly results in fewer complications. *Ann Thorac Surg* 2008; 85: 231–235.

CHAPTER 12

Radiotherapy in the treatment of nonsmall cell lung cancer

M.Q.F. Hatton, J. Martin

Dept of Clinical Oncology, Weston Park Hospital, Sheffield, UK.

Correspondence: M. Hatton, Dept of Clinical Oncology, Weston Park Hospital, Whitham Rd, Sheffield, S10 2SJ, UK.

Radiotherapy plays a major role in the management of nonsmall cell lung cancer (NSCLC). It has an established curative role in the earlier stages of disease when a complete surgical resection cannot be performed. In advanced disease its role is the palliation of symptoms and maintenance of a patient's quality of life, and approximately 70% of cancer patients receive radiation therapy as part of their cancer treatment [1]. Increasingly, radiotherapy is being used in combination treatment with chemotherapy and/or surgery, and the technical advances in imaging, radiotherapy planning and treatment delivery that are occurring have led to a realistic expectation that the outcome from radiotherapy treatment will improve over the coming years. It should be noted at this point that, although chemoradiotherapy is discussed at points in this chapter, the subject is predominantly covered in chapter 14 of this *European Respiratory Monograph (ERM)*.

Principles underlying radiotherapy treatment

The basic principles of irradiation are important in order to understand the potential and the limitations of this modality. Moreover, they may help to explain some of the differences observed between published series and clinical practice. In the early development of radiation treatment it was found that one large dose might have profound effects on tumours but the equally profound effects on normal tissues limited clinical usefulness.

The response to this limitation was the application of the basic radiobiological principles of repair, redistribution, resistance, repopulation and reoxygenation, which led to the development of fractionated treatment. There is little difference in the response of malignant cells and normal cells to ionising radiation: both cell types can repair the sublethal damage inflicted by radiation and are more sensitive to radiation during the mitotic phase of the cell cycle. Hence, the use of multiple small doses favours the cells that are quiescent and able to repair the sublethal damage before the next cell division. This means that radiation will have more effect on rapidly dividing (tumour) cells in comparison with the more slowly dividing normal tissues. In addition, fractionation increases tumour cell killing by allowing the redistribution of tumour cells into more sensitive phases of the cell cycle. Hypoxia protects against the effects of radiation and, as it is a factor that is only present in tumours, it imparts radioresistance to cancer. The fractionation of treatment gives time to improve the oxygenation of tumour cells and reduce the effects of hypoxia.

Eur Respir Mon, 2009, 44, 207–243. Printed in UK - all rights reserved. Copyright ERS Journals Ltd 2009; European Respiratory Monograph; ISSN 1025-448x.

The outcome of treatment will depend on the total dose delivered. Each given dose of radiation destroys a constant fraction of cells; hence, the dose required to control a tumour increases with tumour size and the number of cells present. The majority of patients with NSCLC referred for radiation have large tumours, explaining the low rate of local control. For example, MORITA *et al.* [2] reported a 38% risk of local failure at 5 yrs for tumours <3 cm, and 68% for tumours >5 cm. This influence of tumour size is documented in other series [3–9]. There are other well documented prognostic factors that also influence radiotherapy decisions and the outcome of treatment, including performance status, weight loss and tumour stage. For example, the spread to hilar nodes will approximately halve a 5-yr survival rate of 62% for T1N0 tumours to 34% for T1N1 disease [10].

Both normal and malignant tissues have sigmoid dose–response relationships. A certain radiation dose must be given before a response is seen and tissues (normal and malignant) respond soon after treatment is begun. A maximal reaction can be expected between 3 and 4 weeks after initiating therapy. These factors have led to the classical radiation schedule delivering 1 fraction·day^{-1} (usually 1.8–2 Gy), 5 days·week^{-1} over 5–7 weeks. After these schedules came into widespread use, the evidence started to develop in the 1970s that total dose is important. It was the Radiation Therapy Oncology Group (RTOG) trial that reported 3-yr survival rates of 6, 10 and 15% after doses of 40, 50 and 60 Gy, respectively [3], that set the standard of 60 Gy in 30 fractions over 6 weeks. This schedule has been the control for a number of the subsequent radiotherapy studies.

Radiation toxicity

The use of higher radiation doses remains a challenge for the radiotherapist, due to the tolerance of several vital normal tissues (lung, heart and the spinal cord) that must be taken into account. Most side-effects are predictable and are categorized as early and late by their speed of onset. The early effects tend to be seen in tissues that are turning over rapidly, *e.g.* oesophagitis and skin reactions, and generally resolve in the weeks that follow treatment. Late treatment effects (*e.g.* pulmonary fibrosis and radiation myelitis) develop in the months that follow irradiation and are of much more concern, being irreversible and with the potential to cause profound problems for the patient. It is the risk of these late effects that currently limits the dose delivered in lung cancer treatments.

Total dose is the main determinant, but the risk of late effects is raised by increasing treatment volume and fraction size. Statistical models have been devised to predict normal tissue complications probabilities [11, 12], and an acceptable dose level is one that has a <5% probability of late complications developing during the 5 yrs that follow treatment. However, deciding on an appropriate dose for routine clinical practice has been complicated by different investigators reporting different tolerance doses for individual organs [13]. There are numerous reasons for this, as the nature and severity of the radiation reactions will be dependent on fitness of the patient, presence of comorbidities and the heterogeneous dose distribution across the organ or normal tissue at risk.

Progress in radiation treatment has centred around reduction of the risk of the late effects, primarily by the application of new technologies to reduce the volume of normal tissue being treated but maintaining (or increasing) tumour dose.

Radiation technology

The ability to give high doses of radiation to lung tumours needs accurate delineation of the cancer and knowledge of its position throughout the planning and treatment process. The quality of treatment planning and delivery has an important effect on the outcome of patients treated for NSCLC. Analysis of a series of RTOG trials demonstrated that protocol deviations have negative effects on local control and survival, by showing a fall in 2-yr survival from 33 to 14% if the treatment had been delayed by 5 days [14]. The study reported results of treatments that used two-dimensional (2D) planning with set-up checked by conventional simulation, using diagnostic-quality X-rays at exactly the orientation of the treatment beam portals in order to show target localisation and geometric coverage. These techniques were generally based on field size, with poor definition of anatomical and tumour boundaries, and can only give limited information about the true radiation dose being delivered to the cancer and surrounding normal tissues (fig. 1).

In the 1990s, developments in imaging and computing led to 3D conformal radiation therapy, which aimed at tailoring the high-dose volume to the target volume while delivering a low dose to the normal tissues. These technical advances that are required to deliver the 3D conformal treatment have continued since the turn of the century with the development of 4D planning, which can account for tumour movement over the breathing cycle and the delivery of stereotactic body radiotherapy for early stage NSCLC. The remainder of this section highlights and illustrates the most important areas in which progress is occurring.

Accurate delineation of the tumour and surrounding normal structures. Computed tomography (CT) offered a big advance on conventional simulation in the identification of the gross tumour, involved nodes and adjacent normal structures. For lung cancer, the use of both lung- and soft-tissue window settings is needed for the most accurate delineation of the gross tumour volume (GTV). The use of CT scanning data for target localisation enabled improved geometric accuracy compared with conventional planning, and revealed errors in targeting in 49% of patients planned conventionally, with 30–50% having the treatment plans altered as a result [15].

However, a number of limitations remain in, for example, the separation of collapsed normal lung from tumour, definition of involved lymph nodes on size criteria and identification of functional areas of normal tissue. Studies with various functional

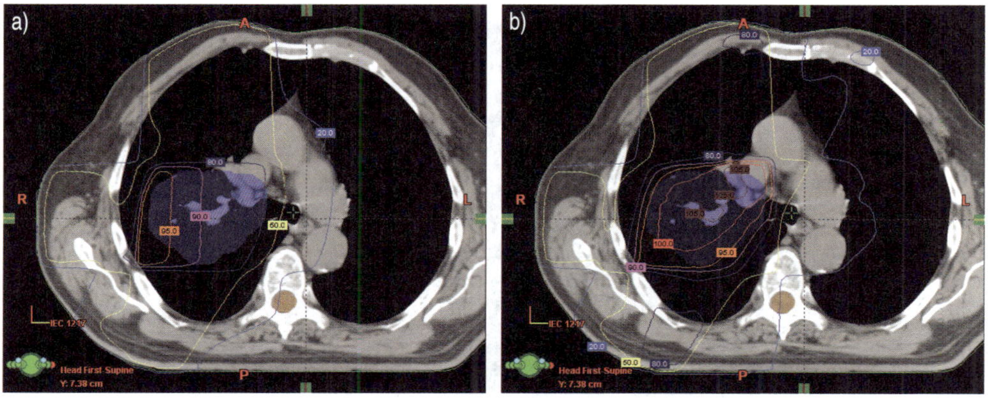

Fig. 1. – An illustration of the radiation dose distribution (isodeses given in percentage: 20, 50, 80, 90, 95 and 100 as marked) using a standard three-field plan. a) The dose distribution achieved when using two-dimensional planning techniques without correction for lung inhomogeneity. Note that the prescribed dose (100%) is not achieved and the marked dose gradient across the planning target volume (PTV) (shaded blue). b) The improved PTV coverage achieved with three-dimensional planned conformal treatment using a convolution algorithm (AAA) that includes a lung correction.

imaging techniques look to overcome some of these limitations, with positron emission tomography (PET) in particular being adopted into routine practice. A large body of evidence has established PET/CT in the staging of lung cancer [16], and the use of PET has been shown to modify the radiation fields in 22–62% of cases [17]. A reduction in GTV by better identification of atelectasis has been reported in 15–23% of cases [18, 19]. However, it is as likely that the GTV will increase with the more accurate identification of local nodal involvement [19]. Although very useful in tumour localisation, caution is still needed before using PET/CT to provide an exact delineation between tumour and normal tissue. There is debate over the correct threshold values to use and further work is needed on the co-registration of PET and CT planning images.

Patient (tumour) immobilisation. Intuitively it is clear that patient set-up errors and organ motion will have significant effects on the delivery and outcome for the radiation treatment of lung cancer. The development of portal imaging on treatment machines (fig. 2) has improved the verification of beam position and enhanced the ability to detect and correct systematic set-up errors in the average position of the patient during a course of treatment. Random errors that occur around this average beam position can be addressed and reduced by immobilisation and careful daily positioning of the patient.

CT planning introduces another stage into the treatment process and adds to the potential problems of reproducibility, with the patient requiring careful set-up on the scanner, simulator and linear accelerator. The process of "virtual simulation" integrates the CT data by scanning the patient in treatment position with laser localisation, which is similar to that on the treatment machine. The 3D CT data are used to generate digitally reconstructed radiographs, beam's eye view and room views (fig. 3), to allow the visualisation of the treatment portals and the relationship of the target to critical structures [20]. The development of techniques that permit co-registering of images onto the CT planning scan allows information from other forms of scanning (such as magnetic resonance imaging (MRI) and PET) to be accurately incorporated into the planning process [21].

The problem of tumour motion can be addressed by limiting respiratory movement and studies have identified a number of techniques that can do this: abdominal compression [22], voluntary breath-hold [23] or active breathing control (ABC) [24].

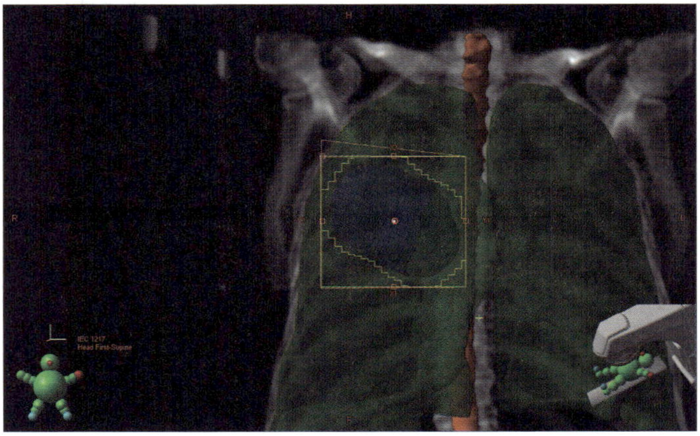

Fig. 2. – The digitally reconstructed radiograph for the anterior field of the plan illustrated in figure 1. The room view (bottom right) indicates patient treatment position. The planning target volume (PTV; blue) and normal tissues have been superimposed, and the beam's eye view demonstrates the use of multileaf collimators to conform the treatment field to the PTV and spare the normal tissues.

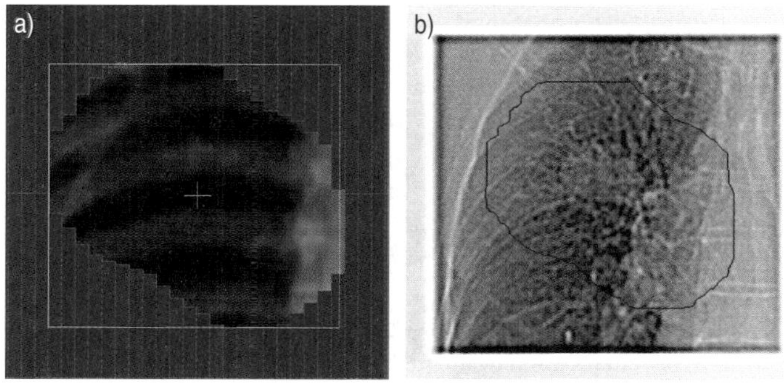

Fig. 3. – Beam's eye view for the anterior field seen in figure 3 of a) a digitally reconstructed radiograph and b) an electronic portal image for the treatment field, giving bone and soft-tissue details to confirm beam position.

Alternatively, treatment can be "gated" and given during a defined part of the respiratory cycle [25, 26]. Another approach is the use of 4D CT planning [27], which identifies the position of the tumour throughout the respiratory cycle and defines an internal tumour volume, which is then used to plan the treatment.

When these techniques are applied, treatment verification becomes crucial in ensuring that the planned treatment is actually the treatment delivered to the tumour. For image-guided radiotherapy (IGRT), a CT is performed with the patient in position before the treatment, and the 3D image produced can then be verified to confirm the anatomical tumour location [28, 29].

Dose prescription. The radiotherapy treatments aim to treat a planning target volume (PTV), which is derived by expanding the GTV into a clinical target volume (CTV), which then includes areas of likely microscopic disease. The CTV is then expanded into the PTV to allow for day-to-day variations in set-up and tumour movement and to ensure that the tumour is always within the treatment fields and receives the prescribed dose. The International Commission on Radiation Units and Measurements (ICRU) reference point for prescription dose (reports 50 and 62) should be the centre of the PTV, and the planning process should ensure that homogeneity is between 95% and 107% of the ICRU reference point across the rest of the PTV. Equally important are the normal structures, as it is late damage done to the organs at risk, particularly lungs and spinal cord, which limits the dose that can be delivered to the tumour.

3D conformation of beam shape and orientation. Virtual simulation allows 3D conformal techniques to better target the tumour (figs 3 and 4) with more accurately placed radiation beams that are then shaped to fit the profile of the target using multileaf collimators (MLCs). This spares normal tissue from treatment and, by reducing the dose to the critical organs, allows dose escalation to the tumour, increasing the chance of local control.

3D dose calculation. Radiotherapy planning is dependent on algorithms that model the dose distribution of the treatment beams and modern planning systems are able to take this information and account for the distribution of the radiation dose in three dimensions. Over time, these systems have been giving a more accurate estimation of the true dose distribution, as they incorporate corrections for tissue inhomogeneity, scattered dose and increased penumbra width in lung tissue. The correction for tissue

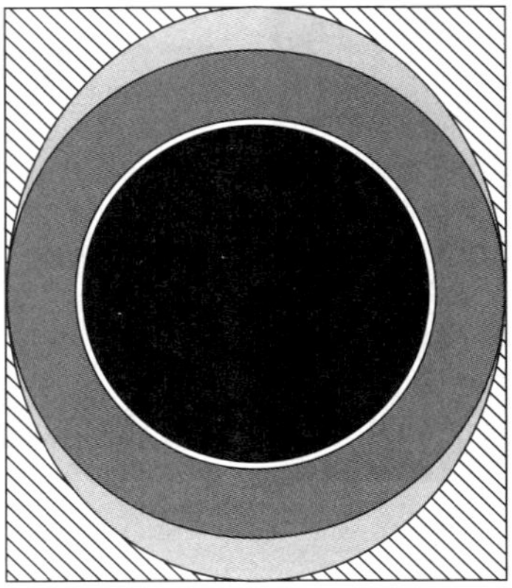

Fig. 4. – A schematic beam's eye view illustration of a 6-cm spherical tumour (■). Margins of 1.25 cm laterally and 2 cm superior/inferiorly are added to create the planning target volume (PTV). A rectangular field representing two-dimensional (2D) treatment (▧) is compared with a 3D conformal field (▒). In this example, the rectangular and conformal field areas are 85 and 67 cm^2, so the conformal technique reduces the irradiated area by more than 20%. Using 4D planning and image guidance to reduce the added margin for the PTV to 1.25 cm (▩) in all directions, the area irradiated is 57 cm^2, 33% less than the original rectangular field.

inhomogeneity is particularly important in the lung (fig. 1), whose density is approximately 30% of the soft tissues. This means less attenuation of the beam and a higher percentage dose at any given depth. In addition, the accurate calculation of dose within the lungs has to take into account the increased distance electrons can travel and deposit dose away from the treatment field, and the reduction of scatter dose back from the low-density tissue that surrounds a tumour in lung.

Plan evaluation. The 3D planning systems create dose–volume histograms (DVHs) by calculating the dose for each pixel on the CT scan. This information can be used to give a graphical representation of the dose (fig. 5) across the PTV as well as normal tissues, including lung, oesophagus, heart and spinal cord. The DVH can be used to evaluate different treatment plans and aid selection of the most appropriate on the basis of the coverage of the PTV and sparing of normal tissues. In addition, DVH parameters have shown predictive ability for radiation pneumonitis, which is the major dose-limiting toxicity [30]. A number of parameters have been found to be predictive, including total mean lung dose and volume of lung receiving >5, 14, 20 or 30 Gy (*V*5, *V*14, *etc.*), with the *V*20 value (*i.e.* volume of lung receiving 20 Gy or more) being the best validated [31]. DVHs can also be used to demonstrate doses to other organs and confirm that treatment is keeping within the dose constraints recommended on the basis of literature evidence, *e.g.* the radiation myelitis risk is ~1% at 50 Gy.

Computer-controlled treatment delivery. High-dose fractionated, conformal radiotherapy treatment requires a complex process of treatment verification and delivery on the linear accelerator. Newer treatment approaches like intensity-modulated radiotherapy (IMRT) greatly add to the complexity of treatment delivery, with their requirement for a significantly higher number of treatment beams often in non-coplanar beam arrangements. The rapid, safe and accurate delivery of this complex 3D therapy is reliant on a high degree of computer technology.

A number of developments have been required to make 3D conformal therapy a routine treatment option. Automatic set-up allows the treatment machine to move by

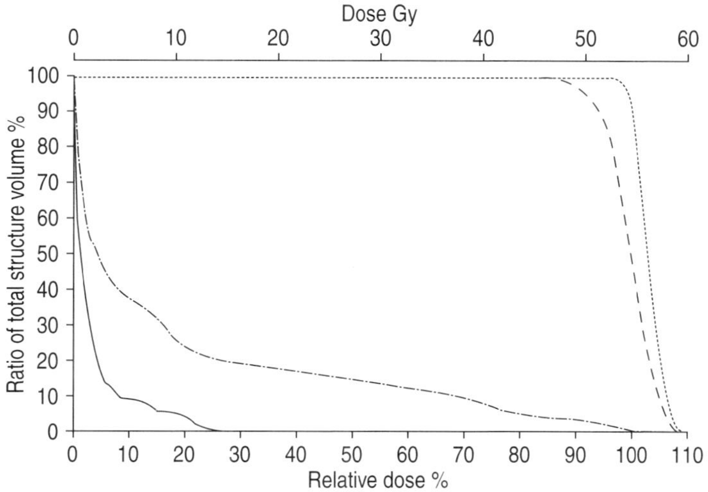

Fig. 5. – Dose–volume histogram (DVH) for the treatment plan illustrated in figure 1 and showing the dose to normal critical structures (——), the gross tumour volume (GTV; ······) and planning target volume (– – – –). The DVH confirms that normal tissue tolerances are not exceeded, and the volume of lung receiving 20 Gy or more (18.5%) is calculated using the combined volumes of both lungs excluding the GTV (· – · – ·).

itself from one field to the next and automatically adjust the rotation of its major components to assume the shape and orientation of the next field; this markedly increases treatment efficiency. Another development is the MLC, which consists of a series of individually motorised opposed metal leaves housed in the linear accelerator. These can be automatically programmed to assume a wide variety of shapes in seconds and allow fields to have complex shapes so that radiation can conform to the shape of the target volume. They replace the time-consuming and labour-intensive customised block technique. In addition, these developments will reduce the risk of human error, as does the computerised transfer of planning information from the planning system straight to the linear accelerator.

Curative radiotherapy

Surgery remains the cornerstone of curative treatment in NSCLC but only 20–30% of patients would have resectable disease after careful staging procedures and one third of these patients presenting with localised NSCLC are considered unsuitable for surgery. In this context, radiotherapy has been developed as an alternative loco-regional treatment. In the 1970s a study by the RTOG evaluated total radiation doses of 40, 50 and 60 Gy delivered at 2-Gy fractions and demonstrated a dose–response effect with better response rates and 2-yr survivals associated with higher dose [3]. This established an international standard radical radiotherapy schedule of 60 Gy over 6 weeks. Small escalations of dose (64–66 Gy) using these conventional fractionations in routine practice have not led to improved local tumour control or survival. This outcome can be related to both a high rate of appearance of distant metastases and a failure to eradicate the local disease. Re-evaluation by bronchoscopy after radical treatment with thoracic radiation has shown persistent local tumour in 85% of patients [32].

Patient selection

Radical radiotherapy is indicated for early (stage I and II) NSCLC when the patient declines surgery or is medically inoperable. It can also be used for locally advanced stage III disease, although the results of treatment with conventional fractionation alone are disappointing. A number of factors have been shown to predict for an increased chance of long-term survival following radical radiotherapy and should be considered when selecting patients for treatment. The importance of tumour size has already been discussed [3–9], with smaller lesions having a higher probability of local control. Good performance status (World Health Organization (WHO) 0 or 1) and minimal weight loss (<10%) are also predictive of long-term survival and are factors that should play a role in patient selection.

The other factor in patient selection is co-existing morbidities, particularly in the lung. It needs to be remembered that long-term fibrosis from radiotherapy may result in an unacceptable level of pulmonary restriction. Those with poor respiratory function need to be treated with caution. There are no published guidelines to indicate the lower limit of pulmonary function needed for radical radiotherapy treatment but it is widely accepted that those with a forced expiratory volume in 1 s or diffusing capacity of the lung for carbon monoxide of <50% predicted value should be treated with caution.

Early stage disease

There have been no randomised trials addressing the benefit of radical radiotherapy in stage I/II NSCLC and selected results for radical radiotherapy are documented in table 1. These results from series published in the 1980s and 1990s report 5-yr survivals ranging 6–50%. Evidence that these radiotherapy series are reporting an improvement in outcome comes from the comparison of their results with a fully staged, but untreated, group of patients with T2N0 NSCLC, who had a median survival of 17 months with no 3-yr survivors [45]. Further supporting evidence from patients treated between 1998 and 2001 (4,357 patients) comes from the Surveillance Epidemiology and End Results (SEER) data, which confirmed a significantly better survival from patients with stage I/II disease who received radiotherapy when compared with untreated patients (stage 1 median survival 21 *versus* 14 months) [46]. Although survival rates at 5 yrs were not significantly different (11 *versus* 10%), the study concluded that there was an observed improvement in median survival of 5–7 months when radiotherapy had been given.

These radiotherapy results are certainly lower than those achieved by surgery, which was reporting 5-yr survivals of 50–60%. The patients with early stage disease are considered for radiotherapy because they are unfit for or refuse surgical treatment. As these patients will have higher rates of concomitant illness and radiological rather than surgical staging, a direct comparison of surgical and radiotherapy outcomes cannot be made. Retrospective analysis suggests that, when an anatomical resection is not possible, limited surgery and radiotherapy offer equivalent results [47]. Although surgery remains the treatment of choice for patients with small localised tumours, this position may be challenged in the coming years with the application of conformal treatment techniques, dose escalation and altered fractionation schedules.

Locally advanced disease

Some selected results for radical radiotherapy in stage III disease are documented in table 2. There was a small survival advantage shown in a randomised trial comparing with no treatment. This was performed in 1968, with doses and techniques that now would be

Table 1. – Reported survival for early nonsmall cell lung cancer treated with radiation alone

First author [ref.]	Year	Stage	Patients n	Median survival months	5-yr survival %
COOPER [33]	1985	T1–3	72		6
HAFFTY [34]	1988	I	43	28	21
NOORDIJK [4]	1988		50	27	16
ZHANG [35]	1989	I, II	44	>36	32
BURT [36]	1990	T1–3 N0	133		27
		T1 N0	29		50
SANDLER [37]	1990	I	77	20	10
TALTON [38]	1990	T1-3 N0	77	16	17
DOSORETZ [39]	1992	T1–2	152	17	10
KASKOWITZ [40]	1993	T1–2	53	21	6
SLOTMAN [41]	1994	I	47	20	15
GAUDEN [42]	1995	I	347	28	27
GRAHAM [43]	1996	T1 N0	35	~16	29
		T1 N0 no weight loss	25		40
KROL [44]	1996	I	108	~24	15
		I (<4 cm)	89		
MORITA [2]	1997	T1–2	149	27	22

considered suboptimal [53]. There have been no trials comparing palliative and radical dose of radiotherapy, and most series have reported a 2-yr survival of ~15% and documented a tail of long-term survivors. A review of 26 series containing 4,796 patients treated to a dose >40 Gy demonstrated an exponential survival curve with 7% alive at 5 yrs [54].

Current radiation practice

The most important aim of radical radiotherapy treatment in NSCLC is to gain local control of the disease within the thorax. The early reports for radiotherapy treatment are documented in tables 1 and 2 and it is clear from a number of these reports that poor outcome can be related to both a high rate of distant metastases and a failure to eradicate the local disease. The rates of local recurrence reported will depend on the investigations undertaken following treatment. Where re-evaluation after radical treatment with thoracic radiation included bronchoscopy, persistent local tumour was identified in 85% of patients [32]. As expected, the failure of local control has been shown to have an impact on survival. In the RTOG study, the 3-yr survival rate fell from 22% in those who had the disease controlled within the thorax to 10% in those who

Table 2. – Survival and local control in selected phase III trials for locally advanced lung cancer treated with radiotherapy alone

First author [ref.]	Year	Patients n	Treatment Gy/weeks/fractions	2-yr survival %	5-yr survival %
PEREZ [3]	1986	378	60/6/30		5
DURCI [48]	1991	81		24	9
ARRIAGADA [32]	1991	177	65/6.5/32	14	
SCHAAKE-KONING [49]	1992	110	55/7/20 (split)	13	
WÜRSCHMIDT [5]	1994	206	>60/>6/>25	36	5
COX [14]	1994	219	>55/>6/>30	33	7
		185 (good prognosis)			15
SAUSE [50]	1995	152	60/6/30	19	5
SAUNDERS [51]	1999	224	60/6/30	21	
BALL [52]	1999	51	60/6/30	26	

relapsed locally [3]. Over the past 20 yrs, three key advances have been made in the physical basis of radiation oncology: conformal radiotherapy, IMRT and IGRT. Conformal radiotherapy is now standard practice in the UK and delivers treatment with MLCs and modern planning systems. IMRT requires additional planning system optimisation and sequencing algorithms and is in routine use for cancer treatment at other sites and is starting to be considered for NSCLC. IGRT requires additional hardware for repeat imaging in treatment rooms; the investment in this equipment is starting to be made in UK centres.

Conformal radiotherapy

Most of the trials referred to in tables 1 and 2 reported results of treatments that used 2D planning, with treatment limited by the dose received by normal tissues adjacent to the tumour. Conformal radiotherapy treatment essentially means that the delivery of radiation conforms to the anatomical configuration of the tumour in three dimensions. The main advantage of conformal treatment is the ability to spare the surrounding normal tissue, reducing the dose to the organs at risk and hence the risk of significant toxicity. This advantage has been felt to be self-evident and it is difficult to find randomised data to show improved outcome for 3D conformal radiotherapy over 2D planned and delivered treatment. The published evidence comes from retrospective analysis [55] and from dose escalation studies. For example, KONG *et al.* [56] were able to apply conformal techniques and deliver doses of 103 Gy while maintaining an acceptable toxicity level.

Elective nodal irradiation

The practice of elective nodal irradiation (ENI) evolved on the basis of the knowledge of the pattern of spread for NSCLC and the likelihood of mediastinal lymph nodes that are "normal" by CT criteria containing microscopic disease. Treatment planning would include these nodes in the CTV and ENI would plan to deliver a radiation dose that would be sufficient to sterilise the microscopic disease. However, over the past few years there has been a move away from ENI, as the main factor limiting thoracic radiotherapy is the volume of lung to be irradiated and the practice of ENI can significantly increase this volume.

Radiotherapy planning studies demonstrated that, by avoiding ENI and limiting the irradiation to the known area of disease (GTV), the amount of normal lung spared allows a dose escalation of 30% without an increase in the risk of radiation pneumonitis [57]. In addition, most studies of conformal radiotherapy have continued to show that local failure occurred within the area of the GTV rather than loco-regional nodes. Some specific studies have reported the outcome of radiotherapy when ENI has been omitted. In one, 132 patients with predominately stage III disease reported an increase in the median dose delivered to 70 Gy with a 2-yr rate of elective nodal control of 92%, but 60% still relapsed within the GTV [58]. Similar figures have been reported for stage I/II disease, with very low rates of mediastinal relapse [59, 60] and no evidence of any compromise of survival. More recently, PET scanning has come into widespread use in the staging of NSCLC and studies have confirmed the safety of confining the radiotherapy to the PET-positive mediastinal lymph node areas [61].

Chemoradiotherapy

Radical radiotherapy remains the mainstay of treatment for inoperable NSCLC, but its curative potential is low, as most patients will die with disseminated disease.

Consequently, it is reasonable to use systemic therapy to treat micrometastases. These small tumours are likely to be more chemosensitive, due to organised microvasculature with resultant better perfusion and oxygenation. In addition, many chemotherapy agents have a radiation-sensitising effect and offer potential benefits in local control.

In NSCLC, neoadjuvant, concomitant and adjuvant chemotherapy have well documented survival benefits and combined treatment is commonly used in locally advanced disease. These benefits and toxicities for conventionally fractionated radiotherapy were established in the NSCLC Collaborative Group meta-analysis [62]. In this meta-analysis, the addition of neoadjuvant cisplatin-based chemotherapy to conventional radical radiotherapy gave a 2-yr survival benefit of 4% with selected trials showing an improvement of ~10% for this sequential approach [9, 50, 63]. This translates into an increase in median survival of 3–4 months (from 10 months to 13–14 months). Concomitant chemoradiotherapy has pushed median survival to around 16 months [64] by improving local control and reducing the risks of metastatic disease. Meta-analysis of the 14 trials that have compared concurrent treatment with radiotherapy alone confirmed the improvement in 2-yr survival with a hazard ratio (HR) of 0.93 (95% confidence interval (CI) 0.72–0.98) in favour of concurrent treatment. The comparison of sequential with concurrent treatment produced a similar HR in favour of the concurrent treatment (0.86, 95% CI 0.78–0.95) [65].

Trials that have reported on the addition of adjuvant or consolidation chemotherapy to concurrent schedules have suggested that median survivals can be taken past 16–17 months in carefully selected patients with stage III NSCLC [66]. However, it needs to be remembered that the potential toxicity from these approaches can be significant, and the performance status, age and comorbidities will exclude a high number of patients from this form of treatment. For these patients, accelerated radiotherapy schedules like continuous hyperfractionated accelerated radiotherapy (CHART) may be more appropriate [67].

The other approach is to use cytotoxic agents as radiosensitisers. Typically, chemotherapy drugs are administered at low doses during the radiotherapy course, with the aim of optimising local disease control. The evidence that this could be a useful approach comes from a randomised trial in which daily low-dose cisplatin was added to a radiotherapy schedule and shown to produce a significantly better 2-yr survival of 26% that was due to an improvement in local control [49]. However, it should be noted that a split course radiotherapy schedule was used and the chemotherapy may simply have compensated for the tumour repopulation that would have occurred in the rest period in the radiation schedule.

Other studies have shown the feasibility of using other drugs (carboplatin, paclitaxel and gemcitabine) as radiation sensitisers [68–70]. However, the phase III trials, particularly the recently closed Gemcitabine and Radiotherapy in NSCLC (GRIN) study, which compared radiosensitising with concurrent weekly 100 $mg \cdot m^{-2}$ gemcitabine with hypofractionated 55 Gy in 20 fractions over 4 weeks, failed to reach the recruitment target needed to demonstrate any significant improvement in outcome [70]. The main concern over these approaches is the possibility of increased toxicity, in particular the risk of pneumonitis; results are eagerly awaited.

Developments in radiation treatment

Intensity-modulated radiotherapy

IMRT extends the capability of 3D conformal treatment. It varies the intensity of the dose within each conformal treatment field, allowing a different radiotherapy dose to be delivered to the same tumour volume during a single exposure. This heterogeneous dose distribution allows the formation of concave isodoses that can improve tumour coverage and sparing of the normal tissue (fig. 6). In some situations, when a critical organ like the spinal cord is in close proximity to the tumour, this reduction in dose justifies the extra resources required to deliver IMRT [71]. By sparing normal tissue, IMRT offers the opportunity for relatively safe dose escalation: feasibility studies have shown an increase of between 16 and 35% in mean dose compared with standard conformal treatment, with a reduced dose to surrounding critical structures [72, 73]. These dosimetric studies are supported by a retrospective comparison that suggested that incidence of grade III or greater pneumonitis was less for patients treated with IMRT compared with those treated using 3D plans (8 *versus* 32%) [74].

Reports of treatment outcome for patients with NSCLC treated with IMRT techniques have started appear in the literature. These studies have delivered conventional doses of treatment (60–66 Gy) to a variety of stages, including patients with recurrent disease [74–76]. Lower rates of toxicity are reported [74] with median survival times of 25–38 months [75, 76]. One study focused on more elderly patients with stage I/II disease and omitted ENI. It is this study that reported a median survival of 38 months with low rates of recurrence in the uninvolved mediastinal nodes [76].

A further reason to consider IMRT in the radical treatment of NSCLC is to reduce symptomatic radiation pneumonitis and fibrosis. In patients with NSCLC, the remaining normal lung is often intertwined with the diseased lung, and delivering a high radiation dose to the target while sparing this normal lung can be challenging. Lung function is not evenly distributed, and it has been shown clinically that radiating through regions of reduced function initially has resulted in greater preservation of diffusion capacity [77]. Single photon emission CT lung perfusion scans have been used to identify areas of highly functional lung and assign these areas as regions to avoid during lung IMRT planning [78], with IMRT planning better able to spare functional regions compared with 3D conformal planning. Similar potential for modifying lung cancer radiotherapy plans using IMRT to reduce the dose to normal functioning lung has been shown using the ventilation images from 4D CT [79] and hyperpolarised helium MRI scanning [21].

There are disadvantages to IMRT that mean that it will not benefit all NSCLC patients undergoing radical treatment. It is resource intensive and requires the time and effort of a multidisciplinary team of radiographers, physicists and clinicians. The situations in which IMRT is likely to find a role will require sharp dose gradients between tumour and normal tissue and thus IMRT will be more susceptible to patient set-up errors and respiratory movement. These errors could adversely affect outcome by geographical miss and underdosage of the target volume. A further concern is that, although IMRT reduces the high doses given to critical normal tissues, it does so by employing extra fields, which means that larger volumes of normal tissue may be exposed to lower radiation doses, which, in lung, raises a concern of late radiation damage.

Dose escalation

A second approach to improving local control rates is to escalate the radiotherapy dose to the tumour. As discussed earlier in this chapter, safe radiation dose escalation is now feasible with modern 3D CT-based planning techniques [56, 80, 81]. In addition to the application of conformal radiotherapy techniques, the omission of ENI can reduce the dose to surrounding normal tissue. McGibney *et al.* [82] suggested that a combination of 3D conformal radiotherapy and omission of ENI could allow escalation

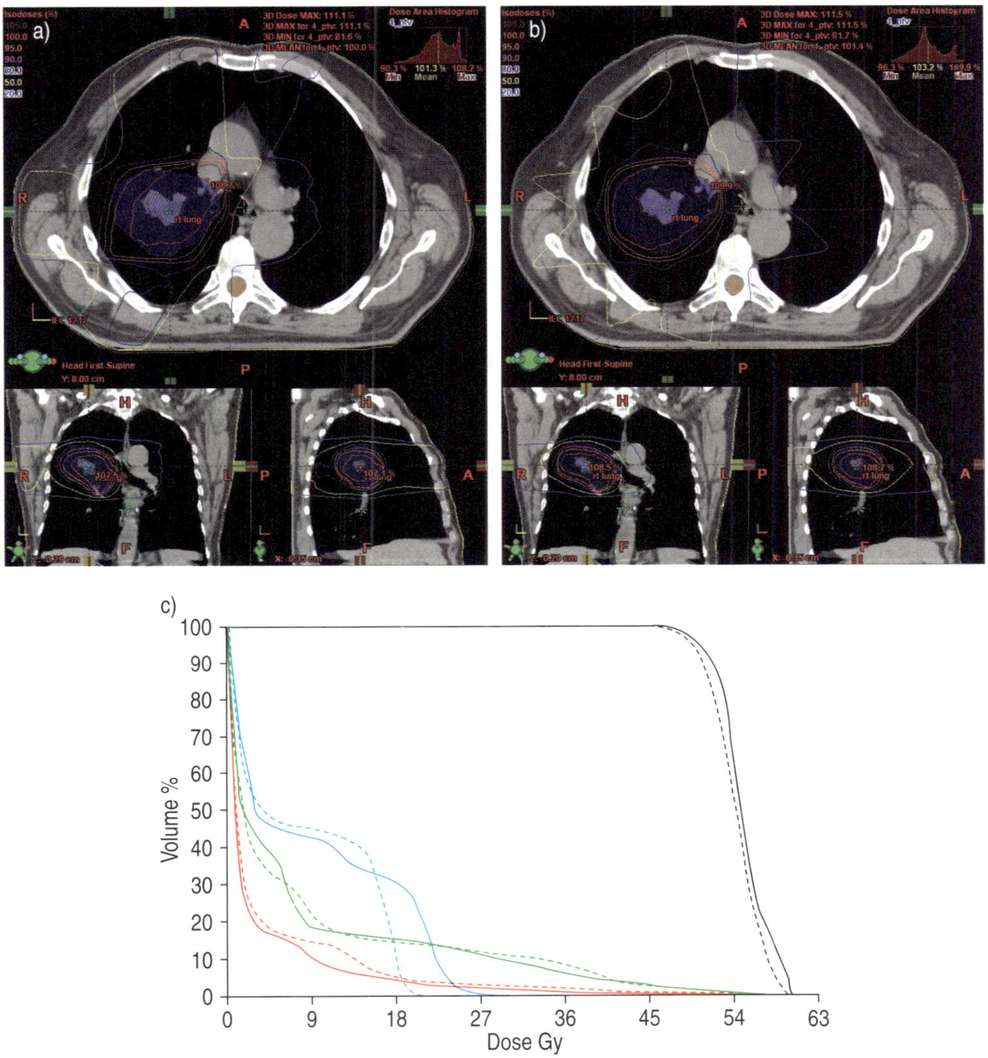

Fig. 6. – Radiation dose distribution comparison of a) a three-dimensional (3D) conformal plan with b) an intensity-modulated radiotherapy (IMRT) plan, illustrating the improved coverage of the planning target volume (PTV; blue) when IMRT planning is used. Tranverse (top), frontal (left) and sagittal (right) views are shown for each type of planning. c) This is confirmed on the dose–volume histogram, which also indicates that this is achieved at the cost of some increase in dose to the normal tissue. ——: IMRT; - - - -: 3D conformal; black: PTV; blue: oesophagus; green: lung; red: heart.

of a radiotherapy schedule (CHART) while maintaining optimal tumour coverage. Interestingly, radiotherapy planning studies have also shown that, when ENI is not intentionally given, the mediastinum is often adequately treated by single phase treatment to known disease alone [58].

Initial dose escalation studies concentrated on the delivery of extra fractions and these studies confirmed that a significantly higher dose could be delivered. Three studies increased the numbers of daily fractions and extended the duration of treatment. In all three studies, patients were assigned into escalation schedules on the basis of predicted lung toxicity. In the study conducted by KONG *et al.* [56] in Ann Arbor (MI, USA), the radiotherapy was administered daily using 2.1 Gy per fraction over treatment times of 6–10 weeks, with patients allocated into five ascending dose bins on the basis of predicted normal lung toxicity. The trial was stopped when recruitment into the maximum dose bin of 103 Gy was complete [56]. The RTOG 9311 study used three sequential dose escalation schedules, which were followed based on V_{20} values and gave 2.15 Gy fractions in an overall treatment time of up to 9 weeks. They reported safe escalation to 83.8 Gy in patients with a V_{20} <25% (90.3 Gy resulted in the dose-related death of two patients) and to 77.4 Gy in patients with V_{20} values of 25–36%. The study was abandoned for the third group where the V_{20} was >37%, due to poor accrual [83]. The third study was reported by a group from the Memorial Sloan-Kettering Cancer Centre (New York, NY, USA), who used 1.8-Gy or 2.0-Gy daily fractions delivered to sequentially higher dose levels with a limit of normal tissue complication probabilities set at <25% and escalated to a dose of 84 Gy [84].

In these studies and others there are indications that higher radiation doses were associated with improved outcomes [56, 85], with subset analysis reporting that survival was statistically better if >80 Gy was delivered [84]. Long-term toxicity follow-up in the three studies has confirmed that such an approach is safe, with acceptable levels of pulmonary toxicity. However, this approach significantly extends the overall treatment time and it has become increasing recognised that there is an accelerated tumour clonogen proliferation, which becomes clinically relevant for NSCLC approximately 3–4 weeks after initiation of radiotherapy [86–88]. Therefore, fractionation techniques that can avoid prolongation of treatment time are attractive, and dose escalation for this alternative fractionation is discussed briefly in the section about hypofractionation, later in this chapter.

Dose escalation for conventionally fractionated radiotherapy has also been reported in the context of chemoradiotherapy treatment. There have been four phase I/II trials reported, which culminated in a fifth study that was a randomised phase II study in which induction chemotherapy was followed by concurrent chemoradiotherapy using a radiation dose of 74 Gy and either carboplatin/paclitaxel or gemcitabine [19]. The gemcitabine arm was closed early due to high rates of pulmonary toxicity, but the toxicity rates in the 43 patients on the carboplatin/paclitaxel arm were more acceptable and a median survival rate of 24 months was reported.

Fractionation

Fractionation is aimed at taking advantage of the five radiobiological principles: reoxygenation, repair, redistribution, resistance and repopulation. This has led to a conventional radiation schedule delivering 1 fraction·day^{-1} (usually 1.8–2 Gy), 5 days·week^{-1} for 6–7 weeks [3]. Several other fractionation schedules have been developed either on an empirical basis or more recently to take advantage of different radiobiological properties of tumour and normal tissues (table 3). The aim of the alteration in fractionation schedules is to try and improve the local control rates, and the results of CHART, which is discussed below, do illustrate that acceleration of treatment schedules can lead to an improvement in local control that feeds through to a reduction in distant metastasis and an improvement in survival.

Split course. A split-course schedule uses daily fractions for 1–2 weeks with a rest period of 2–4 weeks, to allow recovery of the normal tissues, and then treatment is restarted, usually following the same schedule [49]. No study has shown superiority of split-course over continuous regimes [6, 89], and some have demonstrated a negative

Table 3. – Fractionation schedules used in radiotherapy practice

Schedule	Week							Radiation fraction		Weeks n
	1	2	3	4	5	6	7	Size Gy	Dose·day^{-1}	
Conventional	+++++00	+++++00	+++++00	+++++00	+++++00	+++++00	++00000	2	1	6–7
Split course	+++++00	+++++00	0000000	0000000	+++++00	+++++00		>2	1	>5
Hypofractionated	+++++00	+++++00	+++++00	+++++00				>2	1	<5
Hyperfractionated	+++++00	+++++00	+++++00	+++++00	+++++00	+++++00		1–1.3	2	6
	+++++00	+++++00	+++++00	+++++00	+++++00	+++++00				
CHART	+++++++	+++++00						1.5	3	2
	+++++++	+++++00								
	+++++++	+++++00								
HART	+++++00	+++++00	+++0000					1.6	3	2 5
	+++++00	+++++00	+++0000							
	+++++00	+++++00	+++0000							

n: number; CHART: continuous hyperfractionated accelerated radiotherapy; HART: hyperfractionated accelerated radiotherapy. +: day of treatment; o: day of no treatment.

impact on survival or local control with split-course schedules, revealing the major drawback that the rest period allows tumour repopulation. In addition to this, the higher fraction size increases the risk of late damage.

Hypofractionation. A hypofractionated schedule accelerates the schedule, aiming to complete treatment in 4–5 weeks. This is primarily done by increasing the fraction size. Daily treatment schedules of 5 days·week^{-1} are used if the fraction size remains at or below 3 Gy; for larger fraction sizes treatment is given in 3–4 fractions·week^{-1}. These approaches were initially adopted for convenience in departments that lacked treatment capacity or for patients who were living long distances from the radiation treatment units. In addition, some schedules were designed to take advantage of some radiosensitisers, *e.g.* hyperbaric oxygen or misonidazole. A wide variety of hypofractionated schedules have been tested and the published reports for the more extreme hypofractionation schedules using fraction sizes of >3 Gy show a decrease in tumour control, probably due to cell repopulation between fractions, and an increase in late damage [90]. The latter is a direct consequence of the large fraction size, especially in the absence of total dose or volume reduction.

However, it is now recognised that accelerated repopulation of tumour cells can occur 28 days after the start of a course of radiation treatment [87, 88] and there is a place for accelerated hypofractionated treatment within the wide variety of radical radiotherapy regimens in current use. Indeed, in 2001, the regimen of 55 Gy in 20 daily fractions over 4 weeks was the most commonly used fractionation in the UK (A. Price, Edinburgh Cancer Centre, Edinburgh, UK; personal communication). The biologically effective dose of this fractionation is the equivalent of 65 Gy delivered as a conventionally fractionated treatment, and review of its use as a standard treatment for 140 patients with stage I–III NSCLC in our centre showed a 2-yr overall survival of 45% with low levels of grade III/IV toxicity [91]. These results compare well with other published series [59, 92].

There is little published data on the combination of chemotherapy with accelerated hypofractionated radiotherapy [93], and randomised studies are needed to confirm safety and effectiveness. However, the introduction of 3D chemoradiotherapy has allowed dose escalation for these accelerated schedules by limiting the amount of normal tissue irradiated compared with the conventional planning. THIRION *et al.* [94] have reported on giving 72 Gy in 24 3-Gy fractions over 5 weeks to patients with stage I–IIIB

NSCLC and demonstrated that treatment was well tolerated with no reported late grade III/IV toxicities. In a further phase I/II trial in 88 patients to determine the maximum tolerated dose delivered within 6 weeks in patients with NSCLC [95], fraction size was fixed at 2.25 Gy and if more than 30 fractions were prescribed, twice daily fractionation was used. The relative mean lung dose was used to divide patients into five risk groups and safe dose escalation was achieved to 74.25 Gy and 94.5 Gy in the highest and lowest risk groups, respectively. The use of chemotherapy with a schedule of 66 Gy in 24 fractions has been reported by the European Organisation for Research and Treatment of Cancer (EORTC) [68]. This study randomised 158 patients between a sequential treatment (two cycles of cisplatin/gemcitabine) and concurrent treatment with a low dose of daily cisplatin. The study was underpowered and did not detect any significant difference between the two groups with a median and 2-yr survival of 16 months and 37% reported for all the patients entered. It is possible, therefore, with modern planning techniques, to increase the dose prescribed using a hypofractionated regimen while maintaining the benefits of acceleration.

Hyperfractionation. These schedules attempt to take advantage of some radiobiological observations; late effects are directly due to the damage induced to slowly proliferating tissues such as muscle, bone and lung. For these late effects the fraction size is the key factor, with larger fractions increasing the risk of late damage. It is this late damage that can have profound effects on the quality of life and, hence, it is these effects that limit the total radiation dose. In contrast, early acute effects are observed in rapidly proliferating tissues such as the skin, the mucosa and bone marrow, which are influenced more by the daily dose rather than the fraction size. Most tumours act like rapidly proliferating tissue, so by giving several small fractions per day the effect on the tumour may be increased while the risk of late normal tissue effects are decreased. Hyperfractionation may also allow an increase in the total dose if the time interval between the different fractions allows more efficient repair to take place in the normal rapidly proliferating tissues (compared with the tumour).

The classical hyperfractionated schedule uses 2 fractions·day^{-1} of 1–1.2 Gy, separated by a 6-h interval, while keeping the same total dose as the classical once-daily fraction regimens. This approach was investigated by the RTOG with an initial large phase II trial designed to select the optimal total radiation dose. This progressed into a three-arm phase III study comparing the classical schedule of 60 Gy, with 69.6 Gy (with two daily fractions of 1.2 Gy), and induction chemotherapy with cisplatin and vinblastine followed by 60 Gy in 6 weeks [50, 96]. The 1-, 2- and 3-yr survival rates were 46, 19 and 6%, respectively, after 60 Gy, and 51, 24 and 13% after the hyperfractionated schedule. The differences did not reach statistical significance but the number of patients may have been too low to show the small difference expected from an 8% increase in biological total radiation dose. More recently, a single-centre experience of this hyperfractionated schedule confirmed treatment was well tolerated when given alone or with concurrent low dose paclitaxel/carboplatin [69]. They reported medians/5-yr survivals of 29 months/29% and 39 months/36% for the two groups, respectively. These results represented a significant improvement over the historical controls treated with the conventional 60 Gy in 30 fractions.

Accelerated radiotherapy. An increase in total dose using a conventional radiation schedule will also prolong treatment. If repopulation is an important issue, then this increase in treatment time will reduce the efficacy of the extra dose delivered. Accelerated fractionation aims to use hyperfractionation to reduce the duration of treatment with the goal of avoiding tumour repopulation, with evidence suggesting that repopulation starts at 28 days after the beginning of radiotherapy [87, 88].

Ball *et al.* [52] accelerated treatment into a 3-week schedule that gave 60 Gy in twice-daily fractions that maintained the fraction size at 2 Gy. The interim analysis of the first 100 randomised patients showed the expected increase in acute reactions. This was most pronounced in the rates of grade III and IV oesophagitis, which were 9 and 0%, respectively, for the conventional fractionated arm, and 31 and 4% for the accelerated schedule, with six patients requiring dilatation of an oesophageal stricture, demonstrating that the acute and late tolerance of the oesophagus had become the limiting factor for accelerated radiotherapy schedules. Using this twice-daily fractionation and reducing the fraction size to 1.6 Gy, Sibley *et al.* [97] showed dose escalation was feasible using conformal techniques and a dose of 80 Gy in 5 weeks was reached. A further phase I/II dose study escalated dose according to the risk of radiation pneumonitis with three risk groups defined on the basis of V_{20} values. Twice-daily fractions of 1.8 Gy were given and a dose of 68.4 Gy over 25 days was reached [98]. These two studies confirm that dose escalation for accelerated treatment is possible and response rates and 2-yr survivals offer some encouragement.

CHART. There has been one large published randomised trial that completed its target accrual and that directly compared an accelerated schedule with a conventional fractionated schedule in the radical treatment of NSCLC. The schedule used was CHART [51]. This schedule further accelerated treatment by continuing the radiotherapy through the weekend, so that treatment was completed in 12 days (54 Gy in 1.5-Gy fractions given three times daily with a minimum inter-fraction interval of 6 h). A randomised trial of 563 patients compared this CHART radiation protocol with a classical radiation schedule of 60 Gy in daily fractions in 6 weeks. The 2-, 3- and 5-yr survival rates were 21, 13 and 7%, respectively, after conventional radiation, and 30, 18 and 12% after CHART. This difference was even more marked for squamous cell carcinoma with 3- and 5-yr figures of 21 and 15% for CHART and 11 and 7% for the control arm. The differences were highly significant and due to an improvement in local control and a 9% reduction of distant metastasis. The acute morbidity, mainly dysphagia, was higher in the CHART group, with moderate or severe dysphagia reported in 49 *versus* 19% for CHART and conventional radiotherapy, respectively. Importantly, no difference was seen between the two arms in late morbidity.

A five-centre observational study has recently reported the results for 583 patients treated with CHART in routine practice [67]. It confirmed that CHART was deliverable, with 99% of patients completing the treatment and <1% suffering any grade IV/V toxicity. This series reported a median survival of 16.2 months and 2- and 3-yr survivals of 33.6 and 20%, respectively, which suggests that the survivals reported in the original CHART study can be reproduced in day-to-day practice.

The 10% improvement in 2-yr survival documented in the CHART trial is comparable with the improvement seen by the addition of chemotherapy to more conventionally fractionated radiotherapy regimes. Unfortunately, the Induction Chemotherapy and CHART (INCH) trial, which aimed to assess benefits of additional chemotherapy [99], has closed early, so it is not known if there are any additional benefits to adding chemotherapy to these accelerated schedules. However, the median survival of ~17 months for patients with stage III disease seen with concomitant chemoradiotherapy schedules [64, 66] means that this approach is becoming established as standard treatment. However, results suggest that CHART has a place in the treatment of NSCLC [67], particularly for the elderly and other patients who may not have the reserve to cope with combined chemoradiotherapy treatment.

Despite this evidence base, CHART has not been widely adopted as a standard schedule, in the UK or elsewhere. This is mainly due to the difficulty of weekend working, which has led to the development of accelerated, hyperfractionated radiotherapy schedules that avoid treatment over the weekend. CHART weekend-less (CHARTWEL) was developed at Mount Vernon Hospital (Northwood, UK) and delivered a dose escalation of 60 Gy over an 18-day period, maintaining the three-times-daily treatment with 1.5-Gy fractions that are delivered 5 days·week^{-1}. The phase II trial reported on 88 patients treated with this dose, of whom 33 had received induction chemotherapy [80]. Most reported grade I/II oesophagitis, but late toxicity rates were low with one case of grade III pneumonitis documented. Good loco-regional control rates were reported (55% for CHARTWEL alone, 72% with induction chemotherapy) and both arms had a 2-yr survival rate in the region of 45%.

However, randomised trials comparing these schedules with conventionally fractionated treatment have been reported but have not shown the clear advantages seen in the CHART trial. The Eastern Cooperative Oncology Group (ECOG) 2597 trial gave two cycles of induction chemotherapy as standard and then randomised between hyperfractionated accelerated radiotherapy (HART; 57.6 Gy in 1.5-Gy fractions three times daily for 2.5 weeks) and conventional radiotherapy (64 Gy in 32 daily fractions). The trial was closed early due to slow accrual, but results were encouraging and showed a 15% improvement in favour of HART in 2- and 3-yr survival, although this was not statistically significant due to the small numbers recruited [100]. However, a trial comparing a similar European regimen, CHARTWEL (60 Gy), with conventional fractionation of 66 Gy in 33 fractions did complete its planned recruitment and has shown no difference in survival [101]. This has only been published in abstract form so detailed analysis of the results is awaited.

The role of and evidence from combined chemoradiotherapy treatment, particularly in locally advanced disease, is discussed in chapter 14 of this *ERM*. The benefits and toxicities for the combination of chemotherapy and conventionally fractionated radiotherapy are well established, and a similar evidence base needs to be developed for the accelerated radiotherapy schedules over the next few years and then randomised trials are needed in order to establish whether the potential advantages of accelerated chemoradiotherapy schedules translate into meaningful clinical benefits.

Stereotactic body radiotherapy

In clinical practice, the application of the technical developments in radiotherapy includes stereotactic body radiotherapy (SBRT), which is the term coined to indicate precise positioning and imaging for radiation delivery. In lung cancer, SBRT indicates hypofractionated radiotherapy and has been reserved for the treatment of small tumours where only a limited volume of normal lung is treated. The radiotherapy dose delivered by conformal treatment is limited by toxicity of normal tissues, particularly lung, necessarily included in the target volume to account for microscopic tumour extension and tumour and patient movement. The SBRT techniques further reduce the volume of normal lung included in the high dose volume by more accurate imaging and target registration and by techniques that minimise tumour and patient movement.

Studies have identified a number of techniques that can reduce respiratory tumour movement: a stereotactic body frame with abdominal compression [22, 102], voluntary breath-hold [23, 103] or ABC [24]. Additionally, the effect of motion can also be minimised by gating treatment to part of the respiratory cycle [25, 26], tracking the moving tumour [104] or imaging the tumour with respiratory-correlated (4D) CT with high dose delivered to the mean tumour position [27]. The accuracy of treatment can be improved by aiding patient set-up and confirming anatomical tumour location using image guidance, including cone beam CT [28, 105–107], in-room CT performed before each fraction [29, 108] and 3D tracking of fiducials during treatment [109].

The potential advantages of the SBRT approach are a shorter overall treatment time, which minimises accelerated repopulation, dose escalation with a higher biologically effective dose, and patient convenience. Elevating the biologically effective dose will have implications for organs at risk, as doses that are derived from schedules of 2 Gy per fraction may not translate to altered fractionation schedules if they do not take into account overall treatment time. Dose constraints for organs at risk have been reported for most studies and set using the linear quadratic model [12], which provides limited data on tolerances of spinal cord and lung in hypofractionated treatment. This uncertainty is reflected in calculation of biologically effective doses that indicate a two-fold difference in the range of organs at risk dose constraints accepted [13] in the schedules used in table 3.

Table 4 summarises the published reports for SBRT for NSCLC, and a consensus view of an expert panel has been produced that does indicate a number of principles for this form of treatment [125]. However, there have been no phase III studies of SBRT and evidence comes from single- and multicentre phase I/II studies and retrospective reviews [111–123, 126] and studies using heavy particle therapy or a single fraction of photon therapy [124, 127–129]. As expected with an emerging technology, these studies report a variety of immobilisation techniques, tumour motion assessment, added margins in generating the PTV, and beam arrangements. The techniques are best applied to peripheral T1 and T2 tumours. The median tumour diameter is often <3 cm [114], although a number of studies do not specify their upper limit for tumour size. The studies report on a large range of doses (18–90 Gy), doses per fraction (3–30 Gy), and fractions (1–22) given over 1–27 days [111–124, 126]. The most widely reported regimens were in the ranges 30–48 Gy in 3–4 fractions and 48–60 Gy in 5–10 fractions. It is important to note the reduced dose prescribed for central tumours, *e.g.* a prescription of 60 Gy in eight fractions for peripheral tumours is reduced to 48 Gy in eight fractions [112]. However, the optimum dose-fractionation for the SBRT of localised NSCLC has not been defined, although a retrospective review of 245 patients with stage I disease

Table 4. – Reported survival, local control and toxicity in 15 published reports of stereotactic body radiotherapy for early-stage nonsmall cell lung cancer

First author [ref.]	Patients n	Median follow-up months	Total dose Gy	Fractions n	Actual 2-yr survival %	Progression-free 2-yr survival %	Toxicity pneumonitis grade I %
UEMATSU [29]	50	36	50–60	5–10	77		0
FUKUMOTO [110]	22	24	48–60	8	50		0
LEE [111]	9	18	30–40	3–4		90	0
ONIMARU [112]	25	18	48–60	8	47	85	0
TIMMERMAN [113]	37	15	24–60	3			19
ONISHI [114]	245	24	18–75	1–22	70	87	7
WULF [115]	20	11	30–37.5	3	32	92	3
HOYER [116]	49		45	3	47	85	
NAGATA [117]	45	30	48	4	90 stage 1A 72 stage 1B	97 100	4
BEITLER [118]	75	17	30–90	4–12	45		3
XIA [119]	43	27	50	10	78	95	5
FRANKS [120]	22	8	45–60	3–10			5
BAUMANN [121]	138	33	30–48	2–4	65	91	1
ZIMMERMANN [122]	68	17	24–40	3–5	71	88	29
FARIA [123]	32	21	52.5	15	56		3
HOF [124]	42	15	19–30	1	65	49	0

reported better local control and survival rates when the biological effective dose was >100 Gy compared with <100 Gy (local recurrence rates 8.1 *versus* 26.4%, and 3-yr survival 88.4 *versus* 69.4%) [114]. A similar analysis for single fraction treatment reached the same conclusion [124].

The outcome for SBRT is summarised in table 4 and local control rates are in the region of 90% with 2-yr survival rate of 65%. The acute toxicities of a flu-like reaction and oesophagitis are transient and the rates of pulmonary fibrosis and other late toxicities appear low, particularly when treatment avoids including the mediastinum and other central structures in the chest in the PTV. However, as toxicity assessment was only retrospective in most studies, the data on the apparent safety of SBRT should be treated with caution.

Although these results are encouraging, it is clear that the range of outcomes reported reflects big differences in patient selection and comorbidity that confound any comparison of these results with those reported for 3D conformal radiotherapy and surgery.

Particle therapy in lung cancer

The current literature on treatment using proton or carbon ion therapy is limited to reports from a few centres, although the technology is starting to become more widely available. In principle, by using charged particles for radiotherapy it should be possible to design and deliver better dose distributions than those achieved with photons, because the dose given to the tissues deeper than the target approaches zero within millimetres. This results in a smaller dose to a smaller volume of normal tissues and reduces the risk of radiation injury; this has been demonstrated with planning studies. However, these dose distribution properties will leave treatment very sensitive to the changes in depth that occur along the beam path with breathing, and this is one of the significant technical issues that has not yet been fully addressed.

Clinical experience is limited to 214 patients treated with protons [128] and carbon ion therapy [129]. With proton therapy, phase I/II studies have reported 2-yr local control rates of 80–95%, with overall 2-yr survival of 74–84% and grade III toxicity seen in ~10% of patients [128]. The experience of carbon ion treatment is limited to a single-institution phase II study report outcome of different fractionation regimes, with local tumour control rates between 77 and 95% and 5-yr survivals between 42 and 50%. These data suggest some promise for particle therapy but well designed clinical trials and prospective studies are needed in order to demonstrate whether they offer any significant improvement over other high-precision radiotherapy techniques.

Radiotherapy and surgery

Radiotherapy and surgery are the two potentially curative modalities of treatment in NSCLC. The reasons for local failure give a rationale for combining the two modalities. For surgery, local failure occurs because microscopic disease cannot be detected by staging investigations and/or identified at the time of surgery. Local recurrence will occur when this microscopic disease has extended beyond the anatomical boundaries of excision or is present in loco-regional lymph nodes. In radiotherapy, local failure occurs at the site of bulk disease. This is partly due to factors like hypoxia, which increases the inherent radioresistance of the tumour cell. However, it is mainly down to tumour size, because, as discussed earlier, a set dose of radiation will destroy a constant fraction of cells. With the normal tissue constraints that set the limit for the total dose of radiation given, local control rates will fall with increasing numbers of cancer cells, *i.e.* tumour size [2]. Therefore, potentially combining the two modalities overcomes their individual weaknesses: the surgery removes the bulk disease and radiation treatment targets the likely areas of microscopic disease where the numbers of cells are small and hypoxia unlikely to be a factor. This section primarily reviews the use of radiotherapy as an adjuvant to surgery, but the section does touch upon the choice of surgery or radiotherapy following induction chemotherapy and considers trimodality treatment, when all three treatment modalities are combined.

Pre-operative radiotherapy

The pre-operative irradiation approach has not been widely studied but does offer the following theoretical advantages: 1) eradication of microscopic disease beyond the margins of resection; 2) tumour shrinkage, creating more accessible tissue planes for resection; and 3) downstaging of tumours, possibly rendering them resectable.

Balanced against this is the concern of an increased surgical morbidity following the initial radiotherapy and loss of staging information in the resected specimen. The early evidence from randomised trials in the USA showed these concerns to be real, with the two large studies of pre-operative radiotherapy for "operable" NSCLC showing no improvement in survival [130, 131] and an increase in post-operative complications that had a detrimental effect on survival for those patients who received radiotherapy. However, it should be questioned whether this data collected in the 1960s and 1970s is applicable to patients today. These trials were conducted before CT staging was routinely available and 20% were found to have unresectable tumours at the time of operation; the subsequent introduction of routine CT and PET scanning has greatly reduced this "open and shut" rate. The combination of these improvements in staging with those seen in surgical technique and peri-operative care has greatly reduced post-operative mortality when radiation has been given as part of induction treatment [132].

The other potential use for pre-operative radiotherapy is as a downstaging procedure for NSCLC that is unresectable, but the evidence for this approach is limited to a few small series. In a prospective phase II study, WEIDEN *et al.* [133] used surgical staging to confirm unresectability due to T4 tumour extension or N2 disease. Radiotherapy was given to a dose of 44 Gy in 22 fractions over 4.5 weeks and definitive surgery followed 1 month later. 32 patients entered the study and 13 came to surgery, with 11 (34%) having their disease resected; three post-operative deaths were reported [133]. Other small retrospective series have suggested better resectability rates for stage III disease [134] and superior sulcus (Pancoast) tumours, with a 34% 5-yr survival reported for the latter [135].

Currently, there is no reason to advocate pre-operative irradiation in daily practice, although the debate has moved on to consider a role for trimodality therapy, *i.e.* induction chemoradiotherapy followed by surgery. The feasibility of this approach has been tested by a South West Oncology Group (SWOG) study [136], which reported on 126 patients treated with two cycles of cisplatin/etoposide with concurrent radiotherapy to a dose of 45 Gy in 25 fractions over 5 weeks. Those with a response or stable disease were offered surgery 3–5 weeks later. Eighty eight per cent were eligible for surgery and in 83% the disease proved respectable, with pathological examination showing that 21% had no residual disease and in a further 37% there were only microscopic foci present. Local relapse rates were 11%, and a 26% 3-yr survival was reported.

Pancoast tumours

The SWOG group then performed a further phase II study using the same chemoradiotherapy induction schedule in a highly selected group of patients with superior sulcus tumours. The study again confirmed feasibility and reported on 110 patients who had undergone pre-treatment investigation that included mediastinoscopy to confirm T3/4 N0 disease [132]. Again, the successful resection rate following the induction treatment was high (75%) and treatment mortality was reduced to ~5%, probably reflecting the more rigorous selection of patients. The local relapse rate was low (9%) and a median survival of 33 months was reported (94 months in those whose resections were pathologically complete). These results compare very well with previous series of pre-operative radiotherapy and surgery and indicate a role for trimodality therapy in this carefully selected group of patients. Other groups have moved on to intensify the induction regime [137], but it is not clear if higher radiation doses will improve outcome or be safe in the multi-institutional setting.

Radiotherapy or surgery in stage III disease

Although trimodality therapy may have a role in well selected patients with Pancoast tumours, the 10% treatment-related mortality reported in the study by ALBAIN *et al.* [136] raises the question whether surgery adds risk or benefit to chemoradiotherapy in the management of stage III disease.

The 1995 meta-analysis established a 5-yr survival rate of 15% for the combination of platinum-based chemotherapy and radiotherapy [62], and this combination is considered the treatment of choice for stage III NSCLC. The addition of surgery has been subject to randomised phase III studies that have focused on patients with stage IIIA N2 node positive disease. These trials tested the theory that selected patients with "low burden" disease would benefit from surgery to reduce the high local failure seen with chemoradiotherapy treatment [138]. The first trial to fully report took 579 patients with pathologically proven N2 disease and randomised the 332 responders to surgery or radiotherapy consolidation [139]. The median survival was 16.4 *versus* 17.5 months, respectively (HR 1.06, 95% CI 0.84–1.35), and 5-yr figures were also similar (16 *versus* 14%). These findings are supported by the North American Intergroup 0139 trial [140], which used the SWOG chemoradiotherapy schedule outlined earlier and then randomised responders to resection or further chemoradiotherapy, which took the total radiation dose to 61 Gy. 396 patients were randomised, and they had median survivals of 23.6 *versus* 22.2 months (HR 0.87, 95% CI 0.70–1.10) and 5-yr survivals of 27.2 *versus* 20.3%.

Although there was no difference in the survival for either of these trials, both reported a higher initial mortality in the surgical arm (8 *versus* 2% in the Intergroup study), particularly in the patients who required pneumonectomy. In both, the relapse patterns were as predicted, with higher rates of local recurrence in the radiation-treated group, and the Intergroup study gave a hint that 5-yr survival might be improved by surgical treatment. However, in view of the low morbidity of treatment, radiotherapy should be considered the preferred loco-regional treatment for this group of patients following chemotherapy, and further studies are needed to define the subgroups for which surgery may offer an additional benefit.

Post-operative radiotherapy

Despite several randomised trials over the past 40 yrs and a recent meta-analysis published in 1998, post-operative radiotherapy (PORT) remains a very controversial area. The results of the different randomised trials are summarised in table 5. These trials were heterogeneous in terms of patient selection, surgery, radiation technique and other parameters, and taken individually none of those trials showed any benefit for survival. A number of trials, including the Lung Cancer Study Group trial and the Medical Research Council (MRC) trial [147, 148], showed an improvement in local control and triggered the PORT Meta-analysis Group to examine individual patient data from 2,128 patients from nine randomised trials that compared PORT with surgery alone, using an intention-to-treat analysis [153]. The median follow-up time for the surviving patients included in the meta-analysis was 3.9 yrs and the overall results of the PORT meta-analysis indicated that PORT had a significant detrimental effect on survival. There were 707 deaths among 1,056 patients assigned to the PORT arm *versus* 661 deaths among 1,072 patients included in the surgery-alone arm. This represented a 21% relative increase in the risk of death or an absolute decrease in survival of 7% at 2 yrs, reducing the overall survival from 55 to 48% (mortality HR 1.21, 95% CI 1.08–1.34; p=0.001).

Further analysis showed that the deleterious effects of PORT in terms of overall survival were predominantly among patients with stage I/II disease who had a complete resection and no mediastinal involvement (either pN0 or pN1). The value for patients with stage III N2 disease was equivocal, as in this group of patients the analysis showed a 24% relative reduction of the local recurrence rate, although no survival advantage was demonstrated. In addition, there is a significant concern about the applicability of these results to the modern radiotherapy techniques in current use. The meta-analysis included trials that delivered treatment with suboptimal dose distributions, for example treating with just one radiotherapy field per day (*i.e.* an anterior field one day and posterior field the next), which may have reduced the effectiveness of the radiation. In addition, it should be noted that seven out of the nine trials included patients treated with Cobalt-60 equipment, which is now known to increase morbidity [154].

The results of the meta-analysis led to a significant decrease in the use of PORT around the turn of the century. For example, using the SEER database in the USA, the use of PORT fell from 65 to 37% in patients with resected N2 NSCLC [155]. However, retrospective data from this analysis of the SEER database identified a subgroup of 1,987 patients with resected NSCLC with involvement of N2 nodes and suggested a survival advantage for PORT (HR 0.86, 95% CI 0.76–0.96) [156]. Further retrospective data from the Mayo Clinic (Rochester, MN, USA) also demonstrated a survival

Table 5. – Lung cancer: trials of post-operative thoracic radiotherapy

First author [ref.]	Radiation Gy/weeks	Patients n	Pathology	Surgery	Patient selection	Survival p-value
Paterson [141]	45/4	202	All	P	N- N+	NS
Bangma [142]	45/5	73	All	All	N- N+	NS
Van Houtte [143]	60/6	224	All	All	N-	<0.05¶
Israel [144]	45/4.5	392	S	All	N- N+	NS
Debevec [145]	30/2	74	NSCLC	All	N+	NS
Feng [146]	60/6	366	NSCLC	All	N+	NS
LCSG# [147]	50/5	230	SC	All	N+	NS
Stephens# [148]	40/3	308	NSCLC	All	StageII, III	NS
Lafitte [149]	45–60/4–6	163	NSCLC	All	T2N-	NS
Dautzenberg [150]	60/6	728	NSCLC	All	Stage I–III	0.002¶
Wang [151]	60/6	317	NSCLC	All	Stage II–III	NS
PORT Meta-analysis Trialists Group [152]	56/5.5	106	NSCLC	All	Stage II–III	NS

LCSG: Lung Cancer Study Group; PORT: post-operative radiotherapy; P: pneumonectomy; N-: negative hilar or mediastinal nodes; N+: positive hilar or mediastinal nodes; NS: nonsignificant; S: squamous; NSCLC: nonsmall cell lung cancer; SC: squamous cell carcinoma. #: studies showed better local control in cases of positive mediastinal lymph nodes; ¶: for surgery.

advantage and indicated no detrimental effects when treatment was limited to 50 Gy [157]. Recent phase II studies are beginning to build on this retrospective data in evaluating the safety of the modern techniques. MACHTAY *et al.* [158] reported the treatment of patients with resected stage III N2 disease using conformal radiotherapy techniques. The intercurrent death rate appeared slightly higher in the group given PORT (13.5 *versus* 10%) but this did not reach statistical significance, and subgroup analysis suggested that any increase was confined to the patients who received a dose >54 Gy.

The other significant evolution of treatment since the PORT meta-analysis has been the use of adjuvant chemotherapy. The benefit of adjuvant chemotherapy has been recently confirmed in two meta-analyses and several trials, which now include more than 1,800 randomised patients and show 4–15% absolute improvement in the 5-yr survival [159–163]. These results mean that adjuvant chemotherapy is considered a standard treatment in patients with completely resected lung cancer; however, it should be noted that 20–40% of the patients still have local tumour failure. Studies have tested the feasibility of combining adjuvant chemotherapy with PORT using a concomitant treatment schedule. The RTOG suggested that the addition of paclitaxel and carboplatin led to improvement compared with historical controls, with a reduction in local recurrence rates. Other trials offer similar promising results and a randomised study by KELLER *et al.* [163], which compared PORT with or without concomitant chemoradiotherapy, noted that the loco-regional recurrence within the radiotherapy field was ~13%.

It is important to consider the role of PORT in current practice, as the number of eligible patients with mediastinal nodal involvement is increasing with the improvements seen in thoracic surgery. There is good evidence to indicate that PORT does reduce local recurrence in patients who have had N2 NSCLC resected. This evidence suggests that this benefit may be present in current practice, but any possible survival benefit for PORT in the era of adjuvant chemotherapy remains unproven. These questions need to be addressed in the context of a randomised study, such as the collaborative European study Lung Adjuvant Radiotherapy Trial (Lung ART) [164], which will examine the role of conformal PORT in patients with resected N2 disease.

Palliative radiotherapy

Of patients with NSCLC, 70–80% present with disease that is incurable at the time of diagnosis, and the aim of palliative radiotherapy is the relief of symptoms with minimal discomfort to the patient. This is an important goal, as most patients will have symptoms from the primary tumour or loco-regional spread at the time of presentation or develop them over the course of their illness [165]. It is in the setting of palliation of symptoms to maintain or improve quality of life that radiotherapy is most often used, rather than as the high dose radical treatments discussed so far in this chapter.

There are no randomised trials comparing palliative radiotherapy with supportive care alone in symptomatic patients. There is a significant variation in treatment strategies throughout the world, as protocols have evolved on the basis on local experience when clinicians attempted to palliate while minimising toxicity levels, and the evidence for effectiveness comes from trials comparing different radiotherapy schedules. These trials show a consistency in symptomatic benefit (table 6), but when interpreting the reported results it should be remembered that radiotherapy is rarely used in isolation to improve symptoms, and palliative care interventions like the use of morphine will act to improve pain, dyspnoea and cough. In addition, treatment effects are measured by a variety of techniques and any improvement in symptom severity is subjective both for patient and clinician. It should be noted at this point that in patients without thoracic symptoms a study comparing immediate *versus* deferred radiotherapy showed no difference in survival or quality of life [175], suggesting that treatment may never be needed in a proportion of patients with advanced disease who have no thoracic symptoms at presentation.

There have been a number of randomised controlled trials comparing different fractionation in advanced and metastatic NSCLC [167–182], with symptom palliation rates reported in all but one [179]. The majority reported no difference in symptom control, with the series of MRC trials reporting that over 50% of the patients showed some improvement in symptoms [168–170], and table 6 indicates that haemoptysis and chest pain are more likely to be palliated than dyspnoea. These trials also suggested that local radiotherapy may offer some palliation of systemic symptoms like anorexia, with response rates of up to 66% [168]. The more recent studies using well validated instruments for quality of life assessment, like the EORTC QLQ-C30 with lung LC13 module, support the response rates reported for local symptoms but suggest lower levels for palliation of general symptoms such as fatigue or anorexia [173, 174, 180].

The question the majority of these randomised trials were trying to answer was "What are the most effective and the least toxic regimens?" In the MRC series of trials, 17 Gy in two fractions was compared with either 10 Gy in one fraction, 30 Gy in 10 fractions or 39 Gy in 13 fractions, and in terms of immediate palliation, short regimens with one or two fractions were as effective as longer courses, with a quicker onset of symptom relief. The majority of the other studies support this finding, with only three reporting better palliation being achieved with higher doses [172, 177, 180]. The duration of symptom palliation has proved a difficult end-point to investigate, and only one study has suggested that higher doses have been associated with a longer period of symptom control [181].

In contrast, the MRC studies did suggest that higher radiation doses yield better survival in some groups of patients. There is no survival difference reported in the study focusing on patients with poorer performance status (WHO 2–4) [169], but there was a trend for better survival in good performance status patients (WHO 0 or 1) receiving the higher dose of 30 Gy in 10 fractions in the study comparing this with 17 Gy in two fractions [168]. This trend was confirmed in a third study, which recruited patients with good performance status but locally advanced disease that was too advanced for radical radiotherapy treatment [170]. The comparison was 17 Gy in two fractions with 36–39 Gy in 12–13 fractions, and the longer regime was associated with a modest

Table 6. – Palliative radiotherapy for nonsmall cell lung cancer: symptomatic response rate results of selected randomised trials

First author [ref.]	Patients n	Symptom assessment	Cough	Haemoptysis	Chest pain	Dyspnoea
COLLINS [166]	96		67	87	72	53
SIMPSON [167]	409		55	95	50	37
MRC [168]	369	Clinician	60	84	78	61
MRC [169]	235	Clinician	52	73	66	42
MACBETH [170]	509	Patient	52		65	57
REES [171]	216	Patient	64	95	88	72
ERRIDGE [172]	146		54	92	66	56
SUNDSTRøM [173]	421	Patient	20	80		40
LANGENDIJK [174]	65	Patient	49	79	53	39

Data are presented as percentage unless otherwise stated. MRC: Medical Research Council.

improvement in median survival time (7 *versus* 9 months). Two other trials support this finding in good performance patients, with BEZJAK *et al.* [180] reporting an improvement in median survival (6 *versus* 4.2 months) in a trial comparing 20 Gy in five fractions with a 10-Gy single fraction treatment. This difference was due to the improvement seen in patients with no evidence of metastasis and good performance status. KRAMER *et al.* [181] reported an improvement in 1-yr survival for patients receiving 30 Gy in 10 fractions compared with 16 Gy in two fractions that only reached significance in patients with good performance status. A further trial that showed a survival advantage for the higher dose arm compared 50 Gy in 25 fractions with 40 Gy in 10 fractions, which was given as a split course [179]. This result may simply reflect the disadvantages of prolonged split-course treatment, as the arms are radiobiologically very similar.

These improvements need to be balanced against the toxicity of thoracic radiotherapy. The acute side-effects of tiredness, dysphagia, nausea and oesophagitis are well recognised, and more recently it has been recognised that other acute side-effects occur particularly when using one or two large fractions of treatment [183]. Over 50% of patients report acute chest pain, rigors, sweating and fevers within 24 h of fractions >8 Gy. Although the symptoms are usually short lived, lasting for a few hours and relieved by simple analgesia, the chest pain in particular can cause significant anxiety. There is the expected association between the severity of the acute side-effects and the dose of treatment given, with dysphagia particularly being documented as more severe and prolonged in the higher dose arms of a number of the trials [168–170, 173, 174].

In general, the acute side-effects of thoracic radiotherapy are mild and of more concern are the late toxicity of pulmonary fibrosis and radiation myelopathy. As patients frequently do not survive long enough to develop these late complications, it is likely that the frequency and severity of radiation fibrosis is underestimated in the literature. However, analysis of the three MRC studies has given an estimated risk of radiation myelitis at 2 yrs of 2.2% for 17 Gy in two fractions and 2.5% for 39 Gy in 13 fractions [184].

In conclusion, radiation therapy has a definite role in the palliative management of patients with lung cancer. Hypofractionated regimens appear to give results as good as conventional regimes, and have social and economic advantages. The evidence suggests that, if patients are of poor performance status (WHO 2–4), palliation is effectively achieved in one or two fractions. Patient with good performance status and locally advanced disease will gain a small survival advantage from higher dose treatment. There is an increasing tendency to treat this good performance group of patients with palliative chemotherapy, although the relatively little data that exist suggest a lower response rate for thoracic symptoms when chemotherapy is used [185]. There are no randomised comparisons between the two approaches and as yet little data on how to combine the two treatments with clinical trials in order to test the timing, dose and fractionation of palliative radiotherapy before or after a planned chemotherapy treatment.

Summary

There is a well established role for radiation treatment in the management of nonsmall cell lung cancer. As a single modality it is indicated as a radical treatment option for patients with loco-regional disease that is unresectable disease (or for patients who decline surgery) and deemed unsuitable for chemotherapy. For these patients the evidence points towards some advantages for accelerated treatment regimes such as continuous hyperfractionated accelerated radiotherapy, and the research effort should be directed towards dose escalation and the application of the new technologies. As a single modality, radiotherapy also maintains an important role, in combination with all other aspects of palliative care, in the control of symptoms and maintenance of quality of life.

A multimodality approach is now the standard for the management of most presentations of lung cancer and the combination of chemoradiotherapy is established in the radical treatment of nonsmall cell lung cancer. How best these two modalities are combined in palliative treatment is an area for further research. The benefits of the combination of radiotherapy and surgery are less clear-cut, as are any benefits from a trimodality approach with input from all three treatment disciplines.

Keywords: Combined modality treatment, nonsmall cell lung cancer, radiotherapy.

Statement of interest
None declared.

Acknowledgements. The authors thank C. Bragg (Weston Park Hospital, Sheffield, UK) for the preparation of the illustrations.

References

1. Patterson CJ, Hocking M, Bond M, *et al.* Retrospective study of radiotherapy for lung cancer in patients aged 75 years and over. *Age Ageing* 1998; 27: 515–518.
2. Morita K, Fuwa N, Suzuki Y, *et al.* Radical radiotherapy for medically inoperable non-small cell lung cancer in clinical stage I: a retrospective analysis of 149 patients. *Radiother Oncol* 1997; 42: 31–36.
3. Perez CA, Stanley K, Grundy G, *et al.* Impact of irradiation technique and tumor extent in tumor control and survival of patients with unresectable non-oat cell carcinoma of the lung: report by the Radiation Therapy Oncology Group. *Cancer* 1982; 50: 1091–1099.
4. Noordijk EM, vd Poest Clement E, Hermans J, *et al.* Radiotherapy as an alternative to surgery in elderly patients with resectable lung cancer. *Radiother Oncol* 1988; 13: 83–89.
5. Würschmidt F, Bünemann H, Bünemann C, *et al.* Inoperable non-small cell lung cancer: a retrospective analysis of 427 patients treated with high-dose radiotherapy. *Int J Radiat Oncol Biol Phys* 1994; 28: 583–588.
6. Gouders D, Maingon P, Rodrigus P, *et al.* Exclusive radiotherapy for inoperable stage I non small cell lung cancer (NSCLC): a multicentric study. *Lung Cancer* 2000; 29: Suppl. 1, 166.
7. Martel MK, Strawderman M, Hazuka MB, *et al.* Volume and dose parameters for survival of non-small cell lung cancer patients. *Radiother Oncol* 1997; 44: 23–29.
8. Armstrong JG, Burman C, Leibel S, *et al.* Three-dimensional conformal radiation therapy may improve the therapeutic ratio of high dose radiation therapy for lung cancer. *Int J Radiat Oncol Biol Phys* 1993; 26: 685–689.

9. Dillman RO, Seagren SL, Propert KJ, *et al.* A randomized trial of induction chemotherapy plus high-dose radiation *versus* radiation alone in stage III non-small-cell lung cancer. *N Engl J Med* 1990; 323: 940–945.
10. Muers M, Thatcher N, Wells F, *et al.* The Effective Management of Lung Cancer. 2nd Edn. London, Aesculapius Medical Press, 2003.
11. Lyman JT. Complication probability as assessed from dose–volume histograms. *Radiat Res Suppl* 1985; 8: S13–S19.
12. Zaider M, Amols HI. Practical considerations in using calculated healthy-tissue complication probabilities for treatment-plan optimization. *Int J Radiat Oncol Biol Phys* 1999; 44: 439–447.
13. Kehwar TS, Bhardwaj AK. Methods to calculate normal tissue complication and tumour control probabilities for fractionated inhomogeneous dose distribution of intensity-modulated radiation therapy. *J Radiother Pract* 2008; 7: 151–157.
14. Cox JD, Pajak TF, Asbell S, *et al.* Interruptions of high-dose radiation therapy decrease long-term survival of favorable patients with unresectable non-small cell carcinoma of the lung: analysis of 1244 cases from 3 Radiation Therapy Oncology Group (RTOG) trials. *Int J Radiat Oncol Biol Phys* 1993; 27: 493–498.
15. Tepper JE, Padikal TN. The role of computed tomography in treatment planning. *In*: Bleehen NM, Glastein E, Haybittle JL, eds. Radiation Therapy Planning. New York, Marcel Dekker, 1983; pp. 139–158.
16. Deniaud-Alexandre E, Touboul E, Lerouge D, *et al.* Impact of computed tomography and 18F-deoxyglucose coincidence detection emission tomography image fusion for optimization of conformal radiotherapy in non-small-cell lung cancer. *Int J Radiat Oncol Biol Phys* 2005; 63: 1432–1441.
17. Nestle U, Kremp S, Schaefer-Schuler A, *et al.* Comparison of different methods for delineation of 18F-FDG PET-positive tissue for target volume definition in radiotherapy of patients with non-small cell lung cancer. *J Nucl Med* 2005; 46: 1342–1348.
18. Bradley J, Thorstad WL, Mutic S, *et al.* Impact of FDG-PET on radiation therapy volume delineation in non-small-cell lung cancer. *Int J Radiat Oncol Biol Phys* 2004; 59: 78–86.
19. De Ruysscher D, Wanders S, Minken A, *et al.* Effects of radiotherapy planning with a dedicated combined PET-CT-simulator of patients with non-small cell lung cancer on dose limiting normal tissues and radiation dose-escalation: a planning study. *Radiother Oncol* 2005; 77: 5–10.
20. McJury M, Fisher PM, Pledge S, *et al.* The impact of virtual simulation in palliative radiotherapy for non-small-cell lung cancer. *Radiother Oncol* 2001; 59: 311–318.
21. Ireland RH, Bragg CM, McJury M, *et al.* Feasibility of image registration and intensity-modulated radiotherapy planning with hyperpolarized helium-3 magnetic resonance imaging for non-small-cell lung cancer. *Int J Radiat Oncol Biol Phys* 2007; 68: 273–281.
22. Wulf J, Hädinger U, Oppitz U, *et al.* Stereotactic radiotherapy of targets in the lung and liver. *Strahlenther Onkol* 2001; 177: 645–655.
23. Onishi H, Kuriyama K, Komiyama T, *et al.* CT evaluation of patient deep inspiration self-breath-holding: how precisely can patients reproduce the tumor position in the absence of respiratory monitoring devices? *Med Phys* 2003; 30: 1183–1187.
24. Panakis N, McNair H, Christian JA, *et al.* Defining the margins in the radical radiotherapy of non-small cell lung cancer (NSCLC) with active breathing control (ABC) and the effect on physical lung parameters. *Radiother Oncol* 2008; 87: 65–73.
25. Giraud P, Yorke E, Ford EC, *et al.* Reduction of organ motion in lung tumors with respiratory gating. *Lung Cancer* 2006; 51: 41–51.
26. Ford EC, Mageras GS, Yorke E, *et al.* Evaluation of respiratory movement during gated radiotherapy using film and electronic portal imaging. *Int J Radiat Oncol Biol Phys* 2002; 52: 522–531.
27. Wolthaus JW, Schneider C, Sonke JJ, *et al.* Mid-ventilation CT scan construction from four-dimensional respiration-correlated CT scans for radiotherapy planning of lung cancer patients. *Int J Radiat Oncol Biol Phys* 2006; 65: 1560–1571.

28. Guckenberger M, Meyer J, Vordermark D, *et al.* Magnitude and clinical relevance of translational and rotational patient setup errors: a cone-beam CT study. *Int J Radiat Oncol Biol Phys* 2006; 65: 934–942.
29. Uematsu M, Shioda A, Suda A, *et al.* Intrafractional tumor position stability during computed tomography (CT)-guided frameless stereotactic radiation therapy for lung or liver cancers with a fusion of CT and linear accelerator (FOCAL) unit. *Int J Radiat Oncol Biol Phys* 2000; 48: 443–448.
30. Graham MV, Purdy JA, Emami B, *et al.* Clinical dose–volume histogram analysis for pneumonitis after 3D treatment for non-small cell lung cancer (NSCLC). *Int J Radiat Oncol Biol Phys* 1999; 45: 323–329.
31. Clenton SJ, Fisher PM, Conway J, *et al.* The use of lung dose–volume histograms in predicting post-radiation pneumonitis after non-conventionally fractionated radiotherapy for thoracic carcinoma. *Clin Oncol (R Coll Radiol)* 2005; 17: 599–603.
32. Arriagada R, Le Chevalier T, Quoix E, *et al.* ASTRO (American Society for Therapeutic Radiology and Oncology) plenary: Effect of chemotherapy on locally advanced non-small cell lung carcinoma: a randomized study of 353 patients. GETCB (Groupe d'Etude et Traitement des Cancers Bronchiques), FNCLCC (Féderation Nationale des Centres de Lutte contre le Cancer) and the CEBI trialists. *Int J Radiat Oncol Biol Phys* 1991; 20: 1183–1190.
33. Cooper JD, Pearson G, Todd TR, *et al.* Radiotherapy alone for patients with operable carcinoma of the lung. *Chest* 1985; 87: 289–292.
34. Haffty BG, Goldberg NB, Gerstley J, *et al.* Results of radical radiation therapy in clinical stage I, technically operable non-small cell lung cancer. *Int J Radiat Oncol Biol Phys* 1988; 15: 69–73.
35. Zhang HX, Yin WB, Zhang LJ, *et al.* Curative radiotherapy of early operable non-small cell lung cancer. *Radiother Oncol* 1989; 14: 89–94.
36. Burt PA, Hancock BM, Stout R. Radical radiotherapy for carcinoma of the bronchus: an equal alternative to radical surgery? *Clin Oncol (R Coll Radiol)* 1989; 1: 86–90.
37. Sandler HM, Curran WJ Jr, Turrisi AT 3rd. The influence of tumor size and pre-treatment staging on outcome following radiation therapy alone for stage I non-small cell lung cancer. *Int J Radiat Oncol Biol Phys* 1990; 19: 9–13.
38. Talton BM, Constable WC, Kersh CR. Curative radiotherapy in non-small cell carcinoma of the lung. *Int J Radiat Oncol Biol Phys* 1990; 19: 15–21.
39. Dosoretz DE, Katin MJ, Blitzer PH, *et al.* Radiation therapy in the management of medically inoperable carcinoma of the lung: results and implications for future treatment strategies. *Int J Radiat Oncol Biol Phys* 1992; 24: 3–9.
40. Kaskowitz L, Graham MV, Emami B, *et al.* Radiation therapy alone for stage I non-small cell lung cancer. *Int J Radiat Oncol Biol Phys* 1993; 27: 517–523.
41. Slotman BJ, Njo KH, Karim AB. Curative radiotherapy for technically operable stage I nonsmall cell lung cancer. *Int J Radiat Oncol Biol Phys* 1994; 29: 33–37.
42. Gauden S, Ramsay J, Tripcony L. The curative treatment by radiotherapy alone of stage I non-small cell carcinoma of the lung. *Chest* 1995; 108: 1278–1282.
43. Graham PH, Gebski VJ, Langlands AO. Radical radiotherapy for early nonsmall cell lung cancer. *Int J Radiat Oncol Biol Phys* 1995; 31: 261–266.
44. Krol AD, Aussems P, Noordijk EM, *et al.* Local irradiation alone for peripheral stage I lung cancer: could we omit the elective regional nodal irradiation? *Int J Radiat Oncol Biol Phys* 1996; 34: 297–302.
45. Vrdoljak E, Mise K, Sapunar D, *et al.* Survival analysis of untreated patients with non-small-cell lung cancer. *Chest* 1994; 106: 1797–1800.
46. Wisnivesky JP, Bonomi M, Henschke C, *et al.* Radiation therapy for the treatment of unresected stage I–II non-small cell lung cancer. *Chest* 2005; 128: 1461–1467.
47. Yendamuri S, Komaki RR, Correa AM, *et al.* Comparison of limited surgery and three-dimensional conformal radiation in high-risk patients with stage I non-small cell lung cancer. *J Thorac Oncol* 2007; 2: 1022–1028.

48. Durci ML, Komaki R, Oswald MJ, *et al.* Comparison of surgery and radiation therapy for non-small cell carcinoma of the lung with mediastinal metastasis. *Int J Radiat Oncol Biol Phys* 1991; 21: 629–636.
49. Schaake-Koning C, van den Bogaert W, Dalesio O, *et al.* Effects of concomitant cisplatin and radiotherapy on inoperable non-small-cell lung cancer. *N Engl J Med* 1992; 326: 524–530.
50. Sause WT, Scott C, Taylor S, *et al.* Radiation Therapy Oncology Group (RTOG) 88-08 and Eastern Cooperative Oncology Group (ECOG) 4588: preliminary results of a phase III trial in regionally advanced, unresectable non-small-cell lung cancer. *J Natl Cancer Inst* 1995; 87: 198–205.
51. Saunders M, Dische S, Barrett A, *et al.* Continuous, hyperfractionated, accelerated radiotherapy (CHART) *versus* conventional radiotherapy in non-small cell lung cancer: mature data from the randomised multicentre trial. *Radiother Oncol* 1999; 52: 137–148.
52. Ball D, Bishop J, Smith J, *et al.* A randomised phase III study of accelerated or standard fraction radiotherapy with or without concurrent carboplatin in inoperable non-small cell lung cancer: final report of an Australian multi-centre trial. *Radiother Oncol* 1999; 52: 129–136.
53. Roswit B, Patno ME, Rapp R, *et al.* The survival of patients with inoperable lung cancer: a large-scale randomized study of radiation therapy *versus* placebo. *Radiology* 1968; 90: 688–697.
54. Katz HR, Alberts RW. A comparison of high-dose continuous and split-course irradiation in non-oat-cell carcinoma of the lung. *Am J Clin Oncol* 1983; 6: 445–457.
55. Fang LC, Komaki R, Allen P, *et al.* Comparison of outcomes for patients with medically inoperable stage I non-small-cell lung cancer treated with two-dimensional *vs* three-dimensional radiotherapy. *Int J Radiat Oncol Biol Phys* 2006; 66: 108–116.
56. Kong FM, Ten Haken RK, Schipper MJ, *et al.* High-dose radiation improved local tumor control and overall survival in patients with inoperable/unresectable non-small-cell lung cancer: long-term results of a radiation dose escalation study. *Int J Radiat Oncol Biol Phys* 2005; 63: 324–333.
57. Belderbos JSA, Lebesque JV, Barillot I. Normal tissue complication probabilities for irradiation of NSCLC patients with and without elective nodal irradiation. *Lung Cancer* 1997; 18: 126.
58. Rosenzweig KE, Sim SE, Mychalczak B, *et al.* Elective nodal irradiation in the treatment of non-small-cell lung cancer with three-dimensional conformal radiation therapy. *Int J Radiat Oncol Biol Phys* 2001; 50: 681–685.
59. Cheung PC, Mackillop WJ, Dixon P, *et al.* Involved-field radiotherapy alone for early-stage non-small-cell lung cancer. *Int J Radiat Oncol Biol Phys* 2000; 48: 703–710.
60. Bradley JD, Wahab S, Lockett MA, *et al.* Elective nodal failures are uncommon in medically inoperable patients with stage I non-small-cell lung carcinoma treated with limited radiotherapy fields. *Int J Radiat Oncol Biol Phys* 2003; 56: 342–347.
61. De Ruysscher D, Wanders S, van Haren E, *et al.* Selective mediastinal node irradiation based on FDG-PET scan data in patients with non-small-cell lung cancer: a prospective clinical study. *Int J Radiat Oncol Biol Phys* 2005; 62: 988–994.
62. Chemotherapy in non-small cell lung cancer: a meta-analysis using updated data on individual patients from 52 randomised clinical trials. Non-small Cell Lung Cancer Collaborative Group. *BMJ* 1995; 311: 899–909.
63. Le Chevalier T, Arriagada R, Tarayre M, *et al.* Significant effect of adjuvant chemotherapy on survival in locally advanced non-small-cell lung carcinoma. *J Natl Cancer Inst* 1992; 84: 58.
64. Vokes EE, Herndon JE 2nd, Kelley MJ, *et al.* Induction chemotherapy followed by chemoradiotherapy compared with chemoradiotherapy alone for regionally advanced unresectable stage III non-small-cell lung cancer: Cancer and Leukemia Group B. *J Clin Oncol* 2007; 25: 1698–1704.
65. Rowell NP, O'Rourke NP. Concurrent chemoradiotherapy in non-small cell lung cancer. *Cochrane Database Syst Rev* 2004; 4: CD002140.
66. Hanna NH, Neubauer M, Ansari R, *et al.* Phase III trial of cisplatin (P) plus etoposide (E) plus concurrent chest radiation (XRT) with or without consolidation docetaxel (D) in patients (pts) with inoperable stage III non-small cell lung cancer (NSCLC): HOG LUN 01-24/USO-023. *J Clin Oncol* 2007; 25: Suppl. 18, 7512.

67. Din OS, Lester J, Cameron A, *et al.* Routine use of continuous, hyperfractionated, accelerated radiotherapy for non-small-cell lung cancer: a five-centre experience. *Int J Radiat Oncol Biol Phys* 2008; 72: 716–722.
68. Belderbos J, Uitterhoeve L, van Zandwijk N, *et al.* Randomised trial of sequential *versus* concurrent chemo-radiotherapy in patients with inoperable non-small cell lung cancer (EORTC 08972-22973). *Eur J Cancer* 2007; 43: 114–121.
69. Jeremić B, Milicić B. From conventionally fractionated radiation therapy to hyperfractionated radiation therapy alone and with concurrent chemotherapy in patients with early-stage nonsmall cell lung cancer. *Cancer* 2008; 112: 876–884.
70. Price A, Gemcitabine and Radiotherapy in NSCLC (GRIN). A phase III study of radical radiotherapy with or without gemcitabine in patients with T1-2 N0-1 M0 non-small cell lung cancer (NSCLC). ISRCTN61727489. Information available from http://www.controlled-trials.com/ISRCTN61727489
71. Liu HH, Wang X, Dong L, *et al.* Feasibility of sparing lung and other thoracic structures with intensity-modulated radiotherapy for non-small-cell lung cancer. *Int J Radiat Oncol Biol Phys* 2004; 58: 1268–1279.
72. Marnitz S, Stuschke M, Bohsung J, *et al.* Intraindividual comparison of conventional three-dimensional radiotherapy and intensity modulated radiotherapy in the therapy of locally advanced non-small cell lung cancer: a planning study. *Strahlenther Onkol* 2002; 178: 651–658.
73. Schwarz M, Alber M, Lebesque JV, *et al.* Dose heterogeneity in the target volume and intensity-modulated radiotherapy to escalate the dose in the treatment of non-small-cell lung cancer. *Int J Radiat Oncol Biol Phys* 2005; 62: 561–570.
74. Yom SS, Liao Z, Liu HH, *et al.* Initial evaluation of treatment-related pneumonitis in advanced-stage non-small-cell lung cancer patients treated with concurrent chemotherapy and intensity-modulated radiotherapy. *Int J Radiat Oncol Biol Phys* 2007; 68: 94–102.
75. Sura S, Gupta V, Yorke E, *et al.* Intensity-modulated radiation therapy (IMRT) for inoperable non-small cell lung cancer: the Memorial Sloan-Kettering Cancer Centre (MSKCC) experience. *Radiother Oncol* 2008; 87: 17–23.
76. Yu HM, Liu YF, Yu JM, *et al.* Involved-field radiotherapy is effective for patients 70 years old or more with early stage non-small cell lung cancer. *Radiother Oncol* 2008; 87: 29–34.
77. Abratt RP, Willcox PA, Smith JA. Lung cancer in patients with borderline lung functions – zonal lung perfusion scans at presentation and lung function after high dose irradiation. *Radiother Oncol* 1990; 19: 317–322.
78. Lavrenkov K, Christian JA, Partridge M, *et al.* A potential to reduce pulmonary toxicity: the use of perfusion SPECT with IMRT for functional lung avoidance in radiotherapy of non-small cell lung cancer. *Radiother Oncol* 2007; 83: 156–162.
79. Yaremko BP, Guerrero TM, Noyola-Martinez J, *et al.* Reduction of normal lung irradiation in locally advanced non-small-cell lung cancer patients, using ventilation images for functional avoidance. *Int J Radiat Oncol Biol Phys* 2007; 68: 562–571.
80. Saunders MI, Rojas A, Lyn BE, *et al.* Dose-escalation with CHARTWEL (continuous hyperfractionated accelerated radiotherapy week-end less) combined with neo-adjuvant chemotherapy in the treatment of locally advanced non-small cell lung cancer. *Clin Oncol (R Coll Radiol)* 2002; 14: 352–360.
81. Arriagada R, Komaki R, Cox JD. Radiation dose escalation in non-small cell carcinoma of the lung. *Semin Radiat Oncol* 2004; 14: 287–291.
82. McGibney C, Holmberg O, McClean B, *et al.* Dose escalation of CHART in non-small cell lung cancer: is three-dimensional conformal radiation therapy really necessary? *Int J Radiat Oncol Biol Phys* 1999; 45: 339–350.
83. Bradley J, Graham MV, Winter K, *et al.* Toxicity and outcome results of RTOG 9311: a phase I–II dose-escalation study using three-dimensional conformal radiotherapy in patients with inoperable non-small-cell lung carcinoma. *Int J Radiat Oncol Biol Phys* 2005; 61: 318–328.

84. Rosenzweig KE, Fox JL, Yorke E, *et al.* Results of a phase I dose-escalation study using three-dimensional conformal radiotherapy in the treatment of inoperable nonsmall cell lung carcinoma. *Cancer* 2005; 103: 2118–2127.
85. Rengan R, Rosenzweig KE, Venkatraman E, *et al.* Improved local control with higher doses of radiation in large-volume stage III non-small-cell lung cancer. *Int J Radiat Oncol Biol Phys* 2004; 60: 741–747.
86. Fowler JF, Chappell R. Non-small cell lung tumors repopulate rapidly during radiation therapy. *Int J Radiat Oncol Biol Phys* 2000; 46: 516–517.
87. Withers HR, Taylor JMG, Maciejewski B. The hazard of accelerated tumor clonogen repopulation during radiotherapy. *Acta Oncol* 1988; 27: 131–146.
88. Maciejewski B, Withers HR, Taylor JMG, *et al.* Dose fractionation and regeneration in radiotherapy for cancer of the oral cavity and oropharynx: tumor dose–response and repopulation. *Int J Radiat Oncol Biol Phys* 1989; 16: 831–843.
89. Perez CA, Bauer M, Edelstein S, *et al.* Impact of tumor control on survival in carcinoma of the lung treated with irradiation. *Int J Radiat Oncol Biol Phys* 1986; 12: 539–547.
90. Cox JD. Large dose fractionation (hypo-fractionation). *In*: Proceedings of National Conference on Radiation Oncology Cancer 1985; 55S: 2105–2111.
91. Pemberton LS, Din OS, Fisher PM, *et al.* Accelerated radical radiotherapy for non-small cell lung cancer using two common regimens: a single-centre retrospective study of outcome. *Clin Oncol (R Coll Radiol)* 2009; 21: 161–167.
92. Lester JF, Macbeth FR, Brewster AE, *et al.* CT-planned accelerated hypofractionated radiotherapy in the radical treatment of non-small cell lung cancer. *Lung Cancer* 2004; 45: 237–242.
93. Maguire K, Kelly V, Page R, *et al.* Enhanced local control and survival with UK fractionation schedule for concurrent chemoradiation in NSCLC. *Proc Am Soc Clin Oncol* 2003; 22: 2657.
94. Thirion P, Holmberg O, Collins CD, *et al.* Escalated dose for non-small-cell lung cancer with accelerated hypofractionated three-dimensional conformal radiation therapy. *Radiother Oncol* 2004; 71: 163–166.
95. Belderbos JSA, Heemsbergen WD, De Jaeger K, *et al.* Final results of a phase I/II dose escalation trial in non-small-cell lung cancer using three-dimensional conformal radiotherapy. *Int J Radiat Oncol Biol Phys* 2006; 66: 126–134.
96. Cox JD, Azarnia N, Byhardt RW, *et al.* A randomized phase II/III trial of hyperfractionated radiation therapy with total doses of 60.0 Gy to 79.2 Gy: possible survival benefit with $\geq$69.6 Gy in favorable patients with Radiation Therapy Oncology Group stage III non-small-cell lung carcinoma. Report of Radiation Therapy Oncology Group 83–11. *J Clin Oncol* 1990; 8: 1543–1555.
97. Maguire PD, Marks LB, Sibley GS, *et al.* 73.6 Gy and beyond: hyperfractionated, accelerated radiotherapy for non-small-cell lung cancer. *J Clin Oncol* 2001; 19: 705–711.
98. De Ruysscher D, Wanders R, Van Haren E, *et al.* HI-CHART: a phase I/II study on the feasibility of high-dose continuous hyperfractionated accelerated radiotherapy in patients with inoperable non-small-cell lung cancer. *Int J Radiat Oncol Biol Phys* 2008; 71: 132–138.
99. Hatton M. INCH. A trial of induction chemotherapy followed by continuous hyperfractionated accelerated radiotherapy (CHART) *versus* CHART alone in patients with inoperable non-small cell lung cancer. MRC LU23, ISRCTN63027630. Information available from http://www.ctu.mrc.ac.uk/studies/inch.asp
100. Belani CP, Wang W, Johnson DH, *et al.* Phase III study of the Eastern Cooperative Oncology Group (ECOG 2597): induction chemotherapy followed by either standard thoracic radiotherapy or hyperfractionated accelerated radiotherapy for patients with unresectable stage IIIA and B non-small-cell lung cancer. *J Clin Oncol* 2005; 23: 3760–3767.
101. Baumann M, Herrmann T, Koch R, *et al.* Continuous hyperfractionated accelerated radiotherapy – weekend less (CHARTWEL) *versus* conventionally fractionated (CF) radiotherapy in

non-small-cell lung cancer (NSCLC): first results of a phase III randomised multicentre trial (ARO 971). *Eur J Cancer* 2005; 3: Suppl., 322.

102. Nagata Y, Negoro Y, Aoki T, *et al.* Clinical outcomes of 3D conformal hypofractionated single high-dose radiotherapy for one or two lung tumors using a stereotactic body frame. *Int J Radiat Oncol Biol Phys* 2002; 52: 1041–1046.
103. Kim DJ, Murray BR, Halperin R, *et al.* Held-breath self-gating technique for radiotherapy of non-small-cell lung cancer: a feasibility study. *Int J Radiat Oncol Biol Phys* 2001; 49: 43–49
104. Brown WT, Wu X, Wen BC, *et al.* Early results of CyberKnife image-guided robotic stereotactic radiosurgery for treatment of lung tumors. *Comput Aided Surg* 2007; 12: 253–261.
105. Oelfke U, Tücking T, Nill S, *et al.* Linac-integrated kV-cone beam CT: technical features and first applications. *Med Dosim* 2006; 31: 62–70.
106. Purdie TG, Moseley DJ, Bissonnette JP, *et al.* Respiration correlated cone-beam computed tomography and 4DCT for evaluating target motion in Stereotactic Lung Radiation Therapy. *Acta Oncol* 2006; 45: 915–922.
107. Sidhu K, Ford EC, Spirou S, *et al.* Optimization of conformal thoracic radiotherapy using cone-beam CT imaging for treatment verification. *Int J Radiat Oncol Biol Phys* 2003; 55: 757–767.
108. Onishi H, Kuriyama K, Komiyama T, *et al.* A new irradiation system for lung cancer combining linear accelerator, computed tomography, patient self-breath-holding and patient-directed beam-control without respiratory monitoring devices. *Int J Radiat Oncol Biol Phys* 2003; 56: 14–20.
109. Shirato H, Shimizu S, Kunieda T, *et al.* Physical aspects of a real-time tumor-tracking system for gated radiotherapy. *Int J Radiat Oncol Biol Phys* 2000; 48: 1187–1195.
110. Fukumoto S, Shirato H, Shimzu S, *et al.* Small-volume image-guided radiotherapy using hypofractionated, coplanar, and noncoplanar multiple fields for patients with inoperable stage I nonsmall cell lung carcinomas. *Cancer* 2002; 95: 1546–1553.
111. Lee SW, Choi EK, Park HJ, *et al.* Stereotactic body frame based fractionated radiosurgery on consecutive days for primary or metastatic tumors in the lung. *Lung Cancer* 2003; 40: 309–315.
112. Onimaru R, Shirato H, Shimizu S, *et al.* Tolerance of organs at risk in small-volume, hypofractionated, image-guided radiotherapy for primary and metastatic lung cancers. *Int J Radiat Oncol Biol Phys* 2003; 56: 126–135.
113. Timmerman R, Papiez L, McGarry R, *et al.* Extracranial stereotactic radioablation: results of a phase I study in medically inoperable stage I non-small cell lung cancer. *Chest* 2003; 124: 1946–1955.
114. Onishi H, Araki T, Shirato H, *et al.* Stereotactic hypofractionated high-dose irradiation for stage I nonsmall cell lung carcinoma: clinical outcomes in 245 subjects in a Japanese multi-institutional study. *Cancer* 2004; 101: 1623–1631.
115. Wulf J, Hädinger U, Oppitz U, *et al.* Stereotactic radiotherapy for primary lung cancer and pulmonary metastases: a noninvasive treatment approach in medically inoperable patients. *Int J Radiat Oncol Biol Phys* 2004; 60: 186–196.
116. Hoyer M, Roed H, Hansen AT, *et al.* Prospective study on stereotactic radiotherapy of limited stage non-small cell lung cancer. *Int J Radiat Oncol Biol Phys* 2005; 63: Suppl. 1, S396.
117. Nagata Y, Takayama K, Matsuo Y, *et al.* Clinical outcomes of a phase I/II study of 48 Gy of stereotactic body radiotherapy in 4 fractions for primary lung cancer using a stereotactic body frame. *Int J Radiat Oncol Biol Phys* 2005; 63: 1427–1431.
118. Beitler JJ, Badine EA, El-Sayah D, *et al.* Stereotactic body radiation therapy for nonmetastatic lung cancer: an analysis of 75 patients treated over 5 years. *Int J Radiat Oncol Biol Phys* 2006; 65: 100–106.
119. Xia T, Li H, Sun Q, *et al.* Promising clinical outcome of stereotactic body radiation therapy for patients with inoperable stage I/II non-small-cell lung cancer. *Int J Radiat Oncol Biol Phys* 2006; 66: 117–125.
120. Franks KN, Bezjak A, Purdie TG, *et al.* Early results of image-guided radiation therapy in lung stereotactic body radiotherapy (SBRT). *Clin Oncol (R Coll Radiol)* 2007; 19: Suppl. 3, S10.

121. Baumann P, Nyman J, Lax I, *et al.* Factors important for efficacy of stereotactic body radiotherapy of medically inoperable stage I lung cancer. A retrospective analysis of patients treated in the Nordic countries. *Acta Oncol* 2006; 45: 787–795.
122. Zimmermann FB, Geinitz H, Schill S, *et al.* Stereotactic hypofractionated radiotherapy in stage I (T1-2 N0 M0) non-small-cell lung cancer (NSCLC). *Acta Oncol* 2006; 45: 796–801.
123. Faria SL, Souhami L, Portelance L, *et al.* Absence of toxicity with hypofractionated 3-dimensional radiation therapy for inoperable, early stage non-small cell lung cancer. *Radiat Oncol* 2006; 1: 42.
124. Hof H, Muenter M, Oetzel D, *et al.* Stereotactic single-dose radiotherapy (radiosurgery) of early stage nonsmall-cell lung cancer (NSCLC). *Cancer* 2007; 110: 148–155.
125. Timmerman R, Galvin J, Michalski J, *et al.* Accreditation and quality assurance for Radiation Therapy Oncology Group: multicenter clinical trials using stereotactic body radiation therapy in lung cancer. *Acta Oncol* 2006; 45: 779–786.
126. Uematsu M, Shioda A, Suda A, *et al.* Computed tomography-guided frameless stereotactic radiotherapy for stage I non-small cell lung cancer: a 5-year experience. *Int J Radiat Oncol Biol Phys* 2001; 51: 666–670.
127. Hara R, Itami J, Kondo T, *et al.* Clinical outcomes of single-fraction stereotactic radiation therapy of lung tumors. *Cancer* 2006; 106: 1347–1352.
128. Widesott L, Amichetti M, Schwarz M. Proton therapy in lung cancer: clinical outcomes and technical issues. A systemic review. *Radiother Oncol* 2008; 86: 154–164.
129. Miyamoto T, Baba M, Sugane T, *et al.* Carbon ion radiotherapy for stage I non-small cell lung cancer using a regimen of four fractions during 1 week. *J Thorac Oncol* 2007; 2: 916–926.
130. Warram J. Preoperative irradiation of cancer of the lung: final report of a therapeutic trial. A collaborative study. *Cancer* 1975; 36: 914–925.
131. Shields TW. Preoperative radiation therapy in the treatment of bronchial carcinoma. *Cancer* 1972; 30: 1388–1394.
132. Rusch VW, Giroux DJ, Kraut MJ, *et al.* Induction chemoradiation and surgical resection for superior sulcus non-small-cell lung carcinomas: long-term results of Southwest Oncology Group Trial 9416 (Intergroup Trial 0160). *J Clin Oncol* 2007; 25: 313–318.
133. Weiden PL, Piantadosi S. Preoperative chemotherapy (cisplatin and fluorouracil) and radiation therapy in stage III non-small-cell lung cancer: a phase II study of the Lung Cancer Study Group. *J Natl Cancer Inst* 1991; 83: 266–273.
134. Sherman DM, Neptune W, Weichselbaum R, *et al.* An aggressive approach to marginally resectable lung cancer. *Cancer* 1978; 41: 2040–2045.
135. Paulson DL. Carcinomas in the superior pulmonary sulcus. *J Thorac Cardiovasc Surg* 1975; 70: 1095–1104.
136. Albain KS, Rusch VW, Crowley JJ, *et al.* Concurrent cisplatin/etoposide plus chest radiotherapy followed by surgery for stages IIIA (N2) and IIIB non-small-cell lung cancer: mature results of the Southwest Oncology Group phase II study 8805. *J Clin Oncol* 1995; 13: 1880–1892.
137. Kwong KF, Edelman MJ, Suntharalingam M, *et al.* High-dose radiotherapy in trimodality treatment of Pancoast tumors results in high pathologic complete response rates and excellent long-term survival. *J Thorac Cardiovasc Surg* 2005; 129: 1250–1257.
138. Farray D, Mirkovic N, Albain KS. Multimodality therapy for stage III non-small-cell lung cancer. *J Clin Oncol* 2005; 23: 3257–3269.
139. Van Meerbeeck JP, Kramer GWPM, Van Schil PEY, *et al.* Randomized controlled trial of resection *versus* radiotherapy after induction chemotherapy in stage IIIA-N2 non-small-cell lung cancer. *J Natl Cancer Inst* 2007; 99: 442–450.
140. Albain KS, Swann RS, Rusch VR, *et al.* Phase III study of concurrent chemotherapy and radiotherapy (CT/RT) *vs* CT/RT followed by surgical resection for stage IIIA (pN2) non-small cell lung cancer (NSCLC): outcomes update of North American Intergroup 0139 (RTOG 9309). *J Clin Oncol* 2005; 23: Suppl. 16, 7014.

141. Paterson R, Russell MH. Clinical trials in malignant disease. IV Lung cancer. Value of post-operative radiotherapy. *Clin Radiol* 1962; 13: 141–144.
142. Bangma PJ. Postoperative radiotherapy. *In*: Deeley TJ, ed. Carcinoma of the Bronchus: Modern Radiotherapy. New York, Appleton-Century-Crofts, 1972; pp. 163–170.
143. Van Houtte P, Rocmans P, Smets P, *et al.* Postoperative radiation therapy in lung cancer: a controlled trial after resection of curative design. *Int J Radiat Oncol Biol Phys* 1980; 6: 983–986.
144. Israel L, Bonadonna G, Sylvester R, *et al.* Controlled study with adjuvant radiotherapy, chemotherapy, immunotherapy and chemo-immunotherapy in operable squamous cell carcinoma of the lung. *In*: Muggia FM, Rozencweig M, eds. Lung Cancer: Progress in Therapeutic Research. New York, Raven Press, 1979; pp. 443–452.
145. Debevec M, Bitenc M, Vidmar S, *et al.* Postoperative radiotherapy for radically resected N2 non-small-cell lung cancer (NSCLC): randomised clinical study 1988–1992. *Lung Cancer* 1996, 14: 99–107.
146. Feng QF, Wang M, Wang LJ, *et al.* A study of postoperative radiotherapy in patients with non-small-cell lung cancer: a randomized trial. *Int J Radiat Oncol Biol Phys* 2000; 47: 925–929.
147. Effects of postoperative mediastinal radiation on completely resected stage II and stage III epidermoid cancer of the lung The Lung Cancer Study Group. *N Engl J Med* 1986; 315: 1377–1381.
148. Stephens RJ, Girling DJ, Bleehen NM, *et al.* The role of post-operative radiotherapy in non-small-cell lung cancer: a multicentre randomised trial in patients with pathologically staged T1-2, N1-2, M0 disease. Medical Research Council Lung Cancer Working Party. *Br J Cancer* 1996; 74: 632–639.
149. Lafitte JJ, Ribet ME, Prévost BM, *et al.* Postresection irradiation for T2 N0 M0 non-small cell carcinoma: a prospective, randomized study. *Ann Thorac Surg* 1996; 62: 830–834.
150. Dautzenberg B, Arriagada R, Chammard AB, *et al.* A controlled study of postoperative radiotherapy for patients with completely resected nonsmall cell lung carcinoma. Groupe d'Etude et de Traitement des Cancers Bronchiques. *Cancer* 1999; 86: 265–273.
151. Wang M, Gu XZ, Yin WB, *et al.* Randomised clinical trial of post-operative irradiation after surgery for non-small cell lung cancer. *Chin J Radiat Oncol* 1994; 3: 39–43.
152. PORT Meta-analysis Trialists Group. Postoperative radiotherapy for non-small cell lung cancer. *Cochrane Database Syst Rev* 2005; 2: CD002142.
153. Postoperative radiotherapy in non-small-cell lung cancer: systematic review and meta-analysis of individual patient data from nine randomised controlled trials. PORT Meta-analysis Trialists Group. *Lancet* 1998; 352: 257–263.
154. Phlips P, Rocmans P, Vanderhoeft P, *et al.* Postoperative radiotherapy after pneumonectomy: impact of modern treatment facilities. *Int J Radiat Oncol Biol Phys* 1993; 27: 525–529.
155. Bekelman JE, Rosenzweig KE, Bach PB, *et al.* Trends in the use of postoperative radiotherapy for resected non-small-cell lung cancer. *Int J Radiat Oncol Biol Phys* 2006; 66: 492–499.
156. Lally BE, Zelterman D, Colasanto JM, *et al.* Postoperative radiotherapy for stage II or III non-small-cell lung cancer using the Surveillance, Epidemiology, and End Results database. *J Clin Oncol* 2006; 24: 2998–3006.
157. Sawyer TE, Bonner JA, Gould PM, *et al.* The impact of surgical adjuvant thoracic radiation therapy for patients with nonsmall cell lung cancer with ipsilateral mediastinal lymph node involvement. *Cancer* 1997; 80: 1399–1408.
158. Machtay M, Lee JH, Shrager JB, *et al.* Risk of death from intercurrent disease is not excessively increased by modern postoperative radiotherapy for high-risk resectable non-small-cell lung carcinoma. *J Clin Oncol* 2001; 19: 3912–3917.
159. Arriagada R, Bergman B, Dunant A, *et al.* Cisplatin-based adjuvant chemotherapy in patients with completely resected non-small-cell lung cancer. *N Engl J Med* 2004; 350: 351–360.
160. Hotta K, Matsuo K, Ueoka H, *et al.* Role of adjuvant chemotherapy in patients with resected non-small-cell lung cancer: reappraisal with meta-analysis of randomized controlled trials. *J Clin Oncol* 2004; 22: 3860–3867.

161. Winton T, Livingston R, Johnson D, *et al.* Vinorelbine plus cisplatin *vs* observation in resected non-small-cell lung cancer. *N Engl J Med* 2005; 352: 2589–2597.
162. Sedrakyan A, Van Der Meulen J, O'Byrne K, *et al.* Postoperative chemotherapy for non-small cell lung cancer: a systematic review and meta-analysis. *J Thorac Cardiovasc Surg* 2004; 128: 414–419.
163. Keller SM, Adak S, Wagner H, *et al.* A randomized trial of postoperative adjuvant therapy in patients with completely resected stage II or IIIA non-small-cell lung cancer. Eastern Cooperative Oncology Group. *N Eng J Med* 2000; 343: 1217–1222.
164. Le Pechoux C, Lung ART. Phase III study comparing post-operative conformal radiotherapy to no post-operative radiotherapy in patients with completely resected non-small cell lung cancer and mediastinal N2 involvement. EORTC protocol 22055–08053. Brussels, EORTC, 2008.
165. Aurora R, Milite F, Vander Els NJ. Respiratory emergencies. *Semin Oncol* 2000; 27: 256–269.
166. Collins TM, Ash DV, Close HJ, *et al.* An evaluation of the palliative role of radiotherapy in inoperable carcinoma of the bronchus. *Clin Radiol* 1998; 39: 284–286.
167. Simpson JR, Francis ME, Perez-Tamayo R, *et al.* Palliative radiotherapy for inoperable carcinoma of the lung: final report of a RTOG multi-institutional trial. *Int J Radiat Oncol Biol Phys* 1985; 11: 751–758.
168. Inoperable non-small-cell lung cancer (NSCLC): a Medical Research Council randomised trial of palliative radiotherapy of two fractions or ten fractions. Report to the Medical Research Council by its Lung Cancer Working Party. *Br J Cancer* 1991; 63: 265–270.
169. A Medical Research Council (MRC) randomised trial of palliative radiotherapy with two fractions or a single fraction in patients with inoperable non-small-cell lung cancer (NSCLC) and poor performance status. Medical Research Council Lung Working Party. *Br J Cancer* 1992; 65: 934–941.
170. Macbeth FR, Bolger JJ, Hopwood P, *et al.* Randomized trial of palliative two-fraction *versus* more intensive 13-fraction radiotherapy for patients with inoperable non-small cell lung cancer and good performance status. Medical Research Council Lung Cancer Working Party. *Clin Oncol (R Coll Radiol)* 1996; 8: 167–175.
171. Rees GJ, Devrell CE, Barley VL, *et al.* Palliative radiotherapy for lung cancer: two *versus* five fractions. *Clin Oncol (R Coll Radiol)* 1997; 9: 90–95.
172. Erridge SC, Gaze MN, Price A, *et al.* Symptom control and quality of life in people with lung cancer: a randomised trial of two palliative radiotherapy fractionation schedules. *Clin Oncol (R Coll Radiol)* 2005; 17: 61–67.
173. Sundstrøm S, Bremnes R, Aasebø U, *et al.* Hypofractionated palliative radiotherapy (17 Gy per two fractions) in advanced non-small-cell lung carcinoma is comparable to standard fractionation for symptom control and survival: a national phase III trial. *J Clin Oncol* 2004; 22: 801–810.
174. Langendijk JAA, Ten Velde GP, Aaronson NK, *et al.* Quality of life after palliative radiotherapy in non-small cell lung cancer: a prospective study. *Int J Radiat Oncol Biol Phys* 2000; 47: 149–155.
175. Falk SJ, Girling DJ, White RJ, *et al.* Immediate *versus* delayed palliative thoracic radiotherapy in patients with unresectable locally advanced non-small cell lung cancer and minimal thoracic symptoms: randomised controlled trial. *BMJ* 2002; 325: 465–472.
176. Abratt RP, Shepherd LJ, Salton DG. Palliative radiation for stage 3 non-small cell lung cancer – a prospective study of two moderately high dose regimens. *Lung Cancer* 1995; 13: 137–143.
177. Teo P, Tai TH, Choy D, *et al.* A randomized study on palliative radiation therapy for inoperable non small cell carcinoma of the lung. *Int J Radiat Oncol Biol Phys* 1988; 14: 867–871.
178. Nestle U, Nieder C, Walter K, *et al.* A palliative accelerated irradiation regimen for advanced non-small-cell lung cancer *vs* conventionally fractionated 60 Gy: results of a randomized equivalence study. *Int J Radiat Oncol Biol Phys* 2000; 48: 95–103.
179. Reinfuss M, Glinski B, Kowalska T, *et al.* [Radiotherapy for stage III, inoperable, asymptomatic non-small cell lung cancer. Final results of a prospective randomized study (240 patients)]. *Cancer Radiother* 1999; 3: 475–479.

180. Bezjak A, Dixon P, Brundage M, *et al.* Randomized phase III trial of single *versus* fractionated thoracic radiation in the palliation of patients with lung cancer (NCIC CTG SC.15). *Int J Radiat Oncol Biol Phys* 2002; 54: 719–728.
181. Kramer GW, Wanders SL, Noordijk EM, *et al.* Results of the Dutch national study of the palliative effect of irradiation using two different treatment schemes for non-small-cell lung cancer. *J Clin Oncol* 2005; 23: 2962–2970.
182. Senkus-Konefka E, Dziadziuszko R, Bednaruk-Młyński E, *et al.* A prospective, randomised study to compare two palliative radiotherapy schedules for non-small-cell lung cancer (NSCLC). *Br J Cancer* 2005; 92: 1038–1045.
183. Devereux S, Hatton MQ, Macbeth FR. Immediate side effects of large fraction radiotherapy. *Clin Oncol (R Coll Radiol)* 1997; 9: 96–99.
184. Macbeth FR, Wheldon TE, Girling DJ, *et al.* Radiation myelopathy: estimates of risk in 1048 patients in three randomized trials of palliative radiotherapy for non-small cell lung cancer. The Medical Research Council Lung Cancer Working Party. *Clin Oncol (R Coll Radiol)* 1996; 8: 176–181.
185. Danson S, Middleton MR, O'Byrne KJ, *et al.* Phase III trial of gemcitabine and carboplatin *versus* mitomycin, ifosfamide and cisplatin or mitomycin, vinblastine and cisplatin in patients with advanced nonsmall cell lung cancer. *Cancer* 2003; 98: 542–553.

CHAPTER 13

Neoadjuvant and adjuvant treatment for operable nonsmall cell lung cancer

M. Mukesh, D. Gilligan

Oncology Centre, Addenbrooke's Hospital, Cambridge University Hospitals NHS Trust, Cambridge, UK.

Correspondence: D. Gilligan, Oncology Centre, Addenbrooke's Hospital, Cambridge University Hospitals NHS Trust, Cambridge, CB2 0QQ, UK. E-mail: david.gilligan@addenbrookes.nhs.uk

Lung cancer is the leading cause of cancer death in the western world, with 1.2 million cases worldwide in 2000 and 1.1 million deaths. More than 80% of lung cancer cases are of nonsmall cell histology. Surgery has long been the treatment of choice for operable nonsmall cell lung cancer (NSCLC) and offers the best chance of cure, but overall 5-yr survival rates are disappointing, ranging from 55% for stage I to 20% for stage IIIA [1]. Systemic relapses are common and occur in up to 60% of resected patients [2], suggesting that NSCLC is a systemic disease and there is a role of adjuvant and neoadjuvant treatment in its management. The role of adjuvant and neoadjuvant chemotherapy has been long established in other tumour sites, including breast and colorectal cancer, with improvement in survival rates [3, 4]. In the past there has been a lack of enthusiasm among clinicians for the use of chemotherapy in operable NSCLC, as most of the randomised studies in the 1980s were small and underpowered. Also, patient demographics can be very different from breast and colon cancer, as many patients are elderly and have multiple medical comorbidities and a poorer performance status. In the last decade there has been renewed interest in adjuvant chemotherapy based on new randomised trials and meta-analysis. In this chapter we will look at the role of adjuvant and neoadjuvant chemotherapy in operable NSCLC.

Adjuvant chemotherapy

"Adjuvant" therapy means additional treatment, in this setting given after surgery where all the detectable disease has been removed. The clinical rationale behind adjuvant chemotherapy is that completely resected NSCLC patients are at high risk of systemic relapse, possibly due to occult micrometastases. The aim of adjuvant chemotherapy is to eradicate these occult metastatic deposits.

NSCLC collaborative group 1995

In the 1980s there was no clear consensus for the role of post-operative chemotherapy and it was considered experimental. Most of the studies were small and underpowered, with half recruiting fewer than 100 patients. Hence, for most of them the results were inconclusive or statistically insignificant. In 1995 a meta-analysis was published looking at the role of post-operative chemotherapy by the NSCLC collaborative group (fig. 1) [5]. Data were available for 4,357 patients from 14 trials comparing surgery alone with surgery plus chemotherapy. Five trials used long-term alkylating agents (mainly

Eur Respir Mon, 2009, 44, 244–259. Printed in UK - all rights reserved. Copyright ERS Journals Ltd 2009; European Respiratory Monograph; ISSN 1025-448x.

Trial	No. of events/ No. of patients entered: Surgery plus chemotherapy	No. of events/ No. of patients entered: Surgery	Observed −expected deaths	Variance
Long-term alkylating agents				
MRC LUO2	415/428	209/215	18.22	143.32
VASAG	251/291	128/152	4.50	86.00
EORTC 08741	38/71	36/75	5.82	18.06
VASOG 5	292/424	261/417	20.63	137.53
WPL 7351	25/36	15/36	6.36	9.83
Subtotal	1021/1250	649/895	55.53	394.74
Other drugs				
OLCSG 1a	30/163	28/158	-0.09	14.47
OLCSG 1b	27/41	21/42	6.59	11.36
SGACLC ACTLC 1	70/154	75/152	-6.10	36.12
WJSG 2 (2 and 3)	38/108	49/100	-9.79	21.49
Subtotal	165/466	173/452	-9.39	83.44
Cisplatin based				
LCSG 801	66/140	71/143	-1.81	34.21
OLCSG 1c	5/12	7/16	-0.19	2.93
FLCSG 1	20/54	30/56	-7.79	12.21
SGACLC ACTLC 2	64/165	68/167	-4.80	32.88
IPCR Chiba	11/15	7/14	1.33	4.07
WJSG 2 (1 and 3)	44/115	49/100	-7.66	22.94
LCSG 853	29/94	32/94	-1.65	15.22
JLCSSG	59/111	52/98	0.98	27.38
Subtotal	298/706	316/688	-21.58	151.83
Total	1484/2422	1138/2035	24.57	630.01

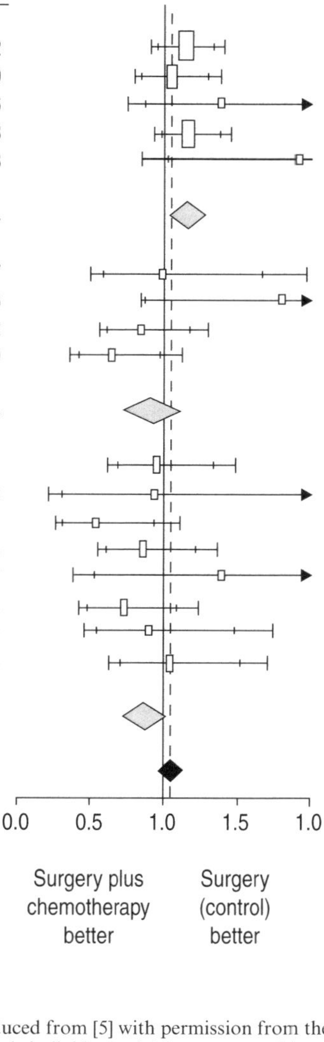

Fig. 1. – Nonsmall cell lung cancer collaborative meta-analysis, 1995. Reproduced from [5] with permission from the publisher. Results of trials of surgery *versus* surgery plus chemotherapy. Each individual trial is represented by a square, the centre of which denotes the hazard ratio (HR) for that trial, with horizontal bars whose extremities denote the 99% confidence interval (CI) and inner bars mark the 95% CI. The size of the square is directly proportional to the amount of information in the trial. The black diamond at the foot of the plot gives the overall HR when the results of all trials are combined, the centre of which denotes the HR and the extremities the 95% CI. Shaded diamonds represent the HR for the various specified categories of chemotherapy. Trials are ordered chronologically by date of start of trial (oldest first) within chemotherapy categories. MRC: Medical Research Council; VASAG: Veterans Administration Surgical Adjuvant Group; EORTC: European Organisation for Research and Treatment of Cancer; VASOG: Veterans Administration Surgical Oncology Group; WPL: Working Party for Lung Cancer (Committee on Surgery and Surgery Consultants); OLCSG Osaka Lung Cancer Study Group; SGACLC ACTLC: Study Group of Adjuvant Chemotherapy for Lung Cancer, Chibu, Japan; WJSG: West Japan Study Group for Lung Cancer Surgery; LCSG: Lung Cancer Study Group; FLCSG: Finnish Lung Cancer Study Group; IPCR Chiba: Institute of Pulmonary Cancer Research, Chiba, Japan; JLCSSG: Japan Lung Cancer Surgical Study Group.

cyclophosphamide and nitrosourea) and eight trials used cisplatin-based combination chemotherapy. The intended dose of cisplatin varied 40–80 mg·m^{-2} per cycle and total dose varied 50–240 mg·m^{-2}. The results showed that adjuvant chemotherapy using alkylating agents were detrimental to survival, with a 15% increase in relative risk of death ($p=0.005$). Cisplatin-based chemotherapy was beneficial, with a 13% reduction in relative risk of death, suggesting an absolute benefit of 3% at 2 yrs and 5% at 5 yrs ($p=0.08$).

Cisplatin-based chemotherapy

Since publication of this meta-analysis there has been renewed interest in adjuvant chemotherapy and new randomised trials have been conducted. Following the favourable reports using cisplatin-based chemotherapy in the 1995 NSCLC meta-analysis, it has been used in five large randomised controlled trials. Some of these have shown improved survival. The International Adjuvant Lung Trial (IALT) randomised 1,867 patients with completely resected stage I–III NSCLC between cisplatin plus vinca-alkaloid or etoposide combination chemotherapy and observation. The primary end-point was overall survival. The results showed an absolute 5-yr survival benefit of 4.1% in the chemotherapy arm (hazard ratio (HR) 0.86; $p=0.04$). 23% of patients experienced grade 3–4 toxicities and seven (0.8%) patients died of chemotherapy toxicity [6]. A recent update with median follow up of 7.5 yrs showed that the beneficial effect of adjuvant chemotherapy is no longer statistically significant for survival (HR 0.91; $p=0.10$). The reason for this is unclear: the use of etoposide could increase the rate of second cancer but this was not seen. However, there were more noncancer-related deaths in the chemotherapy arm after 5 yrs [7].

The National Cancer Institute of Canada (NCIC) JBR.10 trial randomised 482 patients with completely resected stage IB or stage II NSCLC to vinorelbine (25 mg·m^{-2} weekly) plus cisplatin (50 mg·m^{-2} on days 1 and 8) for four cycles or observation. Overall survival was significantly prolonged in the chemotherapy group compared with observation only (94 *versus* 73 months; HR for death 0.69; $p=0.04$). The 5-yr survival rates were 69 and 54%, respectively [8]. Subgroup analysis showed no statistically significant improvement among patients with stage IB NSCLC. Chemotherapy caused febrile neutropenia in 7% of patients and two (0.8%) patients died of chemotherapy toxicity. 17% of patients had grade 3–4 nausea or vomiting during chemotherapy.

The Cancer and Leukemia Group B (CALGB) 9633 study randomised 344 patients, all with completely resected stage IB disease, to either adjuvant chemotherapy with carboplatin (area under the curve 6) and paclitaxel (200 mg·m^{-2}) or observation. Initial results at 4 yrs revealed an absolute survival benefit of 12% when presented in 2004, but subsequent analysis presented in 2006 did not confirm this survival advantage, with a HR of 0.80 ($p=0.10$). The chemotherapy regime was well tolerated and there were no chemotherapy-related deaths. The authors stated that this study was stopped early by the data-monitoring committee and may not have had the power to detect small differences in overall survival that are clinically significant. It is important to note that this study is so far only presented in abstract form [9]. The presentation of these two studies was largely responsible for a major change in practice towards adjuvant chemotherapy in normal clinical practice.

The Adjuvant Navelbine International Trialist Association (ANITA) randomised 840 patients with operated stage IB–IIIA NSCLC to cisplatin (100 mg·m^{-2}) plus vinorelbine (30 mg·m^{-2}) or observation. After a median follow-up of 76 months, the adjusted risk of death was significantly reduced in patients assigned to the chemotherapy arm compared with the control arm (HR for death 0.80; $p=0.017$). Toxicities from chemotherapy mainly included febrile neutropenia in 34 (9%) patients with seven (2%) toxic deaths. 95 (27%) patients suffered World Health Organization (WHO) grade 3–4 nausea or vomiting. The compliance was greater with cisplatin than with vinorelbine. Absolute overall survival improvement at 5 yrs with chemotherapy was 8.6%, which was maintained at 7 yrs [10]. Subgroup analysis indicated that the benefit of adjuvant chemotherapy was mainly in patients with stage II and stage IIIA disease. However, chemotherapy did not improve survival in stage IB disease.

Two other reported trials showed no survival advantage for adjuvant cisplatin chemotherapy. The Adjuvant Lung Cancer Project Italy (ALPI) randomised 1,209 patients with stage I–IIIA operated NSCLC between three cycles of mitomycin C (8 mg·m^{-2} day 1), vindesine (3 mg·m^{-2} days 1 and 8) and cisplatin (100 mg·m^{-2} day 1) (MVP) *versus* observation. The primary end-point was overall survival and secondary end-points were progression-free survival and toxicity. After a median follow-up of 64.5 months, the trial failed to show any statistically significant difference in overall survival or progression-free survival between the two arms (HR 0.96) [11]. One possible explanation for this result could be poor patient compliance, with only 69% patients completing three cycles of MVP due to chemotherapy-related toxicity. Nearly half of them required dose adjustments or omission of some of the regime. Also, DEPIERRE *et al.* [12] had previously reported that pre-operative mitomycin-based chemotherapy was associated with an excess of early deaths. The Big Lung Trial (BLT), a mainly UK-based Medical Research Council trial, reported on 381 NSCLC patients randomised to various platinum-based regimes in the neoadjuvant (4%) and adjuvant (96%) setting. After a median follow-up of 2.9 yrs the trial failed to show any survival advantage with chemotherapy (HR 1.02; p=0.90) [13]. Only 64% of patients received all three cycles of chemotherapy, with 40% requiring dose adjustments. Twenty eight per cent of the patients had grade 3–4 toxicity, mainly haematological (11%), nausea/vomiting (7%) and neutropenic fever (2%). Six patients died of chemotherapy toxicity. Once again, recruitment rates for this study were much lower than anticipated.

With conflicting data from different trials, a meta-analysis can more accurately evaluate the benefits of adjuvant cisplatin chemotherapy. PIGNON *et al.* [14] reported the Lung Adjuvant Cisplatin Evaluation (LACE), a pooled analysis of five randomised trials (fig. 2). The meta-analysis was based on individual patient data of 4,584 patients. The analysis confirmed the previous NSCLC meta-analysis, with cisplatin-based chemotherapy offering a statistically significant survival advantage (HR 0.89; $p<0.005$). This corresponds to an absolute survival benefit of 5.4% at 5 yrs. There was a small increase in non-lung cancer-related death in the adjuvant chemotherapy arm in the first 6 months after randomisation. It was mainly related to chemotherapy toxicity and cardiovascular/pulmonary deaths, possibly due to a detrimental effect of cisplatin. The survival benefits were dependent on stage, with the greatest benefits in stage II and III. The analysis suggested that patients with stage IA may not benefit from chemotherapy. There was a significant interaction between chemotherapy effect and WHO performance status. Chemotherapy effects were increased with better performance status and may be detrimental with performance status of 2. The effect of chemotherapy did not vary significantly with the associated drug used, although the cisplatin plus vinorelbine combination was favourable (p=0.11).

Uracil-tegafur-based chemotherapy

Oral chemotherapy in the form of uracil-tegafur (UFT) has been used as adjuvant chemotherapy in many randomised controlled trials in Japan. The 1995 NSCLC collaborative meta-analysis analysed results of three randomised trials where combination

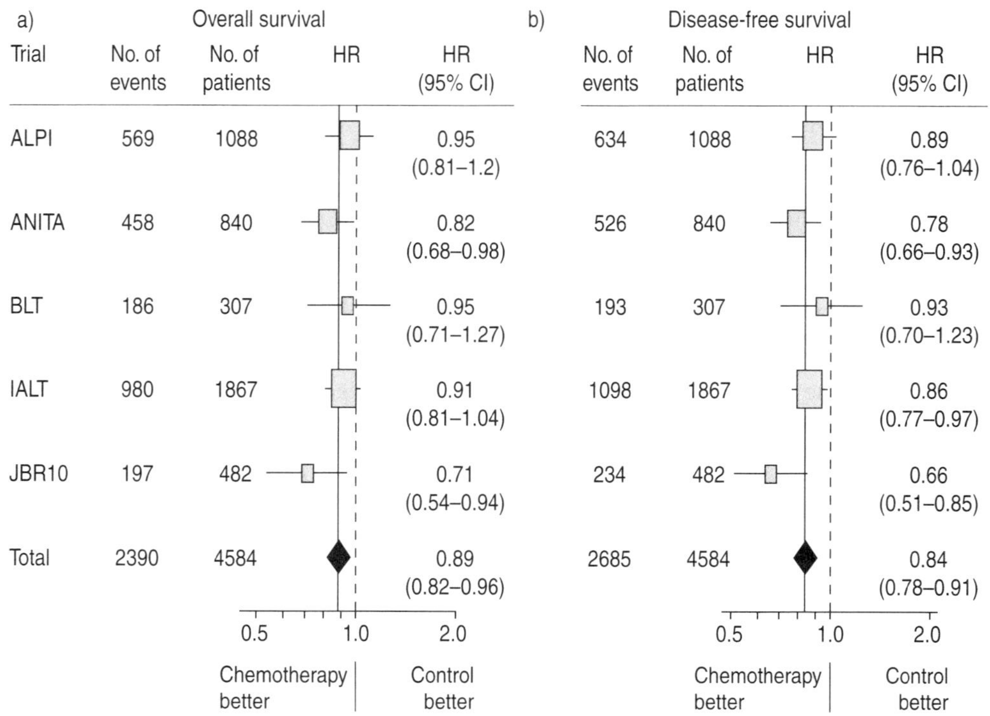

Fig. 2. – Lung Adjuvant Cisplatin Evaluation (LACE) meta-analysis. Reproduced from [14] with permission from the publisher. a) Overall survival: hazard ratio (HR) of death with chemotherapy *versus* control (no chemotherapy). b) Disease-free survival: HR of recurrence or death with chemotherapy *versus* control. HR for individual trials and overall effect are given with 95% confidence interval (CI). The horizontal scale used is a logarithmic scale. ALPI: Adjuvant Lung Cancer Project Italy; ANITA: Adjuvant Navelbine International Trialist Association 01; BLT: Big Lung Trial; IALT: International Adjuvant Lung Trial; JBR10: National Cancer Institute of Canada Clinical Trial Group trial JBR10. Chemotherapy effects: a) logrank statistic 8.5, $p=0.005$; b) logrank statistic 21.1, $p<0.001$. Tests for heterogeneity: a) Chi-squared 4.25, $p=0.37$, $I^2=6\%$; b) Chi-squared 5.16, $p=0.27$, $I^2=23\%$.

chemotherapy using UFT was used in the adjuvant setting [5]. They found a 4% improvement in survival with UFT-based chemotherapy (HR for death 0.89; p=0.30). UFT is an oral fluorouracil (FU) derivative chemotherapeutic drug composed of tegafur and uracil; tegafur is a prodrug of FU and uracil is added to inhibit degradation of FU through inhibition of dihydropyrimidine dehydrogenase, which is the enzyme responsible for FU catabolism. Thus, oral UFT administration can achieve a certain plasma FU concentration for a long time. The West Japan Study Group for Lung Cancer Surgery first reported that the long-term administration of UFT improves post-operative survival in patients with completely resected NSCLC [15]. 323 patients with completely resected primary NSCLC (stage I–III) were randomised into three treatment groups: three cycles of cisplatin plus vindesine and 1-yr oral administration of UFT (CVUft), 1-yr oral administration of UFT only and observation. The 5-yr overall survival was 60.6% in the CVUft arm, 64.1% for the UFT arm and 49% for the observation group. In a subgroup analysis, there was no significant difference in overall survival between the UFT group and the control group among patients with squamous cell carcinoma (p=0.24). In contrast, patients with adenocarcinoma in the UFT group had a significantly better survival than those in the control group (p=0.009). Some other trials using post-operative UFT have shown negative results.

Once again, in order to make more sense of the data across different trials, meta-analysis can be used. HAMADA *et al.* [16] published a meta-analysis to assess the efficacy of post-operative chemotherapy with UFT in NSCLC in 2005. The meta-analysis was based on individual patient data. A total of 2,003 patients from six trials were analysed, comparing surgery alone with surgery plus UFT. Ninety nine per cent of patients were either histologically squamous cell or adenocarcinoma and most were stage I. The meta-analysis showed that the survival rates at 5 and 7 yrs were significantly higher in the surgery plus UFT arm (81.5 and 76.5% in the UFT plus surgery group *versus* 77.2 and 69.5% in the surgery alone group, respectively). The overall HR was 0.74 (p=0.001). Again, UFT was effective, especially in patients with adenocarcinoma histology, but failed to show a statistical advantage in the squamous cell histology. Interestingly, there was no separation of the survival curves at 4 yrs in the meta-analysis. It is unclear from the meta-analysis whether patients with stage II or stage III disease benefit from treatment with UFT and whether treatment for 1 yr is equivalent to treatment for 2 yrs.

Since the meta-analysis, the Japan Lung Cancer Research Group (JLCRG) has published their results. The JLCRG randomised 979 patients with pathological stage I adenocarcinoma of the lung between 2 yrs of UFT and observation [17]. After a median follow-up of 73 months, the difference in overall survival between the two groups was statistically significant in favour of the UFT group (p=0.04). Grade 3 toxic effects occurred in 10 (2%) out of the 482 patients who received UFT.

UFT has a very poor response rate of about 7% in advanced and recurrent NSCLC. So how can the efficacy of UFT in the adjuvant setting be explained? In the post-operative setting, residual lesions requiring control are occult microscopic disease, not bulky tumours. It is postulated that, even if the direct anti-tumour effects of UFT are relatively low, it can be administered for a long time because of its mild toxicity, which results in controlling micrometastases and improving survival. Finally, although the survival improvement has been reported in the post-operative UFT Japanese trials and meta-analysis, there have been no confirmatory trials in the western population, and the routine use of UFT outside a trial setting cannot be recommended.

NSCLC collaborative group 2007

The NSCLC collaborative group updated the 1995 meta-analysis in 2007. Independent data analysis was performed on 8,147 patients from 30 randomised controlled trials. 15 trials used cisplatin without UFT, eight trials used tegafur/UFT without cisplatin and seven trials used tegafur/UFT and cisplatin [18]. The analysis again confirmed the advantage of adjuvant chemotherapy on survival (HR 0.86; p<0.000001), with an absolute survival benefit of 4% (increase from 60 to 64%) at 5 yrs and 5% at 8 yrs. There was a suggestion of a trend in the effect of chemotherapy by stage (p=0.047). There was no evidence that any patient subgroup defined by age or histology benefited more or less with chemotherapy.

Neoadjuvant chemotherapy

"Neoadjuvant" chemotherapy as described in this chapter means treatment given prior to surgery. The rationale of neoadjuvant chemotherapy is to regress the primary cancer in order to facilitate and simplify subsequent surgery, treat occult micrometastatic disease at the time of presentation and also inhibit the release of tumour growth factors at the time of surgery. It does not include treatment given to make an inoperable tumour operable, sometimes referred to as downstaging chemotherapy. As NSCLC is a systemic disease and the majority of patients die of systemic relapse after surgery, there is a clinical rationale to use neoadjuvant treatment. Neoadjuvant chemotherapy has been used in other tumour sites, like oesophageal cancer and bladder cancer, with significant improvements in survival [19].

In NSCLC, interest in this form of treatment was initiated by two trials reported in the 1990s. They reported on the benefits of neoadjuvant chemotherapy in resectable stage IIIA NSCLC. ROSELL *et al.* [20] randomised 60 patients with stage IIIA NSCLC between surgery and three cycles of pre-operative chemotherapy (mitomycin C, ifosfamide and cisplatin) followed by surgery. All patients received mediastinal radiation after surgery. The median period of survival was 26 months in the patients treated with chemotherapy plus surgery, compared with 8 months in the patients treated with surgery alone ($p<0.001$). ROTH *et al.* [21] randomised 60 patients with operable stage IIIA NSCLC between surgery and three cycles of pre-operative chemotherapy (cyclophosphamide, etoposide and cisplatin) followed by surgery. Patients with tumour regression on chemotherapy received an additional three cycles of adjuvant chemotherapy. Patients treated with peri-operative chemotherapy and surgery had an estimated median survival of 64 months compared with 11 months for patients who had surgery alone ($p<0.008$ by log rank test; $p<0.018$ by Wilcoxon test). Both these studies showed significant survival advantages with neoadjuvant chemotherapy, but both trials were stopped prematurely as interim analysis showed clinically meaningful survival difference between the two groups. They were also criticised because patients randomised to the surgery alone arm did not do as well as expected. As a consequence of these studies, larger, collaborative studies were initiated.

The French Thoracic Cooperative Group (FTCG) randomised 355 patients to primary surgery or two cycles of pre-operative chemotherapy (mitomycin, ifosfamide and cisplatin) with two additional post-operative cycles for responding patients [12]. In both arms, patients with pT3 or pN2 disease received thoracic radiotherapy. The results showed a trend towards improved overall survival in the peri-operative chemotherapy arm over surgery (37 *versus* 26 months; $p=0.15$). There were two pre-operative toxic deaths. Post-operative mortality was 6.7% in the chemotherapy arm and 4.5% in the surgery alone arm. It is possible that the survival advantage was secondary to post-operative adjuvant chemotherapy.

The Southwest Oncology Group (SWOG) randomised 354 patients with clinical stage T2N0, T1-2N1 and T3N0-1 NSCLC between surgery and three cycles of pre-operative paclitaxel and carboplatin chemotherapy [22]. The trial failed to show any survival benefit with neoadjuvant chemotherapy (HR 0.88; $p=0.47$). Recently, GILLIGAN *et al.* [23] have reported on the large intergroup (Medical Research Council (MRC)/Nederlandse Vereniging van Artsen voor Longziekten en Tuberculose (NVALT)/ European Organisation for Research and Treatment of Cancer (EORTC)) trial of neoadjuvant chemotherapy. A total of 519 NSCLC patients with clinical stage I–III disease were randomised between surgery and three cycles of platinum-based chemotherapy followed by surgery. Sixty one per cent were stage I, with 31% stage II and 7% stage III. This large neoadjuvant trial in operable NSCLC demonstrated good response rates (49%), but has failed to show a survival benefit with neoadjuvant chemotherapy (HR 1.02; $p=0.86$). One possible explanation for the lack of improvement in survival with pre-operative chemotherapy in this study could be a median survival of 52 months in the surgery alone arm, which is 9–12 months better than would have been expected. Also, the majority of the patients in the trial were stage I NSCLC, the group with the lowest risk of systemic relapse.

The Italian Chemotherapy for Early Stages Trial (ChEST) trial randomised 270 patients with stage IB–IIIA NSCLC between pre-operative cycles of gemcitabine-cisplatin followed by radical surgery and surgery alone [24]. The response rate to chemotherapy was 35%, with 5.5% progressing through chemotherapy. The overall 3-yr survival rate was 60% in the surgery alone group and 67% in the chemotherapy plus surgery group (p=0.053). The trial aimed to enrol 700 patients but was closed prematurely, as was the aforementioned MRC/NVALT/EORTC trial, due to the publication of positive adjuvant studies. However, it demonstrates the efficacy of neoadjuvant chemotherapy in operable NSCLC.

The SWOG, FTCG and MRC/NVALT/EORTC are three large trials of neoadjuvant chemotherapy in operable NSCLC. Although there were a number of differences between the three trials in terms of design and patient characteristics (table 1), they have failed to show improved survival with neoadjuvant chemotherapy.

All of these trials demonstrated that neoadjuvant chemotherapy was feasible with no significant increased post-operative complications. In particular, there was no significant disease progression during chemotherapy and evidence of tumour down-staging is documented. In addition, there appeared to be no detriment to surgery with no delays in the planned resection and no significant increase in post-operative complications in the chemotherapy arm. As some of the later trials had to close because of the emerging adjuvant chemotherapy data, the best evidence for the value of neoadjuvant chemotherapy comes from the systematic review. A meta-analysis performed by Burdett *et al.* [25] looked at data of 988 patients from seven randomised controlled trials and analysed it using the Parmar method (estimating the HR indirectly from other summary statistics or from the Kaplan–Meier curves). Pre-operative chemotherapy improved absolute survival across all stages of disease from 14 to 20% at 5 yrs (HR 0.82; p=0.02). Updating the systematic review with the data from the MRC LU22 trial dilutes the benefit of neoadjuvant chemotherapy (HR 0.88, p=0.07; fig. 3)

Table 1. – Comparison of patients' baseline characteristics and survival in the three large randomised trials of neoadjuvant chemotherapy in resectable nonsmall cell lung cancer

Factor	MRC LU22	FTCG	SWOG
Total patients n	519	355	354
Chemotherapy	Platinum-based	MIC	PC
Pre-operative cycles	3	2	3
Post-operative treatment	None	2 further cycles to responding patients	None
Median age yrs	62–63	60–61	64–65
Male %	72	93	66
Histology %			
Squamous	49	74	38
Adenocarcinoma	27	17	63
WHO PS %			
0	55	64	NA
1	43	34	NA
2	2	2	NA
Stage %			
I	61	37	63
II	31	16	34
III	7	47	4
Overall survival			
Median S months	54	26	40
Median CT+S months	49	37	47
HR	1.02	0.78	0.84
95% CI	0.80–1.31	0.60–1.02	0.60–1.18

MRC: Medical Research Council; FTCG: French Thoracic Cooperative Group; SWOG: Southwest Oncology Group; WHO: World Health Organization; PS: performance status; S: surgery; CT: chemotherapy; HR: hazard ratio; CI: confidence interval; MIC: mitomycin, ifosfamide and cisplatin; PC: paclitaxel and carboplatin; NA: not available.

[23]. The Parmar method is not very accurate and depends on published information. Independent patient data meta-analyses would allow a more reliable estimate and will also allow other outcomes, such as disease-free survival, to be investigated further. An updated independent patient data meta-analysis for neoadjuvant chemotherapy is needed.

Pre-operative *versus* post-operative chemotherapy

There is an ongoing debate about the role of neoadjuvant chemotherapy, especially with adjuvant chemotherapy improving overall survival. Most of the neoadjuvant trials closed to accrual after adjuvant trials results became known, because it was felt by investigators that given the result of the adjuvant studies it would be unethical not to offer chemotherapy to patients who might benefit from it in the adjuvant setting. Given the results of meta-analyses of both adjuvant and neoadjuvant chemotherapy, questions can be raised as to which is best. So far no published trial has directly compared the outcome of pre-operative *versus* post-operative chemotherapy. The numbers required to sufficiently power a trial to answer this question would probably be prohibitive. LIM *et al.* [31] have indirectly compared pre- and post-operative chemotherapy using data from 32 published randomised trials of adjuvant and neoadjuvant chemotherapy in NSCLC. The HR was extracted from the published data or survival curves using the Parmar method. The study concluded that both pre-operative and post-operative chemotherapy yield similar results for overall and disease-free survival (HR 0.99; p=0.91).

In routine clinical practice it is likely that the standard of care will be towards adjuvant chemotherapy in the post-operative setting. Patients treated post-operatively have the advantage of an accurate pathological stage whereas, even with modern staging techniques such as positron emission tomography/computed tomography and endoscopic mediastinal staging (endobronchial and endoscopic ultrasound), tumours can be overstaged and inappropriate treatment given. Patients who are understaged as stage I pre-operatively can be offered post-operative treatment. There may be some circumstances, however, where neoadjuvant chemotherapy is preferred. For instance,

Trial [ref.]	No. of patients CT+S	S	HR (95% CI)
DAUTZENBERG [26]	13	13	1.03 (0.37–2.93)
ROTH [27]	28	32	0.89 (0.42–1.88)
ROSELL [28]	30	30	0.63 (0.32–1.24)
DEPIERRE [12]	179	176	0.83 (0.64–1.07)
JCOG 9209 [29]	31	31	0.75 (0.43–1.30)
SORENSEN [30]	44	46	0.89 (0.49–1.63)
SWOG 9900 [22]	168	167	0.84 (0.60–1.18)
MRC LU22 [23]	258	261	1.02 (0.80–1.31)
Total	751	756	0.88 (0.76–1.01)

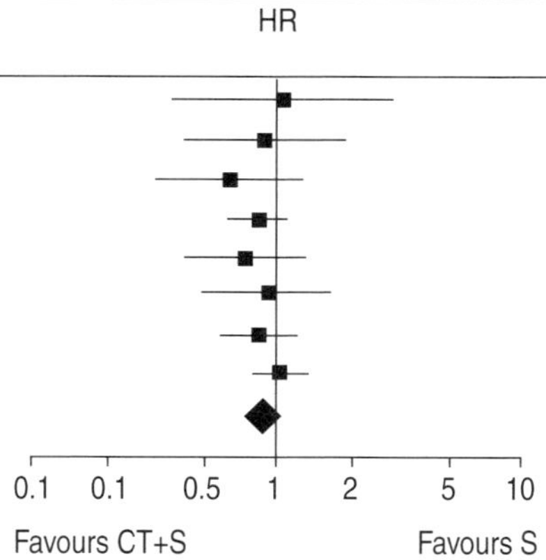

Fig. 3. – Updated meta-analysis of neoadjuvant chemotherapy. Reproduced from [23] with permission from the publisher. CT: chemotherapy; S: surgery; HR: hazard ratio; CI: confidence interval. Test for heterogeneity: Chi-squared 3.04, 7 degrees of freedom, p=0.88, I^2=0%. Test for overall effect: Z=1.78, p=0.07.

if it is felt that there may be a prolonged or difficult recovery from major surgery, then pre-operative treatment is feasible and may be useful in specific cases.

A recent audit in our department demonstrated that adjuvant chemotherapy is feasible in nontrial populations [32]. In a small audit of 50 cases with pathological stages eligible for adjuvant treatment, 12 were not offered treatment due to comorbidity or age >80 yrs, 22 (56%) out of those remaining accepted and of those most (82%) completed at least three cycles of cisplatin-based chemotherapy. Of those that declined, the majority had a prolonged post-operative recovery period or had concerns that pre-dated their surgery.

The neoadjuvant taxol/carboplatin (NATCH) trial is trying to answer this question prospectively. It has completed accrual of 616 patients with resectable stage IA (>2 cm), IB, II and IIIA NSCLC and randomised them between three cycles of neoadjuvant paclitaxel (taxol) plus carboplatin, or surgery alone, or post-operative chemotherapy with the same regimen [33]. The primary end-point is overall survival and the results are awaited. With around 200 patients in each arm, it is unlikely to have sufficient statistical power to enable a direct comparison between adjuvant and neoadjuvant chemotherapy.

Cisplatin versus *carboplatin*

Most of the trials reported have used cisplatin-based regimes and there is no direct comparison between cisplatin and carboplatin in the adjuvant or neoadjuvant setting. Carboplatin-based regimes are easy to administer in the outpatient setting and have a favourable nonhaematological toxicity profile compared with cisplatin-based regimes. If we extrapolate the data from advanced NSCLC, the meta-analysis is suggestive of a slight benefit of cisplatin over carboplatin, especially in combination with new agents [34]. In the adjuvant setting, where the aim is cure, cisplatin-based regimes may be preferred over carboplatin-based regimes. Acute nausea and vomiting are very common after cisplatin. The data from individual trials with cisplatin suggest National Cancer Institute Common Toxicity Criteria grade 3–4 toxicities of up to 17–27% with respect to nausea and vomiting. This can be a major impediment in the administration of subsequent cycles of the regimen, particularly in patients with tender thoracotomy scars. In most studies the administration of 5-hydroxytryptamine 3 antagonist anti-emetics was standard. There are now newer second generation, longer-acting, 5-hydroxytryptamine 3 antagonists and newer anti-emetics such as aprepitant (a selective neurokinin receptor antagonist); therefore, the major toxicity of nausea and vomiting may become less of an issue [35].

Adjuvant chemotherapy in the elderly

There has always been scepticism for use of chemotherapy in the elderly population. This is well reflected in the low number of patients aged over 70 yrs enrolled in clinical trials. This may be due to concerns about efficacy and toxicity of chemotherapy in the elderly patient group. The median age at diagnosis of lung cancer is over 70 yrs; hence, the question of treating the elderly population with adjuvant chemotherapy is important. A retrospective analysis of the NCIC JBR.10 trial was performed in order to evaluate whether elderly patients were able to tolerate platinum-based adjuvant chemotherapy and derive the same survival advantage [36]. There were 327 younger patients and 155 elderly patients. Patients aged >75 yrs had significantly shorter survival than those aged 66–74 yrs (HR 1.95; p=0.02), and patients aged >65 yrs had significantly better survival with chemotherapy *versus* observation (HR 0.61; p=0.04).

The elderly patients received fewer doses of cisplatin and vinorelbine and fewer completed their treatment compared with younger patients. 4.8% of younger and 16.9% of elderly patients died from nonmalignant causes. On the whole, despite receiving less chemotherapy than younger patients, adjuvant chemotherapy improved overall survival in patients aged >65 yrs with acceptable toxicity.

A pooled analysis was performed from the LACE database with survival and toxicities compared between three groups: young (<65 yrs), mid-category (65–69 yrs) and elderly (>70 yrs) [37]. No difference in severe toxicities was observed among the age groups. Elderly patients received smaller total doses of cisplatin. The HR of death for the young patients was 0.82 (95% confidence interval (CI): 0.73–0.92); it was 0.86 (95% CI: 0.70–1.07) for the mid-category and 1.01 (95% CI: 0.78–1.32) for elderly patients (test for trend: p=0.17). More elderly patients died from non-lung cancer-related causes (10% young, 16% mid-category and 20% elderly; p<0.0001). It can be concluded that patients under the age of 70 yrs with a good performance status benefit from adjuvant chemotherapy, but there is little evidence for those aged over 70 yrs, as these patients are underrepresented in clinical trials.

Targeted therapies

Adjuvant cytotoxic chemotherapy has improved survival but 5-yr overall survival is still disappointing. Advances in the knowledge of tumour biology and mechanisms of oncogenesis have allowed us to identify new molecular targets for NSCLC treatment. Targeted therapies are designed to interfere with specific aberrant biological pathways involved in tumourigenesis. This approach has been very successful in other tumour sites: adjuvant herceptin improved the overall survival in breast cancer (HR 0.66; p=0.0115) [38].

The epidermal growth factor receptor (EGFR) is commonly overexpressed in NSCLC and contributes to a number of processes that are important to cancer development and progression, including cell proliferation, apoptosis, angiogenesis and metastatic spread [39]. Gefitinib is an EGFR tyrosine kinase inhibitor that blocks the tumour growth *in vitro*. The NCIC JBR.19 trial randomised 500 patients with resected stage IB–IIIA NSCLC between gefitinib and placebo. Adjuvant chemotherapy was given at the discretion of the treating physician. The trial was closed early after the interim results of the SWOG 0023 trial were reported. The SWOG 0023 trial looked at maintenance gefitinib after completion of concurrent chemoradiotherapy and consolidation chemotherapy for stage IIIB NSCLC. At interim analysis, it was clear that gefitinib therapy did not improve survival and, even more discouraging, the recent update has shown a trend toward a survival disadvantage from the maintenance drug [40]. The results for NCIC JBR.19 are awaited.

Erlotinib is an oral EGFR inhibitor similar to gefitinib. It has shown a good response rate and symptoms relief in advanced stage NSCLC in the NCIC JBR.21 trial [41]. The Randomized Double-blind Trial in Adjuvant NSCLC with Tarceva (RADIANT) trial is a large phase III study to evaluate the role of erlotinib in the adjuvant treatment of patients with resected stage IB–IIIA NSCLC. 975 patients with EGFR-positive tumour tissue tested by either fluorescence in situ hybridisation or immunohistochemistry will be randomised between 2 yrs of daily oral erlotinib (150 $mg \cdot day^{-1}$) and placebo. Patients will be allowed to receive up to four cycles of platinum-based adjuvant chemotherapy prior to randomisation.

Angiogenesis (new vessel formation) stimulates tumour growth, invasion and metastasis, and this process is regulated by vascular endothelial growth factor

(VEGF). Bevacizumab is an anti-VEGF recombinant humanised monoclonal antibody that blocks the binding of all VEGF to the receptors, hence inhibiting all the biological activities of VEGF. The Eastern Cooperative Oncology Group (ECOG) 4599 trial evaluated carboplatin plus paclitaxel with or without bevacizumab in advanced stage NSCLC [42]. The median survival was 10.3 months *versus* 12.3 months (p=0.003), favouring the Bevacizumab-containing arm. As angiogenesis is a key process in tumour growth and progression of microscopic disease, bevacizumab may have a role in the adjuvant setting. The E1505 trial will randomise 1,500 patients with stage IB–IIIA resected NSCLC, stratified by stage, histology, sex and chemotherapy regimen, between bevacizumab and no bevacizumab with cisplatin-based chemotherapy.

The role of targeted therapies in the adjuvant setting is still being evaluated and the results of phase III randomised controlled trials are awaited.

Molecular markers and adjuvant chemotherapy

Better understanding of cancer biology and molecular markers for cancer growth has given hope that it may be possible to identify patients at high risk of systemic relapse and hence most likely to benefit from adjuvant and neoadjuvant chemotherapy. With the overall survival benefit from adjuvant therapy in the order of 5–10%, and the treatment including 3 months of relatively toxic chemotherapy, the ability to identify those most likely to benefit is crucial. The K-RAS protein is a proto-oncogene that regulates other proteins, downstream in the EGFR signalling pathway, that are associated with tumour survival, angiogenesis, proliferation and metastasis. Mutations in K-RAS are found in ~20–30% of NSCLC cases. The NCIC JBR.10 trial prospectively assessed K-RAS status in 450 participants as a predictor of survival, and did not observe a benefit of adjuvant chemotherapy in the subgroup with K-RAS mutations [43].

Increased expression of the excision repair cross complementing (ERCC)1 gene, which is crucial for the repair of the cisplatin DNA adducts, is associated with cisplatin resistance. Increased expression of the ERCC1 gene has been reported to have a negative impact on response and survival in gastric cancer treated with cisplatin and fluorouracil [44]. 761 patients from the IALT study were analysed in order to identify whether ERCC1 expression affects survival in NSCLC. The study found that patients with ERCC1-negative tumours appeared to benefit from adjuvant chemotherapy, whereas patients with ERCC1-positive tumours did not [45]. P27 (KIP-1) protein is a tumour suppressor protein that inhibits cell transition from G1 to S phase of the cell cycle by inhibiting cyclin D and cyclin E. Filipits *et al.* [46] analysed 778 tumour specimens from the IALT trial to determine whether cell cycle regulators are of prognostic and predictive value in patients receiving adjuvant chemotherapy. They reported that patients with P27 (KIP-1)-negative tumours benefited from adjuvant chemotherapy, whereas patients with P27 (KIP-1)-positive tumours did not. This is conceivable, as we know from cellular biology that tumour cells are most sensitive to chemotherapy drugs during G1 and G2 transit phase.

Tsao *et al.* [47] have recently reported identifying a 15-gene signature that is an independent prognostic marker in early stage NSCLC, based on retrospective analysis of RNA isolated from frozen banked tumour tissues of JBR.10 patients. This may help in identifying patients who may benefit from adjuvant chemotherapy. These markers need to be validated in large prospective randomised trials to influence changes in practice. In conclusion, so far no molecular markers have shown a significant relationship with survival, and future studies will be needed to determine whether molecular profiling can identify the patient subgroups most suitable for adjuvant therapy.

Conclusion

Platinum-based adjuvant chemotherapy for resected tumours has become an established part of the management of NSCLC. This development is in line with other major tumour types. The magnitude of the benefit is in keeping with adjuvant treatments for other cancers, such as breast and colorectal, but the evidence to support it has taken longer to emerge. This is due to a number of factors, including the toxicity of the agents used. The administration of cisplatin requires considerable clinical expertise, especially with regard to patient selection. In addition, NSCLC patients tend to be older, may have significant comorbidity and will have recently completed major surgery. Although neoadjuvant chemotherapy is feasible, the pragmatic approach will tend to favour adjuvant, post-operative chemotherapy. Studies show that the benefits are greatest for the more advanced stages (stages II and IIIA) of resectable NSCLC. Adjuvant chemotherapy cannot be routinely recommended for resected stage I tumours.

The interpretation of individual studies can be very misleading. Problems include updated analyses, which may alter the magnitude of treatment effect, and individual trials have suffered from lower than expected recruitment rates and early closure. The use of meta-analysis to determine the overall effect of adjuvant chemotherapy is essential.

Future developments are likely to be based around patient and tumour selection. Although no clear recommendations can be made, molecular profiling of tumours for ERCC1, K-RAS mutations and other changes may avoid unnecessary administration of chemotherapy for those less likely to benefit. Newer targeted agents are still under evaluation but may provide additional therapies that are easier to tolerate in patients who are still recovering from major surgery.

Summary

Lung cancer is the leading cause of cancer death in the western world. Surgical resection remains the treatment of choice for operable nonsmall cell lung cancer (NSCLC). Even after complete resection, systemic relapse is common and hence there is a role for adjuvant and neoadjuvant treatment.

Adjuvant chemotherapy is feasible and improves overall survival in completely resected NSCLC, with cisplatin chemotherapy offering survival advantage of 5% at 5 yrs. Use of alkylating agents is not recommended as they are detrimental to survival. There is a small increase in noncancer-related death with cisplatin chemotherapy; hence, only patients at high risk of systemic relapse should be offered adjuvant treatment. At present, adjuvant chemotherapy is not recommended for stage IA patients and its benefits in stage IB patients are debatable. Adjuvant uracil-tegafur has no confirmatory trials in the western population and, thus, it is not recommended outside the context of a clinical trial. There has been an ongoing debate about neoadjuvant *versus* adjuvant chemotherapy. Neoadjuvant chemotherapy is feasible, with no increase in post-operative complications. It has so far failed to show improvement in overall survival and it is likely that the standard of care is towards adjuvant chemotherapy.

In the adjuvant setting, where the aim is cure, cisplatin-based regimes are preferred over carboplatin-based regimes. One of the main toxicities of cisplatin is nausea and vomiting but, with the use of new anti-emetics, this may be less of an issue. There should be no scepticism about chemotherapy in elderly patients. Patients under the age of 70 yrs with a good performance status benefit from adjuvant chemotherapy,

but there is paucity of data for those over 70.
New knowledge of mechanisms of oncogenesis has allowed us to identify new molecular targets for cancer treatment. So far, no molecular targets have been shown conclusively to have a significant relationship with clinical outcome, particularly survival in NSCLC. Newer targeted agents, including including epidermal growth factor receptor and vascular endothelial growth factor inhibitors, are still under evaluation in phase III clinical trials.

Keywords: Adjuvant, chemotherapy, induction, neoadjuvant, nonsmall cell lung cancer, targeted therapy.

Statement of interest
D. Gilligan has received lecture fees, funding to attend international meetings and consultancy fees from Pierre-Fabre, Eli Lilly, AstraZeneca and Roche Pharmaceuticals.

References

1. Mountain CF. Revisions in the International System for Staging Lung Cancer. *Chest* 1997; 111: 1710–1717.
2. Pisters KMW, Le Chevalier T. Adjuvant chemotherapy in completely resected non-small-cell lung cancer. *J Clin Oncol* 2005; 23: 3270–3278.
3. Eifel P, Axelson JA, Costa J, *et al.* National Institutes of Health Consensus Development Conference Statement: adjuvant therapy for breast cancer, November 1–3, 2000. *J Natl Cancer Inst* 2001; 93: 979–989.
4. NIH consensus conference. Adjuvant therapy for patients with colon and rectal cancer. *JAMA* 1990; 264: 1444–1450.
5. Chemotherapy in non-small cell lung cancer: a meta-analysis using updated data on individual patients from 52 randomised clinical trials. Non-Small Cell Lung Cancer Collaborative Group. *BMJ* 1995; 311: 899–909.
6. Arriagada R, Bergman B, Dunant A, *et al.* Cisplatin-based adjuvant chemotherapy in patients with completely resected non-small-cell lung cancer. *N Engl J Med* 2004; 350: 351–360.
7. Le Chevalier T, Dunant A, Arriagada R, *et al.* Long-term results of the International Adjuvant Lung Cancer Trial (IALT) evaluating adjuvant cisplatin-based chemotherapy in resected non-small cell lung cancer (NSCLC). *J Clin Oncol* 2008; 26: Suppl. 15, 7507.
8. Winton T, Livingston R, Johnson D, *et al.* Vinorelbine plus cisplatin *vs.* observation in resected non-small-cell lung cancer. *N Engl J Med* 2005; 352: 2589–2597.
9. Strauss GM, Herndon JE, Maddaus MA, *et al.* Adjuvant chemotherapy in stage IB non-small cell lung cancer (NSCLC): Update of Cancer and Leukemia Group B (CALGB) protocol 9633. *J Clin Oncol* 2006; 24: Suppl. 18, 7007.
10. Douillard JY, Rosell R, De Lena M, *et al.* Adjuvant vinorelbine plus cisplatin *versus* observation in patients with completely resected stage IB–IIIA non-small-cell lung cancer (Adjuvant Navelbine International Trialist Association (ANITA)): a randomised controlled trial. *Lancet Oncol* 2006; 7: 719–727.
11. Scagliotti GV, Fossati R, Torri V, *et al.* Randomized study of adjuvant chemotherapy for completely resected stage I, II, or IIIA non-small-cell lung cancer. *J Natl Cancer Inst* 2003; 95: 1453–1461.
12. Depierre A, Milleron B, Moro-Sibilot D, *et al.* Preoperative chemotherapy followed by surgery compared with primary surgery in resectable stage I (except T1N0), II, and IIIa non-small-cell lung cancer. *J Clin Oncol* 2002; 20: 247–253.

13. Waller D, Peake MD, Stephens RJ, *et al.* Chemotherapy for patients with non-small cell lung cancer: the surgical setting of the Big Lung Trial. *Eur J Cardiothorac Surg* 2004; 26: 173–182.
14. Pignon JP, Tribodet H, Scagliotti GV, *et al.* Lung adjuvant cisplatin evaluation: a pooled analysis by the LACE Collaborative Group. *J Clin Oncol* 2008; 26: 3552–3559.
15. Wada H, Hitomi S, Teramatsu T. Adjuvant chemotherapy after complete resection in non-small-cell lung cancer. West Japan Study Group for Lung Cancer Surgery. *J Clin Oncol* 1996; 14: 1048–1054.
16. Hamada C, Tanaka F, Ohta M, *et al.* Meta-analysis of postoperative adjuvant chemotherapy with tegafur-uracil in non-small-cell lung cancer. *J Clin Oncol* 2005; 23: 4999–5006.
17. Kato H, Ichinose Y, Ohta M, *et al.* A randomized trial of adjuvant chemotherapy with uracil-tegafur for adenocarcinoma of the lung. *N Engl J Med* 2004; 350: 1713–1721.
18. Stewart LA, Burdett S, Tierney JF, *et al.* Surgery and adjuvant chemotherapy (CT) compared to surgery alone in non-small cell lung cancer (NSCLC): a meta-analysis using individual patient data (IPD) from randomized clinical trials (RCT). *J Clin Oncol* 2007; 25: Suppl. 18, 7552.
19. Allum WH, Fogarty PJ, Stenning SP, *et al.*, Long term results of the MRC OEO2 randomized trial of surgery with or without preoperative chemotherapy in resectable esophageal cancer. American Society of Clinical Oncology Gastrointestinal Cancers Symposium 2008. Abstract 9.
20. Rosell R, Gómez-Codina J, Camps C, *et al.* A randomized trial comparing preoperative chemotherapy plus surgery with surgery alone in patients with non-small-cell lung cancer. *N Engl J Med* 1994; 330: 153–158.
21. Roth JA, Fossella F, Komaki R, *et al.* A randomized trial comparing perioperative chemotherapy and surgery with surgery alone in resectable stage IIIA non-small-cell lung cancer. *J Natl Cancer Inst* 1994; 86: 673–680.
22. Pisters K, Vallieres E, Bunn P, *et al.* S9900: a phase III trial of surgery alone or surgery plus preoperative (preop) paclitaxel/carboplatin (PC) chemotherapy in early stage non-small cell lung cancer (NSCLC): preliminary results. *J Clin Oncol* 2005; 23: Suppl. 16, 7012.
23. Gilligan D, Nicolson M, Smith I, *et al.* Preoperative chemotherapy in patients with resectable non-small cell lung cancer: results of the MRC LU22/NVALT 2/EORTC 08012 multicentre randomised trial and update of systematic review. *Lancet* 2007; 369: 1929–1937.
24. Scagliotti GV, Pastorino U, Vansteenkiste JF, *et al.* A phase III randomized study of surgery alone or surgery plus preoperative gemcitabine-cisplatin in early-stage non-small cell lung cancer (NSCLC): Follow-up data of ChEST. *J Clin Oncol* 2008; 26: Suppl. 15, 7508.
25. Burdett S, Stewart LA, Rydzewska L. A systematic review and meta-analysis of the literature: chemotherapy and surgery *versus* surgery alone in non-small cell lung cancer. *J Thorac Oncol* 2006; 1: 611–621.
26. Dautzenberg B, Benichou J, Allard P, *et al.* Failure of the perioperative PCV neoadjuvant polychemotherapy in resectable bronchogenic non-small cell carcinoma. Results from a randomized phase II trial. *Cancer* 1990; 65: 2435–2441.
27. Roth JA, Atkinson EN, Fossella F, *et al.* Long-term follow-up of patients enrolled in a randomized trial comparing perioperative chemotherapy and surgery with surgery alone in resectable stage IIIA non-small-cell lung cancer. *Lung Cancer* 1998; 21: 1–6.
28. Rosell R, Gómez-Codina J, Camps C, *et al.* Preresectional chemotherapy in stage IIIA non-small-cell lung cancer: a 7-year assessment of a randomized controlled trial. *Lung Cancer* 1999; 26: 7–14.
29. Nagai K, Tsuchiya R, Mori T, *et al.* A randomized trial comparing induction chemotherapy followed by surgery with surgery alone for patients with stage IIIA N2 non-small cell lung cancer (JCOG 9209). *J Thorac Cardiovasc Surg* 2003; 125: 254–260.
30. Sorensen JB, Riska H, Ravn J, *et al.* Scandinavian phase III trial of neoadjuvant chemotherapy in NSCLC stages IB-IIIA/T3. *J Clin Oncol* 2005; 23: Suppl. 16, 7146.
31. Lim E, Harris G, Patel A, *et al.* Preoperative *versus* postoperative chemotherapy in patients with resectable non-small cell lung cancer: systematic review and indirect comparison meta-analysis of randomized trials. *J Clin Oncol* 2008; 26: Suppl. 15, 7546.

32. Treece SJ, Magee L, Gilligan D, *et al.* Adjuvant chemotherapy in non-small cell lung cancer – how feasible is it in a non-trial population? *Clin Oncol (R Coll Radiol)* 2007; 19: 629–630.
33. Felip E, Rosell R, Massuti B, *et al.* The NATCH trial: observations on the neoadjuvant arm. *J Clin Oncol* 2007; 25: Suppl. 18, 7578.
34. Ardizzoni A, Boni L, Tiseo M, *et al.* Cisplatin- *versus* carboplatin-based chemotherapy in first-line treatment of advanced non-small-cell lung cancer: an individual patient data meta-analysis. *J Natl Cancer Inst* 2007; 99: 847–857.
35. de Wit R, Herrstedt J, Rapoport B, *et al.* Addition of the oral NK1 antagonist aprepitant to standard antiemetics provides protection against nausea and vomiting during multiple cycles of cisplatin-based chemotherapy. *J Clin Oncol* 2003; 21: 4105–4111.
36. Pepe C, Hasan B, Winton T, *et al.* Adjuvant chemotherapy in elderly patients: an analysis of National Cancer Institute of Canada Clinical Trials Group and Intergroup BR.10. *J Clin Oncol* 2006; 24: Suppl. 18, 7009.
37. Fruh M, Tribodet H, Pignon J, *et al.* A pooled analysis of the effect of age on adjuvant cisplatin-based chemotherapy for completely resected non-small cell lung cancer (NSCLC). *J Clin Oncol* 2007; 25: Suppl. 18, 7553.
38. Smith I, Procter M, Gelber RD, *et al.* 2-year follow-up of trastuzumab after adjuvant chemotherapy in HER2-positive breast cancer: a randomised controlled trial. *Lancet* 2007; 369: 29–36.
39. Ciardiello F, Tortora G. A novel approach in the treatment of cancer: targeting the epidermal growth factor receptor. *Clin Cancer Res* 2001; 7: 2958–2970.
40. Kelly K, Chansky K, Gaspar LE, *et al.* Phase III trial of maintenance gefitinib or placebo after concurrent chemoradiotherapy and docetaxel consolidation in inoperable stage III non-small-cell lung cancer: SWOG S0023. *J Clin Oncol* 2008; 26: 2450–2456.
41. Bezjak A, Tu D, Seymour L, *et al.* Symptom improvement in lung cancer patients treated with erlotinib: quality of life analysis of the National Cancer Institute of Canada Clinical Trials Group Study BR.21. *J Clin Oncol* 2006; 24: 3831–3837.
42. Sandler A, Gray R, Perry MC, *et al.* Paclitaxel-carboplatin alone or with bevacizumab for non-small-cell lung cancer. *N Engl J Med* 2006; 355: 2542–2550.
43. Tsao M, Zhu C, Livingston R, *et al.* The significance of K-ras mutations in the Intergroup JBR.10 Trial on adjuvant chemotherapy in completely resected early stage non-small cell lung cancer (NSCLC) patients. *Lung Cancer* 2005; 49: Suppl. 2, S41.
44. Metzger R, Leichman CG, Danenberg KD, *et al.* ERCC1 mRNA levels complement thymidylate synthase mRNA levels in predicting response and survival for gastric cancer patients receiving combination cisplatin and fluorouracil chemotherapy. *J Clin Oncol* 1998; 16: 309–316.
45. Olaussen KA, Dunant A, Fouret P, *et al.* DNA repair by ERCC1 in non-small-cell lung cancer and cisplatin-based adjuvant chemotherapy. *N Engl J Med* 2006; 355: 983–991.
46. Filipits M, Pirker R, Dunant A, *et al.* Cell cycle regulators and outcome of adjuvant cisplatin-based chemotherapy in completely resected non-small-cell lung cancer: the International Adjuvant Lung Cancer Trial Biologic Program. *J Clin Oncol* 2007; 25: 2735–2740.
47. Tsao MS, Zhu C, Ding K, *et al.* A 15-gene expression signature prognostic for survival and predictive for adjuvant chemotherapy benefit in JBR.10 patients. *J Clin Oncol* 2008; 26: Suppl. 15, 7510.

CHAPTER 14

Management of locally advanced nonsmall cell lung cancer

M. Edelmann, R.M. Huber

Pneumologie, Dept of Medicine, University of Munich – Campus Innenstadt, Munich, Germany.

Correspondence: R.M. Huber, Division of Respiratory Medicine, Medizinische Klinik Innenstadt, University of Munich, Ziemssenstraße 1, D-80336 Munich, Germany. Fax: 49 8951604905; E-mail: Huber@med.uni-muenchen.de

Lung cancer is still an aggressive tumour entity that is diagnosed late in the natural course of the disease. Therefore, in the largest subgroup of lung cancer, the nonsmall cell lung cancers (NSCLC), up to 40% are in a locally advanced stage at the time of diagnosis. This group includes tumours that are technically difficult to resect either due to their location or local invasion, and tumours that have a poor prognosis due to contralateral mediastinal lymph node metastases (N3 disease) or clinically detectable multilevel mediastinal ipsilateral lymph node involvement (multilevel N2 disease; "bulky" disease; stages IIIA(3) and IIIA(4) according to the American College of Chest Physicians staging system (table 1)). In the "tumour, node, metastasis" (TNM)-staging system they are at least in stage III, ranging from T3 N1 to T4 N3 [1]. Whereas in stage IIIA there is still some discussion regarding radical surgery, stage IIIB disease has until recently usually been accepted as inoperable.

Until recently, radiotherapy alone was the standard therapy, but long-term survival was poor, [2, 3]. With the 5-yr survival in stage IIIB with contralateral lymph node metastases below 10%, this is hardly different from advanced stage disease (table 2). With good performance status and no limiting comorbidities, therapy with curative intent is increasingly possible. The multimodality concept consists of chemotherapy combined with radiotherapy. The benefit of radiochemotherapy must be weighed against the potential for increased toxicity. Several studies were carried out to determine the role of chemotherapy, radiotherapy and the optimal way to apply them. It should be emphasised that choosing the right therapy regimen remains complex. One reason is the heterogeneity of the locally advanced NSCLC group, regarding histology, size and location of the primary tumour, and grade and type of lymph node involvement. Another reason is patient-related factors, such as performance status and the number and severity of comorbidities. Another pitfall lies in the interpretation and comparison of newer studies in NSCLC with older studies, which clearly used different radiotherapy techniques and, at least in part, different chemotherapy regimens. Also, most studies included patients not only recruited from genuinely inoperable stage III NSCLC but also from other nonresectable NSCLC in a variety of other stages, where resection could not be performed for other reasons or the centre decided not to operate due, for example, to functional reasons. The advance in imaging technologies and hence more accurate staging is another problem when it comes to the comparison of older and newer studies. This is particularly true for identifying metastases with positron emission tomography (PET) scans, which can be found in substantial numbers in the more up-to-date reports, and trying to compare with patients that were defined as localised disease

Eur Respir Mon, 2009, 44, 260–270. Printed in UK - all rights reserved. Copyright ERS Journals Ltd 2009; European Respiratory Monograph; ISSN 1025-448x.

Table 1. – American College of Chest Physicians subsets of stage IIIA (N2)

Subset	Features
1	Incidental nodal metastases found on final surgical pathology
2	Single-station nodal metastasis recognised intra-operatively
3	Mediastinal node metastases (single- or multistation) documented pre-operatively (mediastinoscopy or positron emission tomography)
4	Bulky multistation, unresectable N2 disease

in earlier reports when PET was not routinely available. Additionally, metastatic lymph node involvement is detected more frequently nowadays, rendering more "resectable" patients inoperable due to locally advanced disease pre-operatively. Further difficulties can arise from including patients with tumours in different locations and with differing spread within the same TNM classification stage. This may be improved somewhat with the new International Association for the Study of Lung Cancer classification (see chapter 9 of this *European Respiratory Monograph* (*ERM*)). Recent data have also shown the importance of the histology and cell differentiation as a prognostic factor [5] and as an additional descriptor for therapy, at least for advanced disease.

General considerations for the combination of chemotherapy and thoracic radiotherapy

As aforementioned, in locally advanced NSCLC, radiotherapy alone does not confer much of an impact on survival. The median survival in trials of radiotherapy alone was between 9.6 months and 14.5 months [6]. In surgically treated completely resected tumours, local recurrence rates did not increase with increase in stage, but there was a clear rise in systemic recurrences [7]. This is the rationale for combining systemic treatment (chemotherapy) with local treatment (surgery). The same seems to be true for locally advanced tumours treated with radiotherapy alone *versus* combined treatment regimens. Using radical radiotherapy alone, there have been local recurrence rates of only ~27%; however, unfortunately, the extrathoracic relapse was 67 and 77.5% in two studies with radiotherapy alone [8, 9]. Accordingly, in two meta-analyses published in 1995, a significant survival advantage could be demonstrated with combined radio-chemotherapy [10, 11].

Chemotherapy has become potentially important in NSCLC in both resectable and nonresectable presentations [12, 13]. The first trial combined thoracic irradiation with

Table 2. – 5-yr survival rate correlated with stage at time of diagnosis

Stage	TNM	5-yr survival rate %
IA	T1 N0 M0	60
IB	T2 N0 M0	38
IIA	T1 N1 M0	34
IIB	T2 N1 M0	24
	T3 N0 M0	22
IIIA	T3 N1 M0	9
	T1–3 N2 M0	13
IIIB	T4 N0–2 M0	7
	T1–4 N3 M0	3
IV	M1	1

Data taken from [4]. TNM: tumour, node, metastasis.

cisplatin and vinblastine. There was substantial haematological toxicity, but median survival was prolonged by 4 months (13.8 *versus* 9.7 months), and the 3-yr survival rate was nearly doubled with combined treatments (23 *versus* 11%). A further approach combining radiotherapy and chemotherapy evaluated the effects of giving the chemotherapy concomitantly with radiotherapy. This showed the superiority of daily administration of cisplatin on median survival (26 *versus* 13%) [14]. New cytotoxic substances have since become available, so now the regimens can be separated into older combinations that are platinum based, with the addition of older substances like etoposide, and newer combinations that are also platinum based, but include taxanes or vinorelbine as a doublet. The newer substances have equal efficiency with less toxicity and are preferred partners in combination chemotherapy. The combinations of two newer agents without platinum have been shown to be equally potent and have less risk for toxicity than the platinum-based regimens. Non-platinum-based combinations are not adequately tested in chemoradiotherapy trials in locally advanced disease. Another possible choice is cisplatin or carboplatin. Both, when used as doublets in advanced stage disease, have similar 1-yr survival rates. Cisplatin seems to be more active, which can be shown by better overall response. However, cisplatin produces greater grade 3–4 toxicity rates for neutropenia, nausea, vomiting and renal toxicity. Recent data suggest that, in responding patients, cisplatin results in a better outcome with a similar toxicity profile than carboplatin [15]. For radiochemotherapy, cisplatin is the platin of choice and seems well tolerated, although in locally advanced disease the optimal number of courses of chemotherapy remains to be determined.

Due to the diversity in presentation of locally advanced NSCLC in terms of histology or response to therapy, the choice of the right regimen is still a challenge. With respect to these factors and depending on patient status and therapy plan, different options have to be considered. The principal strategies for combining radiotherapy and chemotherapy are outlined in figure 1.

Efficacy of radiochemotherapy and the various approaches

Induction chemotherapy plus radiotherapy versus *radiotherapy alone*

The classic trial of sequential radiochemotherapy, a course of chemotherapy preceding radiation, aimed at enhancing the efficacy of the radiation, was performed by the Cancer and Leukemia Group B (CALGB). Between 1984 and 1987, they

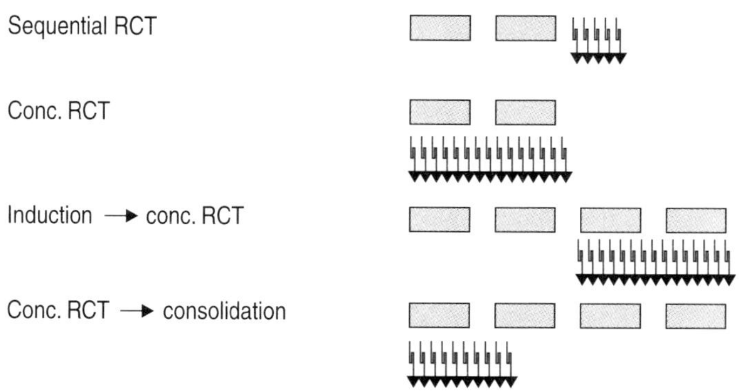

Fig. 1. – Various approaches for combining thoracic radiotherapy (jagged arrows) with chemotherapy ( ). All radiotherapy could possibly be hyperfractionated. RCT: radiochemotherapy; conc.: concomitant.

conducted a study to evaluate a treatment schedule combining chemotherapy and radiation therapy in stage III NSCLC [16]. Patients were randomised to receive either standard radiation therapy alone (6,000 cGy in 30 fractions) or chemotherapy with cisplatin (100 mg·m^{-2}) and vinblastine (5 mg·m^{-2}) followed by radiation. The patients treated with combined radiochemotherapy showed a significant survival benefit over those treated with radiation therapy alone. The benefit of radiochemotherapy in this setting was confirmed with a long-term follow-up study [17]. 7 yrs after completion of the initial CALGB study, 90% of the randomised patients had died, but those who had received combined radiochemotherapy had lived longer (on average 13.7 months) compared with those who had received radiation therapy alone (9.6 months). From the radiochemotherapy arm, 13% of patients were alive at 7-yr follow-up, compared with only 6% from the radiation therapy arm.

SAUSE *et al.* [18], in a confirmatory trial, compared sequential radiochemotherapy (two cycles of cisplatin and vinblastine before radiation therapy) with both standard radiation therapy (2 Gy per daily fraction, total 60 Gy) and hyperfractionated radiation therapy (1.2 Gy per fraction, twice daily, total 69.6 Gy) in the treatment of high performance status NSCLC patients. They found, again, a significant benefit in overall survival in the sequential radiochemotherapy arm compared with both forms of radiation therapy. The survival advantage for hyperfractionated radiotherapy was no better than standard daily radiotherapy following chemotherapy.

A meta-analysis of individual patient data, comparing sequential radiochemotherapy *versus* radiotherapy alone, confirmed the benefit of sequential chemotherapy added to radiotherapy in locally advanced NSCLC *versus* radiotherapy alone. There was a small but significant survival advantage with the sequential strategy (2.7% difference at 3 yrs) [19].

It should be mentioned that radiotherapy is combined in trials of neoadjvant or adjuvant chemotherapy for locally advanced NSCLC tumours, in an effort to render them resectable. Mainly platinum-based regimens have been used in these studies and, in nonrandomised trials, showed improved survival but with increased toxicity, mainly neutropenia. These data are limited due to the heterogeneity of the patients, and so the concept of rendering locally advanced metastatic NSCLC operable is still controversial. More data are available for adjuvant therapy or post-operative radiotherapy in resectable NSCLC, and, for adjuvant therapy after resection of advanced stages (IIIA/B), patient-related factors have to be considered before irradiation is initiated after chemotherapy. Further details can be found in the corresponding chapters of this *ERM*.

Simultaneous radiochemotherapy versus *radiotherapy alone*

Studies have assessed the potential of chemotherapy agents to act as sensitisers when given concurrently with radical radiotherapy. For example, one approach was to investigate weekly or daily doses of cisplatin. One such study compared thoracic radiotherapy alone with radiotherapy and additional weekly doses of 30 mg·m^{-2} cisplatin or with daily application of 6 mg·m^{-2} cisplatin [14]. The daily cisplatin group had a significantly increased overall survival of 54, 26 and 16% at 1, 2 and 3 yrs after diagnosis. Other studies addressed the use of cisplatin *versus* non-platin-containing therapies or full dose combination chemotherapy. Cisplatin seems to be the backbone; whether full dose combination chemotherapy is necessary is not yet decided. Definitive randomised trials are missing.

Many studies have found superiority for chemotherapy with two or more agents and concurrent thoracic radiotherapy [20, 21] compared with induction chemotherapy and sequential radiotherapy. In general, a platin-containing regimen of one or two cytotoxic or biological substances, augmented by radical irradiation up to doses of 74 Gy (at least 60 Gy, mostly 66 Gy) [12, 18], showed a significant increase in median survival times of ~4 months over single modality treatment, in these heterogeneous stage IIIA/B patients. The median survival with concurrent radiochemotherapy was ~13.9 months. The overall survival rates were increased by 15, 13 and 12% at 1, 2 and 3 yrs, suggesting that concurrent treatment should become the standard. Another decision to be made is choosing the best chemotherapy regimen. A meta-analysis of 1,500 patients showed a clear advantage for cisplatin over other partners of a two- or three-drug regimen in the first 2 yrs of treatment, by reducing the death rate by 24 and 30% *versus* 5 and 18% [22]. However, at 3 yrs, this advantage disappears. Patient-related factors have to be considered, as the platin-containing regimens have more severe, potentially life-threatening side-effects when compared with the non-platin regimens. Another point is quality of life, which can be affected more by the platinum-based therapies. To date, there is no regimen widely accepted by oncologists and radiotherapists, so the only recommendation is to treat patients in the context of randomised controlled trials examining chemotherapy regimens.

Another meta-analysis of 14 randomised studies comparing concurrent radiochemotherapy with radiotherapy alone showed significant benefit with concurrent radiochemotherapy. Patients treated with concurrent radiochemotherapy had a reduction in overall risk of death at 2 yrs (risk reduction (RR) 0.93, 95% confidence interval (CI) 0.88–0.98; p=0.01) and an increase in progression-free survival at 2 yrs (RR 0.84, 95% CI 0.72–0.98; p=0.03) compared with patients treated with radiation alone [23]. At the World Lung Cancer Conference 2007 a further meta-analysis was presented, using individual patient data comparing concomitant radiochemotherapy *versus* radiotherapy alone [19]. The benefit of concomitant radiochemotherapy in locally advanced NSCLC *versus* radiotherapy alone was confirmed. There were statistically significant effects on survival with the concomitant strategy (survival difference 3.2% at 3 yrs). A summary of these three meta-analyses regarding the efficacy of radiotherapy, induction chemotherapy and simultaneous chemotherapy are summarised in tables 3 and 4.

Induction chemotherapy versus *concomitant chemotherapy*

As there a several advantages and disadvantages with induction and concomitant radiochemotherapy, direct comparison of both approaches was needed. In 1999, FURUSE *et al.* [25] published data showing that concurrent radiochemotherapy (mitomycin, vindesine and cisplatin with concurrent radiation in 2-Gy daily fractions to total 56 Gy (split course)) was superior to sequential treatment with two cycles of chemotherapy followed by the same radiation dose. Median survival was 16.5 months, with 15.8% survival at 5 yrs with concomitant chemoradiotherapy, significantly longer than survival after sequential radiochemotherapy (13.3 months, 8.9% at 5 yrs). Several further randomised trials are being performed and full results are awaited.

Table 3. – Efficacy of sequential and concomitant radiochemotherapy in comparison with radiotherapy alone

	Sequential *versus* radiotherapy	Concomitant *versus* radiotherapy
Survival benefit[#]	0.88 (0.82–0.94) p<0.001	0.87 (0.81–0.95) p<0.001
Absolute survival benefit at 3 yrs	2.7%	3.2%

Data taken from [19]. #: hazard ratio (95% confidence interval).

Table 4. – Comparison of the efficacy of concomitant *versus* sequential radiochemotherapy

Parameter	Concomitant *versus* sequential			Notes
	HR	95% CI	p-value	
Overall survival	0.84	0.74–0.95	0.004	5.7% absolute benefit at 3 yrs
Progression-free survival	0.90	0.79–1.01	0.07	2.9% absolute benefit at 3 yrs
Loco-regional progression	0.77	0.62–0.95	0.01	6.0% absolute reduction at 3 yrs
Distant progression	1.04	0.86–1.25	0.69	

Data taken from [24]. HR: hazard ratio; CI: confidence interval.

A recent meta-analysis, only available as an abstract, comparing concomitant *versus* sequential radiochemotherapy, showed that concomitant radiochemotherapy improved survival in patients with locally advanced NSCLC, compared with sequential radiochemotherapy, by 5.7% at 3 yrs [24].

Induction chemotherapy plus concomitant chemoradiotherapy

Combining induction and simultaneous radiochemotherapy has theoretical advantages for local and systemic control and does not necessarily increase toxicity. Induction chemotherapy primarily controls systemic disease and concurrent chemotherapy sensitises the local tumour and increases the efficacy of radiotherapy. However, there have been several trials with different regimens, varying randomisation approaches and conflicting results. An upfront use of paclitaxel and carboplatin before multimodality standard platinum-based chemotherapy had no significant influence on overall survival, if the randomisation was done upfront without taking into account whether there was an effect on the tumour (*e.g.* complete or partial remission or stable disease) of induction chemotherapy [20]. However, in one randomised trial in patients with stable disease or better after induction chemotherapy, adding concurrent chemotherapy with weekly paclitaxel resulted in low toxicity and clearly superior progression-free survival [21].

Consolidation chemotherapy

In advanced NSCLC and in the adjuvant setting following curative resection, the overall survival can be increased by applying chemotherapy. There are data demonstrating that at least four cycles of chemotherapy are needed. In the classical radiochemotherapy trials, only two cycles of chemotherapy or its equivalent were used. Therefore, the question remains whether more chemotherapy would be beneficial. One approach is to apply consolidation chemotherapy with two to three cycles after concomitant radiochemotherapy. Recent data suggest that a consolidation regime of single agent docetaxel after multimodality therapy with cisplatin and etoposide and thoracic radiotherapy resulted in good local control and survival [26]. This study used concurrent cisplatin and etoposide with the radiotherapy, followed by docetaxel, whereas another used concurrent cisplatin and etoposide and radiotherapy followed by more cisplatin and etoposide. The resulting median survival was 27 months (95% CI 18–43) *versus* 15 months (95% CI 10–22). The survival rates at 3 yrs were 40% (95% CI 24–55) *versus* 17% (95% CI 7–27). Unfortunately, a randomised trial could not confirm the benefit of the consolidation chemotherapy with docetaxel [27] after concurrent radiochemotherapy with cisplatin and etoposide. It is not clear whether these results are due to the increased toxicity of docetaxel or consolidation *per se* does not work. A German randomised trial that is still recruiting, using vinorelbine and cisplatin for the concurrent radiochemotherapy part and for consolidation, may answer this question.

Toxicity of combining radiotherapy and chemotherapy

Effective treatment and tumour control comes with side-effects. In chemotherapy, all rapidly dividing cell systems are damaged, including the bone marrow and all epithelial cells, mostly in the gastrointestinal and urogenital tract, resulting in pancytopenia, febrile neutropenia, epithelial ulcers and loss of taste and defence functions. Oedema and alopecia are also common side-effects. The short-term effects, such as nausea and vomiting, can be controlled by proper use of modern anti-emetic medication. In the longer term, fatigue and neuropathies can be very important. Patients with poor performance status, older age and advanced disease are more prone to develop complications. The role of granulocyte-stimulating factors, commonly used in high-dose regimens in haemato-oncology, is controversial. In combination with radiotherapy the disadvantages prevail. The use of erythropoietin also has shown disadvantages, such as an increased rate of thromboembolic complications. Therefore, routine use to prevent haematological toxicity is not recommended.

Radiation therapy comes with its own side-effects but can also aggravate the side-effects of chemotherapy. The three-dimensional planning system and application of radiation by leaf-collimators can reduce the damage of surrounding normal tissues enormously, but collateral damage can still occur. There is discussion concerning the overall dose that can be tolerated by normal lung tissue, and it seems that more than 20 Gy to normal lung can lead to pneumonitis and lung fibrosis [13]. Therefore, most regimens try to restrict the overall dose, which should not be applied to more than 30–40% of the lungs, to 20 Gy (known as the V_{20} rule). The common treatment-related effects are oesophagitis and oesophageal ulcers, especially in patients with mediastinal disease and those who need extensive field size radiotherapy. Local supportive care, consisting of local anaesthetics, artificial saliva solution and antifungal drugs as needed, is used for thoracic radiotherapy. Concurrent chemotherapy increases the local toxicity, depending on the choice of regimen and the irradiation protocol. Gemcitabine increases pulmonary toxicity and can only be given at a markedly reduced dose with radiotherapy. There was one randomised phase II trial that compared three different cisplatin doublets, which were given for two cycles as induction chemotherapy and then concurrently with radiotherapy for further two cycles [28]. The substances used with cisplatin (80 $mg \cdot m^{-2}$ at day 1) were vinorelbine, paclitaxel and gemcitabine (table 5). Efficacy was quite comparable, but there was a clear difference for toxicity. Gemcitabine, despite the markedly reduced dose during radiotherapy, demonstrated a higher toxicity for neutropenia, thrombocytopenia and oesophagitis. Paclitaxel had an increased toxicity for neutropenia and oesophagitis in comparison with vinorelbine (table 6). This trial suggested the use of vinorelbine and cisplatin in concurrent radiochemotherapy treatment.

Another point to consider is patient-related comorbidities. Reduced pulmonary function can limit the application of radiotherapy; some chemotherapeutic agents also can impair pulmonary function. Renal insufficiency can occur in patients with chemotherapy, especially platinum-based regimens. Many substances are excreted by the kidneys. Pemetrexed is contraindicated in patients with a reduced glomerular filtration rate of <40 $mL \cdot min^{-1}$, and other substances that are eliminated *via* the kidneys may remain active for longer with aggravated side-effects in the presence of renal dysfunction [7]. Some substances are metabolised in the liver and can be applied safely in these patients. However, for docetaxel, doses should be reduced in hepatic insufficiency. If a pleural effusion is present, metothrexate and pemetrexed should be avoided, as they accumulate in these fluids.

Table 5. – Chemotherapy regimens and dosages in Cancer and Leukemia Group B 9431

Arm	Treatment	Day											
		1	8	15	22	29	36	43	50	57	64	71	78
All	Cisplatin	80			80			80			80		
I	Gemcitabine	1250	1250		1250	1250		600	600		600	600	
II	Paclitaxel	225			225			135			135		
III	Vinorelbine	25	25	25	25	25		15	15		15	15	
All	XRT							66 Gy#					

Data, taken from [28], are given in mg·m^{-2} unless otherwise stated. XRT: percutaneous thoracic radiotherapy. #: starting at day 43, daily until day 78, continuously.

A recent meta-analysis using individual patient data, which compared concomitant *versus* sequential radiochemotherapy, looked at toxicity [24]. Concomitant chemotherapy substantially increased oesophageal toxicity compared with sequential chemotherapy (RR 4.9, 95% CI 3.1–7.8; $p<0.0001$). Pulmonary acute toxicity showed no significant difference between concomitant and sequential chemotherapy (RR 0.69, 95% CI 0.42–1.12; $p=0.13$).

With consolidation chemotherapy, advantages were not seen in terms of improved survival and one explanation could be the increased toxicity with consolidation chemotherapy. In a German trial using vinorelbine and cisplatin, interim analyses do not show increased toxicity at present.

Overall acute toxicity increases with radiochemotherapy, especially oesophagitis in the concomitant approach. However, in well selected patients with a careful approach, concomitant radiochemotherapy results in good local control and survival.

Further developments

Biological agents

In addition to established cytotoxic chemotherapy, the growing knowledge of tumour metabolism and its meticulous regulation by signalling pathways has led to a new class of antitumour agents known as biologicals [29]. Certain pathway dysregulations are known for NSCLC. The most investigated is a family of membrane proteins that can induce cell growth, the epidermal growth factor receptor (EGFR; also called HER1 or erbB1). The EGFR activity is restricted in normal cells, but in NSCLC the intracellular negative feedback mechanism is not working, due to malignant transformation following amplification, overexpression or mutation of tumour suppressor or amplification genes. As an effect of radiotherapy an upregulation of EGFR occurs. Small trials with tyrosine-kinase inhibitors showed promising results. The EGFR antibody cetuximab, which has been approved for other solid cancers, has shown a therapeutic effect in combination with radiotherapy for head and neck tumours. Trials integrating cetuximab in radiochemotherapy regimens for lung cancer are on the way. Other biological agents are likely to be tested in combination with radiochemotherapy.

Optimisation of radiotherapy

There are many technical developments in thoracic radiotherapy, *e.g.* intensity-modulated approaches and stereotactic radiotherapy, which are described in chapter 16 of this *ERM* and should also be studied in radiochemotherapy approaches.

Table 6. – Toxicities of the different chemotherapy regimens in Cancer and Leukemia Group B 9431

Regimen	Neutropenia %	Thrombocytopenia %	Oesophagitis %
Vinorelbine+cisplatin	25	0	24
Paclitaxel+cisplatin	48	6	40
Gemcitabine+cisplatin	51	55	52

Data taken from [28].

Conclusions and practical approach

Patients with locally advanced NSCLC should be treated in a multidisciplinary team of respiratory physicians/oncologists, pathologists, radiologists, radiotherapists and surgeons, in order to achieve the best potential outcomes. In addition, treatment in specialised centres shows beneficial effects for most cancers. As most of the patients already are in stage IIIB with widespread metastatic lymph node involvement (N3), surgery is not recommended. Depending on patient-related factors, such as performance status, mobility and comorbidities, radiochemotherapy is recommended.

For patients in stage IIIB without malignant pleural effusion, or inoperable stage IIIA and good performance status without major comorbidities, platinum-based concomitant radiochemotherapy is the treatment of choice. In patients with performance status >2, this approach should only be considered cautiously; induction chemotherapy or induction chemotherapy in combination with low-dose simultaneous chemotherapy seem to be possible alternatives. The perfect chemotherapeutic partners for simultaneous full-dose radiochemotherapy are not yet determined, but it seems to be clear that gemcitabine should be avoided due to increased toxicity. At the moment a good choice is the combination of vinorelbine and cisplatin, but the older regimen of cisplatin and etoposide is also widely used. The radiotherapy should be given in once-daily fractions, as hyperfractionation with two doses a day showed no additional benefit, but increased toxicity.

Summary

In nonsmall cell lung cancers (NSCLC), up to 40% of patients present with locally advanced disease with involvement of the hilar and mediastinal lymph nodes. The term locally advanced includes tumours at stage IIIB and inoperable tumours at stage IIIA. The primary intention in these patients is curative treatment with multimodality therapy, including chemotherapy and thoracic radiotherapy. However, the benefit of combined radiochemotherapy must be weighed against the potential for increased toxicity. If the individual patient and tumour characteristics allow an intense treatment approach, simultaneous radiotherapy/chemotherapy is the probable standard of care. Biological agents such as tyrosine-kinase inhibitors and the importance of subtypes of NSCLC are being evaluated for integration into the management of these tumours.

Keywords: Locally advanced, nonsmall cell lung cancer, stage IIIA, stage IIIB, therapy.

Statement of interest

R.M. Huber performed various trials in radiochemotherapy partly with support from Sanofi Aventis, Pierre Fabre and Bristol Myers Squibb.

References

1. Toschi L, Cappuzzo F, Jänne PA. Evolution and future perspectives in the treatment of locally advanced non-small cell lung cancer. *Ann Oncol* 2007; 18: Suppl. 9, ix150–ix155.
2. Litzky LA. The pathology of non-small cell lung carcinoma. *In*: Fishman AP, Elias JA, Fishman JA, *et al.*, eds. Fishman's Pulmonary Diseases and Disorders. 4th Edn. McGraw-Hill Medical, New York, 2008; pp. 1831–1850.
3. Mehra R, Treat J. Treatment of non-small-cell lung cancer: chemotherapy. *In*: Fishman AP, Elias JA, Fishman JA, *et al.*, eds. Fishman's Pulmonary Diseases and Disorders. 4th Edn. McGraw-Hill Medical, New York, 2008; pp. 1867–1882.
4. Mountain CF. Revisions in the International System for Staging Lung Cancer. *Chest* 1997; 111: 1710–1717.
5. Ciuleanu TE, Brodowicz T, Belani CP. Maintenance pemetrexed plus best supportive care (BSC) *versus* placebo plus BSC: a phase III study. *J Clin Oncol* 2008; 26: Suppl. 15, 8011.
6. Ball D, Matthews J, Worotniuk V, *et al.* Longer survival with higher doses of thoracic radiotherapy in patients with limited non-small cell lung cancer. *Int J Radiat Oncol Biol Phys* 1993; 25: 599–604.
7. Stinchcombe TE, Socinski MA Considerations for second-line therapy of non-small cell lung cancer. *Oncologist* 2008; 13: Suppl. 1, 28–36.
8. Arriagada R, Komaki R, Cox JD. Radiation dose escalation in non-small cell carcinoma of the lung. *Semin Radiat Oncol* 2004; 14: 287–291.
9. Perez CA, Pajak TF, Rubin P, *et al.* Long-term observations of the patterns of failure in patients with unresectable non-oat cell carcinoma of the lung treated with definitive radiotherapy. Report by the Radiation Therapy Oncology Group. *Cancer* 1987; 59: 1874–1881.
10. Marino P, Preatoni A, Cantoni A. Randomized trials of radiotherapy alone *versus* combined chemotherapy and radiotherapy in stages IIIa and IIIb nonsmall cell lung cancer. A meta-analysis. *Cancer* 1995; 76: 593–601.
11. Chemotherapy in non-small cell lung cancer: a meta-analysis using updated data on individual patients from 52 randomised clinical trials. Non-small Cell Lung Cancer Collaborative Group. *BMJ* 1995; 311: 899–909.
12. Scagliotti G. Optimizing chemotherapy for patients with advanced non-small cell lung cancer. *J Thorac Oncol* 2007; 2: Suppl. 2, S86–S91.
13. Rigas JR, Kelly K. Current treatment paradigms for locally advanced non-small cell lung cancer. *J Thorac Oncol* 2007; 2: Suppl. 2, S77–S85.
14. Schaake-Koning C, van den Bogaert W, Dalesio O, *et al.* Effects of concomitant cisplatin and radiotherapy on inoperable non-small-cell lung cancer. *N Engl J Med* 1992; 326: 524–530.
15. Bunn PA Jr, Thatcher N. Systemic treatment for advanced (stage IIIb/IV) non-small cell lung cancer: more treatment options; more things to consider. Conclusion. *Oncologist* 2008; 13: Suppl. 1, 37–46.
16. Dillman RO, Seagren SL, Propert KJ, *et al.* A randomized trial of induction chemotherapy plus high-dose radiation *versus* radiation alone in stage III non-small-cell lung cancer. *N Engl J Med* 1990; 323: 940–945.
17. Dillman RO, Herndon J, Seagren SL, *et al.* Improved survival in stage III non-small-cell lung cancer: seven-year follow-up of cancer and leukemia group B (CALGB) 8433 trial. *J Natl Cancer Inst* 1996; 88: 1210–1215.

18. Sause W, Kolesar P, Taylor S, *et al.* Final results of phase III trial in regionally advanced unresectable non-small cell lung cancer: Radiation Therapy Oncology Group, Eastern Cooperative Oncology Group, and Southwest Oncology Group. *Chest* 2000; 117: 358–364.
19. Rolland E, Le Chevalier T, Auperin A, *et al.* Sequential radio-chemotherapy (RT-CT) *versus* radiotherapy alone (RT) and concomitant RT-CT *versus* RT alone in locally advanced non-small cell lung cancer (NSCLC): two meta-analyses using individual patient data (IPD) from randomised clinical trials (RCTs). *J Thor Oncol* 2007; 2: Suppl. 4, S309.
20. Govindan R, Bogart J, Vokes EE. Locally advanced non-small cell lung cancer: the past, present, and future. *J Thorac Oncol* 2008; 3: 917–928.
21. Huber RM, Flentje M, Schmidt M, *et al.* Simultaneous chemoradiotherapy compared with radiotherapy alone after induction chemotherapy in inoperable stage IIIA or IIIB non-small-cell lung cancer: study CTRT99/97 by the Bronchial Carcinoma Therapy Group. *J Clin Oncol* 2006; 24: 4397–4404.
22. Blanke C, Ansari R, Mantravadi R, *et al.* Phase III trial of thoracic irradiation with or without cisplatin for locally advanced unresectable non-small-cell lung cancer: a Hoosier Oncology Group protocol. *J Clin Oncol* 1995; 13: 1425–1429.
23. Rowell NP, O'Rourke NP. Concurrent chemoradiotherapy in non-small cell lung cancer. *Cochrane Database Syst Rev* 2004; 4: CD002140.
24. Auperin A, Rolland E, Curran WJ, *et al.* Concomitant radio-chemotherapy (RT-CT) *versus* sequential RT-CT in locally advanced non-small cell lung cancer (NSCLC): a meta-analysis using individual patient data (IPD) from randomised clinical trials (RCTs). *J Thor Oncol* 2007; 2: Suppl. 4, S310.
25. Furuse K, Fukuoka M, Kawahara M, *et al.* Phase III study of concurrent *versus* sequential thoracic radiotherapy in combination with mitomycin, vindesine, and cisplatin in unresectable stage III non-small-cell lung cancer. *J Clin Oncol* 1999; 17: 2692–2699.
26. Gandara DR, Chansky K, Albain KS, *et al.* Consolidation docetaxel after concurrent chemoradiotherapy in stage IIIB non-small-cell lung cancer: phase II Southwest Oncology Group Study S9504. *J Clin Oncol* 2003; 21: 2004–2010.
27. Hanna N, Neubauer M, Yiannoutsos C, *et al.* Phase III study of cisplatin, etoposide, and concurrent chest radiation with or without consolidation docetaxel in patients with inoperable stage III non-small-cell lung cancer: the Hoosier Oncology Group and US Oncology. *J Clin Oncol* 2008; 26: 5755–5760.
28. Vokes EE, Herndon JE 2nd, Crawford J, et al. Randomized phase II study of cisplatin with gemcitabine or paclitaxel or vinorelbine as induction chemotherapy followed by concomitant chemoradiotherapy for stage IIIB non-small-cell lung cancer: cancer and leukemia group B study 9431. *J Clin Oncol* 2002; 20: 4191–4198.
29. Ranson M. ZD1839 (Iressa): for more than just non-small cell lung cancer. *Oncologist* 2002; 7: Suppl. 4, 16–24.

CHAPTER 15

Chemotherapy in advanced nonsmall cell lung cancer

E. Quoix

Correspondence: E. Quoix, Service de Pneumologie, Nouvel Hôpital Civil, Hôpitaux universitaires de Strasbourg, 1, Place de l'hôpital, 67091 Strasbourg cedex, France. E-mail: elisabeth.quoix@chru-strasbourg.fr

Introduction

Lung cancer is the first cause of death from cancer in males in the developed and developing world. It is also the first cause of death by cancer in females in the USA since the end of the 1980s, and the third most common cause of death in Europe.

Approximately 40% of nonsmall cell lung cancer (NSCLC) are metastatic at the time of diagnosis and among the locally advanced disease, which together represents ~30% of cases, some are not irradiable (wet stage IIIB, *i.e.* with a pleural effusion) and are to be treated as if stage IV. Those lung cancers with metastatic pleural and/or pericardial effusion will in any case be classified as stage IV in the next primary tumour, regional lymph nodes, and metastatic involvement (TNM) classification system [1].

Thus, ~50% of all NSCLC patients can be considered to have advanced disease at diagnosis with no treatment benefit from any loco-regional treatment, either surgery (except the very rare cases with a single metastasis, *e.g.* in the brain, which can be resected together with the primary tumour) or mediastinal radiation therapy, except for palliative purpose.

Chemotherapy as become standard in advanced NSCLC since the meta-analysis of clinical trials comparing best supportive care (BSC) to BSC and platin-based chemotherapy and published in 1995 [2].

Questions regarding chemotherapy in advanced NSCLC

Is polychemotherapy better than single agent?

Several clinical trials compared cisplatin plus another drug with a single agent [3–7] or cisplatin plus a second drug with cisplatin alone [8–12]. All these trials demonstrated a higher response rate in the combined arm compared with the single agent arm, but a survival benefit in the combined arm was only observed in some of the trials [3, 5, 9, 11, 12]. The benefit of survival was confined to patients with PS 0 or 1 in two of these [3, 5].

Comparisons of triplets *versus* doublets (mitomycin + ifosfamide + cisplatin *versus* gemcitabine + cisplatin [13]; or cisplatin + vinorelbine *versus* vinorelbine + cisplatin + ifosfamide [14]; or cisplatin + gemcitabine *versus* cisplatin + gemcitabine + vinorelbine [15]) was not in favour of the triplet as there were more toxicity and no improvement in response rate or survival was found.

Eur Respir Mon, 2009, 44, 271–283. Printed in UK - all rights reserved. Copyright ERS Journals Ltd 2009; European Respiratory Monograph; ISSN 1025-448x.

A meta-analysis of all randomised controlled trials performed between 1980–2001 (65 trials, 13,601 patients in total) confirmed that two agents do better than one with regards to response rate and survival benefit, but the use of three agents results in a better response rate but no survival benefit [16].

Is a platin salt mandatory as a component of the doublet?

Platin salts and especially cisplatin have toxicities that are difficult to manage. For example, immediate nausea and vomiting can be avoided at the expense of the use of an anti-nauseant aprepitant plus a 5-hydroxytryptamine receptor type 3 (5HT3) antagonist together with corticosteroids, whereas delayed nausea and vomiting are more difficult to treat. Renal toxicity requires hyperhydration for cisplatin, which can be difficult or impossible to provide in patients with cardiac insufficiency. Ototoxicity is somewhat unpredictible and may appear after only one cycle. Peripheral neurotoxicity precludes the use of cisplatin in patients who already have a peripheral neuropathy, for example due to diabetes mellitus.

Thus, several studies compared platin-based doublets with doublets without platin salts (mostly gemcitabine + taxanes) [15, 17–20] with no definite conclusions. A meta-analysis of phase III trials comparing platinum-based *versus* nonplatinum based regimens was conducted with the 1-yr survival rate as the primary objective. A total of 14 trials (among which, seven had gemcitabine/taxane as the experimental arm) were identified, but only 11 were finally analysed, two trials having platin-based triplets, and one, for which no updated data could be obtained, was discarded. The meta-analysis included 4,602 patients and concluded that platin-based doublets resulted in a significant reduction in the risk of death at 1 yr, a lower risk of being refractory to chemotherapy with no added toxicity [21]. One further trial was published recently, comparing two regimens (carboplatine + gemcitabine and gemcitabine + paclitaxel) in 512 patients. The two regimens were equally active with more myelotoxicity in the carboplatin + gemcitabine group and more neurotoxicity and alopecia in the gemcitabine + paclitaxel group [22]. Platin-based doublets remain the recommendation for first-line therapy [23].

Is cisplatin better than carboplatin?

Carboplatin is far easier to manage than cisplatin. Its toxicity is mainly haematological and the dose is generally adapted to renal function (Calvert or Chatelut method). The combination of carboplatin + paclitaxel is the standard doublet used in the USA, whereas in Europe cisplatin-based doublets are preferred. There have been some clinical trials comparing cisplatin with carboplatin, which showed conflicting results [24, 25]. A meta-analysis of these trials confirms a small but definite advantage to cisplatin-based doublets [26]. However, benefit of cisplatin-based doublet remains confined to patients with performance status (PS) 0-1 as those with PS 2 do not benefit from this combination [27].

Which platin-based doublet to use?

During the 1990s there were some very important clinical trials comparing various doublets. For example in the Southwest Oncology Group study [28], which compared cisplatin + vinorelbine with carboplatin + paclitaxel, there was no significant difference in survival. In the Eastern Cooperative Oncology Group study [29], four regimens were compared: cipslatin + paclitaxel; cisplatin + docetaxel; cisplatin + gemcitabine; and carboplatin + paclitaxel. The survival curves were similar (fig. 1). Comparison of carboplatin + paclitaxel or cisplatin + gemcitabine with the reference arm cisplatin + vinorelbine, did not show any significant difference in the outcome between the three arms [30]. The TAX 326 study was a paired comparison of cisplatin + docetaxel with cisplatin + vinorelbine and carboplatin + docetaxel, using the same reference arm [31]. There was a significantly longer survival for the cisplatin + docetaxel arm compared with cisplatin + vinorelbine. A noninferiority trial was recently conducted comparing overall survival in patients treated with cisplatin + gemcitabine *versus* cisplatin + pemetrexed [32]. There was no significant difference between the two arms. Table 1 summarises the outcome of the patients treated with platin-based doublets in the main phase III trials over the previous 10 yrs.

There was a meta-analysis suggesting that docetaxel-based doublets might provide a longer survival [33] and another one suggesting that gemcitabine + platin-salt might be the best [34].

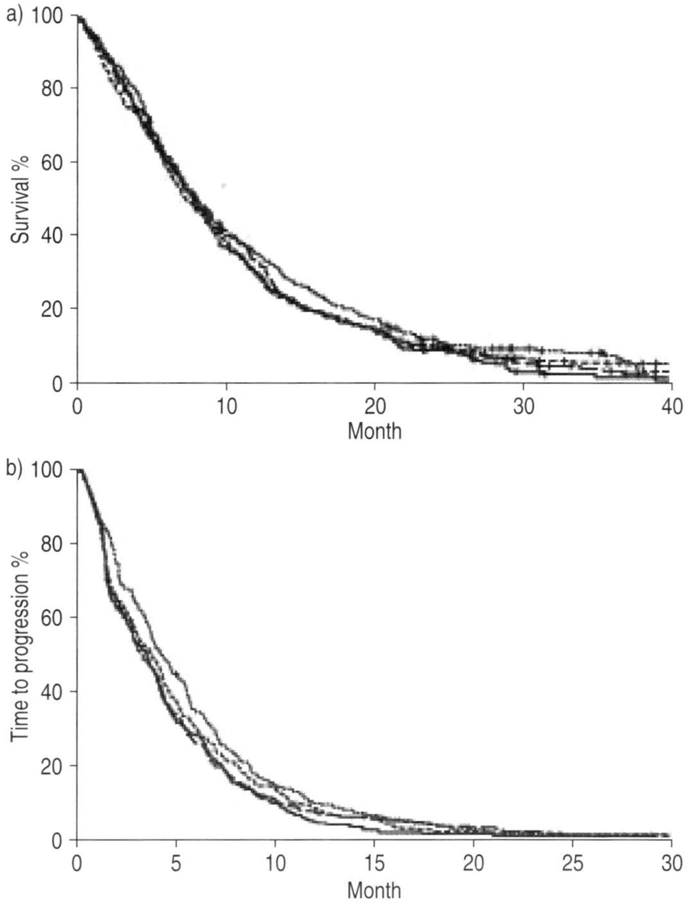

Fig. 1. – Overall a) survival and b) time to progression curves in the Eastern Cooperative Oncology Group study comparing four platin-based doublets as first-line therapy for patients with advanced nonsmall cell lung cancer. Figure reproduced from [29] with permission from the publisher.

Table 1. – Phase III trials comparing different platin-based doublets outcomes

First author [ref.]	Year	Arms	N	RR %	TTP months	MST months	1-yr survival %
KELLY [28]	2001	C+VNR	202	30	4	8.1	36
		Ca+T	206	31	4	8.6	38
SCHILLER [29]	2002	C+T	288	21	3.4	7.8	31
		C+D	289	17	3.7	7.4	31
		C+G	288	22	4.2#	8.1	36
		Ca+T	290	17	3.6	8.1	34
SCAGLIOTTI [30]	2002	C+VNR	203	30	4.6	9.5	37
		C+G	205	30	5.3	9.8	37
		Ca+T	204	31	5.5	9.9	43
FOSSELLA [31]	2003	C+D	408	31.6	5	11.3+	46
		Ca+D	406	23.9	4.6	9.4	38
		C+VNR	404	24.5	5.2	9.9	41
SCAGLIOTTI [32]	2008	C+G	863	30.6	5.1	10.3	41.9
		C+P	862	28.2	4.8	10.3	43.5

N: number of points; RR: response rate; TTP: time to progression; MST: median survival time; C: cisplatin; VNR: vinorelbine; Ca: carboplatine; T: taxol; D: docetaxel; G: gemcitabine; P; pemetrexed; #: significantly longer TTP; +: significantly longer survival compared with C+VNR.

The conclusion is that chemotherapy has reached a plateau and the differences between the different doublets are mainly related to profile toxicities and costs.

A point worthy of note is that the addition of bevacizumab to paclitaxel and carboplatin in selected patients (nonsquamous cell carcinoma histology, no haemoptysis, no brain metastases), improves survival with a median survival time surpassing 1 yr for the first time [35]. This is discussed further in chapter 16 of this current *European Respiratory Monograph*.

Duration of treatment

In clinical trials performed during the 1980s and the 1990s, chemotherapy was often given until disease progression [3] or for a maximum of eight cycles [12] whereas in the recent trials, the number of cycles was six for stable or responding patients [11, 28, 32, 35].

In 1997, the American Society of Clinical Oncology recommendations were to not deliver more than eight cycles of chemotherapy [36]. In 2004, the recommendation for duration of chemotherapy for stage IV NSCLC was that first-line platinum-based chemotherapy should be administered for no more than six cycles [23].

There have been randomised trials comparing different durations of treatment. The first trial compared six cycles of mitomycin, vinblastin and cisplatin with three cycles in 308 patients [37]. There was no advantage from using six cycles of treatment with regards to response rate, time to progression (TTP) or overall survival. A second trial compared 230 patients, who received four cycles, with carboplatin and paclitaxel or continuous treatment until disease progression [38], and again no benefit was seen for those patients beyond four cycles. A third trial compared three to six cycles of carboplatin and vinorelbine in 297 patients with, once again, no benefit for the six cycles arm [39]. The most recent trial compared four to six cycles of cisplatin-based chemotherapy (either one of paclitaxel, docetaxel or gemcitabine + cisplatin) in 452 patients [40] with no difference for response rate or survival. However there was an advantage for TTP. In an editorial published in the same journal at this date, SOCINSKI and STINCHCOMBE [41] stated that at this time in which, effective second- or third-line therapies exist, targeted therapies are more frequently becoming involved in first-, second- or third-line therapies. The problem might be when should we give these second- and third-line regimes? Maybe after induction therapy rather than exposing patients to a long duration of a toxic platin-based doublet.

Maintenance therapy has also been investigated. A trial conducted in locally advanced NSCLC (two cycles of mitomycin, ifosfamide and cisplatin, followed by irradiation) or stage IV disease (four cycles of the same chemotherapy) with in both cases maintenance therapy with vinorelbine for 6 months in responding patients, did not demonstrate any benefit in favour of the maintenance arm [42]. A phase III trial comparing induction chemotherapy with cisplatin + gemcitabine (maximum of four cycles) followed either by gemcitabine as maintenance therapy (until progression or discontinuation at the patient/physician request) or best supportive care was performed in 354 patients of which 206 could be randomised. There was a significant increase in the response rate, longer TTP and a nonsignificant trend to longer survival in the maintenance arm. At this time the French Intergroup of Thoracic Oncology is performing a randomised study comparing in patients treated with four cycles of cisplatin + gemcitabine as induction chemotheray, a maintenance therapy with gemcitabine, or with erlotinib, or just simple follow-up. In the three arms, pemetrexed is to be administered at progression. To date 550 out of the 621, targeted recruitment, has been included.

A tailored approach for the treatment of advanced NSCLC?

Histology. In the recent non-inferiority phase III trial comparing cisplatin + pemetrexed to cisplatin + gemcitabine in 1,725 patients [32], no significant difference in overall survival was shown with a median survival time (MST) of 10.3 months in both arms. However, in a subset analysis, it appears that patients with adenocarcinoma or large cell carcinoma fared better with pemetrexed than gemcitabine (MST 12.6 months versus 10.9, and 10.4 *versus* 6.7 respectively) whereas patients with squamous cell histology did better with gemcitabine (MST 10.8 *versus* 6.7 months). Of note, following this single trial demonstrating differences between chemotherapy regimens effect according to histology (and only in a preplanned subset analysis), the European Medicines Agency (EMEA) Committee for Medicinal Products for Human Use has approved the use of pemetrexed (Alimta®; Eli Lilly and Company, Indianapolis, IN, USA) for nonsquamous cell carcinoma as the first-line treatment of advanced disease.

Gene expression. A strong association between the genes ribonucleotide reductase subunit 1 (*RRM1*) and excision repair cross-complementing (*ERCC1*) and therapeutic benefit from gemcitabine and platinum has been described by several authors during the last few years. Both genes are critical components of DNA synthesis and DNA damage repair pathways. In a feasibility phase II trial [43], patients with low expression of both *RRM1* and *ERCC1* were treated with gemcitabine and carboplatin, whereas patients with low expression of *RRM1* and high expression of *ERCC1* were treated with gemcitabine and docetaxel; patients with high expression of *RRM1* and low expression of *ERCC1* were treated with docetaxel + carboplatin and finally those with high expression of *RRM1* and *ERCC1* were treated with docetaxel and vinorelbine. This tailored treatment was possible in a series of 53 patients amongst 85 preselected and 60 eligible individuals. The best treatment response across these four treatments was a partial response in 23 patients 44% (95% confidence interval (CI), 31–59%), and stable disease in 23 patients 44% (31–59%). The 1-yr survival rate was 59%, and the 1-yr progression-free survival (PFS) rate was 14%. The MST was 13.3 months (95% CI, 11.5–

<24 months) and the median PFS was 6.6 months (95% CI, 4.7–8.8 months). In another retrospective analysis, a significant correlation between outcome and *RRM1* and *ERCC1* expression was found in 61 of 70 patients amongst which 43 were treated with cisplatin + gemcitabine [44]. However, in another recent publication no correlation between the level of expression of *ERCC1* and response rate, toxicity or survival was found [45]. These discrepancies could be linked to the methodologies used for analysis of these enzymes. A phase III study has been conducted comparing in 346 patients, customised chemotherapy according to the level of expression of *ERCC1* (low expression=treatment with cisplatin + docetaxel, high expression=treatment with gemcitabine and docetaxel) to standard chemotherapy with cisplatin and docetaxel [46]. The response rate was 39.3% in the control arm and 50.7% in the genotypic arm (p=0.02). More is needed to discover if there is a genuine link between these genes and responses to chemotherapeutic agents.

Betatubulin expression class III detected by immunohistochemistry on tumour tissue is correlated with reduced response rates and inferior survival with anti-microtubule agents (taxanes, vinorelbine). Besides being a predictive factor of poor response to taxanes and vinorelbine, high betatubulin expression class III could be also a prognostic factor by itself [47]. Development of antimicrotubules agents such as epothilone that would overcome this mechanism of resistance to taxanes is underway.

Specific patient populations

PS 2 patients

Those patients experience significantly more severe toxicity, a lower response rate and shorter survival benefit [27, 48]. They do not benefit from cisplatin-based chemotherapy. Carboplatin-based chemotherapy [49, 50] seems to be feasible, but there is no specific study randomising single agent therapy *versus* carboplatine-based chemotherapy in PS 2 patients. The only data comes from a randomised study comparing paclitaxel with carboplatin + paclitaxel in PS 0–2 patients with a preplanned subset analysis of PS 2 patients, showing a longer survival in the combination treatment arm [50]. A phase II study comparing gemcitabine and carboplatine with gemcitabine alone, in 90 PS 2 patients, showed no clinical benefit for the combined arm and more toxicity [51]. Thus, there is no clear cut recommendation for the treatment of PS 2 patients with advanced NSCLC [52].

The use of targeted therapies as first-line therapy has been discussed for these frail patients. However, a randomised trial comparing carboplatin + paclitaxel with erlotinib as frontline therapy, showed better results for chemotherapy for both response rate and TTP. There was also a nonsignificant trend toward a longer survival with chemotherapy [53]. The recommendation for unselected patients with PS 2 is that the first-line of treatment should remain as chemotherapy, although the optimal approach is not defined [54]. Currently there is no recommendation for PS 3 patients who do not seem to benefit from any chemotherapy.

Elderly patients

Lung cancer incidence increases considerably with age, and as the aged population is also increasing in the developed world, lung cancer in the elderly has become a serious public health problem. The cut-off point to define "elderly" is somewhat variable: generally speaking it is 65 yrs of age in epidemiological studies [55], whereas it is

70 yrs of age in most clinical trials (but not all) [56]. Patients aged >65 yrs represent ~50% of all patients with lung cancer and patients >70 yrs ~30%.

Elderly patients are under represented in clinical trials making any statement about the best treatment according to geriatric status very difficult [57]. Most of the experience was drawn from retrospective analyses of clinical trials with no upper limit of age in which the elderly patients included were almost certainly highly selected and not representative of the general population. The first trial demonstrating the value of chemotherapy in patients aged >70 yrs with stage IIIB/IV NSCLC was published in 1999 [58]. This study compared vinorelbine alone with BSC in 190 patients. The response rate was 19.7% in the vinorelbine arm and MST was 28 weeks compared with 21 in the BSC arm. The 1-yr survival rate was 32% in the vinorelbine arm *versus* 14% in the BSC arm. Moreover, quality of life was superior in the chemotherapy arm. Gemcitabine is the second drug most studied in elderly patients with quite a number of phase II studies demonstrating its efficacy in this subpopulation of patients [59–61]. The combination of vinorelbine and gemcitabine *versus* monotherapy by either of these two agents did not provide any benefit in a study involving 700 patients [62]. Also, the combination with carboplatine and paclitaxel was found to be highly effective and safe in a phase II study [63]. This approach is now being investigated in a randomised trial comparing single agent therapy (vinorelbine or gemcitabine) with the combination of carboplatin and paclitaxel (French Intergroup of Thoracic Oncology) with 374 patients included to date.

Single agent therapy is the recommendation of the American Society of Clinical Oncology [23] and also of the American College of Chest Physicians (with a limitation to 70–79-yr-old category) with a statement that carboplatin-based doublet might be given to good performance status patients [54].

Salvage therapy

Unfortunately the majority if not all patients experience disease progression either during induction treatment or after obtaining a response or stabilisation of their tumour. The median TTP for stage IIIB/IV patients treated with chemotherapy is between 3–6 months after the beginning of chemotherapy [28, 29, 35].

Docetaxel

The first drug which was approved for second-line therapy was docetaxel after two randomis ed trials performed in patients who relapsed after platin-based chemotherapy. The first one [64] compared docetaxel 100 mg·m^{-2} every 3 weeks with BSC in 204 patients. From these patients, one quarter had received two previous lines of chemotherapy. After inclusion of 49 patients, toxicity was found to be too severe and the dosage of docetaxel was reduced to 75 mg·m^{-2} for the 55 additional patients. A significant survival advantage over BSC was demonstrated with this dosage, moreover, quality of life and symptom control were better in the chemotherapy arms. For example, patients treated with docetaxel required fewer analgesics and less palliative radiation therapy [65]. Also, cost-effectiveness for patients treated with docetaxel at the dosage of 75 mg·m^{-2} was considered within the acceptable range of health care expenditure.

The second study compared 75 mg·m^{-2} with 100 mg·m^{-2} with a third arm, consisting in a treatment either with vinorelbine or ifosfamide [66]. There was no significant difference in survival between the three arms, whereas time to progression was longer in the docetaxel arms and 1-yr survival rate higher in the docetaxel arm at the dose of 75 mg·m^{-2}.

Pemetrexed

The second drug to be registered in this setting is pemetrexed, which was compared with a non-inferiority phase III trial to docetaxel for patients who relapsed after platin-based chemotherapy [67]. The first trials performed with Pemetrexed showed considerable myelotoxiciy and mucositis. Vitamin supplementation (folate 350–1,000 $\mu g \cdot day^{-1}$ and vitamin B12 1,000 µg every 9 weeks) reduced this toxicity considerably. The randomised trial was designed for patients having received only one previous regimen of chemotherapy. The trial did not meet the statistical endpoint of non-inferiority of survival for pemetrexed for the fixed margin method, but attained it with the method of per cent retention. Survival curves were very similar. Haematological toxicity was significantly less important in the pemetrexed arm and nonhaematological toxicities were similar in both arms.

Targeted therapies

Although this chapter is strictly devoted to chemotherapy, it will simply cite the third registered therapy for relapsed advanced NSCLC, which is erlotinib following a phase III randomised trial, comparing erlotinib with BSC in 731 patients who relapsed after at least one regimen of chemotherapy and who were not eligible for further chemotherapy [68].

There was a significant gain in survival for patients treated with erlotinib that was observed in all subsets of patients, even if squamous cell carcinoma, smoking and male sex were adverse prognostic factors.

Beyond second- and third-line therapy?

Three agents are now registered for second- and/or third-line purpose (erlotinib can be given either as second-line therapy for selected patients (females, adenocarcinoma, nonsmokers) or as third-line therapy). A significant percentage of patients failing after third-line therapy are still in good performance status and demanding treatment. However, the response rates and disease control rates that can be expected decline as the number of lines increases [69]. There is, therefore, an unmet need for new therapeutic approaches as the number of patients who could benefit from further chemotherapy is increasing.

Table 2. – Results obtained with registered second- or third-line therapies

First author [ref.]	Year	N	Drug	RR %	MST months	1-yr survival %
Shepherd [64]	2000	49	D 100	7.1	5.9	19
		55	D 75	7.1	7.5	37
		100	BSC		4.6	11
Fossella [66]	2000	125	D 100	5.5	5.5	21
		125	D 75	5.7	5.7	32
		123	VNR/Ifo	5.6	5.6	19
Hanna [67]	2004	276	D 75	8.8	7.9	29.7
		265	P	9.1	8.3	29.7
Shepherd [68]	2005	494	E	8.9	6.7	31
		247	BSC		4.7	21

N: number of points; RR: response rate; MST: median survival time; D: docetaxel; BSC: best supportive care; VNR: vinorelbine; Ifo: ifosfamide; P: pemetrexed; E: erlotinib.

Conclusion

Time for nihilism toward the treatment of advanced lung cancer is (should be) over. Platin-based doublets are now the standard treatment for advanced NSCLC in PS 0–1 patients and result in a response rate of around 25 to 30%, a TTP of 4–6 months and a MST of 8–11 months. It seems that there is now a plateau for results with chemotherapy alone, as different doublets result in similar outcomes, so the choice is dictated by the toxicity profile according to the patients characteristics. There is a trend towards a reduction of the number of cycles for induction therapy with, as a consequence, less toxicity and better quality of life.

Elderly and PS 2 patients are now candidates for modified chemotherapy (single agent or carboplatin-based doublet). Results that can be expected in PS 2 patients are inferior to those obtained in PS 0–1 patients.

Second- and third-line therapy are well standardised. There is an unmet need for further chemotherapy beyond third-line as a significant proportion of patients remain with an acceptable PS after third-line treatment. The recent introduction of targeted therapies either in the first-line setting in combination with platin-based doublet (bevacizumab and cetuximab) or in the second-or third-line setting (erlotinib) resulted in an improvement of survival with a MST beyond 1 yr. The tailored approach of chemotherapy either according to histology or to gene expression is another development of paramount importance which is only just beginning.

Summary

There is no dispute that chemotherapy is the standard treatment for advanced stage (IIIB (wet) and IV) nonsmall cell lung cancer.
The best chemotherapy regimen for patients with performance status (PS) 0–1, no renal or cardiac insufficiency is a platin-based doublet. The drug combined with platin salt maybe any of the new generation drugs (vinorelbine, taxotere, taxol, gemcitabine, pemetrexed) with similar results regarding survival benefit, the differences being essentially the toxicity profiles. Carboplatin, which is less toxic than cisplatin, may be used instead of cisplatin, with a slightly less efficacy (probably not clinically important). Tailored treatment approach is a new concept with adaptation of platin-based doublets to the histology of the tumour (gemcitabine is no more recommended for adenocarcinoma and pemetrexed is not recommended for squamous cell carcinoma). Also gene expression (*ERCC1, RRM1*, β-tubulin class III, *etc.*) might become of primary importance for customised chemotherapy.
The recommended number of cycles is four to six for stable or responding patients. At the current time there is no indication in favour of any maintenance therapy.
For patients with PS 2, a combination of carboplatin and paclitaxel is feasible, but there is no direct comparison with single agent therapy and thus no clear-cut recommendation.
In elderly patients the recommended first-line chemotherapy is a single agent, the most extensively studied being vinorelbine and gemcitabine.
Second-line therapy is now well established, with docetaxel or pemetrexed being the recommended choices. Targeted therapies can be used either as second-line therapy (female, nonsmokers, adenocarcinomas) or third-line therapy.
There is no recommendation beyond third-line regarding any chemotherapy/targeted therapy scheme and this remains an unmet need.

Keywords: Advanced, chemotherapy, first-line, metastatic, nonsmall cell lung cancer, second-line.

Statement of interest
None declared.

References

1. Rami-Porta R, Ball D, Crowley J, *et al.* The IASLC Lung Cancer Staging Project: proposals for the revision of the T descriptors in the forthcoming (seventh) edition of the TNM classification for lung cancer. *J Thorac Oncol* 2007; 2: 593–602.
2. Non-small Cell Lung Cancer Collaborative Group. Chemotherapy in non-small cell lung cancer: a meta-analysis using updated data on individual patients from 52 randomised clinical trials. *BMJ* 1995; 311: 899–909.
3. Le Chevalier T, Pujol JL, Douillard JY, *et al.* A three-arm trial of vinorelbine (Navelbine) plus cisplatin, vindesine plus cisplatin, and single-agent vinorelbine in the treatment of non-small cell lung cancer: an expanded analysis. *Semin Oncol* 1994; 21: Suppl. 10, 28–33.
4. Einhorn LH, Loehrer PJ, Williams SD, *et al.* Random prospective study of vindesine versus vindesine plus high-dose cisplatin versus vindesine plus cisplatin plus mitomycin C in advanced non-small-cell lung cancer. *J Clin Oncol* 1986; 4: 1037–1043.
5. Elliott JA, Ahmedzai S, Hole D, *et al.* Vindesine and cisplatin combination chemotherapy compared with vindesine as a single agent in the management of non-small cell lung cancer: a randomized study. *Eur J Cancer Clin Oncol* 1984; 20: 1025–32.
6. Depierre A, Chastang C, Quoix E, *et al.* Vinorelbine versus vinorelbine plus cisplatin in advanced non-small cell lung cancer: a randomized trial. *Ann Oncol* 1994; 5: 37–42.
7. Rosso R, Salvati F, Ardizzoni A, *et al.* Etoposide *versus* etoposide plus high-dose cisplatin in the management of advanced non-small cell lung cancer. Results of a prospective randomized FONICAP trial. Italian Lung Cancer Task Force. *Cancer* 1990; 66: 130–134.
8. Sculier JP, Paesmans M, Thiriaux J, *et al.* Phase III randomized trial comparing cisplatin and carboplatin with or without ifosfamide in patients with advanced non-small-cell lung cancer. European Lung Cancer Working Party. *J Clin Oncol* 1998; 16: 1388–1396.
9. Wozniak A, Crowley JJ, Balcerzak SP, *et al.* Randomized trial comparing cisplatin with cisplatin plus vinorelbine in the treatment of advanced non-small-cell lung cancer: a Southwest Oncology Group study. *J Clin Oncol* 1998; 16: 2459–2465.
10. Gatzemeier U, von Pawel J, Gottfried M, *et al.* Phase III comparative study of high-dose cisplatin *versus* a combination of paclitaxel and cisplatin in patients with advanced non-small-cell lung cancer. *J Clin Oncol* 2000; 18: 3390–3399.
11. Sandler AB, Nemunaitis J, Denham C, *et al.* Phase III trial of gemcitabine plus cisplatin *versus* cisplatin alone in patients with locally advanced or metastatic non-small-cell lung cancer. *J Clin Oncol* 2000; 18: 122–130.
12. von Pawel J, von Roemeling R, Gatzemeier U, *et al.* Tirapazamine plus cisplatin versus cisplatin in advanced non-small-cell lung cancer: A report of the international CATAPULT I study group. Cisplatin and Tirapazamine in Subjects with Advanced Previously Untreated Non-Small-Cell Lung Tumors. *J Clin Oncol* 2000; 18: 1351–1359.
13. Crino L, Scagliotti GV, Ricci S, *et al.* Gemcitabine and cisplatin versus mitomycin, ifosfamide, and cisplatin in advanced non-small-cell lung cancer: A randomized phase III study of the Italian Lung Cancer Project. *J Clin Oncol* 1999; 17: 3522–3530.
14. Souquet PJ, Tan EH, Rodrigues Pereira J, *et al.* GLOB-1: a prospective randomised clinical phase III trial comparing vinorelbine-cisplatin with vinorelbine-ifosfamide-cisplatin in metastatic non-small-cell lung cancer patients. *Ann Oncol* 2002; 13: 1853–1861.
15. Alberola V, Camps C, Provencio M, *et al.* Cisplatin plus gemcitabine versus a cisplatin-based triplet versus nonplatinum sequential doublets in advanced non-small-cell lung cancer: a Spanish Lung Cancer Group phase III randomized trial. *J Clin Oncol.* 2003; 21: 3207–3213.

16. Delbaldo C, Michiels S, Syz N, *et al.* Benefits of adding a drug to a single-agent or a 2-agent chemotherapy regimen in advanced non-small-cell lung cancer: a meta-analysis. *JAMA* 2004; 292: 470–484.
17. Georgoulias V, Papadakis E, Alexopoulos A, *et al.* Platinum-based and non-platinum-based chemotherapy in advanced non-small-cell lung cancer: a randomised multicentre trial. *Lancet* 2001; 357: 1478–1484.
18. Pujol JL, Choma D, Jacot W, *et al.* Platinum-free gemcitabine-based combinations: an alternative to conventional chemotherapy of non-small-cell lung cancers? *Bull Cancer* 2002; 89 Spec S85–90.
19. Smit EF, van Meerbeeck JP, Lianes P, *et al.* Three-arm randomized study of two cisplatin-based regimens and paclitaxel plus gemcitabine in advanced non-small-cell lung cancer: a phase III trial of the European Organization for Research and Treatment of Cancer Lung Cancer Group–EORTC 08975. *J Clin Oncol* 2003; 21: 3909–3917.
20. Pujol JL, Breton JL, Gervais R, *et al.* Gemcitabine-docetaxel *versus* cisplatin-vinorelbine in advanced or metastatic non-small-cell lung cancer: a phase III study addressing the case for cisplatin. *Ann Oncol* 2005; 16: 602–610.
21. Pujol JL, Barlesi F, Daures JP. Should chemotherapy combinations for advanced non-small cell lung cancer be platinum-based? A meta-analysis of phase III randomized trials. *Lung Cancer* 2006; 51: 335–345.
22. Kosmidis PA, Kalofonos HP, Christodoulou C, *et al.* Paclitaxel and gemcitabine versus carboplatin and gemcitabine in patients with advanced non-small-cell lung cancer. A phase III study of the Hellenic Cooperative Oncology Group. *Ann Oncol* 2008; 19: 115–122.
23. Pfister DG, Johnson DH, Azzoli CG, *et al.* American Society of Clinical Oncology treatment of unresectable non-small-cell lung cancer guideline: update 2003. *J Clin Oncol* 2004; 22: 330–353.
24. Rosell R, Gatzemeier U, Betticher DC, *et al.* Phase III randomised trial comparing paclitaxel/carboplatin with paclitaxel/cisplatin in patients with advanced non-small-cell lung cancer: a cooperative multinational trial. *Ann Oncol* 2002; 13: 1539–1549.
25. Paccagnella A, Favaretto A, Oniga F, *et al.* Cisplatin *versus* carboplatin in combination with mitomycin and vinblastine in advanced non small cell lung cancer. A multicenter, randomized phase III trial. *Lung Cancer* 2004; 43: 83–91.
26. Ardizzoni A, Boni L, Tiseo M, *et al.* Cisplatin- *versus* carboplatin-based chemotherapy in first-line treatment of advanced non-small-cell lung cancer: an individual patient data meta-analysis. *J Natl Cancer Inst* 2007; 99: 847–857.
27. Soria JC, Brisgand D, Le Chevalier T. Do all patients with advanced non-small-cell lung cancer benefit from cisplatin-based combination therapy? *Ann Oncol* 2001; 12: 1667–1670.
28. Kelly K, Crowley J, Bunn PA Jr, *et al.* Randomized phase III trial of paclitaxel plus carboplatin *versus* vinorelbine plus cisplatin in the treatment of patients with advanced non-small-cell lung cancer: a Southwest Oncology Group trial. *J Clin Oncol* 2001; 19: 3210–3218.
29. Schiller JH, Harrington D, Belani CP, *et al.* Comparison of four chemotherapy regimens for advanced non-small-cell lung cancer. *N Engl J Med* 2002; 346: 92–98.
30. Scagliotti GV, De Marinis F, Rinaldi M, *et al.* Phase III randomized trial comparing three platinum-based doublets in advanced non-small-cell lung cancer. *J Clin Oncol* 2002; 20: 4285–4291.
31. Fossella F, Pereira JR, von Pawel J, *et al.* Randomized, multinational, phase III study of docetaxel plus platinum combinations versus vinorelbine plus cisplatin for advanced non-small-cell lung cancer: the TAX 326 study group. *J Clin Oncol* 2003; 21: 3016–3024.
32. Scagliotti GV, Parikh P, von Pawel J, *et al.* Phase III study comparing cisplatin plus gemcitabine with cisplatin plus pemetrexed in chemotherapy-naive patients with advanced-stage non-small-cell lung cancer. *J Clin Oncol* 2008; 26: 3543–3551.
33. Douillard JY, Laporte S, Fossella F, *et al.* Comparison of docetaxel- and vinca alkaloid-based chemotherapy in the first-line treatment of advanced non-small cell lung cancer: a meta-analysis of seven randomized clinical trials. *J Thorac Oncol.* 2007; 2: 939–946.

34. Le Chevalier T, Scagliotti G, Natale R, *et al.* Efficacy of gemcitabine plus platinum chemotherapy compared with other platinum containing regimens in advanced non-small-cell lung cancer: a meta-analysis of survival outcomes. *Lung Cancer* 2005; 47: 69–80.
35. Sandler A, Gray R, Perry MC, *et al.* Paclitaxel-carboplatin alone or with bevacizumab for non-small-cell lung cancer. *N Engl J Med* 2006; 355: 2542–2550.
36. Clinical practice guidelines for the treatment of unresectable non small cell lung cancer. Adopted on May 16, 1997 by the American Society of Clinical Oncology. *J Clin Oncol* 1997; 15: 2996–3018.
37. Smith I, O'Brien ME, Talbot DC, *et al.* Duration of chemotherapy in advanced non-small-cell lung cancer: a randomized trial of three versus six courses of mitomycin, vinblastine, and cisplatin. *J Clin Oncol* 2001; 19: 1336–1343.
38. Socinski MA, Schell MJ, Peterman A, Bakri K, Yates S, Gitten R, *et al.* Phase III trial comparing a defined duration of therapy *versus* continuous therapy followed by second-line therapy in advanced-stage IIIB/IV non-small-cell lung cancer. *J Clin Oncol* 2002; 20: 1335–1343.
39. von Plessen C, Bergman B, Andresen O, *et al.* Palliative chemotherapy beyond three courses conveys no survival or consistent quality-of-life benefits in advanced non-small-cell lung cancer. *Br J Cancer* 2006; 95: 966–973.
40. Park JO, Kim SW, Ahn JS, Suh C, Lee JS, Jang JS, *et al.* Phase III trial of two *versus* four additional cycles in patients who are nonprogressive after two cycles of platinum-based chemotherapy in non small-cell lung cancer. *J Clin Oncol* 2007; 25: 5233–5239.
41. Socinski MA, Stinchcombe TE. Duration of first-line chemotherapy in advanced non small-cell lung cancer: less is more in the era of effective subsequent therapies. *J Clin Oncol* 2007; 25: 5155–5157.
42. Westeel V, Quoix E, Moro-Sibilot D, *et al.* Randomized study of maintenance vinorelbine in responders with advanced non-small-cell lung cancer. *J Natl Cancer Inst* 2005; 97: 499–506.
43. Simon G, Sharma A, Li X, *et al.* Feasibility and efficacy of molecular analysis-directed individualized therapy in advanced non-small-cell lung cancer. *J Clin Oncol* 2007; 25: 2741–2746.
44. Ceppi P, Volante M, Novello S, *et al.* ERCC1 and RRM1 gene expressions but not EGFR are predictive of shorter survival in advanced non-small-cell lung cancer treated with cisplatin and gemcitabine. *Ann Oncol* 2006; 17: 1818–1825.
45. Booton R, Ward T, Ashcroft L, *et al.* ERCC1 mRNA expression is not associated with response and survival after platinum-based chemotherapy regimens in advanced non-small cell lung cancer. *J Thorac Oncol* 2007; 2: 902–906.
46. Cobo M, Isla D, Massuti B, *et al.* Customizing cisplatin based on quantitative excision repair cross-complementing 1 mRNA expression: a phase III trial in non-small-cell lung cancer. *J Clin Oncol* 2007; 25: 2747–2754.
47. Seve P, Lai R, Ding K, *et al.* Class III beta-tubulin expression and benefit from adjuvant cisplatin/vinorelbine chemotherapy in operable non-small cell lung cancer: analysis of NCIC JBR.10. *Clin Cancer Res* 2007; 13: 994–999.
48. Sweeney CJ, Zhu J, Sandler AB, *et al.* Outcome of patients with a performance status of 2 in Eastern Cooperative Oncology Group Study E1594: a Phase II trial in patients with metastatic nonsmall cell lung carcinoma. *Cancer* 2001; 92: 2639–2647.
49. Langer CJ, O'Byrne KJ, Socinski MA, *et al.* Phase III trial comparing paclitaxel poliglumex (CT-2103, PPX) in combination with carboplatin *versus* standard paclitaxel and carboplatin in the treatment of PS 2 patients with chemotherapy-naive advanced non-small cell lung cancer. *J Thorac Oncol* 2008; 3: 623–630.
50. Lilenbaum RC, Herndon JE 2nd, List MA, *et al.* Single-agent versus combination chemotherapy in advanced non-small-cell lung cancer: the cancer and leukemia group B (study 9730). *J Clin Oncol* 2005; 23: 190–196.
51. Kosmidis PA, Dimopoulos MA, Syrigos K, *et al.* Gemcitabine versus gemcitabine-carboplatin for patients with advanced non-small cell lung cancer and a performance status of 2: a prospective randomized phase II study of the Hellenic Cooperative Oncology Group. *J Thorac Oncol* 2007; 2: 135–140.

52. Pfister DG, Johnson DH, Azzoli CG, *et al.* American Society of Clinical Oncology treatment of unresectable non-small-cell lung cancer guideline: update 2003. *J Clin Oncol* 2004; 22: 330–353.
53. Lilenbaum R, Axelrod R, Thomas S, *et al.* Randomized phase II trial of erlotinib or standard chemotherapy in patients with advanced non-small-cell lung cancer and a performance status of 2. *J Clin Oncol* 2008; 26: 863–869.
54. Socinski MA, Crowell R, Hensing TE, *et al.* Treatment of non-small cell lung cancer, stage IV: ACCP evidence-based clinical practice guidelines (2nd edition). *Chest* 2007; 132: Suppl. 3, 277S–289S.
55. Earle CC, Tsai JS, Gelber RD, *et al.* Effectiveness of chemotherapy for advanced lung cancer in the elderly: instrumental variable and propensity analysis. *J Clin Oncol* 2001; 19: 1064–1070.
56. Hotta K, Ueoka H, Kiura K, *et al.* An overview of 48 elderly-specific clinical trials of systemic chemotherapy for advanced non-small cell lung cancer. *Lung Cancer* 2004; 46: 61–76.
57. Yee KW, Pater JL, Pho L, *et al.* Enrollment of older patients in cancer treatment trials in Canada: why is age a barrier? *J Clin Oncol* 2003; 21: 1618–1623.
58. Effects of vinorelbine on quality of life and survival of elderly patients with advanced non-small-cell lung cancer. The Elderly Lung Cancer Vinorelbine Italian Study Group. *J Natl Cancer Inst.* 1999; 91: 66–72.
59. Shepherd FA, Abratt RP, Anderson H, *et al.* Gemcitabine in the treatment of elderly patients with advanced non-small cell lung cancer. *Semin Oncol* 1997; 24: Suppl. 7, S7-50–S7-55.
60. Ricci S, Antonuzzo A, Galli L, *et al.* Gemcitabine monotherapy in elderly patients with advanced non-small cell lung cancer: a multicenter phase II study. *Lung Cancer* 2000; 27: 75–80.
61. Quoix E, Breton JL, Ducolone A, *et al.* First line chemotherapy with gemcitabine in advanced non-small cell lung cancer elderly patients: a randomized phase II study of 3-week *versus* 4-week schedule. *Lung Cancer* 2005; 47: 405–412.
62. Gridelli C, Perrone F, Gallo C, *et al.* Chemotherapy for elderly patients with advanced non-small-cell lung cancer: the Multicenter Italian Lung Cancer in the Elderly Study (MILES) phase III randomized trial. *J Natl Cancer Inst* 2003; 95: 362–372.
63. Pujol JL, Milleron B, Molinier O, *et al.* Weekly paclitaxel combined with monthly carboplatin in elderly patients with advanced non-small cell lung cancer: a multicenter phase II study. *J Thorac Oncol* 2006; 1: 328–334.
64. Shepherd FA, Dancey J, Ramlau R, *et al.* Prospective randomized trial of docetaxel versus best supportive care in patients with non-small-cell lung cancer previously treated with platinum-based chemotherapy. *J Clin Oncol* 2000; 18: 2095–2103.
65. Shepherd FA, Fossella FV, Lynch T, *et al.* Docetaxel (Taxotere) shows survival and quality-of-life benefits in the second-line treatment of non-small cell lung cancer: a review of two phase III trials. *Semin Oncol* 2001; 28: Suppl. 2, 4–9.
66. Fossella FV, DeVore R, Kerr RN, *et al.* Randomized phase III trial of docetaxel versus vinorelbine or ifosfamide in patients with advanced non-small-cell lung cancer previously treated with platinum-containing chemotherapy regimens. The TAX 320 Non-Small Cell Lung Cancer Study Group. *J Clin Oncol* 2000; 18: 2354–2362.
67. Hanna N, Shepherd FA, Fossella FV, *et al.* Randomized phase III trial of pemetrexed versus docetaxel in patients with non-small-cell lung cancer previously treated with chemotherapy. *J Clin Oncol* 2004; 22: 1589–1597.
68. Shepherd FA, Rodrigues Pereira J, Ciuleanu T, *et al.* Erlotinib in previously treated non-small-cell lung cancer. *N Engl J Med* 2005; 353: 123–132.
69. Massarelli E, Andre F, Liu DD, Ciuleanu TD, *et al.* A retrospective analysis of the outcome of patients who have received two prior chemotherapy regimens including platinum and docetaxel for recurrent non-small-cell lung cancer. *Lung Cancer* 2003; 39: 55–61.

CHAPTER 16

Targeted therapy in nonsmall cell lung cancer

D.F. Heigener, M. Reck, U. Gatzemeier

Dept of Thoracic Oncology, Krankenhaus Grosshansdorf, Grosshansdorf, Germany.

Correspondence: D.F. Heigener, Dept of Thoracic Oncology, Krankenhaus Grosshansdorf, Woehrendamm 80, 22927 Grosshansdorf, Germany. E-mail: D.Heigener@kh-grosshansdorf.de

Besides conventional chemotherapy, with the success of imantinib in the treatment of chronic myeloid leukaemia and gastrointestinal stromal tumours, as well as rituximab in lymphomas, a class of drugs emerged in oncology, the so-called "targeted therapies". The term is somewhat misleading, because every antineoplastic therapy has its target. The difference can best be described by the fact that most conventional chemotherapeutic agents act in the nucleus by inhibiting division of any rapidly dividing cells, whereas the so-called "targeted" agents inhibit pathways outside the nucleus (or even outside the cancer cell) that are crucial for malignant proliferation. Two pathways are currently of particular interest: the epidermal growth factor receptor (EGFR)-mediated pathway in the tumour cell and the vascular endothelial growth factor receptor (VEGFR)-mediated pathway in the endothelial cell, responsible for blood supply of the tumour. Both pathways can be inhibited at multiple steps.

Other approaches are vaccination against tumour-specific antigens or activation of apoptosis-promoting pathways.

EGFR

Malignant growth is promoted by the uncontrolled production and autocrine secretion of specific molecules, *e.g.* epidermal growth factor (EGF) by cancer cells and enhanced expression of matching receptors on their cell-surface (*i.e.* EGFR) [1]. There are four subtypes of transmembrane growth factor receptors: EGFR, HER2, HER3 and HER4. If a ligand binds to the extra cellular domain of EGFR, it couples with another EGFR, forming a homodimer, or with either HER2, -3 or -4, forming a heterodimer. This process leads to phosphorylation of the intracellular domain of the receptor. This activates multiple pathways, leading to cell cycle progression and anti-apoptotic signals (fig. 1).

The pathways can be inhibited in several ways: 1) at the extracellular domain of EGFR by monoclonal antibodies (*e.g.* cetuximab); 2) at the intracellular tyrosine kinase domain by tyrosine kinase inhibitors (TKIs; erlotinib, gefitinib and vandetanib); and 3) at the Raf kinase step by multikinase inhibitors (*e.g.* sorafenib).

Biomarkers

EGFR-blocking agents are more effective in terms of response and progression-free survival (PFS) in some subgroups of patients that can be described clinically

Eur Respir Mon, 2009, 44, 284–298. Printed in UK - all rights reserved. Copyright ERS Journals Ltd 2009; European Respiratory Monograph; ISSN 1025-448x.

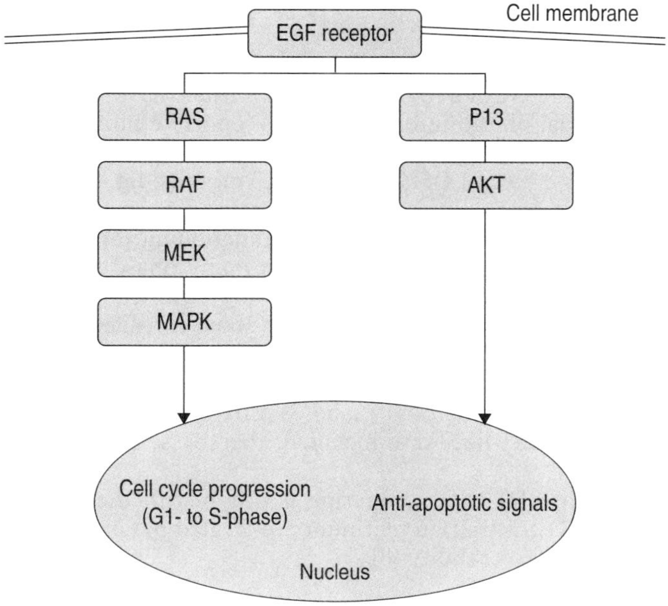

Fig. 1. – The epidermal growth factor (EGF) receptor pathways. MAPK: mitogen-activated protein kinase; MEK: MAPK kinase.

(*i.e.* female, Asian, never-smokers or adenocarcinoma) or in terms of tumour biology (such as mutations in exons 18 to 21 in the EGFR gene or high gene copy number measured with fluorescence in situ hybridisation). However, this phenomenon was investigated mainly in a retrospective manner, and the early studies lacked a control arm with another therapeutic agent. The question that could not be answered was whether these stated clinical and biological characteristics were either predictive (*i.e.* these factors predict a response to a special therapy) or prognostic (*i.e.* these factors influence the prognosis regardless of the subsequent therapy). An answer to this question came from the INTEREST trial, showing that patients with the abovementioned clinical and biological markers had prolonged survival compared with their counterparts, regardless of whether they were given the targeted agent gefitinib or the conventional chemotherapeutic agent docetaxel. There was only an advance in PFS but not overall survival (OS) with gefitinib in patients with exon 19 deletions. This shows that those factors seem to be mainly of prognostic nature [2].

Significant predictors of poor outcome with TKI therapy are Ras mutations. Ras is a guanosine triphosphate (GTP)-binding protein that acts downstream of EGFR. Mutation in its gene resulting in aberrant signalling renders upstream EGFR inhibition useless, thereby explaining the lack of efficacy of EGFR TKIs in this setting [3]. EGFR and K-Ras mutations mutually exclude each other.

Thus, the question of predictive clinical factors and biomarkers is not fully answered yet. Patient characteristics (especially smoking status) and biomarkers should be recorded in every forthcoming trial. However, this goal is not easy to reach because, especially in metastatic disease, the available tissue is often restricted to small biopsies or even fine-needle aspirates not suitable for extensive biomarker testing.

TKIs

Erlotinib and gefitinib. The landmark trials in TKIs, discussed in this section, are shown in table 1. In pre-treated patients several trials have been performed. In a randomised phase III trial of erlotinib *versus* best supportive care in pre-treated patients with nonsmall cell lung cancer (NSCLC; BR.21), erlotinib proved to be better in terms of response (8.9 *versus* <1%) and OS (6.7 *versus* 4.7 months; fig. 2) [4]. There was also a significant improvement in quality of life with erlotinib regarding main symptoms (cough, dyspnoea and pain) as well as physical functioning [5]. The biologically very similar drug gefitinib showed promising results in many phase II studies [6]; however, this could not be proven in a phase III trial showing significant advantages solely for Asians and never-smokers [7]. However, there are some considerations to make: 1) the placebo arm in this study performed unexpectedly well; 2) the dosage of gefitinib (250 mg·day^{-1}) was not the maximum tolerable dose (which is >700 mg·day^{-1}) as in the BR.21 trial with erlotinib (150 mg·day^{-1}); and 3) only primary progressive patients (*i.e.* failure <12 weeks) after first-line were included, thereby selecting the most aggressive tumours.

In a randomised phase III trial comparing gefitinib with the approved second-line agent docetaxel (INTEREST trial) in platinum pre-treated patients, gefitinib proved not to be inferior, with better tolerability [8].

Table 1. – Landmark trials with tyrosine kinase inhibitors

Trial	First author [ref.]	Design	Patients n	RR %	OS	p-value for OS	Message
BR.21[#]	Shepherd [4]	E	488	8.9	6.7 months	<0.001	E works in second-line
		Placebo	243	<1	4.7 months		
ISEL[#]	Thatcher [7]	G	1129	NA	5.6 months	0.087	G does not show a significant advantage in this population
		Placebo	563	NA	5.1 months		
INTEREST[¶]	Douillard [8]	G	733	9.1	7.6 months	0.3257	G and D are equally effective
		D	733	7.6	8.0 months		
TALENT[+]	Gatzemeier [9]	CG + E	580	31.5	43 weeks	0.49	E does not improve outcome with first-line chemotherapy in the overall population
		CG	579	29.9	44.1 weeks		
TRIBUTE[+]	Herbst [10]	CP + E	526	21.5	10.6 months	0.95	E does not improve outcome with first-line chemotherapy in the overall population
		CP	533	19.3	10.5 months		
INTACT I	Giaccone [11]	CG + 500 mg G	330	50.3	9.9 months	0.76	G does not improve outcome with first-line chemotherapy
		CG + 250 mg G	336	51.2	9.9 months		
		CG + placebo	324	47.2	10.9 months		
INTACT II	Herbst [12]	CP + 500 mg G	342	30	8.7 months	0.64	G does not improve outcome with first-line chemotherapy
		CP + 250 mg G	342	30.4	9.8 months		
		CP + placebo	341	28.7	9.9 months		

RR: response rate; OS: overall survival; ISEL: Iressa Survival Evaluation in Lung Cancer; INTEREST: Iressa in Nonsmall Cell Lung Cancer (NSCLC) Trial Evaluating Response and Survival *versus* Taxotere; TALENT: Tarceva Lung Cancer Investigation; TRIBUTE: Tarceva Responses in Conjunction with Paclitaxel and Carboplatin; INTACT: Iressa NSCLC Trial Assessing Combination Treatment; E: erlotinib; G: gefitinib; NA: not available; D: docetaxel; CG: cisplatin/gemcitabine; CP: carboplatin/paclitaxel. [#]: pre-treated patients; [¶]: platinum-pre-treated patients; [+]: first-line.

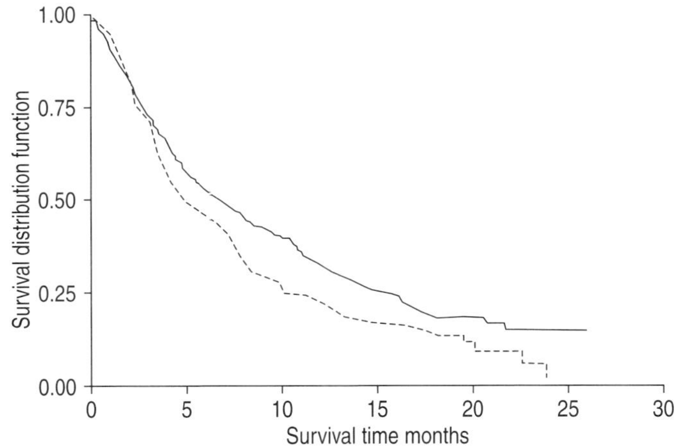

No. at risk						
Placebo 243	20	3	0	0	0	0
Erlotinib 488	115	27	2	1	0	0

Fig. 2. – Erlotinib (——) *versus* placebo (– – – –), showing overall survival. No.: number. Reproduced from [4] with permission from the publisher.

EGFR TKIs have been tested as first-line treatment in advanced disease concurrently with chemotherapy. In the TALENT trial comparing cisplatin/gemcitabine with cisplatin/gemcitabine plus erlotinib in first-line treatment, there was no significant difference in OS or time to progression between the groups. However, the subgroup of never-smokers had a better median survival, but the number (n=8) was too small for statistical analysis [9].

In the TRIBUTE trial comparing carboplatin/paclitaxel with carboplatin/paclitaxel plus erlotinib in first-line therapy of advanced NSCLC, it could be shown that never-smokers had a survival benefit of additional erlotinib compared with placebo, although there was no statistical significant difference in OS in the entire population [10].

Also, gefitinib was tested in this setting in two trials. INTACT I was a three-arm trial comparing cisplatin and gemcitabine with either 500 mg of gefitinib, 250 mg of gefitinib or placebo daily. There was no difference in PFS or OS between the three arms [11]. INTACT II had the same design, but the chemotherapy was carboplatin and paclitaxel instead of cisplatin and gemcitabine. Again there was no benefit to adding gefitinib to chemotherapy [12].

The fact that simultaneous chemotherapy plus EGFR TKI does not work in the majority of patients may be due to the different mechanism of action. The cytostatic effect of erlotinib causing cell cycle arrest might render the cells insensitive to the cytotoxic effect of chemotherapy. Trials with maintenance erlotinib after chemotherapy are ongoing.

The major side-effect of gefitinib and erlotinib is an acneiform rash developing within 2 weeks of initiation of therapy. There is a clear correlation between the extent of the rash and tumour response. The rash may diminish spontaneously over a few weeks. Urea-containing ointments, topical steroids or systemic antibiotics (*i.e.* doxycycline 100 mg·day^{-1}) are helpful, however many patients (especially on erlotinib) need dose reductions to control this side-effect. Other side-effects are diarrhoea (~5–10% of patients), liver enzyme elevation and interstitial lung disease (ILD). The latter usually manifests with cough, fever and bilateral interstitial shadowing on a chest radiograph.

It is reported to be fatal in 34% of cases. Treatment consists of high-dose corticosteroids [13, 14]. It occurs particularly in patients of East Asian ethnicity and was noted in ~1% of patients in a phase II trial of gefitinib [15]. There were no excess cases of ILD with erlotinib in the BR.21 study [4]; however, anecdotal case reports of ILD with erlotinib have been published [16].

Second generation TKIs. Many patients develop resistance to first generation TKIs, although they initially had a response. This is partly due to inherited, activating mutations in the EGFR gene or amplification of the MET oncogene, resulting in continuous signalling despite the presence of gefitinib or erlotinib. However, in 30–50% of cases, other, yet unknown mechanisms of resistance develop [17].

One promising agent to overcome activating mutations is BIBW 2992, an irreversible EGFR/HER2 TKI. In an enriched population with different EGFR mutations including activating mutations, 50% response rate and 87.5% disease control rate was achieved. The main toxicities were skin rash and diarrhoea, as with reversible TKIs. There is now a phase II/III trial ongoing, evaluating the agent in patients who have failed on erlotinib or gefitinib due to activating mutations [18].

Monoclonal antibodies

Cetuximab is a monoclonal antibody blocking EGFR on its extracellular domain. This results in interruption of the signalling pathways downstream, and downregulation of the receptor by internalisation and cleavage of the antibody–receptor complex from the cell surface. Another mechanism of action proposed is an antibody-dependent, cell-mediated cytotoxicity [19]. A phase III trial with 1,125 chemonaive patients with stage IIIB/IV NSCLC whose tumours were "EGFR positive" in immunhistochemistry (~80% of those screened) was recently presented in abstract form [20]. The addition of cetuximab to a platinum doublet (cisplatin and vinorelbine) followed by cetuximab maintenance showed significantly but small prolongation of OS (11.3 *versus* 10.1 months) compared with cisplatin and vinorelbine alone. However, PFS was similar (4.8 months in both groups). Interestingly, only Caucasian patients had an additional benefit from cetuximab (OS 10.5 *versus* 9.1 months), whereas Asians, although they had a significantly better OS regardless of therapy, had no additional benefit from the drug [20]. Another phase III trial compared carboplatin/taxane (paclitaxel or docetaxel according to the investigator's decision) with or without cetuximab. 676 patients were randomised. Preliminary results showed no difference in PFS; OS data are pending [21]. The main side-effect, as with EGFR TKIs, is severe skin toxicity occurring in 10% of patients.

VEGFR

In 1972, Folkman *et al.* [22] found that, from a certain size, a tumour cannot be supplied by diffusion alone but needs its own blood supply, a phenomenon termed "angiogenic switch". They postulated the existence of a factor secreted by the tumour to attract blood vessels to invade it [22]. This factor, called tumour angiogenic factor (TAF), was later identified as vascular endothelial growth factor (VEGF). The corresponding receptors on the endothelial cell are named VEGFR 1–3. VEGFR1, whose role in angiogenesis is not clear, has a binding affinity for VEGF 10 times higher than VEGFR2. However, its signal transducing capability is extremely weak. VEGFR2 is the major signalling receptor responsible for angiogenetic effects. VEGFR3 is responsible for lymphangiogenesis [23]. The idea of inhibiting this pathway led to the development of a monoclonal antibody (bevacizumab) that binds VEGF before it can dock on VEGFR and thereby inhibits blood vessel invasion of the tumour. However, although bevacizumab has proven effective in a variety of tumours, its mechanism of action is not that simple. Indeed, it does not only interrupt blood vessel supply leading to cell apoptosis in the tumour, but also "normalises" the aberrant tumour vasculature and thereby optimises the transport of cytotoxic agents and oxygen (as a radiosensitiser) into the tumour [24].

TKIs

As with EGFR, the intracellular domain of the receptor can be blocked with TKIs, as virtually all of them are multitargeted (also called multikinase or "dirty" inhibitors). There are many TKIs with VEGFR-blocking potential in clinical testing. Selected ones are shown in table 2. However, none is approved yet. The ones tested in advanced clinical trials will be briefly discussed in this section.

Vandetanib. Vandetanib has inhibitory effects on VEGFR and EGFR. It is not yet approved but is showing promising results. In a phase II trial, 168 pre-treated patients received either gefitinib or vandetanib with the option to cross over after disease progression. The PFS was significantly better with vandetanib (11 *versus* 8.1 weeks) [25]. In another three-arm, phase II trial, patients received 100 mg vandetanib, 300 mg vandetanib or placebo, all in combination with docetaxel in the second-line setting. The PFS was significantly better with 100 mg vandetanib *versus* placebo (18.7 *versus* 12 weeks) [26]. Rash is not that severe with this drug, maybe due to its lower affinity to EGFR. Other side-effects include QT prolongation, hypertension and the hand-foot-syndrome.

Sorafenib. The VEGF pathway, as well as the Raf kinase pathway downstream of EGFR (fig. 1), is inhibited by another multikinase TKI, sorafenib. Sorafenib is approved for second-line treatment of metastatic renal cell cancer, hepatocellular carcinoma and gastrointestinal stromal tumour (GIST). It mainly inhibits VEGF but has inhibitory potential on Raf as well. In a single-arm phase II trial, 55 patients received sorafenib. 59% achieved stable disease. Those patients had a PFS of 23.7 weeks

Table 2. – Vascular endothelial growth factor receptor (VEGFR)-blocking tyrosine kinase inhibitors

Name	Targets	Development	Side-effects
Sorafenib	VEGFR2, VEGFR3, Raf, PDGFR, KIT, FLT3	First-line phase III	Nausea/vomiting, hypertension, skin toxicity
Sunitinib	VEGFR1, VEGFR2, PDGFR, KIT, FLT3	First-line phase III	Nausea/vomiting, skin toxicity, hypertension, diarrhoea
Vandetanib	VEGFR2, VEGFR3, EGFR, RET	Second-line phase III	Diarrhoea, rash, QT prolongation
Vatalanib	VEGFR1, VEGFR2, VEGFR3, PDGFR, KIT, FMS	Second-line phase II	Nausea/vomiting, probably haemorrhage
Axitinib	VEGFR1, VEGFR2, VEGFR3, PDGFR, KIT	Second-line phase II	Nausea/vomiting, skin toxicity, hypertension
BIBF 1120	VEGFR1, VEGFR2, VEGFR3, PDGFR, FGFR	Second-line phase II	Nausea/vomiting, fatigue, abdominal pain

PDGFR: platelet-derived growth factor receptor; FLT: fms-related tyrosine kinase; EGFR: epidermal growth factor receptor; RET: "rearranged during transfection" proto-oncogene; QT: QT time in ECG; FGFR: fibroblast growth factor receptor.

[27]. In another phase II discontinuation trial, sorafenib showed promising results in an enriched, heavily pre-treated NSCLC population. All patients received the drug for 2 months. Those with partial remission continued on the drug, those with progression dropped out of the study. Patients with stable disease were randomised to sorafenib or placebo. In this study, PFS was significantly better for the sorafenib-treated patients (3.6 *versus* 1.9 months) [28]. There are two first-line trials with platinum doublets with or without sorafenib. The Evaluation of Sorafenib, Carboplatin and Paclitaxel Efficacy in NSCLC (ESCAPE) trial compared paclitaxel, carboplatin and sorafenib with carboplatin, paclitaxel and placebo. The accrual was stopped early as it became clear that the trial would not meet its primary end-point of improving OS. The outcome of patients with squamous histology even had excess mortality with sorafenib. The second trial, NSCLC Research Experience Utilizing Sorafenib (NEXUS), using the same design with cisplatin and gemcitabine as chemotherapy, is ongoing. However, patients with squamous histology will no longer be accrued, due to the results of the ESCAPE trial.

Sunitinib. Sunitinib is a multitargeted inhibitor of VEGFR, platelet-derived growth factor receptor (PDGFR), KIT and FMS. It is approved for first-line therapy of metastatic renal cell carcinoma and GIST. A phase II study in 63 pre-treated NSCLC patients showed a disease control rate of 52.5% with 23.9 weeks median survival [29]. In a phase I trial, previously untreated patients were given cisplatin and gemcitabine in combination with sunitinib. Dose-limiting toxicities were not observed and further testing is warranted [30]. Hypertension, fatigue, mucositis and diarrhoea are major side-effects of this agent.

BIBF 1120. BIBF 1120 is another TKI with VEGFR-, PDGFR- and fibroblast growth factor receptor (FGFR)-inhibiting properties. In a phase II study, 74 pre-treated patients with NSCLC received the drug. The disease control rate was 47% and the median PFS was 1.6 months, warranting further testing. The drug has a favourable toxicity profile, with abdominal pain, nausea and vomiting occurring in some patients [31].

Monoclonal antibodies

Bevacizumab. The landmark trials of bevacizumab are detailed in table 3. Bevacizumab is a monoclonal humanised antibody against VEGF. Its mechanism of action is described earlier in this chapter. In a phase III trial comparing carboplatin, paclitaxel and bevacizumab with carboplatin and paclitaxel alone in advanced NSCLC, the three-drug combination has shown to prolong both PFS and OS significantly. Median OS was prolonged to more than 1 yr for the first time in the treatment of NSCLC (fig. 3) [32].

A second trial, comparing cisplatin and gemcitabine alone with cisplatin, gemcitabine and bevacizumab in two doses (either 15 or 7.5 $mg \cdot m^{-2}$), showed significantly improved PFS for both bevacizumab arms over cisplatin and gemcitabine alone; however, OS was not significantly better for bevacizumab in this trial [33].

Major side-effects include pulmonary haemorrhage, seen in a phase-II study, especially in squamous histology. Therefore, squamous histology was omitted in all phase III trials. Another concern is intracranial haemorrhage, especially in patients with brain metastases. However, a recent study showed that bevacizumab might be safely used in those patients with brain metastases [34]. Other side-effects are hypertension, which can be managed with standard antihypertensive agents, and proteinuria, which is generally mild, seldom necessitating change of bevacizumab dose.

Table 3. – Phase III trials with bevacizumab (B)

Trial	First author [ref.]	Design	Patients n	RR %	PFS months	OS months	p-value	Message
ECOG 4599	SANDLER [32]	CP + B CP	434 444	35 15	6.2 4.5	12.3 10.3	0.003#	B significantly improved survival when added to CP
AVAiL	MANEGOLD [33]	CG + 7.5 mg·kg^{-1} B CG + 15 mg·kg^{-1} B CG	345 351 347	34 30 20	6.7 6.5 6.1	Data pending	0.002¶	B significantly improved PFS but not OS, with CG, even in a lower dose (7.5 mg·kg^{-1})

RR: response rate; PFS: progression-free survival; OS: overall survival; ECOG: Eastern Cooperative Oncology Group; AVAiL: AVAstin in Lung cancer; CP: carboplatin/paclitaxel; CG: cisplatin/gemcitabine. #: for OS; ¶: for 7.5 mg·kg^{-1} B *versus* placebo, for PFS.

Other drugs

Aflibercept. A soluble receptor of VEGFR 1 and 2 is aflibercept (also called "VEGF trap"), which binds to VEGF with high affinity. Aflibercept has shown promising activity in a phase II study as a single agent showing three partial remissions in 33 heavily pre-treated patients [35]. The main side-effects in this small group were dyspnoea, chest pain and hypertension. No major bleeding occurred. Aflibercept is now being tested with docetaxel *versus* docetaxel alone in the second-line setting.

Enzastaurin. The serine-threonine kinase inhibitor enzastaurin acts downstream of VEGF at a molecule called protein kinase (PK)Cβ, as well as in the P13/AKT pathway. In a phase II study with 55 patients with pre-treated, advanced NSCLC, the drug achieved an OS of 8.4 months and a 6-month PFS rate of 13%. The trial did not meet its primary end-point (6-month PFS rate of 20%) [36]; however, enzastaurin is being tested in further trials including combination therapy with pemetrexed in the second-line setting.

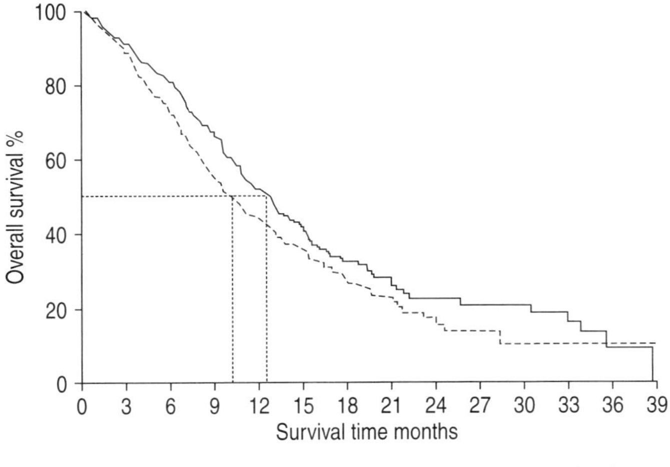

Fig. 3. – Carboplatin/paclitaxel with (——) and without (– – – –) bevacizumab, showing overall survival. ·····: median overall survival. Reproduced from [32] with permission from the publisher.

Other targets

Mapatumumab

Mapatumumab is a fully humanised agonistic antibody to a receptor called tumour necrosis factor (TNF)-related apoptosis-inducing ligand (TRAIL-R1). This receptor belongs to the TNF-α cytokine system. Activation of this receptor leads to cell death *via* apoptosis mediated by enzymes called caspases. Since TRAIL-R1 receptors are expressed on various cancer cells, it is an attractive target for treatment.

In a phase I trial, mapatumumab was given in combination with gemcitabine and cisplatin to patients with solid malignancies including patients with lung cancer. 49 patients were enrolled and the dose-limiting toxicities were those related to the chemotherapy with cisplatin and gemcitabine. There were no excess toxicities related to mapatumumab. Nine patients achieved a partial response and 13 achieved disease stabilisation [37]. A phase II/III trial has just started in the first-line setting for mapatumumab in combination with carboplatin and paclitaxel.

Vaccination

There are many approaches to stimulate the host defence against cancer cells. Recent advantages in the understanding of the immune system and modern engineering techniques have led to some successful vaccination strategies, some of which will be discussed in this section.

Melanoma-associated antigen A3 immunotherapy. Melanoma-associated antigen (MAGE)-A3 is a tumour-specific antigen not expressed in normal cells. It is found in ~35% of NSCLC patients in stages IB to IIB and 48% in stage III. A vaccine against this antigen was developed that shows some evidence of activity in patients with melanoma.

In a phase II study, 1,089 resection specimens of patients with stage pIB or pII NSCLC were screened for the antigen. Of these, 363 were positive. Of these, 182 entered the study and were randomised in a 2:1 design: 122 patients received MAGE-A3 intramuscularly every 3 weeks for a total of five injections followed by eight injections every 3 months; 60 patients received placebo. The agent was well tolerated, with only three patients experiencing grade III adverse events attributed to the vaccination and only one withdrawal. The recurrence rates for MAGE-A3 and placebo were 30.6 and 43.3%, respectively, after a median follow-up of 28 months. Deaths occurred in 21.3 and 31.6%, respectively. Disease-free survival and OS showed a trend towards better outcome with the vaccine ($p=0.093$ and $p=0.088$, respectively) [38]. These encouraging results led to another trial that is in progress with four cohorts: vaccination concurrent with adjuvant chemotherapy, after adjuvant chemotherapy, without adjuvant chemotherapy and after chemoradiation (thereby including the most common adjuvant settings).

TG 4010. Mucin (MUC)-1 is a tumour-associated antigen. TG 4010 is a vaccination consisting of a recombinant vector (a highly attenuated virus called vaccinia virus Ankara) coding for MUC-1 and interleukin (IL)-2. In a recently presented trial, 148 patients with advanced disease (stage IIIB with pleural effusion or stage IV) were randomised to receive cisplatin, gemcitabine and TG 4010 (the latter until disease progression) or cisplatin and gemcitabine alone. The primary end-point was PFS at 6 months, which was 44% in the vaccination arm and 35% in the control arm ($p=0.13$). The response rate was significantly better with vaccination (43 *versus* 27%; $p=0.03$).

Long-term survival data are not yet published. Side-effects were minimal, including injection site reactions and abdominal pain [39].

L-BLP25. Another vaccine against MUC-1 is L-BLP25 (Stimuvax®), a liposome vaccine targeted to the extracellular core peptide of MUC-1. In a randomised phase II trial including patients with stage III/IV NSCLC who responded or were at least stable after chemotherapy, patients were randomised to vaccination *versus* observation. The vaccine was administered weekly for 8 weeks, with maintenance therapy every 6 weeks thereafter if feasible. All patients received a single infusion of cyclophosphamide before vaccination to reduce activity of suppressor T-cells. Median OS was 17.4 months for vaccination *versus* 13.0 months for control ($p=0.66$). In the subgroup of IIIB patients the median survival has not been reached and results are pending [40]. Additionally, this agent was well tolerated, with flu-like symptoms as the main side-effect.

PF-3512676. Toll-like receptors (TLRs) regulate antigen-specific innate immunity. TLR-9 is a receptor expressed on B- and T-lymphocytes. Activation is believed to reduce immune tolerance, thereby enhancing the recognition of tumour-associated antigens. PF-3512676 is a TLR-9 agonist In a phase II trial, 112 chemonaive patients with stage IIIB/IV NSCLC received carboplatin and paclitaxel with or without concurrent vaccination. There was a trend for improved survival in the vaccination arm, justifying two further phase III studies. In one trial, PF-3512676 was combined with cisplatin and gemcitabine (CGP) and compared with cisplatin and gemcitabine alone (CG) in chemonaive patients with advanced NSCLC. In an interim analysis, injection-site reactions occurred in 62% of patients in the CGP arm (8% grade III or IV). There was no increment in either OS (CGP: 120 deaths; CG: 118 deaths) or PFS (CGP: 4.9 months; CG: 5.1 months). Due to additional toxicity and lack of incremental efficacy, the trial was terminated [41]. The other trial had a similar design, but with a different chemotherapy: carboplatin and paclitaxel. Again, no increment in OS or PFS for vaccination was detected in an interim analysis, resulting in termination of the study [42].

Current recommendations on the use of targeted drugs

Adjuvant and neoadjuvant treatment

There is no targeted agent approved in adjuvant and neoadjuvant treatment; however, some phase III trials are under way. One approach is maintenance therapy after surgery and adjuvant chemotherapy with erlotinib for up to 2 yrs (Randomized Double-Blind Trial in Adjuvant NSCLC with Tarceva (RADIANT) trial).

As aforementioned, the adjuvant setting theoretically seems to be ideal for vaccination strategies: the tumour burden is extremely low allowing immunological control of residual disease. However, phase III data of this approach are lacking and trials are ongoing.

Treatment of locally advanced disease

Chemoradiotherapy is the mainstay of therapy in locally advanced disease. There is no targeted drug approved in this setting as yet. Cetuximab might be an attractive combination partner with radiotherapy, as shown in head and neck cancer. To date, there are some feasibility studies showing that this might work. After platinum-containing induction chemotherapy, 12 patients with locally advanced NSCLC received concomitant radiation (64 Gy in 32 fractions) and weekly cetuximab. Nine patients completed the schedule and eight were alive after 1 yr. One patient had a grade III pneumonitis. This is an acceptable result and further studies of this approach are warranted [43].

Adjuvant treatment with gefitinib after chemoradiation was tested in the Southwest Oncology Group (SWOG) S0023 trial. Patients with previously untreated stage III NSCLC received concomitant cisplatin and etoposide with thoracic irradiation of up to 61 Gy followed by three cycles of consolidation with docetaxel. Those patients who did not progress after this schedule were randomised to either gefitinib or placebo until disease progression. The trial was terminated early after accrual of 243 patients, as it became clear that it would not meet its primary end-point. At a median follow-up of 27 months, the OS was 23 months for gefitinib and 35 months for placebo. Toxicity-related deaths were 2% for gefitinib and 0% for placebo. The increment in deaths in the gefitinib group was due to tumour progression for an unknown reason [44]. Thus, adjuvant EGFR TKI therapy in stage III cannot be recommended.

Palliative treatment

First-line. The only approved targeted drug to date in first-line palliative treatment is bevacizumab in combination with platinum-based therapy in advanced NSCLC with nonsquamous histology. As previously stated, the presence of brain metastases might not be an exclusion criterion according to current studies. Therapy should include up to six cycles of combination therapy followed by bevacizumab maintenance; however, the optimal duration of bevacizumab therapy is not known. Bevacizumab has a high response rate and is feasible for patients with a high tumour burden. There is only mild subjective toxicity, so treatment is well accepted by the patients.

Cetuximab has also been shown to improve survival in combination with a platinum doublet, compared with the doublet alone. It is likely to be approved for first-line therapy in EGFR-positive patients. It might also be a good choice for patients with squamous histology where bevacizumab is not approved. One must keep in mind that skin toxicity can be tremendous.

Our conclusion is that cetuximab or bevacizumab can be considered as a third agent in combination with a platinum doublet in first-line treatment. Cetuximab can be safely used in patients with haemoptysis and all histological subtypes, including squamous cell cancers, where bevacizumab is not approved. Bevacizumab can be used in all nonsquamous subtypes in the absence of bleeding. Unless further trials clarify this issue, decisions should be made on an individual basis.

Concurrent admission of VEGFR or EGFR TKIs to a platinum doublet is restricted to clinical trials as well as sequential administration of those drugs. Vaccination is performed in clinical trials only and has also not entered clinical routine yet.

Second- and third-line. Monotherapy with erlotinib and gefitinib in the second- or third-line setting is as effective as chemotherapy (*i.e.* with docetaxel). In our opinion, current data do not support the practice of precluding patients with squamous histology or smoking history from treatment with these drugs. Ras mutational status as a potentially predictive factor has to be investigated further.

There is to date no indication for combination therapy in the second-line setting; however, many studies combining chemotherapy with a targeted agent are under way.

Treatment of the elderly

It is common sense that age alone should not preclude patients from effective chemotherapy. Additionally, in the elderly with good performance status, a platinum doublet is the standard therapy in advanced disease. However, due to the fact that elderly people tend to have more comorbidity and a poor performance status, alternatives are clearly needed.

A randomised phase II trial is currently under way investigating whether erlotinib is a reasonable alternative to first-line carboplatin/vinorelbine in patients aged $\geq$70 yrs. Recruitment was completed in 2008.

In a retrospective subgroup analysis, the addition of bevacizumab to a platinum doublet showed excess toxicity without obvious improvement, compared with a platinum doublet alone [45]. According to those data, bevacizumab should not be given to elderly patients on a routine basis; however, prospective studies are needed to clear this issue.

Summary

There are numerous targeted approaches under investigation, and mentioning them all is beyond the scope of this chapter. The only approved substances are erlotinib, bevacizumab and gefitinib; the latter not in Europe. Cetuximab has proven to be effective as additional treatment in the first-line setting of advanced disease and is awaiting approval. Beyond that, we have to await many phase III trials for further effective drugs. Combination trials of agents with different targets (*e.g.* epidermal growth factor receptor and vascular endothelial growth factor receptor) are under way.

Keywords: Epidermal growth factor receptor, monoclonal antibodies, targeted therapy, tyrosine kinase inhibitors, vaccination, vascular endothelial growth factor.

Statement of interest

D.F. Heigener received speaking fees from Roche, manufacturer of some targeted therapies mentioned in this chapter. M. Reck received honoraria and reimbursement for attending conferences from Roche, Lilly and Pierre Fabre. He received speakers' honoraria from Roche, Lilly, Merck, Pfizer and AstraZeneca, and consulting fees from Roche, Lilly, Pfizer, Merck and AstraZeneca. U. Gatzemeier received honoraria and reimbursement for attending conferences from Roche, AstraZeneca, Bayer, Merck and Lilly. He received speakers' honoraria from Novartis, GlaxoSmithKline, Lilly, Roche, AstraZeneca, Bayer and Pierre Fabre, and consulting fees from Roche, Lilly, Novartis, Merck and AstraZeneca.

References

1. Sporn MB, Todaro GJ. Autocrine secretion and malignant transformation of cells. *N Engl J Med* 1980; 303: 878–880.
2. Douillard JY, Hirsh V, Mok TS, *et al.* Molecular and clinical subgroup analyses from a phase III trial comparing gefitinib with docetaxel in previously treated non-small cell lung cancer (INTEREST). *J Clin Oncol* 2008; 26: Suppl. 15, 8001.

3. Eberhard DA, Johnson BE, Amler LC, *et al.* Mutations in the epidermal growth factor receptor and in KRAS are predictive and prognostic indicators in patients with non-small-cell lung cancer treated with chemotherapy alone and in combination with erlotinib. *J Clin Oncol* 2005; 23: 5900–5909.
4. Shepherd FA, Rodrigues Pereira J, Ciuleanu T, *et al.* Erlotinib in previously treated non-small-cell lung cancer. *N Engl J Med* 2005; 353: 123–132.
5. Bezjak A, Tu D, Seymour L, *et al.* Symptom improvement in lung cancer patients treated with erlotinib: quality of life analysis of the National Cancer Institute of Canada Clinical Trials Group Study BR.21. *J Clin Oncol* 2006; 24: 3831–3837.
6. Kris MG, Natale RB, Herbst RS, *et al.* Efficacy of gefitinib, an inhibitor of the epidermal growth factor receptor tyrosine kinase, in symptomatic patients with non-small cell lung cancer: a randomized trial. *JAMA* 2003; 290: 2149–2158.
7. Thatcher N, Chang A, Parikh P, *et al.* Gefitinib plus best supportive care in previously treated patients with refractory advanced non-small-cell lung cancer: results from a randomised, placebo-controlled, multicentre study (IRESSA Survival Evaluation in Lung Cancer). *Lancet* 2005; 366: 1527–1537.
8. Kim ES, Hirsh V, Mok T, *et al.* Gefitinib *versus* docetaxel in previously treated non-small-cell lung cancer (INTEREST): a randomised phase III trial. *Lancet* 2008; 372: 1809–1818.
9. Gatzemeier U, Pluzanska A, Szczesna A, *et al.* Phase III study of erlotinib in combination with cisplatin and gemcitabine in advanced non-small-cell lung cancer: the Tarceva Lung Cancer Investigation Trial. *J Clin Oncol* 2007; 25: 1545–1552.
10. Herbst RS, Prager D, Hermann R, *et al.* TRIBUTE: a phase III trial of erlotinib hydrochloride (OSI-774) combined with carboplatin and paclitaxel chemotherapy in advanced non-small-cell lung cancer. *J Clin Oncol* 2005; 23: 5892–5899.
11. Giaccone G, Herbst RS, Manegold C, *et al.* Gefitinib in combination with gemcitabine and cisplatin in advanced non-small-cell lung cancer: a phase III trial – INTACT 1. *J Clin Oncol* 2004; 22: 777–784.
12. Herbst RS, Giaccone G, Schiller JH, *et al.* Gefitinib in combination with paclitaxel and carboplatin in advanced non-small-cell lung cancer: a phase III trial – INTACT 2. *J Clin Oncol* 2004; 22: 785–794.
13. Endo M, Johkoh T, Kimura K, *et al.* Imaging of gefitinib-related interstitial lung disease: multi-institutional analysis by the West Japan Thoracic Oncology Group. *Lung Cancer* 2006; 52: 135–140.
14. Sessa C, Hansen HH. Appendix: Chemotherapy. *In*: Hansen HH, ed. Textbook of Lung Cancer. 2nd Edn. London, Informa Healthcare, 2008; pp. 275–329.
15. Fukuoka M, Yano S, Giaccone G, *et al.* Multi-institutional randomized phase II trial of gefitinib for previously treated patients with advanced non-small-cell lung cancer (The IDEAL 1 Trial). *J Clin Oncol* 2003; 21: 2237–2246.
16. Liu V, White DA, Zakowski MF, *et al.* Pulmonary toxicity associated with erlotinib. *Chest* 2007; 132: 1042–1044.
17. Riely GJ. Second-generation epidermal growth factor receptor tyrosine kinase inhibitors in non-small cell lung cancer. *J Thorac Oncol* 2008; 3: Suppl. 2, 146–149.
18. Yang C, Shih J, Chao T, *et al.* Use of BIBW 2992, a novel irreversible EGFR/HER2 TKI, to induce regression in patients with adenocarcinoma of the lung and activating EGFR mutations: preliminary results of a single-arm phase II clinical trial. *J Clin Oncol* 2008; 26: Suppl. 15, 8026.
19. Ciardiello F, Tortora G. EGFR antagonists in cancer treatment. *N Engl J Med* 2008; 358: 1160–1174.
20. Pirker R, Sczcesna A, von Pawel J, *et al.* FLEX: a randomized, multicenter, phase III study of cetuximab in combination with cisplatin/vinorelbine (CV) *versus* CV alone in the first-line treatment of patients with advanced non-small cell lung cancer (NSCLC). *J Clin Oncol* 2008; 26: Suppl. 15, 3.

21. Lynch T, Patel T, Dreisbach L, *et al.* A randomized multicenter phase III study of cetuximab (Erbitux®) in combination with Taxane/Carboplatin *versus* Taxane/Carboplatin alone as first-line treatment for patients with advanced/metastatic non-small cell lung cancer (NSCLC): B3-03. *J Thorac Oncol*, 2: Suppl. 4, S340–S341.
22. Folkman J, Merler E, Abernathy C, *et al.* Isolation of a tumor factor responsible for angiogenesis. *J Exp Med* 1971; 133: 275–288.
23. Kerbel RS. Tumor angiogenesis. *N Engl J Med* 2008; 358: 2039–2049.
24. Duda DG, Jain RK, Willett CG. Antiangiogenics: the potential role of integrating this novel treatment modality with chemoradiation for solid cancers. *J Clin Oncol* 2007; 25: 4033–4042.
25. Natale RB, Bodkin D, Govindan R, *et al.* Vandetanib *versus* gefitinib in patients with advanced non-small-cell lung cancer: results from a two-part, double-blind, randomized phase II study. *J Clin Oncol* 2009; [Epub ahead of print PMID: 19332730].
26. Heymach JV, Johnson BE, Prager D, *et al.* Randomized, placebo-controlled phase II study of vandetanib plus docetaxel in previously treated non small-cell lung cancer. *J Clin Oncol* 2007; 25: 4270–4277.
27. Gatzemeier U, Blumenschein G, Fosella F, *et al.* Phase II trial of single-agent sorafenib in patients with advanced non-small cell lung carcinoma. *J Clin Oncol* 2006; 24: Suppl. 18, 7002.
28. Schiller JH, Lee JW, Hanna NH, *et al.* A randomized discontinuation phase II study of sorafenib *versus* placebo in patients with non-small cell lung cancer who have failed at least two prior chemotherapy regimens: E2501. *J Clin Oncol* 2008; 26: Suppl. 15, 8014.
29. Socinski MA, Novello S, Brahmer JR, *et al.* Multicenter, phase II trial of sunitinib in previously treated, advanced non-small-cell lung cancer. *J Clin Oncol* 2008; 26: 650–656.
30. Reck M, Frickhofen N, Gatzemeier U, *et al.* A phase I dose escalation study of sunitinib in combination with gemcitabine + cisplatin for advanced non-small cell lung cancer (NSCLC). *J Clin Oncol* 2007; 25: Suppl. 18, 18057.
31. Von Pawel J, Kaiser R, Eschbach C, *et al.* A double blind phase II study of BIBF 1120 in patients suffering from relapsed advanced non-small cell lung cancer (NSCLC). *J Clin Oncol* 2007; 25: Suppl. 18, 7635.
32. Sandler A, Gray R, Perry MC, *et al.* Paclitaxel-carboplatin alone or with bevacizumab for non-small-cell lung cancer. *N Engl J Med* 2006; 355: 2542–2550.
33. Reck M, von Pawel J, Zatloukal P, *et al.* Phase III trial of cisplatin plus gemcitabine with either placebo or bevacizumab as first-line therapy for nonsquamous non-small-cell lung cancer: AVAil. *J Clin Oncol* 2009; 27: 1227–1234.
34. Akerley WL, Langer CJ, Oh Y, *et al.* Acceptable safety of bevacizumab therapy in patients with brain metastases due to non-small cell lung cancer. *J Clin Oncol* 2008; 26: Suppl. 15, 8043.
35. Massarelli E, Miller VA, Leighl NB, *et al.* Phase II study of the efficacy and safety of intravenous (IV) AVE0005 (VEGF Trap) given every 2 weeks in patients (Pts) with platinum- and erlotinib-resistant adenocarcinoma of the lung (NSCLA). *J Clin Oncol* 2007; 25: Suppl. 18, 7627.
36. Oh Y, Herbst RS, Burris H, *et al.* Enzastaurin, an oral serine/threonine kinase inhibitor, as second- or third-line therapy of non-small-cell lung cancer. *J Clin Oncol* 2008; 26: 1135–1141.
37. Oldenhuis C, Mom C, Sleijfer S, *et al.* A phase I study with the agonistic TRAIL-R1 antibody, mapatumumab, in combination with gemcitabine and cisplatin. *J Clin Oncol* 2008; 26: Suppl. 15, 3540.
38. Vansteenkiste J, Zielinski M, Linder A, *et al.* Final results of a multi-center, double-blind, randomized, placebo-controlled phase II study to assess the efficacy of MAGE-A3 immunotherapeutic as adjuvant therapy in stage IB/II non-small cell lung cancer (NSCLC). *J Clin Oncol* 2007; 25: Suppl. 18, 7554.
39. Ramlau R, Westeel V, Papai, *et al.* Randomized phase IIb trial evaluating the therapeutic vaccine TG4010 (MVA-MUC1-IL2) as an adjunct to chemotherapy in patients with advanced non-small cell lung cancer (NSCLC). *J Clin Oncol* 2008; 26: Suppl. 15, 8023.
40. Bradbury PA, Shepherd FA. Immunotherapy for lung cancer. *J Thorac Oncol* 2008; 3: Suppl. 2, S164–S170.

41. Manegold C, Thatcher N, Benner RJ, *et al.* Randomized phase III trial of gemcitabine/cisplatin with or without PF-3512676 as first line treatment of advanced non-small cell lung cancer (NSCLC). *J Clin Oncol* 2008; 26: Suppl. 15, 8017.
42. Hirsh V, Boyer M, Rosell R, *et al.* Randomized phase III trial of paclitaxel/carboplatin with or without PF-3512676 as first line treatment of advanced non-small cell lung cancer (NSCLC). *J Clin Oncol* 2008; 26: Suppl. 15, 8016.
43. Hughes S, Liong J, Miah A, *et al.* A brief report on the safety study of induction chemotherapy followed by synchronous radiotherapy and cetuximab in stage III non-small cell lung cancer (NSCLC): SCRATCH study. *J Thorac Oncol* 2008; 3: 648–651.
44. Kelly K, Chansky K, Gaspar LE, *et al.* Phase III trial of maintenance gefitinib or placebo after concurrent chemoradiotherapy and docetaxel consolidation in inoperable stage III non-small-cell lung cancer: SWOG S0023. *J Clin Oncol* 2008; 26: 2450–2456.
45. Ramalingam SS, Dahlberg SE, Langer CJ, *et al.* Outcomes for elderly, advanced-stage non small-cell lung cancer patients treated with bevacizumab in combination with carboplatin and paclitaxel: analysis of Eastern Cooperative Oncology Group Trial 4599. *J Clin Oncol* 2008; 26: 60–65.

CHAPTER 17

Treatment of limited disease-small cell lung cancer

D. De Ruysscher*, C. Pöttgen#, H.J.M. Groen¶, S.M. Bentzen+

*Dept of Radiation Oncology (Maastro Clinic), University Medical Center Maastricht, GROW Research Institute, Maastricht and ¶Dept of Pulmonary Diseases, University Medical Center Groningen, Groningen, The Netherlands, #Dept of Radiotherapy, University of Duisburg-Essen, Essen, Germany, and +Dept of Human Oncology, University of Wisconsin School of Medicine and Public Health, Madison, WI, USA.

Correspondence: D. De Ruysscher, Dept of Radiation Oncology (Maastro Clinic), University Medical Center Maastricht, GROW Research Institute, Dr. Tanslaan 12, NL-6229 ET Maastricht, The Netherlands. Fax: 31 884455773; E-mail: dirk.deruysscher@maastro.nl

Small cell lung cancer (SCLC) accounts for 10–15% of all lung cancers [1], and this disease is characterised by rapid growth, with volume doubling times of approximately 30 days and early seeding of distant metastases [2]. Approximately 20% of SCLC patients present with so-called limited disease (LD) and are potentially amenable to treatment with curative intent.

The definition of LD-SCLC varies across studies and time eras. The first, still widely used, staging system for SCLC was introduced in the 1950s by the Veterans' Administration Lung Study Group (VALSG) and divided SCLC into two subgroups: limited and extensive disease [3]. LD was defined as tumours confined to one hemithorax, although local extension and ipsilateral, supraclavicular nodes could also be present provided they could be encompassed in the same radiation portal as the primary tumour. No extrathoracic metastases could be present. All other disease was classified as extensive disease (ED). In 1989, the International Association for the Study of Lung Cancer (IASLC) introduced changes to the VALSG staging system, suggesting that LD should be expanded to include tumours limited to one hemithorax with regional lymph node metastases, including hilar, ipsilateral and contralateral mediastinal, and ipsilateral and contralateral supraclavicular nodes [4]. They also recommended that patients with ipsilateral pleural effusion, regardless of whether cytology is positive or negative, be considered to have LD if no extrathoracic metastases were detected. The "tumour, node, metastasis" (TNM) staging systems [5, 6] are also applicable to SCLC, but have been used less frequently in clinical practice, although recently the use of the TNM system has been advocated [7]. As the definition of LD-SCLC has varied between clinical trials, and inclusion criteria such as the size of the mediastinal lymph nodes along with patient characteristics also vary, outcome comparisons between trials is very difficult.

As the overwhelming majority of patients with LD-SCLC have subclinical systemic disease at the time of presentation, chemotherapy has become an essential part of the treatment. The current agents of choice and the possible future role of targeted agents will be discussed in this chapter.

A logical question is whether the addition of a local treatment affects survival. Surgery is in most cases not possible because of the local extent of the tumour or lymph nodes, but might be considered in rare, early stages [8]. For the majority of patients, chest radiotherapy is the most important local therapy.

Eur Respir Mon, 2009, 44, 299–309. Printed in UK - all rights reserved. Copyright ERS Journals Ltd 2009; European Respiratory Monograph; ISSN 1025-448x.

Two meta-analyses have shown a 5.4% improvement in 3-yr overall survival in patients who received chest irradiation in addition to chemotherapy *versus* chemotherapy alone [9, 10]. However, the 5-yr survival remained disappointingly low at 10–15%. The two meta-analyses provide evidence that chemotherapy should be supplemented with chest irradiation. The best way to combine the two modalities will be addressed.

As brain metastases are common in LD-SCLC after primary treatment, the role of prophylactic cranial irradiation (PCI) has been investigated in depth. These items will be discussed in the following paragraphs.

Systemic treatment

The most effective agents in SCLC are alkylating agents (cisplatin, carboplatin, ifosfamide and cyclophosphamide), antimitotic agents (vincristine and paclitaxel) and topoisomerase inhibitors (etoposide, irinotecan, topotecan and doxorubicin). In both ED- and LD-SCLC, the chemotherapy schedule of first choice is the combination of a platinum drug and etoposide (see chapter 18). In LD-SCLC the most common choice is cisplatin and etoposide (PE). This schedule has been compared with cyclophosphamide, etoposide and vincristine (CEV) in a prospective randomised trial by the Norwegian Lung Cancer Study Group [11]. A total of 436 eligible patients were randomised to chemotherapy with PE (n=218) or CEV (n=218). Of the whole group, 214 had LD and 222 had ED. The PE group received five cycles of etoposide at 100 mg·m^{-2} *i.v.* and cisplatin at 75 mg·m^{-2} *i.v.* on day 1, followed by oral etoposide 200 mg·m^{-2}·day^{-1} on days 2–4. The CEV group received five courses of epirubicin at 50 mg·m^{-2}, cyclophosphamide at 1,000 mg·m^{-2} and vincristine at 2 mg, all *i.v.*, on day 1. In addition, patients with LD received chest radiation concurrently with cycle three of the chemotherapy, and those achieving a complete remission (CR) received PCI. The 2-yr and 5-yr survival rates in the PE arm (14 and 5%) were significantly higher (p=0.0004) than those in the CEV arm (6 and 2%). Among patients with LD, the median survival time was 14.5 months *versus* 9.7 months, in the PE and CEV arms, respectively (p=0.001). The 2-yr and 5-year survival rates of 25 and 10% in the PE arm compared with 8 and 3% in the CEV arm (p=0.0001). Quality-of-life assessments revealed no major differences between the randomised groups. PE is thus superior to CEV in patients with LD-SCLC.

To improve outcome, several drugs have been added and new regimens have been explored. Paclitaxel added to standard cisplatin and etoposide and thoracic radiotherapy did not give any added benefit [12]. This is in line with the results from three randomised trials in ED-SCLC that did not show improved median survival rates from adding paclitaxel. Adding gemcitabine or epirubicin has also been disappointing. Novel systemic approaches with tamoxifen also failed to demonstrate any benefit in phase III studies [13].

Among the new agents, topoisomerase II inhibitors such as irinotecan and topotecan were an exception, with excellent results in Japanese but not in Caucasian patients (see chapter 18 in this *European Respiratory Monograph*). Unfortunately, several combinations with topoisomerase I and II inhibitors, cisplatin and thoracic radiotherapy did not yield impressive results [14, 15]. Other approaches to improving outcome in LD-SCLC have included dose-intense regimens using either growth factors or stem-cell support [16–18]. However, all these trials only showed very modest gains in outcome.

We thus conclude that cisplatin and etoposide is the recommended chemotherapy regimen to combine with thoracic radiotherapy in the treatment of limited-stage SCLC.

Thoracic radiotherapy

SCLC is very responsive to radiotherapy, with rapid tumour shrinkage seen in the majority of patients. However, >30% of the patients develop local tumour progression, even with the best available concurrent chemoradiation regimen [19]. Thus, although SCLC is very radioresponsive, it is not easily controlled locally.

Important questions to be addressed are as follows. 1) What is the optimal radiation dose and fractionation? 2) What are the target volumes? 3) What is the best timing, sequencing and overall treatment time? These items have been also reviewed previously [20].

What is the optimal radiation dose and fractionation?

The effect of the radiation dose on local tumour control was studied in only one phase III trial. In this study, patients were randomised between 25 Gy in 10 fractions in 2 weeks or 37.5 Gy in 15 fractions in 3 weeks. The 2-yr local recurrence rate was 80% for the lower *versus* 63% for the higher dose ($p<0.05$). However, according to the linear-quadratic model with an assumed α/β ratio of 10 Gy for the tumour and no proliferation in 15 days, even the highest dose of 37.5 Gy in 15 fractions over 3 weeks is only equivalent to 39 Gy in daily fractions of 2 Gy, a dose which is still low.

We therefore have to consider data from nonrandomised, retrospective and prospective studies, to evaluate the effect of higher doses on local control. From literature review, it seems that the major improvement in local control is achieved when the dose is increased from 35 to 40 Gy, with possibly a modest gain of 10% with a further escalation to 50 Gy, mostly delivered in fractions ranging from 2 to 3 Gy [20]. With doses of <40 Gy, local control ranged from 0 to 31%; with doses of 40 Gy, local control was 57–77%; with 45 Gy, it was 58–84%; with 50 Gy, it was 58–75%; and with doses of >60 Gy local control ranged from 53 to 96%. However, these data should be taken with a pinch of salt as they are derived from studies with a wide variety in the irradiated volume, the overall treatment time and the type and sequence of chemotherapy.

In a small phase II study using an alternating radiation/chemotherapy schedule, the radiation dose was escalated from 45 to 65 Gy but a better local control rate was not found with the higher doses [20]. The local control was 58% with a dose of 45 Gy, 75% by giving 50 Gy, and ranged from 53 to 62% when >60 Gy was delivered. However, because an alternating schedule was used, it is not possible to extrapolate the conclusions about the effect of dose escalation to continuous radiation programmes. In Radiation Therapy Oncology Group (RTOG) 97-12, a phase I study, it was established that the maximal tolerated dose of accelerated radiation, delivered with concurrent cisplatin and etoposide, was 61.2 Gy in 5 weeks [21].

At the present time, it is not possible to draw definitive conclusions regarding radiation dose–response effects in LD-SCLC.

Little is known about the fractionation sensitivity of SCLC compared with that of the critical normal tissues. Thus, it is not clear whether an improved efficacy:toxicity ratio could be obtained by decreasing the dose per fraction below 1.8 Gy, *e.g.* employing a hyperfractionated regimen.

What are the target volumes?

The appropriate target volume was investigated in only one randomised trial by the Southwest Oncology Group (SWOG), where 466 patients with LD-SCLC were stratified according to their response to induction chemotherapy.

Patients having obtained a CR were randomised to wide-volume radiation followed by chemotherapy, or to further chemotherapy only. Wide-volume fields included the pre-chemotherapy tumour plus the mediastinum and a margin with "all surrounding abnormal-appearing lung" to a dose of 30 Gy in 10 fractions in 2 weeks. After a rest period of 2 weeks, 30 Gy in 12 fractions in 2.5 weeks was delivered to the post-chemotherapy tumour volume with a margin of 2 cm. Patients with a partial remission (PR) or stable disease (SD) were randomised to either wide-volume radiotherapy followed by further chemotherapy or reduced-field radiotherapy followed by further chemotherapy. Reduced-volume radiation fields included only the post-chemotherapy tumour volume with a margin of 2 cm. The dose and fractionation was the same as used in the wide-field arm. Patients with disease progression after induction chemotherapy (9% of the total number) were excluded from the study. From the 191 patients who obtained a PR or SD after chemotherapy, 93 received wide-volume radiotherapy and 98 reduced-volume radiotherapy. The local recurrence was 32 and 28%, respectively, a nonsignificant difference. Patients with a CR after chemotherapy who were irradiated had a 50% local recurrence rate, while this was 72% for those without radiotherapy ($p<0.01$). Interestingly, the median survival of patients achieving a CR with thoracic radiotherapy after a PR or SD after chemotherapy (65 out of 191; 34%) was 18 months, which is similar to the 18.5 months median survival of the group with a CR after chemotherapy.

Several nonrandomised analyses of the influence of the irradiated volume on local control have been made. A higher incidence of local recurrence was found when "inadequate" fields were treated, compared with "adequate" fields [20]. In contrast to these older studies, in which no modern treatment planning was available, more recent studies found no difference in local control whether the pre- or post-chemotherapy volume was treated. Data from the Mayo Clinic (Rochester, MN, USA) showed that all intrathoracic recurrences were within the radiation field, although half of the patients were treated to the pre-chemotherapy volume and half to the post-chemotherapy volume [20]. It was also found that 86% of the intrathoracic recurrences appeared in the post-chemotherapy volume [20].

Although no firm conclusions can be drawn, there is some evidence from nonrandomised studies that irradiating the post-chemotherapy tumour volume results in local control rates which are comparable with larger volumes.

In nonsmall cell lung cancer (NSCLC), elective irradiation of mediastinal lymph nodes has gradually been replaced by the treatment of pathological nodes on computed tomography (CT) or positron emission tomography (PET) only, whereby radiation volumes could be reduced and hence toxicity diminished. In LD-SCLC, only one prospective study has been carried out in which only CT-positive mediastinal lymph nodes were included in the gross tumour volume (GTV) [22]. 27 patients were treated with concurrent carboplatin, etoposide and chest irradiation (45 Gy delivered in 30 *b.i.d.* fractions). Three patients developed an isolated nodal failure (crude rate 11%, 95% confidence interval (CI) 2.4–29%), all of them in the ipsilateral supraclavicular fossa. Because of the higher than expected isolated nodal recurrence rates, the study was terminated early. Since 18-fluorodeoxyglucose PET scans have a higher accuracy than CT scans also in SCLC, irradiation of only PET-positive nodes would be a possibility allowing omission of elective nodal irradiation in the future [23].

At present, the safety of selective nodal irradiation in NSCLC should not be extrapolated to patients with LD-SCLC until more data are available. In the meantime, elective nodal irradiation should only be omitted in clinical trials.

What is the best timing, sequencing and overall treatment time?

Many phase III studies have investigated the timing of chest radiation in LD-SCLC [19, 24]. When all studies were considered, the delivery of early *versus* late thoracic irradiation did not influence the survival. However, when the most active chemotherapy regimen (platinum-based) were administered concomitantly with chest radiotherapy, long-term survival was increased at the expense of a higher incidence of severe, though transient oesophagitis. At 5 yrs, the survival was significantly higher when chest radiotherapy was given early, *i e.* within 30 days of the initiation of chemotherapy, representing a 5-yr survival rate of 20.2% for early *versus* 13.8% for late thoracic radiotherapy. In a pivotal phase III study, decreasing the overall treatment time of chest radiotherapy from 5 weeks (2 Gy *q.d.*) to 3 weeks (1.5 Gy *b.i.d.*), while keeping the total radiation dose to 45 Gy, increased the 5-yr survival from 16 to 26% [25].

Early, concurrent chemotherapy with accelerated radiation may result in ~30% grade 3 acute oesophagitis, which contrasts with ~15% in early, concurrent, nonaccelerated radiotherapy and ~5% in sequential schedules. Interestingly, lung toxicity appeared not to be influenced by the timing of radiotherapy.

It has been hypothesised that accelerated repopulation is triggered by the first dose of any effective cytotoxic agent and that, in order to obtain local tumour control, the last tumour clonogen should be killed by the end of radiotherapy [26]. It follows from these two assumptions that the long-term survival should decrease with increasing time between the start of any treatment and the end of radiotherapy. A meta-analysis of published data showed superior long-term survival if this time between start of any treatment and end of radiotherapy was kept below 30 days in LD-SCLC (fig. 1).

These results are consistent with accelerated proliferation of tumour clonogens triggered by radiotherapy and/or chemotherapy. As expected, accelerated treatments also cause more toxicity in rapidly proliferating tissues, such as the oesophageal mucosa.

In conclusion, for limited-stage SCLC, current evidence supports the early administration of thoracic radiotherapy with concurrent cisplatin and etoposide chemotherapy.

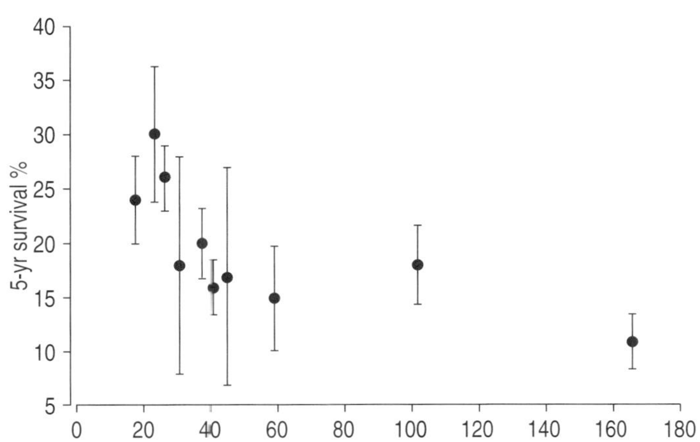

Fig. 1. – The survival at 5 yrs as a function of the SER (start of any treatment to the end of radiotherapy). ● single trial; bars: SE.

Prophylactic cranial irradiation

Brain metastases are a frequent problem in LD-SCLC, being found in 10–14% of cases at the time of presentation. Magnetic resonance imaging (MRI) is more sensitive than CT in detection of brain metastases [27]. During the course of disease, brain metastases will be diagnosed in another 20–25%, with increasing risk with prolonged length of survival. Even after achievement of CR, the cumulative rate of brain metastases (symptomatic and asymptomatic) at 2 yrs approaches >50% [28]. In one half of cases, patients present with multiple lesions.

Since therapeutic whole-brain radiotherapy after diagnosis of brain-only relapse in SCLC yields a response rate of 50% and a median survival of 4.7 months [29], several randomised studies have been undertaken to address what effect PCI had on brain recurrence and survival. These studies consistently demonstrated a reduction in the rate of brain recurrences with PCI but failed to demonstrate a survival benefit (table 1). Obviously, any survival benefit from prophylactic irradiation of a single metastatic site will be diluted by the competing risk of progression in extracranial sites, and it has been shown that the survival advantage from PCI is mainly seen in patients with an overall relatively favourable prognosis [33].

In 1999, the Prophylactic Cranial Irradiation Overview Collaborative Group published a meta-analysis of seven randomised trials, including 987 patients treated with or without PCI [28]. All patients had SCLC without brain metastases at diagnosis and >80% of patients had limited-stage disease.

This group found a statistically significant difference in the relative risk of death with the addition of PCI (relative risk 0.84, 95% CI 0.73–0.97; p=0.01), corresponding to a 5.4% absolute increase in the 3-yr survival rate (15.3% without PCI *versus* 20.7% with PCI). Furthermore, addition of PCI increased the disease-free survival (absolute benefit at 3 yrs of 8.8%) and reduced the cumulative incidence of subsequent brain metastases (relative risk with PCI 0.46, 95% CI 0.38–0.57; p<0.001). Increasing doses of PCI (8 Gy, 24–25 Gy, 30 Gy and 36–40 Gy) decreased the risk of brain metastases (relative risk: 0.76, 0.52, 0.34 and 0.27, respectively; p=0.02, trend test), but the effect on survival did not vary significantly with dose. There was a significant trend towards a greater effect of PCI on the incidence of brain metastases in patients with smaller time intervals (<4 months or 4–6 months *versus* >6 months) between start of induction therapy and randomisation (p=0.01). This is in accordance with a radiation dose–response analysis indicating a nearly linear dose–response relationship in PCI administered within 60 days of the first day of induction therapy [34]. Beyond 60 days after start of induction, higher doses of PCI are required to achieve the same level of brain metastasis risk reduction, with a threshold of 15–20 Gy, possibly reflecting growth of micrometastases. Hence, there is probably a benefit of early *versus* late administration of PCI.

Table 1. – Results of prophylactic cranial irradiation (PCI) in limited disease small cell lung cancer: selected randomised studies with actuarial failure rates

Study [ref.]	Patients n	Dose Gy	CNS failure %		2-yr survival %	
			Control	PCI	Control	PCI
UKCCCR/EORTC [30]	314	8–36	54	38*	19	25
IGR [31]	211	24–30	51	44	16	22
IGR [32]	145	24	67	40*	22	29

CNS: central nervous system; UKCCCR: United Kingdom Coordinating Committee for Cancer Research; EORTC: European Organisation for Research and Treatment of Cancer; IGR: Institut Gustave Roussy, Villejuif, France.

However, the optimal PCI dose and fractionation remain controversial. In the meta-analysis, doses ranged from 8 Gy in one fraction to 40 Gy in 20 fractions [28]. This issue has been examined in a large intergroup phase III trial that has been presented recently [35]. Patients with LD-SCLC in CR after induction chemotherapy were randomised to either standard PCI (25 Gy, 10 daily fractions) or higher PCI dose (36 Gy), delivered by either conventional (18 fractions in 24 days) or accelerated hyperfractionated radiotherapy (24 *b.i.d.* fractions in 16 days), respectively. Between 1999 and 2005, 720 patients were randomised. At 2 yrs, the brain metastasis rate was 30% (95% CI 25–36%) after the standard PCI dose, compared with 24% (95% CI 18–30%) in the higher-dose PCI arms (hazard ratio 0.77, 95% CI 0.55–1.08; p=0.13). Interestingly, overall survival at 2 yrs was 42% (95% CI 37–48%) in the standard PCI dose arm *versus* 37% (95% CI 32–42%) in the higher-dose arms (p=0.02), in association with a chest relapse rate of 40% (95% CI 34–46%) in the standard PCI dose arm *versus* 48% (95% CI 42–54%) in the higher-dose arms (p=0.02), which at a median follow-up of 38 months remains so far biologically unexplained.

Based on these results, the current recommendation of 25 Gy in 2.5-Gy fractions remains the standard of care in LD-SCLC.

Neurotoxicity

Up to now, major arguments against the administration of PCI have been concerns about treatment-related neurotoxicity in long-term survivors. In fact, only few investigators have assessed prospectively the possible neurotoxicity of PCI [36]. In the most recent analysis of 93 patients who underwent formal neurocognitive testing before PCI, 47% had evidence of impaired cognitive function, which is in accordance with results of earlier studies demonstrating baseline cognitive dysfunctions in a significant proportion of patients before randomisation. Despite transient declines in executive functions and language performance at early time-points after PCI, persistent declines in cognitive function were not observed. It should be noted, however, that patients who comply with neurocognitive function tests and quality-of-life assessment at intermediate to long follow-up times are not necessarily comparable to those compliant at baseline [37].

The recent demonstration of the existence of radiosensitive neural progenitor cells in the hippocampal region [38] has stimulated interest in hippocampal-avoidance whole-brain radiation therapy [39] as a strategy for reducing the risk of memory-related neurocognitive decline after irradiation. The role of such techniques for PCI needs to be tested.

Large daily fraction sizes and the use of concomitant chemotherapy are possible co-factors in developing neurological toxicity and should be avoided. Furthermore, competing risk factors for neurocognitive decline (*e.g.* mental stress, paraneoplastic syndromes, small-vessel central nervous system thrombosis and age-related predisposition) should be carefully evaluated.

In summary, PCI should be planned for all patients with LD-SCLC in CR and may be considered for patients with any response to induction therapy. However, it should be used with caution in patients with significant medical comorbidities, poor performance status or impaired neurocognitive function.

Future perspectives

SCLC remains a challenging disease, with most patients dying from distant metastases and a significant proportion with persistent local tumour. A better integration of systemic treatment with thoracic irradiation is still needed, as well as innovative drugs and sophisticated thoracic and cranial irradiation techniques. At present, targeted drugs have failed to improve the prognosis of patients with SCLC but, as time goes by, there is a very high probability that this situation will change. Possibilities include anti-angiogenesis drugs and hypoxic cell sensitisers. Moreover, although, at the time of writing, SCLC stem cells have not been identified, selectively targeting these cells has a high therapeutic potential. The same applies to the integration of molecular imaging data into radiotherapy treatment planning. The advent of sparing the hippocampus brain area with advanced radiation techniques opens perspectives to avoid sensitive volumes within organs. Lastly, identification of predictive and/or prognostic factors on an individual patient basis may allow selection of the right patient for the best-fitted treatment.

Summary

Limited disease small cell lung cancer (LD-SCLC) is a heterogeneous disease, not only for its clinical behaviour, but also for its anatomical extension. In very rare, early cases, LD-SCLC might be treated with surgery and chemotherapy, but as the overwhelming majority of patients present with locally advanced disease, the standard of care is concurrent chest radiotherapy with cisplatin and etoposide chemotherapy followed by prophylactic cranial irradiation (PCI). Newer chemotherapeutic drugs as well as targeted agents have not improved the outcome thus far.

Given concurrently with chest irradiation, cisplatin combined with etoposide, administered every 21 days for 4–5 cycles, have frequently been used.

Thoracic radiotherapy should begin as early as possible during the first chemotherapy cycle. A total radiation dose of 45 Gy is recommended, delivered in a short overall treatment time (<4 weeks). Accelerated therapy increases absolute 5-yr survival rates by 10% compared with longer treatment times, at the expense of an incidence of severe oesophagitis of ~30% that is reversible within a few weeks. Haematological complications and late pulmonary damage may occur but are not more frequent than with less intensive schedules yielding inferior long-term survival. Obviously, only fit patients (World Health Organisation performance status 0–2) with adequate organ function can tolerate this treatment.

As the tumour remission status is difficult to assess due to radiographic changes induced by chemoradiation therapy, patients that show no tumour progression are suitable for PCI. The recommended dose is 25 Gy, given in 10 daily fractions of 2.5 Gy. PCI reduces the risk of brain metastases by ~50%. When delivered after chemotherapy and at the recommended doses and fractionation, PCI did not lead to persistent neurocognitive function decline.

With this treatment strategy, 5-yr survival rates of 25% can be achieved in patients with LD-SCLC.

Keywords: Concurrent chemoradiation, limited-stage small cell lung cancer, prophylactic cranial irradiation, radiotherapy, treatment.

Statement of interest

H.J.M. Groen has received funds for translational research from Pfizer and Roche.

References

1. Jemal A, Siegel R, Ward E, *et al.* Cancer statistics, 2008. *CA Cancer J Clin* 2008; 58: 71–96.
2. Brigham BA, Bunn PA Jr, Minna JD, *et al.* Growth rates of small cell bronchogenic carcinomas. *Cancer* 1978; 42: 2880–2886.
3. Zelen M. Keynote address on biostatistics and data retrieval. *Cancer Chemother Rep* 1973; 4: 31–42.
4. Bunn P, Carbone D, Grim J, *et al.* 5th IASLC Lung Tumor Biology Workshop, August 13–17, 1996, Ermatingen, Switzerland. *Lung Cancer* 1997; 16: 239–257.
5. Greene FL, Compton CC, Fritz AG, *et al.*, eds. American Joint Committee on Cancer Staging Atlas. Chicago, Springer, 2006; pp. 167–176.
6. Sobin LH, Wittekind C, eds. TNM Classification of Malignant Tumours. 6th Edn. New York, Wiley-Liss, 2002.
7. Shepherd FA, Crowley J, Van Houtte P, *et al.* The International Association for the Study of Lung Cancer lung cancer staging project: proposals regarding the clinical staging of small cell lung cancer in the forthcoming (seventh) edition of the tumor, node, metastasis classification for lung cancer. *J Thorac Oncol* 2007; 2: 1067–1077.
8. Eberhardt W, Korfee S. New approaches for small-cell lung cancer: local treatments. *Cancer Control* 2003; 10: 289–296.
9. Pignon JP, Arriagada R, Ihde DC, *et al.* A meta-analysis of thoracic radiotherapy for small-cell lung cancer. *N Engl J Med* 1992; 327: 1618–1624.
10. Warde P, Payne D. Does thoracic irradiation improve survival and local control in limited-stage small-cell carcinoma of the lung? A meta-analysis. *J Clin Oncol* 1992; 10: 890–895.
11. Sundstrøm S, Bremnes RM, Kaasa S, *et al.* Cisplatin and etoposide regimen is superior to cyclophosphamide, epirubicin, and vincristine regimen in small-cell lung cancer: results from a randomized phase III trial with 5 years' follow-up. *J Clin Oncol* 2002; 20: 4565–4672.
12. Ettinger DS, Berkey BA, Abrams RA, *et al.* Study of paclitaxel, etoposide, and cisplatin chemotherapy combined with twice-daily thoracic radiotherapy for patients with limited-stage small-cell lung cancer: a Radiation Therapy Oncology Group 9609 phase II study. *J Clin Oncol* 2005; 23: 4991–4998.
13. McClay EF, Bogart J, Herndon JE 2nd, *et al.* A phase III trial evaluating the combination of cisplatin, etoposide, and radiation therapy with or without tamoxifen in patients with limited-stage small cell lung cancer: Cancer and Leukemia Group B Study (9235). *Am J Clin Oncol* 2005; 28: 81–90.
14. Saito H, Takada Y, Ichinose Y, *et al.* Phase II study of etoposide and cisplatin with concurrent twice-daily thoracic radiotherapy followed by irinotecan and cisplatin in patients with limited-disease small-cell lung cancer: West Japan Thoracic Oncology Group 9902. *J Clin Oncol* 2006; 24: 5247–5252.
15. Han JY, Cho KH, Lee DH, *et al.* Phase II study of irinotecan plus cisplatin induction followed by concurrent twice-daily thoracic irradiation with etoposide plus cisplatin chemotherapy for limited-disease small-cell lung cancer. *J Clin Oncol* 2005; 23: 3488–3494.
16. Pedrazzoli P, Ledermann JA Lotz JP, *et al.* High dose chemotherapy with autologous hematopoietic stem cell support for solid tumors other than breast cancer in adults. *Ann Oncol* 2006; 17: 1479–1488.
17. Lorigan P, Woll PJ, O'Brien ME, *et al.* Randomized phase III trial of dose-dense chemotherapy supported by whole-blood hematopoietic progenitors in better-prognosis small-cell lung cancer. *J Natl Cancer Inst* 2005; 97: 666–674.
18. Ardizzoni A, Tjan-Heijnen VC, Postmus PE, *et al.* Standard *versus* intensified chemotherapy with granulocyte colony-stimulating factor support in small-cell lung cancer: a prospective European Organization for Research and Treatment of Cancer-Lung Cancer Group Phase III Trial-08923. *J Clin Oncol* 2002; 20: 3947–3955.

19. Pijls-Johannesma M, De Ruysscher D, Vansteenkiste J, *et al.* Timing of chest radiotherapy in patients with limited stage small cell lung cancer: a systematic review and meta-analysis of randomised controlled trials. *Cancer Treat Rev* 2007; 33: 461–473.
20. De Ruysscher D, Vansteenkiste J. Chest radiotherapy in limited-stage small cell lung cancer: facts, questions, prospects. *Radiother Oncol* 2000; 55: 1–9.
21. Komaki R, Swann RS, Ettinger DS, *et al.* Phase I study of thoracic radiation dose escalation with concurrent chemotherapy for patients with limited small-cell lung cancer: Report of Radiation Therapy Oncology Group (RTOG) protocol 97-12. *Int J Radiat Oncol Biol Phys* 2005; 62: 342–350.
22. De Ruysscher D, Bremer RH, Koppe F, *et al.* Omission of elective node irradiation on basis of CT-scans in patients with limited disease small cell lung cancer: a phase II trial. *Radiother Oncol* 2006; 80: 307–312.
23. van Loon J, Offermann C, Bosmans G, *et al.* 18FDG-PET based radiation planning of mediastinal lymph nodes in limited disease small cell lung cancer changes radiotherapy fields: a planning study. *Radiother Oncol* 2008; 87: 49–54.
24. Fried DB, Morris DE, Poole C, *et al.* Systematic review evaluating the timing of thoracic radiation therapy in combined modality therapy for limited-stage small-cell lung cancer. *J Clin Oncol* 2004; 22: 4837–4845.
25. Turrisi AT 3rd, Kim K, Blum R, *et al.* Twice-daily compared with once-daily thoracic radiotherapy in limited small-cell lung cancer treated concurrently with cisplatin and etoposide. *N Engl J Med* 1999; 340: 265–271.
26. De Ruysscher D, Pijls-Johannesma M, Bentzen SM, *et al.* Time between the first day of chemotherapy and the last day of chest radiation is the most important predictor of survival in limited-disease small-cell lung cancer. *J Clin Oncol* 2006; 24: 1057–1063.
27. Seute T, Leffers P, ten Velde GPM, *et al.* Detection of brain metastases from small cell lung cancer: consequences of changing imaging techniques (CT *versus* MRI). *Cancer* 2008; 112: 1827–1834.
28. Aupérin A, Arriagada R, Pignon JP, *et al.* Prophylactic cranial irradiation for patients with small-cell lung cancer in complete remission. Prophylactic Cranial Irradiation Overview Collaborative Group. *N Engl J Med* 1999; 341: 476–484.
29. Postmus PE, Haaxma-Reiche H, Gregor A, *et al.* Brain-only metastases of small cell lung cancer; efficacy of whole brain radiotherapy. An EORTC phase II study. *Radiother Oncol* 1998; 46: 29–32.
30. Gregor A, Cull A, Stephens RJ, *et al.* Prophylactic cranial irradiation is indicated following complete response to induction therapy in small cell lung cancer: results of a multicentre randomised trial. United Kingdom Coordinating Committee for Cancer Research (UKCCCR) and the European Organization for Research and Treatment of Cancer (EORTC). *Eur J Cancer* 1997; 33: 1752–1758.
31. Laplanche A, Monnet I, Santos-Miranda JA, *et al.* Controlled clinical trial of prophylactic cranial irradiation for patients with small-cell lung cancer in complete remission. *Lung Cancer* 1998; 21: 193–201.
32. Arriagada R, Le Chevalier T, Borie F, *et al.* Prophylactic cranial irradiation for patients with small-cell lung cancer in complete remission. *J Natl Cancer Inst* 1995; 87: 183–190.
33. Work E, Bentzen SM, Nielsen OS, *et al.* Prophylactic cranial irradiation in limited stage small cell lung cancer: survival benefit in patients with favourable characteristics. *Eur J Cancer* 1996; 32A: 772–778.
34. Suwinski R, Lee SP, Withers HR. Dose–response relationship for prophylactic cranial irradiation in small cell lung cancer. *Int J Radiat Oncol Biol Phys* 1998; 40: 797–806.
35. Le Pechoux C, Hatton M, Kobierska A, *et al.* Randomized trial of standard dose to a higher dose prophylactic cranial irradiation (PCI) in limited-stage small cell cancer (SCLC) complete responders (CR): primary endpoint analysis (PCI99-01, IFCT 99-01, EORTC 22003-08004, RTOG 0212). *J Clin Oncol* 2008; 26: Suppl. 15, LBA7514.
36. Grosshans DR, Meyers CA, Allen PK, *et al.* Neurocognitive function in patients with small cell lung cancer: effect of prophylactic cranial irradiation. *Cancer* 2008; 112: 589–595.

37. Li J, Bentzen SM, Mehta MP, *et al.* Avoiding bias in the prospective evaluation of patients with brain metastases. In reply. *J Clin Oncol* 2007; 25: 4024–4025.
38. Monje ML, Mizumatsu S, Fike JR, *et al.* Irradiation induces neural precursor-cell dysfunction. *Nat Med* 2002; 8: 955–962.
39. Gutiérrez AN, Westerly DC, Tomé WA, *et al.* Whole brain radiotherapy with hippocampal avoidance and simultaneously integrated brain metastases boost: a planning study. *Int J Radiat Oncol Biol Phys* 2007; 69: 589–597.

CHAPTER 18

Management of extensive disease-small cell lung cancer

P.E. Postmus, E.F. Smit

Dept of Pulmonary Diseases, Vrije Universiteit University Medical Centre, Amsterdam, The Netherlands. E-mail: pe.postmus@vumc.nl

Correspondence: P.E. Postmus, Dept of Pulmonary Diseases, Vrije Universiteit University Medical Centre, Amsterdam, The Netherlands. E-mail: pe.postmus@vumc.nl

Small cell lung cancer (SCLC) represents only 15–20% of overall lung cancer, with incidence rates declining among men but continuing to increase among women in most countries [1]. It is characterised by its rapid growth rate, early dissemination to regional lymph nodes and distant sites, and its sensitivity to chemotherapy and radiotherapy [2].

Staging

As the available chemotherapy had only a very limited role in the early years of treatment of SCLC, radiotherapy was the only effective therapy and a staging system came into practice that was fully based on borders for radiotherapy fields. It was introduced in the 1950s by the Veterans' Administration Lung Study Group (VALSG) for use in their randomised clinical trials [3].This simple system divided SCLC into two disease subgroups termed "limited" and "extensive" disease. Limited disease (LD) was characterised by tumours confined to one hemithorax, although local extension and ipsilateral, supraclavicular nodes could also be present if all known disease could be encompassed in the same radiation portal as the primary tumour. No extrathoracic metastases could be present. All other disease was classified as extensive disease (ED).

The introduction of more active chemotherapy created optimism about the future control of SCLC [4] and indeed led to significant improvements in median and 5-yr survival rates in the following years; however, a plateau was reached at the end of the 1980s [5]. At that time, almost universally, a single modality treatment, chemotherapy, was used and therefore the relevance of a more accurate staging did not seem to be an important issue. Staging had little or no impact on choice of therapy and was mainly used as a prognostic factor. This probably explains why it took until 1989 before the International Association for the Study of Lung Cancer (IASLC) issued a consensus report [6] that, for the first time in 30 yrs, introduced changes to the VALSG staging system. This report suggested that LD should be expanded to include tumours limited to one hemithorax with regional lymph node metastases, including hilar, ipsilateral and contralateral mediastinal nodes, and ipsilateral and contralateral supraclavicular nodes. The report also recommended that patients with ipsilateral pleural effusion, regardless of whether cytology is positive or negative, be considered to have LD if no extrathoracic metastases were detected. Accurate staging again became an important issue as radiotherapy was demonstrated to be essential for improving therapeutic outcome [7].

Eur Respir Mon, 2009, 44, 310–317. Printed in UK - all rights reserved. Copyright ERS Journals Ltd 2009; European Respiratory Monograph; ISSN 1025-448x.

In a recent report of the IASLC staging committee [8], a revision of the 1989 staging system was suggested. This was based on data of more than 12,000 patients with SCLC, with information on staging and all with a minimum follow-up of 5 yrs or to the time of death. The most important recommendation of the SCLC staging subcommittee of the IASLC Lung Cancer Staging Project was that tumour, node, metastasis classification (TNM) staging should be applied to SCLC. For prospective staging validation studies, more information must be collected to determine whether there is a difference in prognosis for patients with cytology-negative or -positive pleural effusions and for patients with pericardial effusions. For non-SCLC these effusions are considered as "M1a" and therefore stage IV (*i.e.* extensive) disease [9]. Furthermore, it is needed to determine whether "N3" supraclavicular nodal involvement, whether unilateral or bilateral, should be included in the limited disease category, as part of a radiation field, or in the ED group, as was the situation in the past.

Standard chemotherapy

Combination chemotherapy became standard clinical practice in the 1970s. Most combinations consisted of an alkylating agent, a topoisomerase 2 inhibitor and a mitotic inhibitor such as a vinca alkaloid.

Many attempts to improve the outcome after standard first-line chemotherapy have failed. Examples of these are alternating so-called maintenance chemotherapy, non-cross-resistant regimens, dose intensification, dose-dense regimens, high-dose regimens and late intensification. In several trials, it was demonstrated that a restricted number of courses [4–6] resulted in the same outcome as prolonged treatment, provided appropriate treatment at relapse is administered.

After the re-introduction of thoracic radiotherapy and the positive effects of concurrent chemoradiotherapy, the role of cisplatin became very important for limited disease. The important role of a platinum analogue became clear after a meta-analysis [10] and led to the current standard treatment for all stages of SCLC: 4–6 cycles of etoposide and a platinum analogue, being either cisplatin (for LD and ED) or carboplatin (for ED).

Nevertheless, with these regimens the outcome for ED-SCLC is far from satisfying: an objective response rate of 60–80%, median survival of 9–11 months and 2-yr survival of 1–5% [11].

New chemotherapy developments

As chemotherapy for NSCLC became an important issue during the 1990s, development of new drugs was very much focused on this malignancy and little on SCLC. The evaluation of the so-called third-generation drugs used for NSCLC (*e.g.* topoisomerase-1 inhibitors, taxanes, gemcitabine, anti-metabolites) was performed in SCLC as well, but with a 5–10-yr delay.

Topoisomerase-1 inhibitors

The story of topoisomerase-1 inhibitors for SCLC starts with demonstrated activity of topotecan in relapsed SCLC [12]. In several phase III trials in first-line topotecan in combination with cisplatin was compared with the standard treatment. Although demonstrated to give a comparable outcome either after oral [13] or intravenous administration [14], data were not convincing due to myelotoxicity and most likely will not result in incorporating topotecan in first-line treatment.

For irinotecan, the story is less clear. In a Japanese study, the combination of irinotecan–cisplatin in ED patients was found to be superior to the standard treatment of cisplatin etoposide at an interim analysis, so much so that the data-monitoring committee had to decide to close the study early and conclude the new regimen as superior to the standard [15]. In a non-Japanese population, a mature phase III study failed to demonstrate the superiority of the irinotecan–cisplatin combination [16], although the dose and schedule used was not exactly the same as in the Japanese study. Therefore, an adequately powered study with exactly the same regimens was initiated in a Caucasian population. Apart from considerable differences in toxicity between the Japanese study and the American Southwest Oncology Group study, possibly related to differences of polymorphism in genes encoding for metabolic pathways in the populations [17], this study again failed to demonstrate the superiority of irinotecan–cisplatin [18]. Although, in Japan, the latter regimen might be the standard treatment for ED-SCLC, in Europe, USA and Australia, this will not be the case. This is not very likely influenced by the outcome of a rather small study performed in Europe in which irinotecan–carboplatin resulted in better therapeutic outcome than (oral) etoposide–carboplatin [19].

Taxanes

Of the two available drugs, docetaxel and paclitaxel, only the latter has been evaluated in phase III studies. Adding paclitaxel to carboplatin–etoposide resulted in a better outcome compared with the same combination with vincristine [20], whereas, in a phase III study paclitaxel–cisplatin–etoposide did not improve the outcome and was associated with excessive toxicity despite the use of haematopoietic growth factors [21]. Additionally, in comparison with the old cyclophosphamide–doxorubicin–etoposide regimen it was not superior with respect to overall survival when combined with carboplatin [22]. Overall these results halted the clinical evaluation of paclitaxel in first-line treatment regimens.

Gemcitabine

Initially gemcitabine was evaluated in second- or third-line treatment and not found to be very promising [23]. In a recent study, in combination with carboplatin, it resulted in an outcome comparable to cisplatin–etoposide [24]. This is also not very likely to change current practice.

Pemetrexed

After an initial promising outcome in a randomised phase II study of pemetrexed in combination with carboplatin or cisplatin [25], a very large phase III study with non-inferiority design was launched which, at the advice of the data-monitoring committee, had to be stopped early due to inferior outcome in the carboplatin–pemetrexed arm compared with the control arm which consisted of carboplatin–etoposide at standard dose and schedule [26].

As of the present time, the outcome of several large phase III studies has not resulted in a change of the standard chemotherapy treatment which continues to be a combination of etoposide and either carboplatin or cisplatin.

Other new developments

Targeted agents

As with the third-generation chemotherapeutic agents for NSCLC the new, so-called targeted, therapies are evaluated at a later point in time in SCLC. Outcome of several early studies of these agents have been disappointing [27]. It is symptomatic for the prioritising in drug development strategies that an old drug against one of the new discovered targets (*i.e.* vascular endothelial growth factor) has already gone through phase II and III testing, whereas all newer agents have not been tested at all in SCLC. After a promising randomised phase II study of the older angiogenesis inhibitor thalidomide, in combination with chemotherapy and as maintenance [28], a phase III study was completed which failed to confirm the promising results of the previous study [29].

Radiotherapy

ED-SCLC patients were excluded for many years from the potential benefits of prophylactic cranial irradiation (PCI). In limited-stage disease, PCI became standard after demonstrating a survival benefit in a meta-analysis [30]. For ED this was considered not to be beneficial, probably based on the assumed benefit from whole-brain radiotherapy, if brain metastases became symptomatic [31], or the activity of chemotherapy against brain metastases [32]. Despite these potential palliative possibilities, brain metastases remain a serious problem with excessive morbidity during the final months of life. It was for this reason that the lung cancer group from the European Organisation for Research and Treatment of Cancer started a simple straightforward randomised clinical trial in ED patients with a response after chemotherapy. In the experimental PCI arm, not only was the number of brain metastases significantly reduced but also the survival improved significantly. Therefore for ED patients, responding to chemotherapy, PCI is now part of standard treatment [33].

Second-line therapy

Unfortunately, for most patients with SCLC, both LD and ED, the benefit of first-line therapy is limited and relapse or progression of the disease is the reason to consider second-line therapy. Despite a decades-long history of chemotherapy for SCLC, the proof of benefit of treatment at relapse has been demonstrated only very recently [34]. In this small phase III study, topotecan was found to result in much longer survival compared with best supportive care alone. Based on the selection of cases progressing for >45 days after the first-line therapy the majority of patients treated are the ones classified in a previous study as the sensitive cases [12]. In a recent review [35], a number of guidelines were provided (table 1).

New developments

One of the promising new agents is amrubicin [36], a synthetic anthracycline analogue. Clinical trials using this as first- and second-line therapy are underway.

Table 1. – Guidelines of CHENG *et al.* [35]

The selection of patients for treatment with second-line therapy should be dependent on the treatment-free interval, the extent of response to first-line therapy, residual toxicity from first-line therapy, and the performance status of the patient.
There is insufficient evidence to recommend a specific chemotherapy regimen. Nevertheless, patients who relapse $\geq$3 months after having completed first-line chemotherapy may benefit from re-treatment with the same regimen that induced their initial response.
Topotecan, orally or intravenously, is a possible alternative for patients who initially respond to chemotherapy and who have a response duration of $\geq$45 days.
There is currently no standard second-line chemotherapy regimen for patients who fail to respond to, or who relapse shortly after, first-line therapy.

Treatment of patients with a poor performance status and/or considerable comorbidity

Often older age by itself is considered a reason to administer a less-than-standard first-line therapy. The evidence for such a strategy is not very strong and for that reason upper limits for age have nowadays become abandoned from the list of inclusion criteria for many clinical trials in SCLC. Much more important are prognostic factors, such as performance status and comorbidity. For these patients, a more "patient-tailored" approach might be necessary.

One of the possibilities is to reduce the number of drugs to single-agent therapy. However, in a number of trials the outcome of single-agent therapy was demonstrated to be slightly inferior to combination chemotherapy, although data on toxicity and quality of life were not very different [37–39]. One may question the relevance of a slightly but significantly better survival because preservation of quality of life, especially in these patients, is the main goal of therapy. Also, for these patients, a personal judgment of the treating physician and patient is necessary. Part of a more personalised "patient-tailored" approach could be the reconsideration after one or two cycles of single-agent therapy and, in case of substantial symptomatic benefit due to tumour response, re-evaluation of what might be achieved with continuation of the mild but less effective treatment *versus* changing treatment to a more effective combination chemotherapy.

Future studies

Evaluation of new drugs remains an ongoing attempt to improve survival in SCLC in general. However, it is fair to say that the prospects for this are not very promising at this stage. Partly due to a paucity of better ideas, a new study will be performed to evaluate the role of thoracic irradiation in ED as well [40].

Conclusions

First, TNM staging should become standard for SCLC. Secondly, for ED-SCLC, standard chemotherapy consists of 4–6 cycles of a platinum analogue with etoposide; however, in Japan, etoposide has been replaced by irinotecan. Thirdly, responding ED patients should receive PCI. Finally, second-line treatment is of clinically relevant significance, the only drug specifically licensed for this indication is topotecan. Depending on treatment free interval, re-treatment with the first-line treatment might be a good choice.

Summary

Treatment outcome of extensive disease small cell lung cancer has reached a plateau during the last two decades. The only relevant and recent improvement has come from adding cranial irradiation to patients responding to chemotherapy. New drugs have either not been tested yet in small cell lung cancer or failed to demonstrate any promising result.

Keywords: Chemotherapy, radiotherapy, small cell lung cancer.

Statement of interest
None declared.

References

1. Devesa SS, Bray F, Vizcaino AP, *et al.* International lung cancer trends by histologic type: male:female differences diminishing and adenocarcinoma rates rising. *Int J Cancer* 2005; 117: 294–299.
2. Masters G. The clinical presentation of small cell lung cancer. *In:* Pass HI, Carbone DP, Johnson DH, *et al.*, eds. Lung Cancer: Principles and Practice. Philadelphia, Lippincott Williams & Wilkins, 2005; pp. 304–314.
3. Zelen M. Keynote address on biostatistics and data retrieval. *Cancer Chemother Rep 3* 1973; 4: 31–42.
4. Greco FA, Oldham RK. Current concepts in cancer: small-cell lung cancer. *N Engl J Med* 1979; 301: 355–358.
5. Jänne PA, Freidlin B, Saxman S, *et al.* Twenty-five years of clinical research for patients with limited-stage small cell lung carcinoma in North America. *Cancer* 2002; 95: 1528–1538.
6. Stahel RA, Ginsberg R, Havemann K, *et al.* Staging and prognostic factors in small cell lung cancer: a consensus report. *Lung Cancer* 1989; 5: 119–126.
7. Pignon JP, Arriagada R, Ihde DC, *et al.* A meta-analysis of thoracic radiotherapy for small-cell lung cancer. *N Engl J Med* 1992; 327: 1618–1624.
8. Shepherd FA, Crowley J, Van Houtte P, *et al.* The International Association for the Study of Lung Cancer lung cancer staging project: proposals regarding the clinical staging of small cell lung cancer in the forthcoming (seventh) edition of the tumor, node, metastasis classification for lung cancer. *J Thorac Oncol* 2007; 2: 1067–1077.
9. Postmus PE, Brambilla E, Chansky K, *et al.* The IASLC Lung Cancer Staging Project: proposals for revision of the M descriptors in the forthcoming (seventh) edition of the TNM classification of lung cancer. *J Thorac Oncol* 2007; 2: 686–693.
10. Pujol JL, Carestia L, Daurès JP. Is there a case for cisplatin in the treatment of small-cell lung cancer? A meta-analysis of randomized trials of a cisplatin-containing regimen *versus* a regimen without this alkylating agent. *Br J Cancer.* 2000; 83: 8–15.
11. Ferraldeschi R, Baka S, Jyoti B, *et al.* Modern management of small-cell lung cancer. *Drugs* 2007; 67: 2135–2152.
12. Ardizzoni A, Hansen H, Dombernowsky P, *et al.* Topotecan, a new active drug in the second-line treatment of small-cell lung cancer: a phase II study in patients with refractory and sensitive disease. *J Clin Oncol* 1997; 15: 2090–2096.

13. Eckardt JR, von Pawel J, Papai Z, *et al.* Open-label, multicenter, randomized, phase III study comparing oral topotecan/cisplatin *versus* etoposide/cisplatin as treatment for chemotherapy-naïve patients with extensive-disease small-cell lung cancer. *J Clin Oncol* 2006; 24: 2044–2051.
14. Heigener DF, Freitag L, Eschbach C, *et al.* Topotecan/cisplatin (TP) compared to cisplatin/etoposide (PE) for patients with extensive disease-small cell lung cancer (ED- SCLC): final results of a randomised phase III trial. *J Clin Oncol* 2008; 26: Suppl. 15, 7513.
15. Noda K, Nishiwaki Y, Kawahara M, *et al.* Irinotecan plus cisplatin compared with etoposide plus cisplatin for extensive small-cell lung cancer. *N Engl J Med* 2002; 346: 85–91.
16. Hanna N, Bunn PA Jr, Langer C, *et al.* Randomized phase III trial comparing irinotecan/cisplatin with etoposide/cisplatin in patients with previously untreated extensive-stage disease small-cell lung cancer. *J Clin Oncol* 2006; 24: 2038–2043.
17. Lara P, Redman M, Lenz H, *et al.* Cisplatin (Cis)/etoposide (VP16) compared to cis/irinotecan (CPT11) in extensive-stage small cell lung cancer (E-SCLC): pharmacogenomic (PG) and comparative toxicity analysis of JCOG 9511 and SWOG 0124. *J Clin Oncol* 2007; 25: Suppl. 18, 7524.
18. Natale RB, Lara PN, Chansky K, *et al.* S0124: a randomized phase III trial comparing irinotecan/cisplatin (IP) with etoposide/cisplatin (EP) in patients (pts) with previously untreated extensive stage small cell lung cancer (E-SCLC). *J Clin Oncol* 2008; 26: Suppl. 15, 7512.
19. Hermes A, Bergman B, Bremnes R, *et al.* Irinotecan plus carboplatin *versus* oral etoposide plus carboplatin in extensive small-cell lung cancer: a randomized phase III trial. *J Clin Oncol* 2008; 26: 4261–4267.
20. Reck M, von Pawel J, Macha HN, *et al.* Randomized phase III trial of paclitaxel, etoposide, and carboplatin *versus* carboplatin, etoposide, and vincristine in patients with small-cell lung cancer. *J Natl Cancer Inst* 2003; 95: 1118–1127.
21. Niell HB, Herndon JE 2nd, Miller AA, *et al.* Randomized phase III intergroup trial of etoposide and cisplatin with or without paclitaxel and granulocyte colony-stimulating factor in patients with extensive-stage small-cell lung cancer: Cancer and Leukemia Group B Trial 9732. *J Clin Oncol* 2005; 23: 3752–3759.
22. de Jong WK, Groen HJ, Koolen MG, *et al.* Phase III study of cyclophosphamide, doxorubicin, and etoposide compared with carboplatin and paclitaxel in patients with extensive disease small-cell lung cancer. *Eur J Cancer* 2007; 43: 2345–2350.
23. van der Lee I, Smit EF, van Putten JW, *et al.* Single-agent gemcitabine in patients with resistant small-cell lung cancer. *Ann Oncol* 2001; 12: 557–561.
24. Lee SM, James LE, Qian W, *et al.* Comparison of gemcitabine and carboplatin *versus* cisplatin and etoposide for patients with poor-prognosis small cell lung cancer. *Thorax* 2008; 64: 75–80.
25. Socinski MA, Weissman C, Hart LL, *et al.* Randomized phase II trial of pemetrexed combined with either cisplatin or carboplatin in untreated extensive-stage small-cell lung cancer. *J Clin Oncol* 2006; 24: 4840–4847.
26. Socinski MA, Smit EF, Lorigan P, *et al.* Phase III study of pemetrexed plus carboplatin (PC) *versus* etoposide plus carboplatin (EC) in chemonaïve patients (pts) with extensive-stage disease small cell lung cancer (ED-SCLC): interim results. Presented at the American Society of Clinical Oncology Annual Meeting 2008, abstract NSA.
27. Johnson BE, Rudin CM, Salgia R. Novel and Targeted Agents for Small Cell Lung Cancer. www.asco.org/portal/servlet/filedownload?file=/edbook/2008/lung03.pdf
28. Lee SM, James L, Buchler T, *et al.* Phase II trial of thalidomide with chemotherapy and as maintenance therapy for patients with poor prognosis small-cell lung cancer. *Lung Cancer* 2008; 59: 364–368.
29. Lee SM, Woll P, James LE, *et al.* A phase III randomised, double blind, placebo controlled trial of etoposide/carboplatin with or without thalidomide in advanced small cell lung cancer (SCLC): PRS-04. *J Thorac Oncol* 2007; 2: Suppl. 4, S306–S307.
30. Aupérin A, Arriagada R, Pignon JP, *et al.* Prophylactic cranial irradiation for patients with small-cell lung cancer in complete remission. *N Engl J Med* 1999; 341: 476–484.

31. Postmus PE, Haaxma-Reiche H, Gregor A, *et al.* Brain-only metastases of small cell lung cancer; efficacy of whole brain radiotherapy: an EORTC phase II study. *Radiother Oncol* 1998; 46: 29–32.
32. Postmus PE, Smit EF. Chemotherapy for brain metastases of lung cancer: a review. *Ann Oncol* 1999; 10: 753–759.
33. Slotman B, Faivre-Finn C, Kramer G, *et al.* Prophylactic cranial irradiation in extensive small-cell lung cancer. *N Engl J Med* 2007; 357: 664–672.
34. O'Brien ME, Ciuleanu TE, Tsekov H, *et al.* Phase III trial comparing supportive care alone with supportive care with oral topotecan in patients with relapsed small-cell lung cancer. *J Clin Oncol* 2006; 24: 5441–5447.
35. Cheng S, Evans WK, Stys-Norman D, *et al.* Chemotherapy for relapsed small cell lung cancer: a systematic review and practice guideline. *J Thorac Oncol* 2007; 2: 348–354.
36. Ettinger DS, Jotte RM, Gupta V, *et al.* A phase II trial of single-agent amrubicin (AMR) in patients with extensive disease small cell lung cancer (ED-SCLC) that is refractory or progressive within 90 days of completion of first-line platinum-based chemotherapy. *J Clin Oncol* 2008 26: Suppl. 15, 8041.
37. Girling DJ. Comparison of oral etoposide and standard intravenous multidrug chemotherapy for small-cell lung cancer: a stopped multicentre randomised trial. Medical Research Council Lung Cancer Working Party. *Lancet* 1996; 348: 563–566.
38. Souhami RL, Spiro SG, Rudd RM, *et al.* Five-day oral etoposide treatment for advanced small-cell lung cancer: randomized comparison with intravenous chemotherapy. *J Natl Cancer Inst* 1997; 89: 577–580.
39. White SC, Lorigan P, Middleton MR, *et al.* Randomized phase II study of cyclophosphamide, doxorubicin, and vincristine compared with single-agent carboplatin in patients with poor prognosis small cell lung carcinoma. *Cancer* 2001; 92: 601–608.
40. Eckert F, Müller AC. SCLC extensive disease – treatment guidance by extent or/and biology of response? *Radiat Oncol* 2008; 3: 33.

CHAPTER 19

Malignant pleural disease in primary lung cancer

E. Mishra, H.E. Davies*, Y.C.G. Lee#,¶,+*

**Oxford Centre for Respiratory Medicine, Churchill Hospital, Oxford, UK. #University of Western Australia, ¶Sir Charles Gairdner Hospital, and +Pleural Disease Unit, Lung Institute of Western Australia, Perth, Australia.*

Correspondence: Y.C.G. Lee, University Dept of Medicine, 4/F, G Block, Queen Elizabeth II Medical Centre, Perth WA 6009, Australia. Fax: 61 893462816; E-mail: ycgarylee@hotmail.com

As many as 100,000 patients with lung cancer develop a pleural effusion in Europe every year [1, 2]. Metastasis of lung cancer to the pleura significantly affects staging, prognosis and management and often produces distressing symptoms, impairing quality of life. The diagnosis and management of malignant pleural effusions (MPEs), therefore, form an integral part of medical care for patients with lung cancer.

Lung cancers can affect the pleura in a variety of ways, often generating diagnostic and management challenges. Contrary to common belief, malignant spread to the pleura does not always produce clinically apparent effusions. Conversely, the presence of an effusion does not necessarily imply neoplastic pleural involvement in patients with lung cancer. An MPE is conventionally defined by identification of malignant cells in pleural tissue or fluid. This contrasts with paramalignant effusions, which develop due to indirect effects of cancer in the absence of malignant pleural invasion.

An international survey on management of MPEs revealed significant differences in clinical practice worldwide [3]. This is not surprising, given the wide range of diagnostic and treatment options available, each with its advantages and shortcomings. Although professional guidelines exist, they are often rendered out of date as medical advances and clinical controversies continue to emerge rapidly [4, 5]. This chapter highlights important management strategies and recent developments in malignant pleural disease, especially in the setting of lung cancer.

Incidence

Pleural effusions affect 0.3% of the population per year [6], and up to 70% of all exudative effusions are secondary to malignancy [7]. At *post mortem*, 15% of patients who die of cancer have an MPE [8].

Lung cancer is the commonest cause of an MPE, responsible for one third of all cases, followed by breast cancer (25%), lymphoma (10%), ovarian cancer (5%), gastric cancer (2%) and unknown primaries (7%) [9]. Development of a MPE in lung cancer appears more often with advanced disease and a histological diagnosis of small cell lung cancer [10, 11]. Age and sex are not associated with a higher risk of developing a malignant effusion [2].

The actual incidence of malignant pleural involvement in lung cancer may be underestimated. About half of patients with pleural metastases have "dry pleural

Eur Respir Mon, 2009, 44, 318–335. Printed in UK - all rights reserved. Copyright ERS Journals Ltd 2009; European Respiratory Monograph; ISSN 1025-448x.

dissemination" without a pleural effusion [8]. Even in the absence of visible pleural metastases or an effusion, pleural lavage can reveal tumour cells (presumably from microscopic pleural invasion) in patients with lung cancer. The incidence of positive pleural lavage (3–39%) is dependent on the stage of the tumour [12–14], and can be increased by saline jet washings of the visceral pleura or touch cytology [15, 16]. In one series of 1,279 lung cancer patients undergoing thoracotomy, 4% had a pleural effusion of greater than 100 mL that was not diagnosed pre-operatively. These patients were more likely to be found to have inoperable disease during exploratory thoracotomy [17].

Although the majority of effusions associated with lung cancer are malignant, it should be noted that up to 40% of pleural effusions in lung cancer patients are paramalignant [11, 17]. Hence, histocytological proof should be established before labelling a pleural effusion as malignant.

Prognosis

MPE is a poor prognostic marker, often indicating advanced disease. For patients with lung cancer and MPE, the median survival is only 3 months [18]. This is similar to the median survival (4 months) in another study, which included patients with MPE from any lung or extrapulmonary cancers [19]. The median survival of patients with MPE differs by up to 10-fold between patients with good and poor performance status (Karnofsky score $\geq$70 *versus* $\leq$30 respectively) [19].

In the sixth edition of *TNM Classification of Malignant Tumours*, visceral pleural involvement stages a tumour at T2 and the presence of an MPE is staged at T4 (stage IIIB) [20, 21]. This is due to be revised in the seventh edition, with the presence of an MPE staged at M1a (stage IV), reflecting the advanced nature of the disease when the pleura is involved [22].

Positive pleural lavage cytology is a poor prognostic indicator in patients undergoing resection of lung cancer with curative intent, with a 5-yr survival rate of 28% compared with 70% if negative [12–14]. However, results of pleural lavage are not currently part of the TNM (tumour, node, metastasis) staging system.

In patients with small cell lung cancer, the presence of a pleural effusion without evidence of spread outside the hemithorax is conventionally classified as limited disease. However, patients with small cell lung cancer and an MPE have an intermediate prognosis between those of limited staging (but without an effusion) and patients with extensive disease [23].

In contrast, a paramalignant effusion has no impact on prognosis [11, 17], emphasising the importance of its differentiation from a malignant effusion.

Symptoms and signs

Common symptoms in patients presenting with MPE are breathlessness, cough and chest pain, yet some patients are asymptomatic [24]. Clinical history is unreliable in predicting whether an effusion is malignant or benign. However, symptoms associated with a higher likelihood of an underlying malignancy are as follows: dull (rather than pleuritic) chest pain; work exposure to carcinogens; a shorter history of disease symptoms; severe breathlessness; absence of fevers; and a personal history of cancer [25]. As well as signs of a pleural effusion, patients often have evidence of advanced malignancy, such as cachexia and lymphadenopathy [26].

MPE causes dyspnoea *via* a variety of pathophysiological changes. The extra volume of the pleural fluid is compensated for mainly by an increase in the size of the thoracic cavity, rather than a consequent reduction in lung (or heart) volume. The weight of the pleural fluid can profoundly affect the diaphragm, thus adversely influencing normal respiratory mechanics. Dyspnoea is often more significant in patients whose diaphragm is inverted [27]. For every litre of pleural fluid removed, the forced vital capacity and the forced expiratory volume in 1 s will only increase on average by about 200 mL, and the total lung capacity by about 500 mL [28].

Most patients with moderate or large pleural effusions have abnormal arterial blood gases, primarily a low arterial oxygen tension. The main mechanism underlying this hypoxaemia is an intrapulmonary shunt that does not change significantly after thoracentesis; hence, blood gas results often do not improve and may even deteriorate after fluid evacuation [28].

It should be emphasised that breathlessness in patients with lung cancer and malignant effusions often involves extrapleural factors. Concurrent infection, atelectasis, pulmonary embolism, lymphangitis and pericardial involvement must be considered. The relative contribution of pleural disease can only be assessed upon removal of the pleural fluid.

Pathobiology of pleural metastases

Knowledge of the molecular biology underlying the development of pleural metastases and MPE remains limited, which in part contributes to the relative lack of translational advances and novel therapies.

Spread of malignant cells to the pleura

Malignant cells often spread as tumour emboli from cancer foci in the lung to the parenchymal tissue and subsequently into the pleura. Direct invasion and haematogenous or lymphatic spread can also occur [8, 11, 29]. Following visceral pleura involvement, cells then spread to the parietal pleura either across adhesions or freely through the pleural fluid [8, 29]. Peripheral tumours are more commonly associated with pleural invasion and pleural effusions [30].

Anchoring and proliferation of cancer cells in the pleura

For tumour cells to anchor onto pleural tissues and continue to expand, they need to adhere to the mesothelial surface, be able to proliferate and to avoid immune surveillance. Numerous mediators have been postulated to play a role *in vitro*, although few have been tested in animal models, let alone humans.

Cytokines, such as transforming growth factor (TGF)-β, matrix metalloproteinases (MMPs) and tissue inhibitor of metalloproteinase, are important in the regulation of matrix formation (which aids cancer cell anchoring to pleural tissue). Batimastat, an MMP inhibitor, led to a decrease in the frequency of pleural aspiration in a phase I trial of the treatment of MPE [31].

Angiogenesis

Malignant cells can induce effusion accumulation by releasing pro-angiogenic factors, especially vascular endothelial growth factor (VEGF). VEGF levels are higher in MPEs than in other effusions and relative to matched serum concentrations [32–35]. Cytokines found to stimulate VEGF production by tumour and mesothelial cells in MPEs include TGF-β, interleukin (IL)-6 *via* Stat3 (signal transducer and activator of translation protein), and tumour necrosis factor (TNF)-α *via* nuclear factor (NF)-κB [35–39]. Strategies to antagonise VEGF have shown success in treatment of malignant effusions in animal models [40]. Bevacizumab (a VEGF antagonist) has been used with effect in small series of patients with recurrent pleural effusions [41, 42]; its role in MPEs is under investigation.

Recent preclinical work has presented several other potential therapeutic targets. For example, inhibition of NF-κB in mouse models decreases TNF-α levels in MPE, tumour burden and pleural fluid volume [43]. Also, bisphosphonates prevent adhesion to the extracellular membrane, perhaps by decreasing the levels of adhesion molecules and reducing MMP-9 release into the pleural space, and may have a role in the treatment of MPE. In particular, zoledronic acid, a nitro-bisphosphonate, has shown particular promise in a mouse model of lung cancer-induced MPE: administration of zoledronic acid reduced tumour load, vascular hyperpermeability and *in vivo* fluid accumulation, and improved survival [44]. Other anti-angiogenic approaches, *e.g.* use of endostatin, are being explored [45].

Intrapleural immune defences against spread of malignant cells

The intrapleural immune system defends against invasion of malignant cells, which, in turn, develop mechanisms to overcome this and continue replicating. Mesothelial cells and intrapleural dendritic cells are part of the innate immune response and act as antigen-presenting cells, preventing tumour cell invasion of the pleura. They attract lymphocytes and macrophages to the pleural space *via* intercellular adhesion molecule-1 and Toll-like receptor-2, causing a lymphocytic effusion [46, 47]. Manipulation of the intrapleural immune system offers another experimental therapeutic target for the management of MPE. Potential immunotherapies for MPE include macrophage stimulation by MDP-Lys, a synthetic muramyl dipeptide derivative, and OK-432, a streptococcal preparation that induces a local immune response [48, 49]. New therapies focusing on dendritic cell-based immunotherapy are under phase I clinical assessment in mesothelioma and may be useful for other MPEs.

In response to host defences, malignant cells induce a locally immunosuppressive state in MPEs, triggering high levels of IL-4, IL-10, TGF-α and TGF-β and low levels of IL-2, IL-12, IL-18 and interferon-γ and a T-helper cell type 2 immune response [50, 51]. The CD4+CD25- T-lymphocytes found in MPEs have low tumour cytolytic activity [52]. Tumour-associated macrophages may also be exploited by malignant cells to aid tumour progression *via* release of growth factors and cytokines [53].

Aetiology of MPEs

In health, pleural fluid is filtered from the parietal systemic circulation into the pleural space, and exits *via* lymphatic stomata between mesothelial cells in the parietal pleura. The fluid drains *via* the intercostal lymphatics to the mediastinal lymph nodes [54]. The normal pleural fluid volume is ~8 mL in each pleural space [55]. MPEs accumulate as a result of both increased production and decreased absorption of pleural fluid.

Neovascularisation is common in malignant pleural disease and is, in part, induced by angiogenic factors from tumour cells, particularly VEGF. The new blood vessels are hyperpermeable, which results in leakage of fluid, protein and blood cells, and generation of an exudative, often blood-stained, effusion [30, 56]. YANO *et al.* [30] showed that human adenocarcinoma lung cancer cells frequently caused MPEs in a mouse model, whereas squamous cell cancer cells did not. This is hypothesised to be due to the more peripheral location of adenocarcinoma metastases allowing invasion of the pleura, and to the high levels of VEGF produced by adenocarcinoma cells [30]. In humans, a positive correlation is seen between pleural fluid volume and VEGF levels [34].

Malignant infiltration into lymphatics slows drainage of pleural fluid. *Post mortem* series have shown that the development of an effusion relates to malignant infiltration of mediastinal lymph nodes, not to the extent of pleural involvement by metastases [26, 29]. The usefulness of therapies targeting production of pleural fluid may, therefore, be limited in the presence of extensive lymphatic infiltration.

Investigation of a suspected MPE

Imaging

Chest radiography. A pleural effusion is usually first confirmed on a chest radiograph (CXR), which can reveal as little as 200 mL of fluid. Pleural deposits and thickening may also be seen. Up to 15% of patients with lung cancer have a pleural effusion demonstrable on CXR at diagnosis [57–59]. CXR also allows diagnosis of a trapped lung following pleural fluid drainage and is useful to assess for fluid re-accumulation on follow-up (fig. 1).

Ultrasonography. Thoracic ultrasonography is more sensitive in detecting pleural fluid than CXR (fig. 2). It can also distinguish between pleural fluid and pleural thickening and guide pleural drainage and pleural biopsy, particularly if the effusion is small or loculated [60]. Pleural metastases may be visualised as pleurally based masses that may invade neighbouring structures, or hypoechoic regions of pleural thickening with irregular or indistinct borders [61, 62]. Physician-performed ultrasonography is rapidly gaining acceptance and imaging guidance is recommended by many governing bodies (*e.g.* the National Patient Safety Agency, London, UK) for chest drain insertion [63].

Computed tomography. Up to 25% of patients with lung cancer have a pleural effusion on computed tomography (CT) at the time of presentation [2]. In patients with an undiagnosed pleural effusion, CT should be performed with pleural-phase contrast enhancement to aid detection of pleural abnormalities (fig. 3). Benign pleuritis may produce pleural abnormalities; however, the presence of pleural thickening that is >1 cm wide, nodular, circumferential or extending onto the mediastinal surface [64] suggests malignant pleural disease. In patients with lung cancer without a pleural effusion, subtle pleural thickening or nodularity suggest the presence of pleural metastases. These features are frequently missed prior to thoracotomy [65].

The absence of pleural abnormalities on CT does not exclude pleural metastases, and CT is unable to accurately predict the histological subtype of cancer (such as differentiating between metastatic lung cancer and mesothelioma). It is therefore important that histocytological examination is performed in patients with undiagnosed effusions, particularly those who are candidates for radical treatment.

Positron emission tomography-CT. The role of positron emission tomography (PET) in patients with suspected MPE is not yet established. Pleural inflammation is common in most exudative pleural effusions and is likely to produce radiolabelled

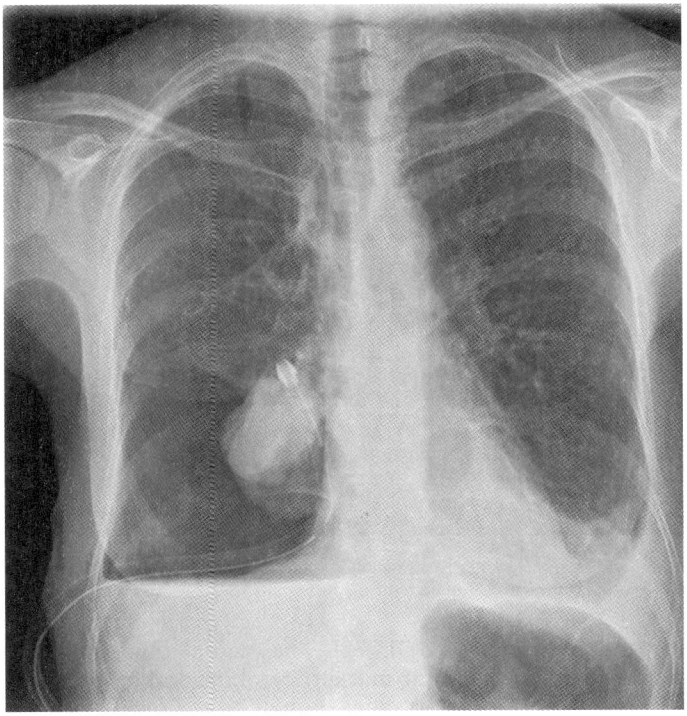

Fig. 1. – Radiographic appearance of trapped right lower lobe following drainage of malignant pleural effusion.

18-fluorodeoxyglucose avidity. Hence, the discriminatory value of PET in separating malignant exudative effusions from benign inflammatory ones is limited.

When applied to patients known to have extrapleural malignancy, a PET-CT result showing focal pleural uptake and activity in the pleural effusion has a sensitivity of 89–100%, specificity of 67–94%, positive predictive value 67–95% and negative predictive value 67–100% for MPE [66–69]. This does not preclude the need for histocytological evidence to confirm the diagnosis of MPE.

Magnetic resonance imaging. Magnetic resonance imaging has few advantages over CT, although it is useful for identifying areas of chest wall involvement by lung cancer [70].

Pleural fluid analysis

Demonstration of malignant cells in the pleural cavity, by cytology or biopsy, defines a malignant effusion and may provide information on the underlying malignancy to guide treatment. No biochemical or tumour markers can reliably determine a malignant effusion.

The appearance of the pleural fluid is not diagnostic. Although haemorrhagic effusions often raise concern about malignancy, only 50% of haemorrhagic effusions turn out to be malignant; conversely, only 10% of MPEs are haemorrhagic. Malignant effusions are usually exudates, although ~5% are transudates, usually a result of concurrent transudative causes (*e.g.* heart failure) [9].

A low pleural fluid pH (<7.3) reflects more extensive tumour load in the pleura, a higher chance of positive pleural fluid cytology, a lower success rate of subsequent

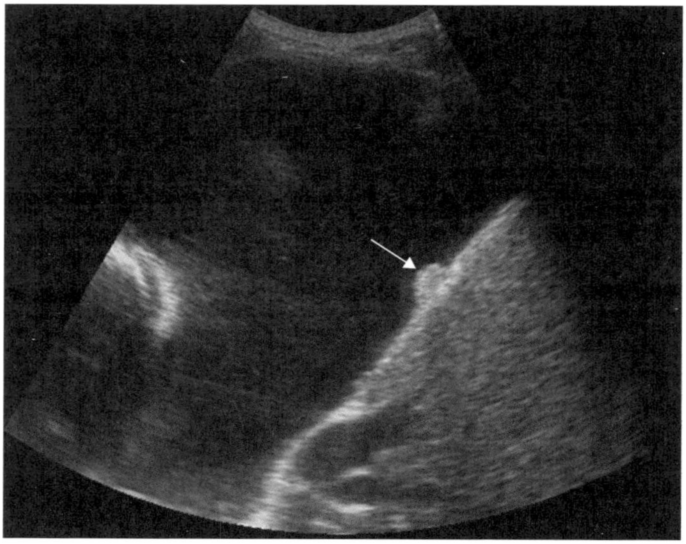

Fig. 2. – Inverted hemidiaphragm secondary to a malignant pleural effusion as a consequence of underlying primary lung adenocarcinoma. Note the presence of malignant diaphragmatic deposit (arrow).

pleurodesis and a poorer prognosis [71, 72]. The pleural fluid glucose level generally parallels the pleural fluid pH. Tumour marker, cytokine and cytogenetic assessment in pleural fluid are not sensitive or specific enough for clinical use [73] and are not recommended.

Pleural fluid should be sent for cytological examination, which has a sensitivity of about 60% for malignancy. The sensitivity is dependent on tumour type, extent and experience of the cytologist. A volume of 20 mL is sufficient [60]. Although repeat thoracentesis can increase the sensitivity of cytological diagnosis, the additional yield decreases with each subsequent sample. Pleural biopsy should be considered if the initial cytological analysis fails to provide a diagnosis.

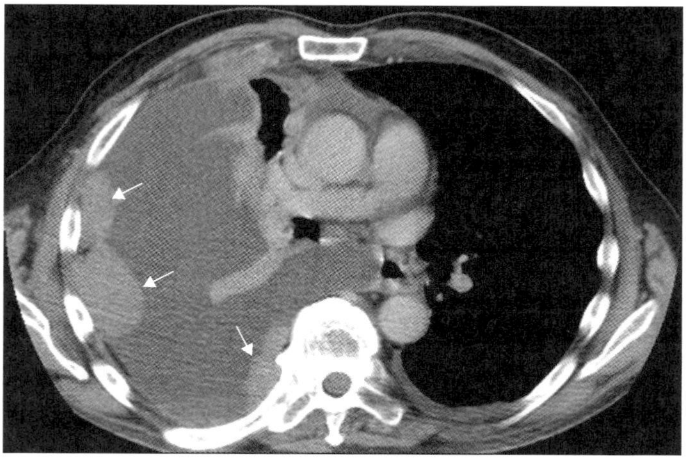

Fig. 3. – Malignant pleural effusion and pleural tumour deposition (arrows).

Blind pleural biopsy is not advocated in the investigation of malignancy because it increases sensitivity by only about 7% over cytological examination alone and carries additional risks of haemorrhage, pain and pneumothorax [60, 74].

Imaging-guided biopsy. If focal pleural nodularity or thickening is present, pleural biopsy guided by CT or ultrasound is superior to blind pleural biopsy [75], with a sensitivity of 76–88% and specificity of 100% regardless of the underlying type of malignancy. Complications include pneumothorax (4.7%), most of which do not require drain insertion, and chest wall haematoma [75–77].

Video-assisted thoracoscopy and thoracotomy. Thoracoscopy is indicated in patients with undiagnosed exudative pleural effusions despite thoracentesis and/or pleural biopsy (fig. 4) [60]. It is also indicated to investigate effusions in patients with lung cancer who would be candidates for radical, potentially curative, treatment. The diagnostic sensitivity of video-assisted thoracoscopy (VATS) for pleural cancer is about 95% and mortality is low (0.35%). Side-effects include subcutaneous emphysema, haemorrhage and empyema. VATS may not be technically feasible in the presence of pleural adhesions. Open thoracotomy has largely been replaced by VATS and is seldom indicated.

Management

The primary objectives of treatment for MPE are symptom control and improvement in quality of life. For patients with an asymptomatic MPE, no intervention is required and patients can remain under observation. However, in the majority of patients with MPE, pleural aspiration is required to achieve symptom relief and, in 70–90% of these, symptomatic re-accumulation following drainage occurs [78]. No clinical or biochemical factors reliably predict which effusions will recur and the choice of subsequent treatment

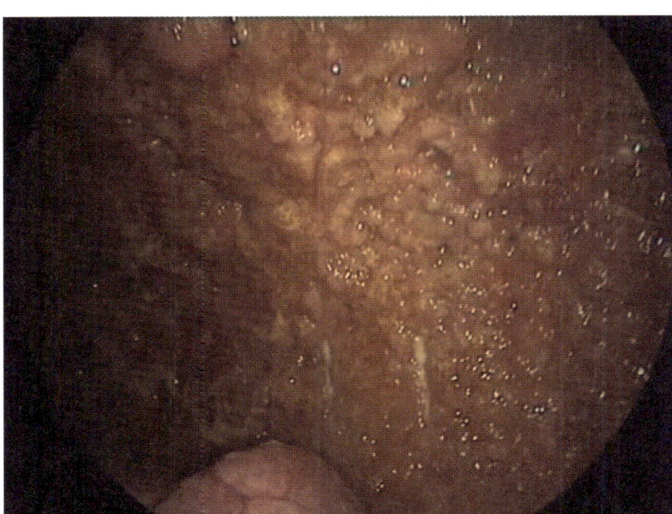

Fig. 4. – Thoracoscopic view into left pleural cavity. The chest wall pleura is diffusely infiltrated with whitish nodular tumour deposits secondary to metastatic lung adenocarcinoma.

should take into account the rate of fluid accumulation, associated symptoms and the patient's prognosis.

Strategies for management of recurrent MPE can grossly fall into three categories: removal of pleural fluid, obliteration of the pleural space to avoid fluid re-accumulation (*i.e.* pleurodesis) or antagonising fluid formation. The latter is a focus of active translational research and may reach clinical practice in the near future.

Removal of pleural fluid

Therapeutic thoracentesis. In lung cancer patients with multiple potential causes of breathlessness, thoracentesis may be the most direct way to establish the relative contribution of the pleural effusion to the dyspnoea. Evacuation of pleural fluid relieves breathlessness by restoring the mechanical advantage of the diaphragmatic muscles. It does not prevent fluid recurrence and only provides short-term symptom relief. Re-expansion pulmonary oedema is a rare but potentially fatal complication when ipsilateral pulmonary oedema occurs following rapid removal of a large volume of pleural fluid, especially if the underlying lung has collapsed for a period of time. The European Respiratory Society (ERS)/American Thoracic Society (ATS) statement recommends monitoring pleural fluid pressure by manometry during the procedure and to stop if the pleural pressure falls below -20 cmH_2O [4]. However, manometry is not widely available and clinicians are advised not to remove more than 1.5 L of fluid on each occasion and to discontinue aspiration if the patient develops dyspnoea, chest pain or cough (signs of rapid pulmonary expansion). In patients with advanced disease, a limited life expectancy (*i.e.* <2 months) or poor performance status, repeated thoracentesis may be appropriate to manage pleural fluid re-accumulation, rather than pleurodesis.

Indwelling pleural or pleuroperitoneal catheters. Long-term indwelling tunnelled pleural catheters are increasingly being used in the management of MPE [79]. They are indicated in patients with recurrent symptomatic effusion and trapped lung (fig. 1), or when pleurodesis has failed. Their potential as an alternative to pleurodesis in the first-line management of MPE is the subject of an ongoing British Lung Foundation clinical trial.

The catheters can be inserted under local anaesthetic in the outpatient setting, and allow patient-controlled ambulatory drainage of the effusion whenever symptoms arise. They are cost effective, provide patients with a sense of control, and improve quality of life [80, 81]. The pleural catheter may be removed once drainage ceases (usually after no pleural fluid is obtained over 6 weeks and imaging confirms no fluid re-accumulation). In one series (n=97), 87% of patients did not require any further pleural procedures on the side of catheter insertion and 70% achieved spontaneous pleurodesis [82]. Complications include pleural infection, catheter blockage or displacement and tumour invasion of the catheter tract (*e.g.* with adenocarcinoma) [80].

Pleuroperitoneal shunts are an alternative to indwelling pleural catheters, although the latter are easier to insert and manage. Pleural fluid is transferred *via* a patient-operated pump into the peritoneal cavity. Presence of ascites is a contraindication for use of a pleuroperitoneal shunt. Complications include shunt occlusion (7.5%) and infection, but malignant peritoneal seeding and ascites are extremely rare [83].

Pleurodesis

Pleurodesis is the iatrogenic fusion of the visceral and parietal pleural surfaces to prevent re-accumulation of pleural fluid or air. Pleurodesis may be either chemical, with instillation of a sclerosing agent *via* a chest drain or thoracoscope, or mechanical, *e.g.* pleurectomy and mechanical abrasion. The latter are often reserved for patients with MPE and an exceptional performance status. For a detailed discussion, see DAVIES and LEE [84].

MPE is the most common indication for pleurodesis but the latter should only be considered in patients who have symptom relief following thoracentesis. Bilateral pleurodesis should not be performed contemporaneously. Contraindications to pleurodesis include a poor prognosis (generally but arbitrarily accepted as <3 months) and failure of apposition of the pleural surfaces (trapped lung). Trapped lung occurs when lung expansion is restricted, either by visceral pleura tumour encasement or by endobronchial obstruction. Creation of pleural fibrosis to bridge the two pleural surfaces is not feasible with underlying trapped lung and attempts at pleurodesis may induce additional visceral thickening, further restricting lung expansion.

There is a wide variation between physicians in the timing of pleurodesis for MPE. Some advocate pleurodesis at diagnosis whereas others delay until symptomatic recurrence has occurred [3]. Early pleurodesis before the development of trapped lung may theoretically allow a higher success rate, although this has not been formally tested.

Numerous compounds have been used for pleurodesis, with talc being the most commonly used agent worldwide. In all comparative trials, talc has shown a superior success rate to other sclerosants, including bleomycin and tetracycline. Successful pleurodesis, often defined as no significant fluid re-accumulation in 30 days, occurs in about 75% of patients in large clinical studies [4].

Talc can be insufflated as a dry powder (poudrage) during thoracoscopy, or instilled *via* a chest tube (talc slurry). In all randomised trials performed to date, no significant advantage has been shown in either delivery method [85, 86]. Conventionally it is believed that poudrage allows a more uniform delivery of talc over the pleural surface, which carries a theoretical advantage of efficacy; however, there is little scientific reason to support this argument. Radioactively labelled talc studies have shown that talc can be distributed well around the pleural cavity as a slurry [87]. Talc acts by inducing an acute inflammatory response, which, if sufficiently intense, results in eventual pleural fibrosis and adhesion formation [85]. As talc is not "glue", even spread of talc over the pleural surface is not necessary.

Common complications include chest pain and fever. However, potentially fatal talc-induced acute respiratory distress syndrome (ARDS) or pneumonitis has been reported [88], and has led to a reappraisal of its use. In a randomised, controlled trial comparing different talc preparations, MASKELL *et al.* [89] found that small particle (<15 μm mean diameter) talc produced more systemic and pulmonary inflammation, with resultant hypoxia, than large particle size graded preparations. A large European study (n=558) of calibrated large particle size talc found no cases of ARDS, but demonstrated significant arterial oxygen desaturation after pleurodesis even using large particle size talc preparations [90]. The UK Medicines and Healthcare Products Regulatory Authority recently reclassified talc as a medicinal product and removed its licensed use as a medical device [91, 92].

Other available pleurodesis agents are less effective than talc [93–95], but may be preferable in patients with significant hypoxia or concomitant respiratory disease. These include cyclines, *e.g.* tetracycline (1,500 mg or 20 $mg \cdot kg^{-1}$) and doxycycline (500 mg), and bleomycin (15–240 units). OK432, a preparation of *Streptococcus pyogenes* type A3, is often used for pleurodesis in Japan, and quinacrine is popular in Scandinavia [96, 97].

New agents are being developed, stimulated by limitations of current pleurodesis agents and a greater understanding of the molecular mechanisms of pleurodesis. TGF-β, a potent mediator of fibrosis, shows promise in animal models, and a recent phase I study utilising intrapleural lipoteichoic acid-T, a novel agent based on a bacterial cell wall motif, confirmed safety for intrapleural administration in humans [98]. This area will be the focus of much future research.

Palliative therapy

For some patients, a noninvasive approach to their pleural effusion is appropriate, *e.g.* those with a grave prognosis or who refuse pleural intervention. Use of sedatives and anxiolytic agents should be used sparingly to afford symptom relief.

Special scenarios of malignant effusion management in lung cancer

Malignant effusions in patients receiving chemotherapy

Controversy exists regarding management approaches of MPE in patients who are undergoing chemotherapy, *e.g.* for small cell lung carcinoma. In a recent survey of pulmonologists, two-thirds favoured withholding pleurodesis and assessing effusion evolution following chemotherapy [3]. However, counter-arguments exist. First, third spacing of chemotherapeutic compounds is known to occur in pleural fluid. Secondly, the persistent pleural fluid may become a site of infection during the neutropenic phase of chemotherapy and empyemas in patients who are immunosuppressed carry a significant mortality and morbidity. Finally, if the chemotherapy is not curative, the effusion is likely to recur when the tumour relapses.

Post-pneumonectomy effusions

Following a pneumonectomy, air fills the residual post-pneumonectomy space (PPS). A number of physiological changes subsequently result in reduction of the hemithorax size with hemidiaphragm elevation, hyperinflation of the contralateral lung and ipsilateral mediastinal herniation. Fluid progressively replaces the air within the PPS, which is slowly reabsorbed. Post-pneumonectomy pleural fluid is seen in up to 60% of patients many years following the procedure [99]. In others, PPS air persists indefinitely, or a fibrothorax, with obliteration of the PPS, develops.

Reversal of mediastinal shift or development of a more convex effusion margin suggest production of increased fluid and usually indicate disease relapse or PPS empyema. Pleural fluid aspiration for pH, culture and cytological examination may secure the diagnosis, and CT or ultrasound imaging can further define underlying pathology.

Paramalignant effusions

Pleural effusions arising as an indirect consequence of lung malignancy in the absence of malignant pleural invasion are termed paramalignant effusions. These may be due to the following: systemic effects, *e.g.* hypoproteinaemia and pulmonary embolism; local effects of the lung cancer, *e.g.* post-obstructive pneumonitis, pneumonia and mediastinal lymph node obstruction; or treatment effects, *e.g.* radiotherapy- and chemotherapy-induced pleural inflammation. Treatment should address the underlying cause.

Chylothorax

Chylothorax should be suspected if "milky" coloured pleural fluid is obtained at thoracentesis. The diagnosis is confirmed on pleural fluid analysis with detection of chylomicrons and/or a triglyceride concentration $>1.24\ \mathrm{mmol \cdot L^{-1}}$ ($110\ \mathrm{mg \cdot dL^{-1}}$).

Chylothoraces develop following disruption of the thoracic duct and result in the accumulation of chyle (lymph rich in chylomicrons) in the pleural cavity. They may arise as a consequence of malignant mediastinal lymphadenopathy (*e.g.* lymphoma or metastatic lung carcinoma) or complicated cardiothoracic surgery (*e.g.* following curative lung resection) [100].

Management should aim to achieve the following. 1) To lessen chyle production and minimise malnutrition with a low-fat, medium-chain fatty acid. Parenteral supplementation may be required. 2) To optimise symptom relief with pleural fluid aspiration. More definitive measures, *e.g.* pleurodesis or indwelling pleural catheter insertion, may be required in refractory cases [101]. 3) To close the thoracic duct defect: radiologically guided percutaneous thoracic duct embolisation or surgical ligation can be considered. Successful closure following octreotide administration, in tandem with a low-fat diet, has also been reported [102].

Future advances

The management of MPEs in lung cancer is relatively neglected and deserves more research, given the number of patients affected and the morbidity caused. The diagnostic pathway must be improved, ideally enabling clinicians to elucidate the cause from a single pleural aspirate without more invasive procedures. The advances of biomarkers and other molecular technologies (*e.g.* DNA profiling), in combination with cytological analysis, may significantly reduce the need for invasive pleural biopsies.

Improved imaging modalities will also provide substantial benefits and, as more mesothelial markers are now identified, tissue-specific imaging modalities may prove feasible for examination of the pleura (and peritoneum). Scanning for specific disease pathologies, such as angiogenic markers, may have important roles in management and research of MPEs. In the more immediate term, better imaging methods are required for accurately staging patients and defining candidates for curative surgery.

Further clarification of the lung cancer staging process is necessary, in order to identify the role of pleural lavage cytology and, in small cell lung cancer, whether a more detailed staging system is required to encompass patients with MPE.

Management of malignant effusion should focus on improving dyspnoea and quality of life, rather than the traditional clinical end-points, *i.e.* radiological re-accumulation of effusions. The natural course of MPEs in lung cancer patients varies and the ability to accurately predict prognosis and treatment response, particularly to pleurodesis, would enable clinicians to tailor treatment appropriately. Additionally, advancement in outpatient management strategies should benefit all patients with a short life expectancy secondary to MPE, whose current treatment options are largely hospital based. The quest for a novel pleurodesis agent that is highly effective and does not cause pain or hypoxaemia or carry a risk of ARDS has begun.

Through a greater understanding of the molecular biology underlying MPE development, and translational research to target essential pathways identified, effective intrapleural chemotherapy preventing fluid formation and arresting malignant invasion of the pleura and lymphatic systems may be achieved.

Conclusion

Involvement of the pleura in lung cancer is common and ranges from MPE to dry pleural dissemination to paramalignant effusion. Identification of malignant pleural disease has key prognostic implications, and thorough investigation is essential for optimal patient management.

Recent advances in cellular biology are leading to improved understanding of how neoplastic cells spread to the pleura and how subsequent pleural effusions form. This knowledge is being exploited with the development of novel treatments, some of which may enter clinical practice over the next few years.

Until treatments exist that can cure or prolong the lives of patients with MPE, the focus of care should be on improvement of patients' quality of life. Few trials to date primarily address this outcome; however, this is changing as clinical research in malignant pleural disease and lung cancer expands.

Summary

Malignant pleural disease is common in patients with lung cancer. Establishing malignant pleural involvement in lung cancer patients often alters management and significantly impacts on staging and prognosis.

Histocytological confirmation should be obtained for suspected malignant pleural effusions to differentiate them from paramalignant effusions. If cytology is negative, imaging-guided biopsy or thoracoscopy should be considered.

Relieving dyspnoea and improving quality of life are the goals of management of malignant effusions. Pleurodesis should be considered in suitable patients. Long-term indwelling pleural catheters are recommended in patients with trapped lung or in whom pleurodesis has failed.

Keywords: Indwelling pleural catheter, malignant pleural effusion, pleurodesis.

Statement of interest

Y.C.G. Lee was the lead investigator of a project involving mesothelin. All ELISAs were provided by CisBio Ltd for free. Y.C.G. Lee is a co-investigator of the multi-centre intrapleural sepsis trial-2, which is funded, in part, by an unrestricted education grant from Roche UK Ltd. Y.C.G. Lee did not receive any personal benefits from these studies.

References

1. Ferlay J, Autier P, Boniol M, *et al.* Estimates of the cancer incidence and mortality in Europe in 2006. *Ann Oncol* 2007; 18: 581–592.
2. Mishra EK, Davies HE, Lee YCG. Pleural effusion in primary lung cancer: prevalence and risk factors. *Thorax* 2008; 63: Suppl. 7, A138.
3. Lee YCG, Baumann MH, Maskell NA, *et al.* Pleurodesis practice for malignant pleural effusions in five English-speaking countries: survey of pulmonologists. *Chest* 2003; 124: 2229–2238.
4. Antony VB, Loddenkemper R, Astoul P, *et al.* Management of malignant pleural effusions. *Eur Respir J* 2001; 18: 402–419.

5. Antunes G, Neville E, Duffy J, *et al.* BTS guidelines for the management of malignant pleural effusions. *Thorax* 2003; 58: Suppl. 2, ii29–ii38.
6. Marel M, Zrustova M, Stasny B, *et al.* The incidence of pleural effusion in a well-defined region. Epidemiologic study in central Bohemia. *Chest* 1993; 104: 1486–1489.
7. Valdes L, Alvarez D, Valle JM, *et al.* The etiology of pleural effusions in an area with high incidence of tuberculosis. *Chest* 1996; 109: 158–162.
8. Rodriguez-Panadero F, Borderas Naranjo F, Lopez Mejias J. Pleural metastatic tumours and effusions. Frequency and pathogenic mechanisms in a post-mortem series. *Eur Respir J* 1989; 2: 366–369.
9. Sahn SA. Pleural diseases related to metastatic malignancies. *Eur Respir J* 1997; 10: 1907–1913.
10. Cerfolio RJ, Bryant AS. Distribution and likelihood of lymph node metastasis based on the lobar location of nonsmall-cell lung cancer. *Ann Thorac Surg* 2006; 81: 1969–1973.
11. Canto A, Ferrer G, Romagosa V, *et al.* Lung cancer and pleural effusion. Clinical significance and study of pleural metastatic locations. *Chest* 1985; 87: 649–652.
12. Enatsu S, Yoshida J, Yokose T, *et al.* Pleural lavage cytology before and after lung resection in non-small cell lung cancer patients. *Ann Thorac Surg* 2006; 81: 298–304.
13. Buhr J, Berghäuser KH, Gonner S, *et al.* The prognostic significance of tumor cell detection in intraoperative pleural lavage and lung tissue cultures for patients with lung cancer. *J Thorac Cardiovasc Surg* 1997; 113: 683–690.
14. Okada M, Sakamoto T, Nishio W, *et al.* Pleural lavage cytology in non-small cell lung cancer: lessons from 1000 consecutive resections. *J Thorac Cardiovasc Surg* 2003; 126: 1911–1915.
15. Ichinose Y, Yano T, Asoh H, *et al.* Diagnosis of visceral pleural invasion in resected lung cancer using a jet stream of saline solution. *Ann Thorac Surg* 1997; 64: 1626–1629.
16. Saito Y, Yamakawa Y, Kiriyama M, *et al.* Diagnosis of visceral pleural invasion by lung cancer using intraoperative touch cytology. *Ann Thorac Surg* 2002; 73: 1552–1556.
17. Ruffini E, Rena O, Bongiovanni M, *et al.* The significance of intraoperative pleural effusion during surgery for bronchogenic carcinoma. *Eur J Cardiothorac Surg* 2002; 21: 508–513.
18. Heffner JE, Nietert PJ, Barbieri C. Pleural fluid pH as a predictor of survival for patients with malignant pleural effusions. *Chest* 2000; 117: 79–86.
19. Burrows CM, Mathews WC, Colt HG. Predicting survival in patients with recurrent symptomatic malignant pleural effusions: an assessment of the prognostic values of physiologic, morphologic, and quality of life measures of extent of disease. *Chest* 2000; 117: 73–78.
20. Sobin LH, Wittekind C, eds. TNM Classification of Malignant Tumours. 6th Edn. New York, Wiley-Liss, 2002; pp. 99–103.
21. Mountain CF. Revisions in the International System for Staging Lung Cancer. *Chest* 1997; 111: 1710–1717.
22. Goldstraw P, Crowley J, Chansky K, *et al.* The IASLC Lung Cancer Staging Project: proposals for the revision of the TNM stage groupings in the forthcoming (seventh) edition of the TNM Classification of malignant tumours. *J Thorac Oncol* 2007; 2: 706–714.
23. Shepherd FA, Crowley J, Van Houtte P, *et al.* The International Association for the Study of Lung Cancer lung cancer staging project: proposals regarding the clinical staging of small cell lung cancer in the forthcoming (seventh) edition of the tumor, node, metastasis classification for lung cancer. *J Thorac Oncol* 2007; 2: 1067–1077.
24. Kolschmann S, Ballin A, Gillissen A. Clinical efficacy and safety of thoracoscopic talc pleurodesis in malignant pleural effusions. *Chest* 2005; 128: 1431–1435.
25. Marel M, Scarontastny B, Melinova L, *et al.* Diagnosis of pleural effusions: experience with clinical studies, 1986 to 1990. *Chest* 1995; 107: 1598–1603.
26. Chernow B, Sahn SA. Carcinomatous involvement of the pleura: an analysis of 96 patients. *Am J Med* 1977; 63: 695–702.
27. Wang LM, Cherng JM, Wang JS. Improved lung function after thoracocentesis in patients with paradoxical movement of a hemidiaphragm secondary to a large pleural effusion. *Respirology* 2007; 12: 719–723.

28. Lee YCG, Noppen M, Light RW. Pleural effusion: transudate *versus* exudate. *In*: Laurent GJ, Shapiro S, eds. Encyclopedia of Respiratory Diseases. Oxford, Elsevier, 2006; pp. 358–362.
29. Meyer PC. Metastatic carcinoma of the pleura. *Thorax* 1966; 21: 437–443.
30. Yano S, Shinohara H, Herbst RS, *et al.* Production of experimental malignant pleural effusions is dependent on invasion of the pleura and expression of vascular endothelial growth factor/vascular permeability factor by human lung cancer cells. *Am J Pathol* 2000; 157: 1893–1903.
31. Macaulay VM, O'Byrne KJ, Saunders MP, *et al.* Phase I study of intrapleural batimastat (BB-94), a matrix metalloproteinase inhibitor, in the treatment of malignant pleural effusions. *Clin Cancer Res* 1999; 5: 513–520.
32. Yeo KT, Wang HH, Nagy JA, *et al.* Vascular permeability factor (vascular endothelial growth factor) in guinea pig and human tumor and inflammatory effusions. *Cancer Res* 1993; 53: 2912–2918.
33. Yanagawa H, Takeuchi E, Suzuki Y, *et al.* Vascular endothelial growth factor in malignant pleural effusion associated with lung cancer. *Cancer Immunol Immunother* 1999; 48: 396–400.
34. Ishimoto O, Saijo Y, Narumi K, *et al.* High level of vascular endothelial growth factor in hemorrhagic pleural effusion of cancer. *Oncology* 2002; 63: 70–75.
35. Zebrowski BK, Yano S, Liu W, *et al.* Vascular endothelial growth factor levels and induction of permeability in malignant pleural effusions. *Clin Cancer Res* 1999; 5: 3364–3368.
36. Cheng D, Lee YCG, Rogers JT, *et al.* Vascular endothelial growth factor level correlates with transforming growth factor-β isoform levels in pleural effusions. *Chest* 2000; 118: 1747–1753.
37. Maeda J, Ueki N, Ohkama T, *et al.* Transforming growth factor-β1 (TGF-β1)- and β2-like activities in malignant pleural effusions caused by malignant mesothelioma or primary lung cancer. *Clin Exp Immunol* 1994; 98: 319–322.
38. Yeh HH, Lai WW, Chen HHW, *et al.* Autocrine IL-6-induced Stat3 activation contributes to the pathogenesis of lung adenocarcinoma and malignant pleural effusion. *Oncogene* 2006; 25: 4300–4309.
39. Stathopoulos GT, Kollintza A, Moschos C, *et al.* Tumor necrosis factor-α promotes malignant pleural effusion. *Cancer Res* 2007; 67: 9825–9834.
40. Grove CS, Lee YC. Vascular endothelial growth factor: the key mediator in pleural effusion formation. *Curr Opin Pulm Med* 2002; 8: 294–301.
41. Hoyer RJ, Leung N, Witzig TE, *et al.* Treatment of diuretic refractory pleural effusions with bevacizumab in four patients with primary systemic amyloidosis. *Am J Hematol* 2007; 82: 409–413.
42. Pichelmayer O, Zielinski C, Raderer M. Response of a nonmalignant pleural effusion to bevacizumab. *N Engl J Med* 2005; 353: 740–741.
43. Stathopoulos GT, Zhu Z, Everhart MB, *et al.* Nuclear factor-κB affects tumor progression in a mouse model of malignant pleural effusion. *Am J Respir Cell Mol Biol* 2006; 34: 142–150.
44. Stathopoulos GT, Moschos C, Loutrari H, *et al.* Zoledronic acid is effective against experimental malignant pleural effusion. *Am J Respir Crit Care Med* 2008; 178: 50–59.
45. Sumi M, Kagohashi K, Satoh H, *et al.* Endostatin levels in exudative pleural effusions. *Lung* 2003; 181: 329–334.
46. Mutsaers SE. Mesothelial cells: their structure, function and role in serosal repair. *Respirology* 2002; 7: 171–191.
47. Gjomarkaj M, Pace E, Melis M, *et al.* Dendritic cells with a potent accessory activity are present in human exudative malignant pleural effusions. *Eur Respir J* 1997; 10: 592–597.
48. Kitsuki H, Katano M, Ikubo A, *et al.* Induction of inflammatory cytokines in effusion cavity by OK-432 injection therapy for patients with malignant effusion: role of interferon-γ in enhancement of surface expression of ICAM-1 on tumor cells *in vivo*. *Clin Immunol Immunopathol* 1996; 78: 283–290.
49. Yanagawa H, Haku T, Takeuchi E, *et al.* Intrapleural therapy with MDP-Lys (L18), a synthetic derivative of muramyl dipeptide, against malignant pleurisy associated with lung cancer. *Lung Cancer* 2000; 27: 67–73.

50. Li R, Ruttinger D, Li R, *et al.* Analysis of the immunological microenvironment at the tumor site in patients with non-small cell lung cancer. *Langenbecks Arch Surg* 2003; 388: 406–412.
51. Yanagawa H, Takeuchi E, Suzuki Y, *et al.* Presence and potent immunosuppressive role of interleukin-10 in malignant pleural effusion due to lung cancer. *Cancer Lett* 1999; 136: 27–32.
52. Chen YQ, Shi HZ, Qin XJ, *et al.* CD4+CD25+ regulatory T lymphocytes in malignant pleural effusion. *Am J Respir Crit Care Med* 2005; 172: 1434–1439.
53. Condeelis J, Pollard JW. Macrophages: obligate partners for tumor cell migration, invasion, and metastasis. *Cell* 2006; 124: 263–266.
54. Wang NS. The preformed stomas connecting the pleural cavity and the lymphatics in the parietal pleura. *Am Rev Respir Dis* 1975; 111: 12–20.
55. Noppen N, De Waele M, Li R, *et al.* Volume and cellular content of normal pleural fluid in humans examined by pleural lavage. *Am J Respir Crit Care Med* 2000; 162: 1023–1026.
56. Matsumori Y, Yano S, Goto H, *et al.* ZD6474, an inhibitor of vascular endothelial growth factor receptor tyrosine kinase, inhibits growth of experimental lung metastasis and production of malignant pleural effusions in a non-small cell lung cancer model. *Oncol Res* 2006; 16: 15–26.
57. Emerson GL, Emerson MS, Sherwood CE. The natural history of carcinoma of the lung. *J Thorac Surg* 1959; 37: 291–304.
58. Storey CF, Knudtson KP, Lawrence BJ. Bronchiolar ("alveolar cell") carcinoma of the lung. *J Thorac Surg* 1953; 26: 331–405.
59. Cohen S, Hossain S. Primary carcinoma of the lung: a review of 417 histologically proved cases. *Chest* 1966; 49: 67–74.
60. Maskell NA, Butland RJA, Pleural Diseases Group Standards of Care Committee British Thoracic Society. BTS guidelines for the investigation of a unilateral pleural effusion in adults. *Thorax* 2003; 58: Suppl. 2, ii8–ii17.
61. Chian CF, Su WL, Soh LH, *et al.* Echogenic swirling pattern as a predictor of malignant pleural effusions in patients with malignancies. *Chest* 2004; 126: 129–134.
62. Mayo PH, Doelken P. Pleural ultrasonography. *Clin Chest Med* 2006; 27: 215–227.
63. National Patient Safety Agency. Rapid Response Report – Risks of Chest Drain Insertion. NPSA/2008/RRR003. 2008. www.npsa.nhs.uk/nrls/alerts-and-directives/rapidrr/risks-of-chest-drain-insertion
64. Leung AN, Muller NL, Miller RR. CT in differential diagnosis of diffuse pleural disease. *AJR Am J Roentgenol* 1990; 154: 487–492.
65. Hwang JH, Song KS, Park SI, *et al.* Subtle pleural metastasis without large effusion in lung cancer patients: preoperative detection on CT. *Korean J Radiol* 2005; 6: 94–101.
66. Toaff JS, Metser U, Gottfried M, *et al.* Differentiation between malignant and benign pleural effusion in patients with extra-pleural primary malignancies: assessment with positron emission tomography-computed tomography. *Invest Radiol* 2005; 40: 204–209.
67. Gupta NC, Rogers JS, Graeber GM, *et al.* Clinical role of F-18 fluorodeoxyglucose positron emission tomography imaging in patients with lung cancer and suspected malignant pleural effusion. *Chest* 2002; 122: 1918–1924.
68. Eramus JJ, McAdams HP, Rossi SE, *et al.* FDG PET of pleural effusions in patients with non-small cell lung cancer. *AJR Am J Roentgenol* 2000; 175: 245–249.
69. Schaffler GJ, Wolf G, Schoellnast H, *et al.* Non-small cell lung cancer: evaluation of pleural abnormalities on CT scans with 18F FDG PET. *Radiology* 2004; 231: 858–865.
70. Hierholzer J, Luo L, Bittner RCSC, *et al.* MRI and CT in the differential diagnosis of pleural disease. *Chest* 2000; 118: 604–609.
71. Sahn SA, Good JT Jr. Pleural fluid pH in malignant effusions. Diagnostic, prognostic and therapeutic implications. *Ann Intern Med* 1988; 108: 345–349.
72. Rodriguez P, Lopez M. Low glucose and pH levels in malignant pleural effusions. Diagnostic significance and prognostic value in respect to pleurodesis. *Am Rev Respir Dis* 1989; 139: 663–667.
73. Liang QL, Shi HZ, Qin XJ, *et al.* Diagnostic accuracy of tumour markers for malignant pleural effusion: a meta-analysis. *Thorax* 2008; 63: 35–41.

74. Prakash UB, Reiman HM. Comparison of needle biopsy with cytologic analysis for the evaluation of pleural effusion: analysis of 414 cases. *Mayo Clin Proc* 1985; 60: 158–164.
75. Adams RF, Gleeson FV. Percutaneous image-guided cutting-needle biopsy of the pleura in the presence of a suspected malignant effusion. *Radiology* 2001; 219: 510–514.
76. Benamore RE, Scott K, Richards CJ, *et al.* Image-guided pleural biopsy: diagnostic yield and complications. *Clin Radiol* 2006; 61: 700–705.
77. Maskell NA, Gleeson F, Davies RJO. Standard pleural biopsy *versus* CT-guided cutting-needle biopsy for diagnosis of malignant disease in pleural effusions: a randomized controlled trial. *Lancet* 2003; 361: 1326–1330.
78. Anderson CB, Philpott GW, Ferguson TB. The treatment of malignant pleural effusions. *Cancer* 1974; 33: 916–922.
79. Davies HE, Lee YC. Indwelling pleural tunnelled catheters: practical aspects. *Turkish Pleural Bulletin* 2008; 2: 8–13.
80. Tremblay A, Michaud G. Single-center experience with 250 tunnelled pleural catheter insertions for malignant pleural effusion. *Chest* 2006; 129: 362–368.
81. Putnam JB Jr, Walsh GL, Swisher SG, *et al.* Outpatient management of malignant pleural effusion by a chronic indwelling pleural catheter. *Ann Thorac Surg* 2000; 69: 369–375.
82. Tremblay A, Mason C, Michaud G. Use of tunnelled catheters for malignant pleural effusions in patients fit for pleurodesis. *Eur Respir J* 2007; 30: 759–762.
83. Genc O, Petrou M, Ladas G, *et al.* The long-term morbidity of pleuroperitoneal shunts in the management of recurrent malignant effusions. *Eur J Cardiothorac Surg* 2000; 18: 143–146.
84. Davies HE, Lee YCG. Pleurodesis. *In*: Light RW, Lee YCG, eds. Textbook of Pleural Diseases. London, Arnold Press, 2008.
85. Dresler CM, Olak J, Herndon JE 2nd, *et al.* Phase III intergroup study of talc poudrage *vs* talc slurry sclerosis for malignant pleural effusion. *Chest* 2005; 127: 909–915.
86. Yim AP, Chan AT, Lee TW, *et al.* Thoracoscopic talc insufflation *versus* talc slurry for symptomatic malignant pleural effusion. *Ann Thorac Surg* 1996; 62: 1655–1658.
87. Mager HJ, Maesen B, Verzijlbergen F, *et al.* Distribution of talc suspension during treatment of malignant pleural effusion with talc pleurodesis. *Lung Cancer* 2002; 36: 77–81.
88. Brant A, Eaton T. Serious complications with talc slurry pleurodesis. *Respirology* 2001; 6: 181–185.
89. Maskell NA, Lee YCG, Gleeson FV, *et al.* Randomized trials describing lung inflammation after pleurodesis with talc of varying particle size. *Am J Respir Crit Care Med* 2004; 170: 377–382.
90. Janssen JP, Collier G, Astoul P, *et al.* Safety of pleurodesis with talc poudrage in malignant pleural effusion: a prospective cohort study. *Lancet* 2007; 369: 1535–1539.
91. Medical and Healthcare Products Regulatory Authority (MHRA). MHRA Statement on Talc Preparations for Pleurodesis. Ref: MDR 10-10/07. London, MHRA, 2007.
92. Davies HE, Lee YCG, Davies RJO. Pleurodesis for malignant pleural effusion: talc, toxicity and where next? *Thorax* 2008; 63: 572–574.
93. Diacon AH, Wyser C, Bolliger CT, *et al.* Prospective randomized comparison of thoracoscopic talc poudrage under local anesthesia *versus* bleomycin instillation for pleurodesis in malignant pleural effusions. *Am J Respir Crit Care Med* 2000; 162: 1445–1449.
94. Fentiman IS, Rubens RD, Hayward JL. A comparison of intracavitary talc and tetracycline for the control of pleural effusions secondary to breast cancer. *Eur J Cancer Clin Oncol* 1986; 22: 1079–1081.
95. Hartman DL, Gaither JM, Kesler KA, *et al.* Comparison of insufflated talc under thoracoscopic guidance with standard tetracycline and bleomycin pleurodesis for control of malignant pleural effusions. *J Thorac Cardiovasc Surg* 1993; 105: 743–747.
96. Kishi K, Homma S, Sakamoto S, *et al.* Efficacious pleurodesis with OK-432 and doxorubicin against malignant pleural effusions. *Eur Respir J* 2004; 24: 263–266.
97. Ukale V, Agrenius V, Hillerdal G, *et al.* Pleurodesis in recurrent pleural effusions: a randomized comparison of a classical and a currently popular drug. *Lung Cancer* 2004; 43: 323–328.

98. Rahman NM, Davies HE, Salzberg M, *et al.* Use of lipoteichoic acid-T for pleurodesis in malignant pleural effusion: a phase I toxicity and dose-escalation study. *Lancet Oncol* 2008; 9: 946–952.
99. Biondetti PR, Fiore D, Sartori F, *et al.* Evaluation of post-pneumonectomy space by computed tomography. *J Comput Assist Tomogr* 1982; 6: 238–242.
100. Le Pimpec-Barthes F, D'Attellis N, Dujon A, *et al.* Chylothorax complicating pulmonary resection. *Ann Thorac Surg* 2002; 73: 1714–1719.
101. Jimenez CA, Mhatre AD, Martinez CH, *et al.* Use of an indwelling pleural catheter for the management of recurrent chylothorax in patients with cancer. *Chest* 2007; 132: 1584–1590
102. Mincher L, Evans J, Jenner MW, *et al.* The successful treatment of chylous effusions in malignant disease with octreotide. *Clin Oncol (R Coll Radiol)* 2005; 17: 118–121.

CHAPTER 20

Endobronchial management of central cancers

F.J.F. Herth

Correspondence: F.J.F. Herth, Dept of Pneumology and Critical Care Medicine, Thoraxklinik am Universitätsklinikum, Amalienstr. 5, D-69126 Heidelberg, Germany. Fax: 49 62213961202; E-mail: Felix.Herth@thoraxklinik-heidelberg.de

Most of the estimated 215,020 new cases of lung cancer diagnosed in the USA in the year 2008 will be in an advanced stage [1]. More than 50% of these patients will have involvement of the central airways [2]. This can be in the form of bulky endobronchial disease, endobronchial extension or extrinsic compression of the airways by the tumour or by lymphadenopathy. Many of these patients have respiratory symptoms due to their disease. Shortness of breath, haemoptysis and cough are often the complaints that bring patients to a physician and to the complex treatment programmes currently used for the management of lung cancer. Some of these patients may benefit from endobronchial intervention as part of the management of their disease [3].

Standard management techniques of lung cancer (surgery, radiation therapy and chemotherapy) measure treatment response, 5-yr survival and recurrence rates. When treating endobronchial disease, the concepts of symptom-free survival, dyspnoea indices and quality-of-life scores also need to be evaluated. Obstruction of the central airways (trachea and mainstem bronchi) can cause worrisome symptoms such as dyspnoea, cough and haemoptysis and, when significant (>50% obstruction), cannot be tolerated for any length of time. This may be either intrinsic or extrinsic to the airway [3].

Some patients become incapacitated by their symptoms of dyspnoea. Many studies not only demonstrate improvement in clinical symptoms and quality of life, but also suggest increased overall survival with the use of endobronchial management techniques [4–8].

Not all endobronchial disease causes complete obstruction of the airways. Sometimes patients have partial obstruction, which often has a less severe symptom complex. As these patients enter treatment programmes, the endobronchial component of their disease, in response to these treatments, can lead to more complicated concerns. External-beam radiotherapy can induce endobronchial inflammation and swelling, further compromising the airways. Radiation or chemotherapy can lead to necrosis of the endobronchial component of the cancer. The inflammation and necrotic tissue can cause further airway compromise by inducing airway obstruction, lung collapse and possible post-obstructive pneumonia. Therefore, endobronchial techniques should be considered throughout the management of lung cancer patients [7, 8].

Lastly, when all management options have been used, end-stage patients will often develop compromise of their airways as the cancer continues to progress. Endobronchial management options may help to relieve some of their symptoms, allowing them freedom from shortness of breath as they go home, in conjunction with hospice or other palliative therapies [3, 9, 10].

Most endobronchial techniques are performed on an outpatient basis. Unless a patient presents with respiratory failure, many of the procedures performed provide

Eur Respir Mon, 2009, 44, 336–348. Printed in UK - European Respiratory Monograph; ISSN 1025-448x.

immediate relief of symptoms. This rapid symptomatic improvement allows patients to return home with an improved quality of life or better prepares them to continue treatment at their local programmes. Although interventional procedures are not definitive therapies, they often provide partial to total relief of the strangling sensation produced by complete airway occlusion.

Interventional pulmonary programmes that include endobronchial procedures need an armamentarium of therapeutic modalities rather than a single invasive approach to manage patients with complicated lung cancer. As each patient's anatomy differs, the manner in which the patient's cancer leads to symptoms varies. Several procedures used in conjunction (*e.g.* laser and stenting) may be necessary to provide the most efficacious management of the disease. Offering a multitude of modalities allows the best selection of approaches for the patient [7, 8].

The following sections discuss a variety of techniques and tools available to the interventionalist. In many cases, no one technique is better than the others and some combination of these techniques often offers the greatest benefit to the patient. The current author suggests that patients with central airway obstruction be managed by specialised centres that offer multiple modalities of therapy and where experts from multiple specialties work as a team [7–9].

Bronchoscopy

Since the inception of flexible fibreoptic bronchoscopy in the late 1960s in Japan and in 1970 in the USA, the flexible bronchoscope has become the most widespread tool for evaluating and diagnosing diseases of the airways and lungs [11]. The rigid bronchoscope, the flexible bronchoscope's predecessor, was in many regards forgotten as a tool until interventional pulmonology evolved in the 1980s. Interventional pulmonologists re-evaluated this tool and found its properties advantageous to the procedures that are currently performed. A survey in 1991 by the American College of Chest Physicians reported that only 8% of responding pulmonologists used a rigid bronchoscope [12].

Overall, the concurrent use of the flexible bronchoscope with the rigid bronchoscope is necessary for the practice of interventional pulmonology. The rigid bronchoscope offers many advantages to the interventional pulmonologist, one of which is the superior control of the airway achieved with its use. Ventilation is performed through the scope itself rather than around the flexible bronchoscope. The larger-bore rigid bronchoscopes allow optical systems, large calibre suction catheters and the laser to pass through the scope simultaneously. Large biopsy forceps are used through the rigid bronchoscope, which can provide more significant tissue biopsies as well as assist in mechanical debulking of lesions. However, the rigid bronchoscope is a more difficult tool to use, which requires additional training. In addition, rigid bronchoscopy is most commonly performed in the operating room with general anaesthesia. Overall, in difficult airway conditions, rigid bronchoscopy is an excellent technique for the management of endobronchial disease [3, 10].

The rigid bronchoscope itself can be used as a tool in the management of endobronchial disease (fig. 1). The distal end of the bronchoscope has a bevelled end. This edge can be used to shear large sections of endobronchial tumour away from the airway wall in a technique often referred to as coring out. In a report on 56 patients with endobronchial obstruction from the trachea to the distal mainstem bronchi, MATHISEN and GRILLO [13] described improvement in 90% of their patients. Only three out of the 56 patients had more than minor bleeding with this procedure. Although this procedure is technically difficult, coring out combined with the use of larger biopsy forceps allows tumour to be quickly resected from the obstructed airway.

Functional evaluation in interventional bronchoscopy

As interventional bronchoscopy moves towards becoming a specialty in its own right, it is essential that global leaders in the field work together to develop standard approaches to the pre-interventional evaluation. These tests and procedures will allow better selection of patients for particular interventions and, potentially, better predictions of outcomes.

In addition, standard protocols, decision trees and management algorithms need to be developed and investigated as they pertain to many post-intervention issues. Studies of outcome measures, in addition to survival, should be well designed and implemented so that practitioners can further justify the performance of these expensive but often life-saving procedures to hospital administrators who are often unwilling to invest in the necessary equipment, as well as to physician groups and third-party payers who may be reluctant to approve patient referrals because of cost-of-care concerns.

Mechanical removal of obstruction

In cases of life-threatening central airway obstruction, rapid mechanical resection of intraluminal, exophytic tumour tissue by rigid bronchoscopy "curettage" and/or forceps resection is a well established technique [10, 14] (fig. 2). Provided functional lung parenchyma can be recruited and the pulmonary artery is open, this procedure may provide instant relief. However, because bleeding is inevitable, which may compromise gas exchange, coagulation methods should be applied prior to mechanical removal. Neodymium:yttrium-aluminium-garnet (Nd:YAG) laser, electrocautery, cryotherapy or other techniques may be used for this purpose. Immediate haemostasis can often be obtained by mechanical airway wall compression using the rigid bronchoscope shaft.

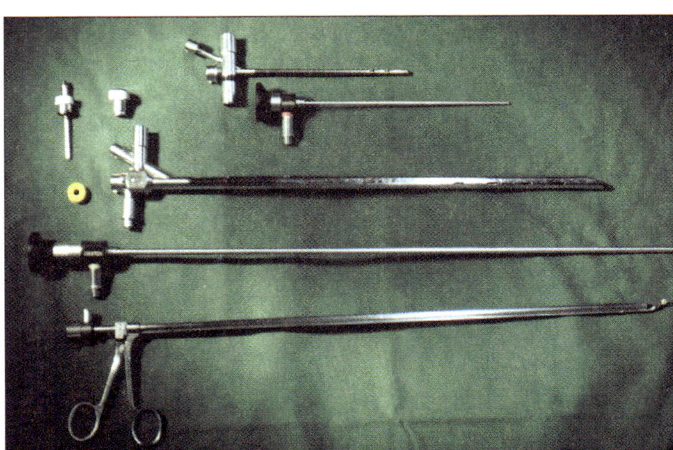

Fig. 1. – Different types of rigid scopes and lenses.

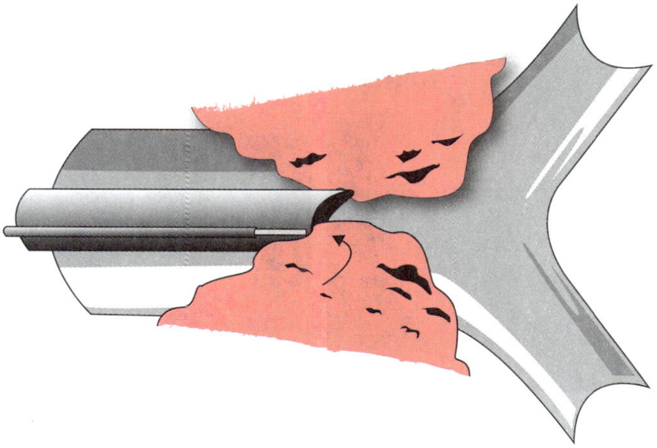

Fig. 2. – Example for a coring out.

Laser therapy

Laser, an acronym coined from light amplification by stimulated emission of radiation, has many medical uses, including the endobronchial management of lung cancer. Several laser types are currently used within the bronchi: Nd:YAG, potassium-titanyl-phosphate (KTP) and carbon dioxide (CO_2). The most common laser used endoscopically is the Nd:YAG, which delivers energy at a wavelength of 1,064 nm. The laser energy can be conducted *via* a quartz monofilament and, thus, can be easily used with either the rigid or flexible bronchoscope. Normally, Nd:YAG is used at 30–60 W, but it has a wide range of power outputs, up to 100 W. Depending on the energy level used, the laser can affect tissue several millimetres to several centimetres in depth [15].

The predominant tissue effects of Nd:YAG lasers are thermal necrosis and photocoagulation. Thermal necrosis uses higher energy levels to destroy tissue. The problem with this approach is the significant vascularity of most lung cancers. In destroying tissue with laser energy, large blood vessels can also be destroyed. These blood vessels can be perforated with the tissue destruction, leading to significant haemorrhage and an increase rather than a decrease in morbidity and mortality with this procedure.

The most commonly used effect of laser energy is photocoagulation. Using lower energy levels, the surface of the tumour is heated, causing shrinkage of the tumour and diminishing the blood flow to that region. By devascularising the tumour, more rapid mechanical debulking can be performed with improved control of bleeding.

Laser therapy can be performed *via* either flexible or rigid bronchoscopy (fig. 3). The majority of interventionalists use rigid bronchoscopy as the predominant tool for the performance of laser procedures when possible. Nd:YAG laser fibres can be passed through the working channel of most flexible bronchoscopes. Using the flexible bronchoscope, laser energy can be delivered to areas that cannot be reached with the rigid bronchoscope [16, 17].

The reported success rate of symptom palliation using laser energy in the endobronchial management of lung cancer is high. Reports of clinical improvement rates range 84–92% following laser bronchoscopy [18–20]. Brutinel *et al.* [21] compared 25 historical controls (*i.e.* patients who would have been candidates for laser management but did not receive it due to the unavailability of the procedure at

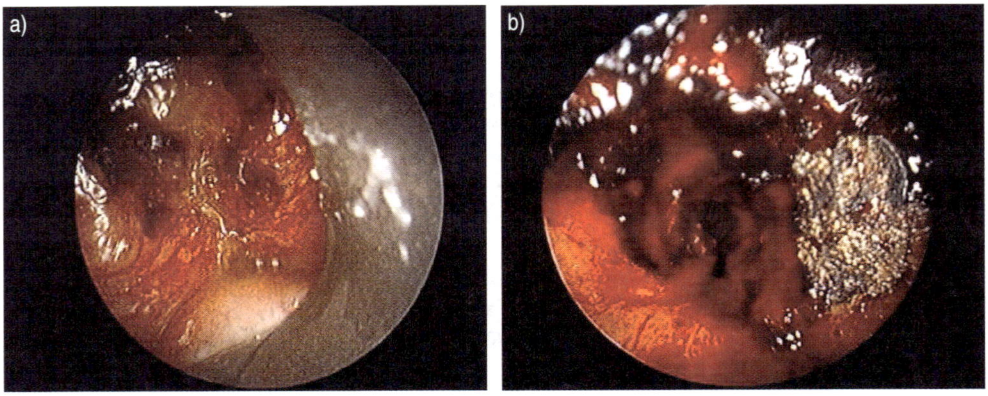

Fig. 3. – Tumour mass in the trachea a) before and b) after laser resection.

the time of their management) with 71 patients treated with laser bronchoscopy as part of the treatment programme. The authors reported 76 and 100% mortality rates at 4 and 7 months, respectively, in the control population. In the group treated with laser bronchoscopy, survival rates at 7 months and 1 yr were 60 and 28%, respectively. Although no definitive randomised studies are available, review of historical studies would suggest improved survival in patients treated with endobronchial techniques.

Cryotherapy

Cryotherapy is another modality for the endobronchial destruction of malignant tissue that obstructs the tracheobronchial tree. This technique uses cold instead of the heat used in laser-based technologies. A probe is placed onto or into an obstructing tumour mass. Liquid nitrogen (-196°C) or nitrous oxide (-80°C) cools the probe tip when performing cryotherapy. This tissue freezing leads to the destruction of all cells in an area of ~1 cm in diameter around the probe tip. Vascular thrombosis occurs with the super-cooling of tissue, minimising the bleeding during resection of the tumour.

The limiting factor to using cryotherapy is that the tissues destroyed with the freezing procedure take time to die and necrose. This requires returning to the lesion to remove the necrosed arterial and, in some cases, repeating treatments. Although cryotherapy is effective at tumour destruction and management, the necessity of repeated procedures makes this a more time-consuming procedure to perform, limiting its usefulness in management of bulky endobronchial disease [22, 23].

Electrocautery

In recent years, the use of electrocautery to treat endobronchial obstruction of central airways has become more popular because the equipment is much less expensive than laser, is available in most hospitals, and the electrocautery probes can be passed through rigid or flexible bronchoscopes. SUTEDJA *et al.* [24] reported 17 patients with central airway obstruction treated with electrocautery *via* a flexible bronchoscope. 15 of the 17 patients had an immediate reopening of the airway. Although physiological parameters did not improve in 11 patients, airway calibre >75% normal was achieved and dyspnoea was relieved. Haemoptysis was also effectively palliated. There were no deaths in this series. The authors comment on the simplicity of the technique and the ability of electrocautery to produce rapid palliation and immediate tumour debulking. VAN BOXEM *et al.* [25] described the tissue effects of bronchoscopic electrocautery and showed that this technique can produce superficial airway damage but also has the potential of damaging deeper cartilaginous layers. The amount of damage seems to correlate with the duration of the coagulation therapy. COULTER and MEHTA [26] also found excellent success rates of 89% in a series of 38 patients who underwent 47 endobronchial electrocautery procedures using flexible bronchoscopy. These authors state that endobronchial electrosurgery has the potential of eliminating the need for laser photo resection in more than one third of patients presenting with central airway obstruction.

The argon plasma coagulator (APC) is a variant of endobronchial electrocautery that uses argon gas passed through a small catheter to act as an electrical conducting medium. This is a noncontact technique that has excellent coagulation properties. The APC machine is much less expensive to purchase than a laser. It has been used to relieve endobronchial obstruction with good results. The instrument is particularly helpful for the palliation of haemoptysis and is said to be relatively safe when treating granulation tissue around airway stents. MORICE *et al.* [27] achieved 100% palliation of haemoptysis in cancer patients using the APC. Patients presenting with airway obstruction had improvement in the degree of airway lumen obstruction, decreasing from a pre-treatment average obstruction of $76 \pm 24.9\%$ to $18.4 \pm 22.1\%$ after APC debulking using flexible bronchoscopy. FREITAG and REICH [28] recently reviewed their experience with the APC and state that APC is the instrument of choice for treating haemoptysis from lesions visible by bronchoscopy.

Endobronchial prosthesis

Endobronchial prosthesis involves stents, which can be used in several clinical situations: intrinsic, extrinsic or mixed endobronchial obstruction. Stents work well in conjunction with other modalities, such as laser and mechanical debulking of tumours. Currently, stents are composed of silastic rubber and metal alloys. Advantages and disadvantages of each are noted in tables 1 and 2.

Silicon stents

Many of the silicon stents in use evolved from the Montgomery T-tube, which was first used in the early 1960s. This T-shaped stent supports the entire trachea with an arm that extends through a permanent tracheostomy. In patients with a patent

Table 1. – Advantages and disadvantages of silicon stents

Advantages	Disadvantages
Removable and replaceable	Potential for migration/dislodgement
No growth through stent	Rigid bronchoscopy needed for placement
Low cost	Possible secretion adherence
Low likelihood of granulation tissue formation	

Table 2. – **Advantages and disadvantages of metalic stents**

Advantages	Disadvantages
Easy to place	Permanent
Good wall/internal diameter relationship	Tumour regrowth (noncovered stents)
Powerful radial force	Possible migration of covered stents
Excellent conformity for irregular tracheal or bronchial walls	Significant granulation tissue stimulation
Good epithelialisation	Epithelialisation affecting wall mechanics and secretion clearance
	Radial force causing necrosis of bronchial wall, erosion, fistulas and perforation

tracheostomy, the Montgomery T-tube remains an excellent tool for the management of endotracheal disease [29].

In 1990, DUMON [30] reported the use of what is now referred to as the Dumon stent (Bryon Corporation, Woburn, MA, USA). Developed in 1987, it is a silastic stent with evenly spaced studs along its outside walls (fig. 4). These studs not only assist in maintaining the placement of the stent in the airway, but also allow the clearance of secretions around the walls of the stent. Although the use of expandable wire mesh stents is increasing, the Dumon stent probably is currently the most common stent used by interventionalists.

The Dumon stent is effective in maintaining the structural integrity when placed endobronchially. Its solid walls prevent tumour growth from re-obstructing airways. Endobronchial tumours are often debulked and then a stent is placed prior to the initiation of radiotherapy or chemotherapy or both. Another advantage of the Dumon stent is the ease of removal. This can be significant when endobronchial procedures are used early in the management of cancer patients. After definitive therapies have been used (radiation or chemotherapy), re-evaluation of the airway can be performed, and the stent can be left in place, removed (if deemed of no further clinical advantage) or replaced with a larger stent that would further improve the calibre and stability of the airway. The disadvantages of the Dumon stent are the potential for migration and the need for a rigid bronchoscope for placement. The migration issue, although often referred to, occurs less often when the stent is placed by an experienced interventional endoscopist [30–34].

Other silastic stents include the Hood stent (Hood Laboratories, Decatur, GA, USA) and the hybrid Rüsch Y stent (Rüsch Inc., Duluth, GA, USA). The Hood stent is similar

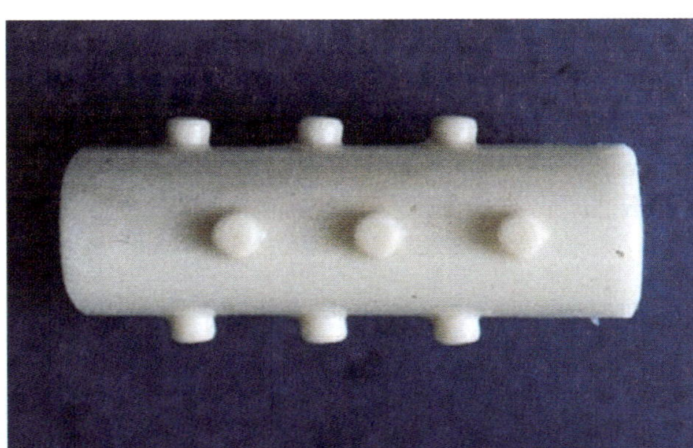

Fig. 4. – The Dumon stent.

to the Dumon stent in design and use. The Rüsch Y stent is a silastic stent with stainless steel c-rings that artificially represent the cartilage. The posterior wall of the stent is made of a thinner silastic plastic to make it more functional, similar to the membranous trachea itself. The three available sizes of this stent are designed to traverse the entire length of the trachea with branches into the right and left mainstem bronchi. The Rüsch Y stent requires rigid bronchoscopy and is difficult to place, remaining uncommon in clinical practice.

Metal stents

Metal stents have been used in the endobronchial management of lung cancer. The advantage of metal stents is the relative ease for placement *via* a flexible bronchoscope with fluoroscopic assistance. This ease of placement allows some bronchoscopists to use these stents as their sole modality in the management of endobronchial disease. However, this practice limits the options to patients that may otherwise be available if all interventional modalities were offered. The wire mesh design of many of the original metal stents did not prevent the tumour from growing through the stent over time. A wrap is applied to the outside of the wire mesh to prevent tumour invasion through the stent. Data that support the use of both of these stents for the endobronchial management of lung cancer is available [35–38].

Most of the metallic stents are made of nitinol, a titanium and nickel alloy, which has little bioreactivity. These stents have excellent inner to outer diameter and conform well to various airway shapes, maintaining an equal pressure along the entire length of the stent. They are available in a variety of lengths and diameters. Overall, the covered versions of the stents are excellent for use in palliation of airway obstruction (fig. 5).

Metal stents epithelialise, as they remain in the airways, thereby becoming incorporated into the wall of the bronchus. The epithelialisation changes the mechanics of the airways with time by making them stiffer, which may lead to further airway complications [39, 40]. Another consideration with the use of metal stents is the fact that, once they are endoscopically placed, their removal is difficult and often impossible. Although uncommon, the risk with the use of metal stents is the erosion that can occur through bronchial/tracheal walls. This is particularly serious when erosion occurs into blood vessels, leading to massive uncontrollable haemoptysis.

Stents are effective tools for the endobronchial management of lung cancer. The choice of stent to use should be made carefully, weighing advantages and disadvantages of each, so that the proper tool is used in all situations. Multiple stent types need to be available to the endoscopist to allow the proper choice for the clinical situation.

Although several new prototypes are being studied, there have been relatively few advances in stent technologies in recent years. Bolliger *et al.* [4] described an improvement in the Polyflex stent (Rüsch AG, Kernen-Rommelshausen, Germany) by the addition of studs on the outer surface to reduce the chance of migration. This silicon stent has some advantages over the Dumon stent, including a thinner stent wall and a better ability to mould to airways of varying diameter.

Photodynamic therapy

Photodynamic therapy (PDT) has received increased attention in recent years. PDT is an important adjunctive modality to the management of endobronchial disease, but it

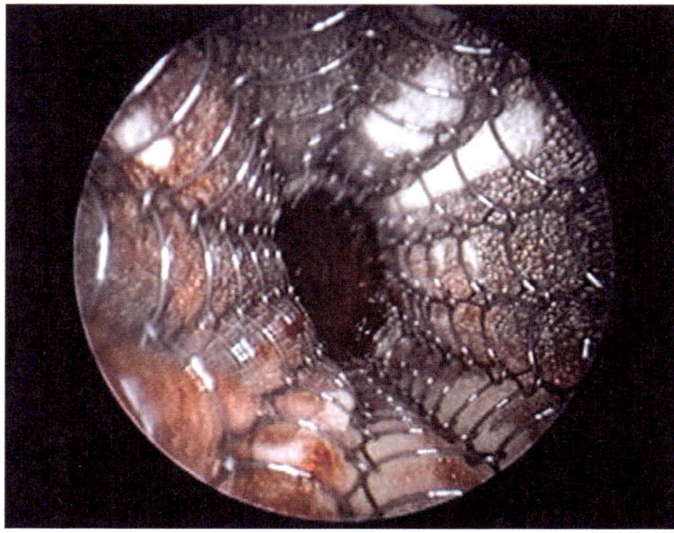

Fig. 5. – Metallic stent in the trachea.

does not replace Nd:YAG lasers, stents and rigid bronchoscopy. PDT also can be used with bulky disease, but most interventionalists feel that it is of limited benefit in this role [41, 42]. The most suitable lesions for PDT are in situ carcinomas or those limited to 4–5 mm of microinvasion [43].

A photosensitising drug is intravenously administered to the patient 48–72 h prior to the procedure. Porfimer sodium (Photofrin) is the most common agent currently used for this. This photosensitiser penetrates all cells systemically. It is not cleared as quickly in cancer cells as in other cells and is, therefore, found in higher concentrations in cancer cells as opposed to the endothelium surrounding the tumour [43, 44]. An argon dye laser is then used to provide the 630-nm wavelength light energy required to activate the intracellular porfimer sodium. The laser energy is transmitted *via* a flexible quartz fibre, which can be used through either a flexible or rigid bronchoscope. The fibre tip can be placed in close proximity to the tumour mass or it can be imbedded into the tumour to provide the energy needed to start the intracellular activation of the porfimer sodium. This reaction leads to cellular destruction by a variety of mechanisms. Tissue necrosis then ensues as the cancer cells die [43–45].

As the neoplastic tissue necrotises, it must be removed by repeated bronchoscopies. Flexible bronchoscopy is commonly performed daily or every other day for up to 1 week to remove the necrotic tissue. The necrosis of a bulky tumour can be dangerous to the patient if the necrotic tissue separates from the bronchial wall and occludes the airway. In some programmes that use only PDT, patients remain intubated following the procedure for 1–2 days due to this concern. If necrotic tissue is removed over the first 24–48 h, a second laser application to the cancer can be performed, thus improving the cancer tissue destruction. PDT is an excellent therapeutic modality for patients with early-stage cancers. It destroys neoplastic tissue effectively and is an outstanding therapeutic modality in carcinoma in situ and microinvasive cancers. PDT is a necessary tool in our armamentarium of endobronchial treatments, but the time delays and multiple steps of management make it a more cumbersome therapy for the management of late-stage endobronchial lung cancer [45].

Endoluminal brachytherapy

Brachytherapy means the direct placement of a highly radioactive source inside a tumour mass. This can be done either by implanting the source directly into the tumour, *via* the natural route (endoluminal brachytherapy) or by placing the source into the tumour bed during tumour resection. Endoluminal brachytherapy employing the afterloading technique with iridium-192 high dose rate (HDR) is largely applied for the curative and palliative treatment of endobronchial tumours due to its tumour-specific and long-lasting effect. Endoluminal brachytherapy using flexible bronchoscopy and an HDR regimen can be performed on an outpatient basis and is not more strenuous for the patient than a diagnostic bronchoscopy. Symptomatic improvement can be achieved in 70–80% of patients and sometimes small tumours can even be cured. The afterloading procedure can be combined with all other modalities of tumour therapy. It can be used as a boost to conventional external irradiation and as a local treatment modality in patients on systemic chemotherapy or as the only local treatment. HDR treatment is usually delivered with 1–6 fractions at an interval of 1–3 weeks and a dose of 3–20 Gy per fraction (at 1 cm from the source axis). In patients previously treated with external beam radiation therapy and in the palliative setting, a regimen of 7–10 Gy (HDR) per fraction and a total of 2–3 fractions per treatment is recommended. However, the optimal dosage and fractionation schemes for the tumour therapy are still un-known and there is need for further studies. In about 10% of the patients, radiation bronchitis occurs, and there may be fatal haemorrhage, possibly related to the therapy and often occurring weeks to months after the actual treatment. This complication could perhaps be avoided through scheduling and dosing of the HDR brachytherapy [46]. Overall, endobronchial brachytherapy is a well tolerated, not very aggressive treatment option, especially in patients with reduced performance status [46]. Endoluminal brachytherapy is therefore a permanent interdisciplinary challenge with the need for a close contact between radiation oncologists and chest physicians.

Conclusion

Modern interventional pulmonology techniques have evolved during the last 25 yrs. These techniques are now mainstream therapies for central airway obstruction resulting from malignant and benign conditions. Recent literature confirms the efficacy and safety of endobronchial therapies developed in the 1980s and 1990s. Although the Nd:YAG laser remains the prototypic therapy for endoluminal disease, there is a trend toward the use of less expensive, more readily available techniques such as electrocautery. A variety of stents are available for management of central airway obstruction resulting from external compression or loss of cartilage support. Whether these techniques should be performed by all pulmonologists or be limited to centres of excellence remains controversial. Certainly all pulmonologists should become familiar with the indications and contraindications of these procedures so that they can be made available to appropriate patients.

Summary

The field of interventional pulmonary medicine is a relatively new area in pulmonary medicine, resulting from technological advances as well as the increasing need for palliative and curative treatment modalities for patients with tracheobronchial, parenchymal and pleural disease. This chapter reviews the advances in endoscopic techniques aimed at the tracheobronchial tree, laser photoresection, electrosurgery, argon plasma coagulation, stent placement, brachytherapy and others, in patients suffering from lung cancer.

Keywords: Bronchoscopy, cryotherapy, electrocautery, interventional pneumology, laser therapy, stents.

Statement of interest
F.J.F. Herth has received travel support to the European Respiratory Society (ERS) Congress from the ERS, and an honorarium to speak at the Postgraduate courses.

References

1. Cancer Facts and Figures, 2008. Atlanta, American Cancer Society, 2008. Available from http://www.cancer.org/docroot/STT/content/STT_1x_Cancer_Facts_and_Figures_2008.asp
2. Luomanen RKJ, Watson WL. Autopsy findings. *In*: Watson WL, ed. Lung Cancer: A Study of Five Thousand Memorial Hospital Cases. St Louis, CV Mosby Co., 1968; pp. 504–510.
3. Ernst A, Feller-Kopman D, Becker HD, *et al.* Central airway obstruction. *Am J Respir Crit Care Med* 2004; 169: 1278–1297.
4. Bolliger CT, Sutedja TG, Strausz J, *et al.* Therapeutic bronchoscopy with immediate effect: laser, electrocautery, argon plasma coagulation and stents. *Eur Respir J* 2006; 27: 1258–1271.
5. Sonett JR, Keenan RJ, Ferson PF, *et al.* Endobronchial management of benign, malignant, and lung transplantation airway stenoses. *Ann Thorac Surg* 1995; 59: 1417–1422.
6. Macha HN, Becker KO, Kemmer HP. Pattern of failure and survival in endobronchial laser resection. A matched pair study. *Chest* 1994; 105: 1668–1672.
7. Beamis JF, Becker HD, Cavaliere S, *et al.* ERS/ATS statement on interventional pulmonology. *Eur Respir J* 2002; 19: 356–373.
8. Ernst A, Silvestri GA, Johnstone D, *et al.* Interventional pulmonary procedures: guidelines from the American College of Chest Physicians. *Chest* 2003; 123: 1693–1717.
9. Beamis JF Jr. Interventional pulmonology techniques for treating malignant large airway obstruction: an update. *Curr Opin Pulm Med* 2005; 11: 292–295.
10. Noppen M, Meysman M, D'Haese J, *et al.* Interventional bronchoscopy: 5-year experience at the Academic Hospital of the Vrije Universiteit Brussel (AZ-VUB). *Acta Clin Belg* 1997; 52: 371–380.
11. Ikeda S. Flexible bronchofiberscope. *Ann Otol Rhinol Laryngol* 1970; 79: 916–923.
12. Prakash UB, Stubbs SE. The bronchoscopy survey. Some reflections. *Chest* 1991; 100: 1660–1667.
13. Mathisen DJ, Grillo HC. Endoscopic relief of malignant airway obstruction. *Ann Thorac Surg* 1989; 48: 469–475.
14. Freitag L, Macha H-N, Loddenkemper R. Interventional bronchoscopic procedures. *In*: Spiro SG, ed. Lung Cancer. *Eur Respir Mon* 2001; 17: 272–304.
15. Dumon JF, Reboud E, Garbe L, *et al.* Treatment of tracheobronchial lesions by laser photoresection. *Chest* 1982; 81: 278–284.

16. Venuta F, Rendina EA, De Giacomo T, *et al.* Nd:YAG laser resection of lung cancer invading the airway as a bridge to surgery and palliative treatment. *Ann Thorac Surg* 2002; 74: 995–998.
17. Diaz-Jimenez JP, Rodriguez AN. Laser bronchoscopy for malignant disease. *In*: Beamis JF, Mathur PN, Mehta AC, eds. Interventional Pulmonary Medicine. New York, Marcel Dekker, 2004; pp. 89–126.
18. van Boxem T, Muller M, Venmans B, *et al.* Nd-YAG laser *versus* bronchoscopic electrocautery for palliation of symptomatic airway obstruction: a cost-effectiveness study. *Chest* 1999; 116: 1108–1112.
19. Mehta AC, Golish JA, Ahmad M, *et al.* Palliative treatment of malignant airway obstruction by Nd-YAG laser. *Cleve Clin Q* 1985; 52: 513–524.
20. Arabian A, Spagnolo SV. Laser therapy in patients with primary lung cancer. *Chest* 1984; 86: 519–523.
21. Brutinel WM, Cortese DA, McDougall JC, *et al.* A two-year experience with the neodymium-YAG laser in endobronchial obstruction. *Chest* 1987; 91: 159–165.
22. Noppen M, Meysman M, Van Herreweghe R, *et al.* Bronchoscopic cryotherapy: preliminary experience. *Acta Clin Belg* 2001; 56: 73–77.
23. Homasson JP. Cryosurgery and electrocautery. *In*: Strausz J, ed. Pulmonary Endoscopy and Biopsy Techniques. *Eur Respir Mon* 1998; 9: 106–123.
24. Sutedja G, van Kralingen K, Schramel FM, *et al.* Fibreoptic bronchoscopic electrosurgery under local anaesthesia for rapid palliation in patients with central airway malignancies: a preliminary report. *Thorax* 1994; 49: 1243–1246.
25. van Boxem T, Westerga J, Venmans BJ, *et al.* Tissue effects of bronchoscopic electrocautery: bronchoscopic appearance and histologic changes of bronchial wall after electrocautery. *Chest* 2000; 117: 887–891.
26. Coulter TD, Mehta AC. The heat is on: impact of endobronchial electrosurgery on the need for Nd-YAG laser photoresection. *Chest* 2000; 118: 516–521.
27. Morice RC, Ece T, Ece F, *et al.* Endobronchial argon plasma coagulation for treatment of hemoptysis and neoplastic airway obstruction. *Chest* 2001; 119: 781–787.
28. Freitag L, Reich L. Argon plasma coagulator. *In*: Beamis JF, Mathur PN, Mehta AC, eds. Interventional Pulmonary Medicine. New York, Marcel Dekker, 2004; pp. 203–213.
29. Montgomery WW. T-tube tracheal stent. *Arch Otolaryngol* 1965; 82: 320–321.
30. Dumon JF. A dedicated tracheobronchial stent. *Chest* 1990; 97: 328–332.
31. Colt HG, Dumon JF. Tracheobronchial stents: indications and applications. *Lung Cancer* 1993; 9: 301–306.
32. Cooper JD, Pearson FG, Patterson GA, *et al.* Use of silicone stents in the management of airway problems. *Ann Thorac Surg* 1989; 47: 371–378.
33. Tojo T, Iioka S, Kitamura S, *et al.* Management of malignant tracheobronchial stenosis with metal stents and Dumon stents. *Ann Thorac Surg* 1996; 61: 1074–1078.
34. Dumon JF, Cavaliere S, Diaz-Jimenez JP, *et al.* Seven-year experience with the Dumon prosthesis. *J Bronchol* 1996; 3: 6–10.
35. Miyazawa T, Yamakido M, Ikeda S, *et al.* Implantation of ultraflex nitinol stents in malignant tracheobronchial stenoses. *Chest* 2000; 118: 959–965.
36. Saad CP, Murthy S, Krizmanich G, *et al.* Self-expandable metallic airway stents and flexible bronchoscopy: long term outcomes analysis. *Chest* 2003; 124: 1993–1999.
37. Herth F, Becker HD, LoCicero J 3rd, *et al.* Successful bronchoscopic placement of tracheobronchial stents without fluoroscopy. *Chest* 2001; 119: 1910–1912.
38. Miyazawa T, Miyazu Y, Iwamoto Y, *et al.* Stenting at the flow-limiting segment in tracheobronchial stenosis due to lung cancer. *Am J Respir Crit Care Med* 2004; 169: 1096–1102.
39. Noppen M, Piérard D, Meysman M, *et al.* Bacterial colonization of central airways after stenting. *Am J Respir Crit Care Med* 1999; 160: 672–677.
40. Freitag L. Tracheobronchial stents. *In*: Strausz J, ed. Pulmonary Endoscopy and Biopsy Techniques. *Eur Respir Mon* 1998; 9: 79–105.

41. Lam S. Photodynamic therapy of lung cancer. *Semin Oncol* 1994; 21: Suppl. 15, 15–19.
42. Sutedja T, Lam S, LeRiche JC, *et al.* Response and pattern of failure after photodynamic therapy for intraluminal stage I lung cancer. *J Bronchol* 1994; 1: 295–298.
43. Furuse K, Fukuoka M, Kato H, *et al.* A prospective phase II study on photodynamic therapy with photofrin II for centrally located early-stage lung cancer. The Japan Lung Cancer Photodynamic Therapy Study Group. *J Clin Oncol* 1993; 11: 1852–1857.
44. Hayata Y, Kato H, Konaka C, *et al.* Photodynamic therapy (PDT) in early stage lung cancer. *Lung Cancer* 1993; 9: 287–294.
45. Vergnon JM, Huber RM, Moghissi K. Place of cryotherapy, brachytherapy and photodynamic therapy in therapeutic bronchoscopy of lung cancers. *Eur Respir J* 2006; 28: 200–218.
46. Ozkok S, Karakoyun-Celik O, Goksel T, *et al.* High dose rate endobronchial brachytherapy in the management of lung cancer: response and toxicity evaluation in 158 patients. *Lung Cancer* 2008; 62: 326–333.

CHAPTER 21

Epidemiology of lung cancer and mesothelioma

J.M. Samet, A.J. Alberg#, J.G. Ford¶*

**Dept of Preventive Medicine, Keck School of Medicine, Institute for Global Health, University of Southern California, Los Angeles, CA, #Dept of Biostatistics, Bioinformatics and Epidemiology, College of Medicine, Medical University of South Carolina, Charleston, SC, and ¶Dept of Epidemiology, Johns Hopkins University, Bloomberg School of Public Health, Baltimore, MD, USA.*

Correspondence: J.M. Samet, Dept of Preventive Medicine, Keck School of Medicine, Institute for Global Health, University of Southern California, 1441 Eastlake Ave, Room 4436, MC 9175, Los Angeles, CA 90089, USA. Fax: 1 3238650127; E-mail: jsamet@usc.edu

The first section of this chapter, on lung cancer, originally appeared in *Chest* in 2007, co-authored by A.J. Alberg, J.G. Ford and J.M. Samet [1]. It is reproduced here, with modifications, with permission from the publisher.

THE EPIDEMIOLOGY OF LUNG CANCER

Epidemiological evidence is the foundation for primary and secondary disease prevention. Epidemiological approaches are used to track the occurrence of disease, to characterise natural history and to identify determinants of disease. The benefits of intervention programmes, whether based in risk factor interventions or screening, are also assessed using epidemiological approaches. For lung cancer, routine mortality statistics confirmed the clinical impression that the disease became more frequent across the first half of the 20th century. Case–control and cohort studies, the epidemiological study designs used to evaluate exposure–disease associations, causally linked smoking to lung cancer in investigations reported from the 1950s onwards [2–4]. As we have continued to follow lung cancer incidence and mortality rates, we have readily shown that their rise and decline parallel past trends of cigarette smoking [5]. The epidemiological evidence and the complementary biological understanding of respiratory carcinogenesis have unassailably supported the conclusion that smoking causes lung cancer. Epidemiological findings are also relevant to patient care, as skilled clinicians weigh alternative diagnoses depending on risk factor profiles of patients.

This chapter provides a summary of the epidemiological evidence on lung cancer, with an emphasis on issues that are currently relevant to prevention. This literature is now extraordinarily large and we have not attempted to conduct a comprehensive review and systematic synthesis. Such syntheses have been periodically carried out by expert review groups, including the committees assembled to prepare the US Surgeon General's reports on smoking and health and other federal documents, and expert committees of other governments and organisations, including the United Kingdom's Royal College of Physicians and Scientific Committee on Tobacco and the World Health Organization's International Agency for Research on Cancer (IARC). Several relevant reports have been recently published, including the 2004 IARC monographs on active and involuntary smoking [6] and the 2004 report of the Surgeon General [7].

Eur Respir Mon, 2009, 44, 349–391. Printed in UK - all rights reserved. Copyright ERS Journals Ltd 2009; European Respiratory Monograph; ISSN 1025-448x.

At the end of the 20th century, lung cancer had become one of the world's leading causes of preventable death [8]. It was a rare disease at the start of that century, but exposures to new aetiological agents and an increasing life span combined to make lung cancer a scourge of the 20th century. While tobacco had been widely used throughout the world for centuries, the present pandemic of lung cancer followed the introduction of manufactured cigarettes with addictive properties, which resulted in a new pattern of sustained exposure of the lung to inhaled carcinogens [9]. German scientists in Nazi Germany conducted some of the earliest research on the links between smoking and lung cancer [10]. By the early 1950s, epidemiological studies in Britain and the USA using the case–control method had shown that cigarettes were strongly associated with the risk of lung cancer [11–13]; this association was corroborated by the pioneering cohort studies of British physicians, veterans in the USA, and volunteers recruited by the American Cancer Society (ACS) [14]. By 1964, the evidence was sufficient to support a conclusion by the US Surgeon General that cigarette smoking caused lung cancer [14]. The Royal College of Physicians had reached the same conclusion 2 yrs previously [15]. Passive smoking, the involuntary inhalation of tobacco smoke by nonsmokers, has also been found to cause lung cancer [16, 17].

While its predominant cause is now well known (tobacco smoking), there are other causes as well, some acting in concert with smoking to synergistically increase risk. The suspicion that radon was a cause of lung cancer in underground miners, raised early in the 20th century, led to what was probably the first occupational respiratory carcinogen to be identified [18]; radon in indoor environments is now considered as the second leading cause of lung cancer in the USA [19]. The list of human occupational causes of lung cancer also includes arsenic, asbestos, chromates, chloromethyl ethers, nickel, polycyclic aromatic hydrocarbons, radon progeny and other agents [20]. Outdoor air pollution, which includes combustion-generated carcinogens, is also considered to contribute to the lung cancer burden in urban dwellers. Indoor air contains several respiratory carcinogens, including radon, asbestos and cigarette smoke. In some developing countries, exposure to fumes from cooking stoves and fires is associated with lung cancer risk. Beginning in the 1970s, associations of diet with lung cancer risk have been vigorously investigated, with the anticipation that dietary micronutrients might be found that modify the high lung cancer risk in smokers.

Even though the epidemiology of lung cancer has been extensively investigated for >50 yrs, there are still active areas of research, some quite relevant to prevention. Investigation of lung cancer and diet continues, using both observational and experimental approaches, and concern remains over the risk of indoor and outdoor pollutants including, for example, radon and diesel emissions. There has also been a need for research to track the risks of smoking over time, as the cigarette has evolved in its design characteristics and yields of tar and nicotine, as assessed by standard protocol using a machine, have declined since the 1950s. The histological characteristics of lung cancer in a number of developed countries, including the USA, have also changed in recent decades such that the frequency of adenocarcinoma has risen and that of squamous cell carcinoma has declined [5]. There is also emerging evidence on genetic determinants of lung cancer risk. A current research approach, termed molecular epidemiology, melds the population and laboratory tools used to address susceptibility to environmental carcinogens. While the evidence from the "traditional" epidemiological approaches conclusively established the carcinogenicity of tobacco smoke, molecular epidemiology should characterise the sequence of molecular and cellular changes as a nonmalignant cell becomes malignant and genetic factors possibly determining susceptibility to tobacco smoke. Biomarkers of exposure, dose, susceptibility and genetic damage may allow epidemiological investigations to uncover specific pathways of human lung carcinogenesis and provide useful intermediate markers for prevention studies.

Patterns of occurrence

Survival

The 5-yr relative survival rate for lung cancer for the period 1995–2001 was 15.7%, reflecting a steady, but slow, improvement from 12.5% in 1974–1976 [21]. The 5-yr relative survival rate varies markedly depending on the stage at diagnosis, from 49% to 16% to 2% for local, regional and distant stage disease, respectively [21]. Stage at diagnosis accounts for the most marked variation in prognosis, but patient characteristics associated with poorer survival also include being older, male and African American [21].

Temporal trends

Because of the high case-fatality rate of lung cancer, incidence and mortality rates are nearly equivalent and, consequently, routinely collected vital statistics provide a long record of the occurrence of lung cancer. We are presently amidst an epidemic of lung cancer that dates to the first half of the last century.

Sex

Lung cancer was rare until the disease began a sharp rise around 1930 that culminated by mid-century with lung cancer becoming the leading cause of cancer death among males [22]. The epidemic among females followed that among males, with a sharp rise in rates from the 1960s to the present, propelling lung cancer to become the most frequent cause of female cancer mortality [22]. As the leading cause of cancer death among females, lung cancer is a major female health issue. Due to historical cigarette-smoking patterns, the epidemic of lung cancer started later in females than males but, in contrast to the situation in males, lung cancer incidence rates in females have not yet begun to consistently decrease [21]. Far more males than females still die from lung cancer each year, but the sex gap in lung cancer mortality is steadily narrowing and will eventually close [23, 24]. This trend is due to historical smoking patterns, with smoking prevalence having peaked approximately two decades earlier among males than females [23, 24].

Examination of time trends of age-specific lung cancer mortality rates in the USA further highlights the differing epidemic patterns in males compared with females. The sex-race specific mortality rates are now almost all decreasing [23]. The rates of lung cancer in the younger age groups have been declining over the last several decades in males and over the last decade in females [23]. As the younger birth cohorts age, their reduced risk of lung cancer foreshadows substantial reductions in the overall occurrence of lung cancer, but the reductions will be greater for males than for females. These patterns are all consistent with population patterns of smoking prevalence over time [23].

Race and ethnicity

The patterns of occurrence of lung cancer by race and ethnicity make lung cancer a relevant disease for those concerned with the health of minorities. Of particular note is that, whereas lung cancer incidence rates are similar among African-American and white females, lung cancer occurrence is ~45% higher among African-American males than among white males [21]. This racial disparity may be partially due to greater susceptibility of African-American smokers to smoking-induced lung carcinogenesis [25]. The higher mortality rates of lung cancer in African Americans compared with white Americans reflect not only their higher incidence rate, but also the poorer survival from lung cancer among African Americans compared with white Americans. The 5-yr relative survival rate was 13% lower in African Americans compared with white Americans during the period 1995–2001 [21]. This racial gap persisted within each stage at diagnosis category, and for males and females [21].

Lung cancer mortality rates among Hispanics, Native Americans and Asians/Pacific Islanders are significantly lower than rates among African Americans and non-Hispanic Whites [26]. Nevertheless, lung cancer poses a considerable public health burden among these groups.

Socioeconomic status

Lung cancer is more likely to occur in the poor and less educated, a pattern that is observed in many countries worldwide. For example, in Canada the risk of lung cancer in both sexes was inversely associated with income, education and social class, even after adjustment for cigarette smoking [27]. In China, those classified as low income had a six-fold increased risk of lung cancer compared with those in the high income category [28]. In the Netherlands, the risk of lung cancer was inversely associated with attained education, an association that was not attributable to occupational exposures [29]. Lower socioeconomic status has also been observed to be associated with later stage at diagnosis [30].

Socioeconomic status is associated with a constellation of interacting determinants of lung cancer risk, such as smoking, diet and exposures to inhaled carcinogens in the workplace and general environment. Lower socioeconomic status is associated with an unfavourable profile for all of these factors. Advancing our understanding of the complex linkages between components of socioeconomic status and lung cancer risk is essential to effectively addressing this social class disparity, and reducing lung cancer rates in the poorer segments of society.

Geographical patterns

Lung cancer is the most commonly diagnosed cancer worldwide [31], but its geographical distribution shows marked regional variation: age-standardised incidence rates range over 60-fold among males and 30-fold among females (fig. 1) [32]. Because of differences in cancer registration between countries, caution is needed in interpreting these data. However, this marked variation in rates cannot be explained on the basis of diagnostic practices and data quality alone. Lung cancer tends to be most common in developed countries, particularly in North America and Europe, and less common in developing countries, particularly in Africa and South America [32, 33]. The low rates of lung cancer in Africa are comparable to rates in the USA in 1930, when rates of lung cancer were under five per 100,000 for both sexes [34]. In contrast, African Americans in the USA, an epicentre, now experience lung cancer incidence rates that are among the highest in the world. As the lung cancer epidemic begins to subside in the developed countries, it is on the rise in the developing world [31].

Within countries, lung cancer incidence among males invariably exceeds that in females by well over 100% in most nations. The international rankings of lung cancer

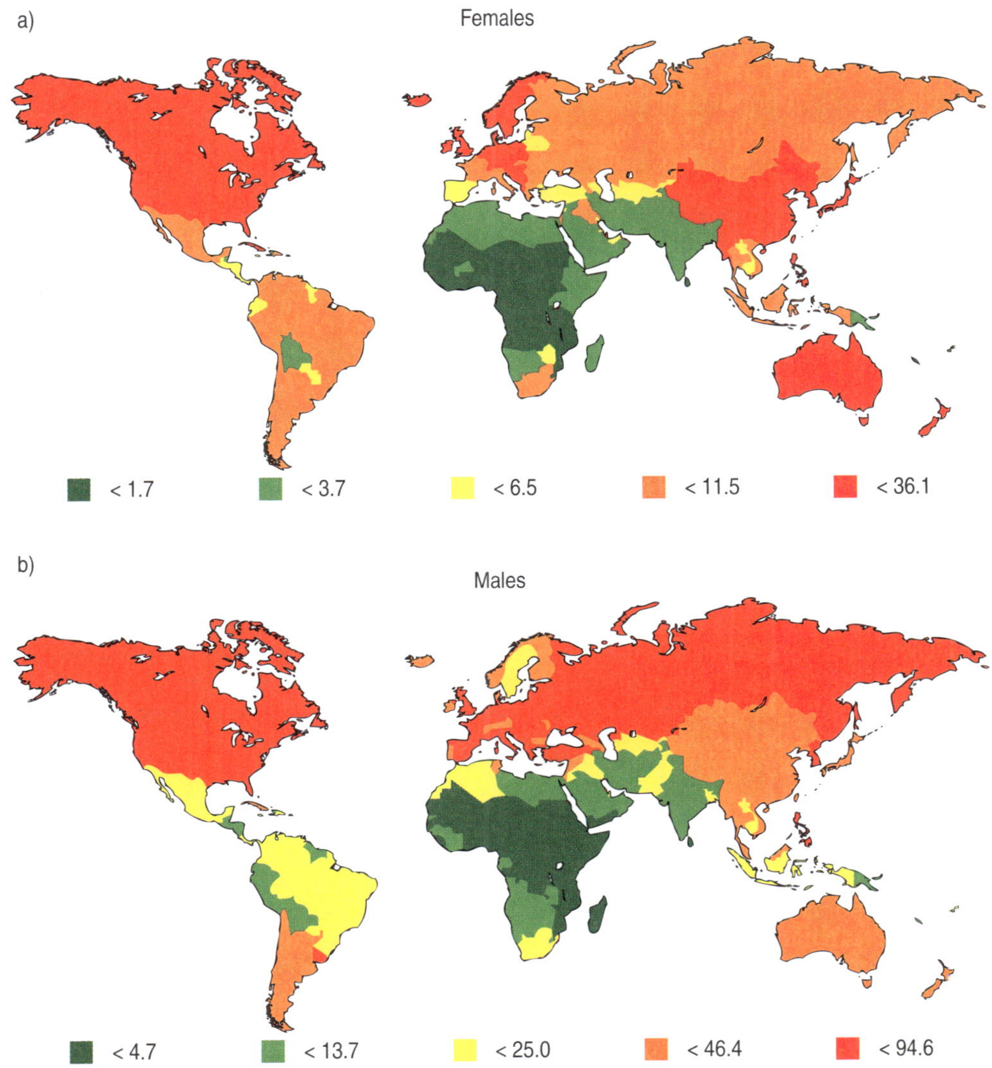

Fig. 1. – Lung cancer in a) females and b) males. Age-standardised incidence rates per 100,000 worldwide in 2002. Reproduced from [32], an open-source publication.

incidence of males and females from the same countries tend to differ only slightly, so that the highest rates of lung cancer occur in the same regions of the world for both sexes.

Substantial geographical variation in lung cancer mortality rates has also been observed within countries. For example, during the period 1997–2001, the age-adjusted lung cancer mortality rates varied more than three-fold between the state with the highest rate (Kentucky: 78 per 100,000) and the state with lowest rate (Utah: 25 per 100,000) [21]. Trends in its regional distribution can provide clues about determinants of lung cancer. In the past, rates tended to be highest in urban areas, which led to conjecture that air pollution might be a cause of the lung cancer epidemic [35]. Later on, several hypotheses [36, 37] were prompted by patterns observed in a systematic review of lung cancer mortality rates in the USA for the period 1950–1969 [38], particularly the rates among males. For example, high rates in coastal areas were postulated to reflect employment in shipyards with attendant asbestos exposure. This hypothesis was then tested in a series of population-based case–control studies that showed that employment in the shipbuilding industry was indeed associated with an excess risk of lung cancer [39]. Another shift then took place in the distribution of lung cancer within the USA, with lung cancer mortality rates among white males becoming highest in the south and lower in the northeast [40]. This temporal fluidity in the geographical variation underscores the need for regular monitoring of lung cancer mortality patterns.

The aetiology of lung cancer

Overview

Although the causes of lung cancer are almost exclusively environmental, there is probably substantial individual variation in susceptibility to respiratory carcinogens. The risk of the disease can be conceptualised as reflecting the joint consequences of the interrelationship between exposure to aetiological (or protective) agents and individual susceptibility to these agents. The "environment" in its broadest sense may influence the risk of disease through direct exposures or indirectly by affecting the likelihood of exposure to exogenous agents. Given lung cancer's multifactorial aetiology, synergistic interactions among risk factors may have substantial consequences for lung cancer risk. These interactions have typically been considered on an agent-by-agent basis, such as, for example, the synergistic effect of cigarette smoking on the lung cancer risk from asbestos exposure [41]. Our emerging understanding of cancer genetics indicates the additional relevance of gene–environment interactions.

Given the many risk factors that have been identified for lung cancer, a practical question is the relative contribution of these factors to the overall burden of lung cancer. The "population attributable risk" approach takes into account the magnitude of the relative risk (RR) associated with an exposure along with the likelihood of exposure in the general population. Because of the interactions between exposures, the combined population attributable risk for diseases such as lung cancer that have a well-characterised set of important risk factors can exceed 100%. As discussed in the following sections, population attributable risk estimates for lung cancer indicate that, in the USA, active smoking is responsible for 90% of lung cancer, occupational exposures to carcinogens for ~9–15%, radon for 10% of lung cancer [19] and outdoor air pollution for perhaps 1–2% [42]. The precise contribution of nutritional factors remains to be determined, but dietary factors have been hypothesised to account for ~20% (range 10–30%) of the lung cancer burden [43].

Environmental and occupational agents

Smoking.

Overview. A single aetiological agent, cigarette smoking is by far the leading cause of lung cancer, accounting for ~90% of lung cancer cases in the USA and other countries where cigarette smoking is common [44]. Compared with never-smokers, smokers who have smoked without quitting successfully have about a 20-fold increase in lung cancer risk at present. Few exposures to environmental agents convey such risks for any disease. In general, trends of lung cancer occurrence closely reflect patterns of smoking, but rates of occurrence lag behind smoking rates by about 20 yrs. Analyses using statistical modelling techniques show a tight association between national mortality rates and smoking [45]. The unequivocal role of cigarette smoking in causing lung cancer is one of the most thoroughly documented causal relationships in biomedical research [9, 46].

The burden of lung cancer attributable to smoking has been extensively documented. Using an attributable risk approach, the annual number of deaths caused in the USA by smoking-related lung cancer during the period 1995–1999 was 122,800 [7]. PETO *et al.* [44] have used a different attributable risk method to quantify the burden of smoking-related deaths from lung cancer in the major developed countries. For 1990 the total in the USA was 127,000, the highest in the world, with country-specific estimates ranging down to 150 for Tajikistan. The total for the developed countries was 457,371 [44]. A staggering future burden of lung cancer has been forecasted for China, where the numbers are predicted to reach several millions by mid-century [47, 48].

Cigar smoking is also an established cause of lung cancer [49]. The lung cancer risks associated with cigar smoking are substantial but less than the risks observed for cigarette smoking, due to differences in smoking frequency and depth of inhalation. The same pattern holds true for pipe smoking [50].

Quantitative risks. The risk of lung cancer among cigarette smokers increases with the duration of smoking and the number of cigarettes smoked per day [51]. This observation has been made repeatedly in cohort and case–control studies. Risk models have been derived to quantitatively estimate how lung cancer risk varies with number of cigarettes smoked, duration of smoking and age. Such models are useful for estimating the future burden of lung cancer under various scenarios of tobacco control. In one widely cited analysis, DOLL and PETO [51] proposed a quantitative model for lung cancer risk based on data from the cohort study of British physicians. This model predicted a stronger effect of duration of smoking than of amount smoked per day. Thus, a tripling of the number of cigarettes smoked per day was estimated to triple the risk whereas a tripling of duration of smoking was estimated to increase the risk 100-fold [52]. These quantitative dimensions of the dose–response relationship between smoking and lung cancer have implications concerning the now widespread smoking among youths. Those starting at younger ages have a greater likelihood of becoming a heavier smoker and remaining a smoker [53]. The exponential effect of duration of smoking on lung cancer risk markedly increases the lifetime risk for those who become regular smokers in childhood and places them at increased risk at younger ages. Prevention approaches that delay the age of onset of smoking in a population could have substantial impact on the incidence of lung cancer by shortening the duration of smoking. In considering the likelihood of lung cancer in a particular patient, clinicians should give more weight to the duration of smoking and less to actual age.

Smoking cessation. Cigarette smokers can benefit at any age by quitting smoking. The likelihood of developing lung cancer decreases among those who quit smoking compared with those who continue to smoke [53]. As the period of abstinence from smoking cigarettes increases, the risk of lung cancer decreases [54]. However, even for periods of abstinence of over 40 yrs the risk of lung cancer among former smokers remains elevated compared with never-smokers [54, 55]. The benefits derived from smoking cessation also depend on the duration of smoking; for a given period of abstinence, the decrease in risk increases as the duration of smoking decreases [54]. In general, studies have shown comparable reductions in risk following cessation regardless of sex, type of tobacco smoked and histological type of lung cancer [56].

The changing cigarette. The composition of cigarettes has evolved considerably since the 1950s. The marketplace has shifted from mainly unfiltered cigarettes to predominantly filtered cigarettes. The filters in use in the USA are predominantly cellulose acetate, while charcoal filters are used extensively in Japan and some other countries [57]. In the mid-1960s, ventilation holes were added to the filter, which dilute the smoke with air drawn through them. However, smokers can readily block the holes with their fingers, which are left unblocked by the machines used to test cigarettes. There have also been substantial changes in the design of the cigarette and in the tobacco used. Reconstituted tobacco has been used increasingly since the 1960s and there have been changes to the cigarette paper and additives used and most cigarettes are more ammoniated in the USA [57].

A concomitant shift toward lowered levels of "tar" and nicotine, as measured by a smoking machine, has occurred [58]. Cigarette "tar" refers to the condensable residue of cigarette smoke, *i.e.* the total particulate matter of cigarette smoke deposited on the machine's filter less the moisture and nicotine. Tar is a complex mixture that includes many chemicals that are cancer initiators and/or promoters [58]. Tar and nicotine yields are measured with a smoking machine according to a standardised protocol established by the Federal Trade Commission (FTC) that specifies such details and puff volume, the frequency of puffing and the length to which the cigarette is to be smoked [59].

Studies using biomarkers of exposure and dose of tobacco smoke components show little relationship of levels of these markers with tar or nicotine yield as measured by the FTC's protocol [59]. These studies have been conducted in both the population context and during smoking in the laboratory setting. For example, COULTAS *et al.* [60] collected saliva for analysis for cotinine level and end-tidal breath samples for measurement of carbon monoxide level in a population sample of New Mexico Hispanics included in a respiratory health survey. After taking account of numbers of cigarettes smoked, biomarker levels were not associated with the yields of tar and nicotine of the current brand smoked. DJORDJEVIC *et al.* [61] evaluated smoking pattern and biomarkers in the laboratory setting, contrasting smokers of medium-yield and low-yield cigarettes. The smokers had greater puff volumes and frequencies than are specified in the FTC protocol and had substantially greater intakes of tar and nicotine than implied by the brand listings. The lack of association of tar and nicotine yields with biomarker levels partially reflects compensatory changes in smoking patterns for those switching from higher- to lower-yield products. The compensation includes blocking of the ventilation holes, more frequent and deeper puffs, and an increase in the number of cigarettes smoked [62].

The gradual reduction in machine-measured tar yield over recent decades would be expected to have reduced smokers' exposures to carcinogens if the FTC test protocol were predictive of carcinogen doses delivered to the lung [58]. However, questions remain as to whether the FTC test method is informative with regard to lung cancer risk or risks of smoking-caused diseases more generally [62, 63]. Epidemiological studies have been carried out to assess whether the seemingly substantial changes in tar and nicotine yield, as measured by the FTC protocol, have resulted in parallel changes in the risk of smoking. Epidemiological studies have been the key source of information, as they can provide direct evidence on the risks of smoking cigarettes, as they are actually smoked during use, including any compensatory behaviour.

For lung cancer and for other diseases, three lines of epidemiological data have been available on changes in products. The first comes from case–control studies that compare the smoking history profiles of persons developing lung cancer with those of controls. The second comes from cohort studies that tracked the risk of lung cancer over time, as the products smoked changed. The third comes from assessment of the temporal changes in age-specific patterns of lung cancer mortality rates in comparison with changes in cigarette characteristics.

The initial evidence came primarily from case–control studies that compared risks in persons who had used filter-tip cigarettes with persons who had smoked nonfiltered cigarettes exclusively [64, 65]. This evidence suggests that filtered cigarettes and cigarettes with lower tar yields slightly reduce the risk of lung cancer associated with cigarette smoking compared with unfiltered cigarettes or those with higher tar yields [66–68]. This comparison could be made among smokers in the 1960s, as there was still a substantial proportion who had not used filter cigarettes at all. For example, in one of the first studies, Bross and Gibson [64] compared lung cancer risk of filter and nonfilter smokers among patients seen at Roswell Park Memorial Cancer Institute (Buffalo, NY, USA); persons were classified as filter cigarette smokers if they had used these products for at least 10 yrs.

The relevant cohort studies are the ACS Cancer Prevention Study (CPS)-I and CPS-II studies and the British physicians cohort. In a 1976 publication, Hammond *et al.* [69] compared mortality risks from lung cancer and other diseases by tar yield of products smoked by participants in the ACS CPS-I. The follow-up interval spanned 1960–1972. Smokers were placed into three categories of products smoked: low yield (<17.6 mg·cigarette^{-1}), high yield (25.8–35.7 mg·cigarette^{-1}) and medium (intermediate). The standardised mortality rate for lung cancer in low- and medium-yield smokers was ~80% of the rate in high-yield smokers. A further analysis of tar yield using the same data set confirmed that risk for lung cancer death increased with tar yield [70].

Further insights have been gained by comparing the risks in the two CPS studies of the ACS; this comparison addresses whether risks have changed, comparing smokers developing disease during 1960–1972 with a similar group developing disease during the initial follow-up of CPS II, in 1980–1986 [71, 72]. If the risk for lung cancer associated with smoking was decreasing over time, the expectation would be that risks for smokers would be less in CPS II than in CPS I. In fact, the opposite was observed, with increasing lung cancer mortality in male and female smokers in CPS II, compared with CPS I [73].

In an analysis with a similar pattern of findings, Doll *et al.* [74] compared the risks of death from lung cancer and other causes during the first and second 20 yrs of the 40-yr follow-up of the British physicians cohort. Lung cancer mortality increased among smokers in the second 20 yrs (1971–1991), even though products smoked during this time period would have had a substantially lower tar and nicotine yield than those smoked during the first 20 yrs (1951–1971). For the first 20 yrs, the annual lung cancer mortality rate among current smokers was 264 per 100,000 and for the second 20 yrs it was 314 per 100,000. In 2004, Doll *et al.* [75] reported the findings at 50 yrs of follow-up and, compared with lifelong nonsmokers, the risk of developing lung cancer was increased four-fold among former smokers and over 14-fold among current smokers; among current smokers the RRs increased from 7.7 to 13.7 to 24.5 among smokers of 1–14, 15–24 and >25 cigarettes·day^{-1}, respectively.

The third line of observational evidence comes from descriptive analyses of age-specific trends of lung cancer mortality [6, 62, 76]. Successive birth cohorts have had differing patterns of exposure to cigarettes of different characteristics and yields. For example, the cohort of persons born between 1930 and 1940 who started to smoke in the 1950s was one of the first to have the opportunity to smoke primarily filter-tipped cigarettes. Subsequent birth cohorts would have had access to the increasingly lower-yield products while earlier cohorts had access initially only to unfiltered cigarettes. Patterns of temporal change in age-specific rates of lung cancer mortality in younger males have been examined, in order to assess whether there has been a decline greater than expected from changing prevalence, duration and amount of smoking, hence indicating a possible effect of cigarette yield.

Data on lung cancer mortality in younger males in the United Kingdom have been interpreted as indicating a possible reduction in lung cancer risk associated with changes in cigarettes [62, 76]. A sharp decline in lung cancer mortality has occurred across recent decades in the United Kingdom in males under 50 yrs of age. The decline seems greater than anticipated from trends in prevalence and other aspects of smoking, such as age of starting and number of cigarettes smoked. A similarly steep decline has not taken place in the USA. Given the ecological nature of the data under consideration, uncertainty remains with regard to their interpretation and alternative explanations have been proposed, including less intense smoking at younger ages in more recent birth cohorts [62].

This discussion highlights the complexity of isolating the precise effect on lung cancer risk of the continually changing cigarette. The data available to evaluate these effects have limitations, particularly in successively capturing the experience of successive birth cohorts in either case–control or cohort studies that were appropriately designed. The United Kingdom mortality data suggest a greater effect of changes in cigarettes than is found in the case–control and cohort studies. As recommended by the Institute of Medicine, surveillance is needed to track the health consequences of the changing cigarette [77].

Several expert panels have recently reviewed the findings. The Institute of Medicine carried out a comprehensive review on various harm reduction strategies for reducing the disease burden caused by smoking, including lower-yield cigarettes [77]. There are also new products in various phases of development that are intended to deliver nicotine without direct combustion of tobacco. The Institute of Medicine report concluded that smoking lower-yield products had not been shown to benefit the health of smokers.

This topic was addressed in the 2004 report of the US Surgeon General, with the conclusion that "Although characteristics of cigarettes have changed during the last 50 yrs and yields of tar and nicotine have declined substantially, as assessed by the Federal Trade Commission's test protocol, the risk of lung cancer in smokers has not declined" [7].

Are females more susceptible to smoking-induced lung cancer? Results of some case–control studies have suggested a potentially higher risk of smoking-associated lung cancer in females compared with males [78, 79], but methodological issues cloud the interpretation of these studies, particularly a lack of focus on the most informative comparisons [80]. Furthermore, the evidence from prospective cohort studies fails to support the notion of a sex differential in susceptibility to lung cancer from smoking [81]. The equal rates of lung cancer mortality in younger males and females in the USA corresponding to a time of equal smoking prevalence also provides evidence against an important sex difference in susceptibility to smoking-induced lung cancer [23]. At present, the evidence against this hypothesis outweighs the evidence in favour of the hypothesis, based on the fact that the results of studies that have compared the RR estimates for males and females for a specific degree of smoking history demonstrate very similar associations [81].

Menthol cigarettes and the high risk of lung cancer among African Americans. The development of menthol cigarettes was targeted specifically at Blacks and females [82, 83]. Blacks are more likely than Whites (69 *versus* 29%) to smoke menthol cigarettes [84]; and the menthol smoke delivery levels of common cigarette brands have increased significantly since the 1980s [85, 86]. This has led to the hypothesis that menthol cigarettes explain the greater susceptibility to lung cancer from cigarette smoking in

Blacks *versus* Whites [25], and thus the disparity in lung cancer risk between Blacks and Whites in the USA, especially among males.

Menthol cigarettes may cause a greater increase in lung cancer risk than non-menthol cigarettes, either by increasing systemic exposure to toxicants from tobacco smoke or by affecting the metabolism of nicotine and/or tobacco smoke carcinogens. Initially, this hypothesis gained currency because of the potential for increased nicotine uptake through the effects of menthol in the respiratory tract. These include the following: an increase in the smoothness of tobacco smoke, which promotes deeper inhalation; stimulation of cold receptors, which results in airway cooling effects that mask the irritation caused by cigarette smoke, promoting deeper inhalation and altered inhalation frequency; further masking of irritation through anaesthetic effects [85, 86]; and increased permeability and diffusibility of smoke constituents [87].

There is limited information on the molecular mechanisms by which mentholation might increase the health risk of smoking. 70–80% of nicotine is metabolised to cotinine, and cytochrome P450 2A6 is responsible for 90% of this conversion [88]. The P450 2A6 gene has multiple functional polymorphisms that vary by race. The observation that menthol competitively inhibits cotinine metabolism by the monkey analogue of a human UDP-glucuronyltransferase (UGT) [89] suggested that inhibition of either CYP2A6 or UGT by menthol might alter nicotine and cotinine metabolism. African-American and Caucasian menthol smokers have similar baseline cotinine levels [90]. Recent human studies have suggested that smoking mentholated cigarettes inhibits nicotine metabolism, so smokers experience higher doses of nicotine for a given level of smoking [88, 90–92]. Menthol inhibits the microsomal oxidation of nicotine to cotinine [91], suggesting that smoking mentholated cigarettes may lead to inhibition of nicotine metabolism. In a randomised crossover study of seven African Americans and seven Caucasians, Benowitz *et al.* [92] found that the systemic intake of nicotine was not affected by mentholation, but smoking mentholated cigarettes inhibited the metabolism of nicotine. By slowing the metabolism of nicotine and thereby reducing the need for nicotine from smoking, menthol may reduce the number of cigarettes smoked per day. A menthol effect might explain why African Americans smoke fewer cigarettes per day than Whites. It may also explain, in part, the variation by race and sex in the correlation between cotinine level and cigarettes smoked per day among smokers of menthol cigarettes [93], possibly reflecting the effect of menthol on nicotine inactivation by P450 2A6 [88].

However, the epidemiological data suggest that, overall, smokers of mentholated cigarettes do not have an increased risk of lung cancer compared with smokers of non-mentholated cigarettes. This evidence is based primarily on hospital-based case–control studies [94–97], but also includes a population-based case–control study [98] and a cohort study within a health maintenance organisation [99]. Furthermore, menthol cigarettes have not been associated with any specific histological subtypes of lung cancer [100].

Evidence that menthol cigarettes might carry greater risks were that, in one case–control study, black male heavy smokers of mentholated cigarettes (>37.5 pack-yrs or $\geq$21 cigarettes·day^{-1}) had a higher risk than white males with similar smoking histories [96], and in the cohort study the RR of lung cancer among males, but not females, was slightly elevated in menthol smokers compared with non-menthol smokers, with a graded increase in lung cancer risk with increasing duration of menthol cigarette use [99].

At present, the evidence does not indicate that menthol cigarettes are an important contributor to the high rates of lung cancer in African Americans. A more definitive answer to this question will emerge if future studies address several methodological challenges, including misclassification of menthol cigarette exposure due to brand ambiguity, potential for selection bias in hospital-based case–control studies, due a lower prevalence of menthol cigarette use among African-American patients at university hospitals used for such studies than in the general population, and lack of information about compensatory mechanisms [101].

Second-hand smoke exposure. Passive smokers inhale a complex mixture of smoke now widely referred to as second-hand smoke (SHS) or environmental tobacco smoke (ETS). Passive smoking was first considered as a possible risk factor for lung cancer in 1981 when two studies were published that described increased lung cancer risk among never-smoking females who were married to smokers. HIRAYAMA [102] reported the findings from a cohort study in Japan that showed that, among nonsmoking females, those whose husbands smoked cigarettes were at higher risk of lung cancer than those whose husbands were nonsmokers. A case–control study in Athens reported by TRICHOPOLOUS *et al.* [103] shortly thereafter replicated this finding. Additional evidence rapidly accrued so that by 1986 two important summary reports were published. The National Research Council reviewed the epidemiological evidence and concluded that nonsmoking spouses who were married to cigarette smokers were about 30% more likely to develop lung cancer than nonsmoking spouses married to nonsmokers and that this relationship was biologically plausible [104]. Almost one quarter of lung cancer cases among never-smokers were estimated to be attributed to exposure to passive smoking [104]. The 1986 Surgeon General's report also judged passive smoking to be a cause of lung cancer [16], an inference corroborated by the 1992 review of the evidence and risk assessment by the US Environmental Protection Agency, which classified ETS as a known human (class A) carcinogen [17]. Estimates indicate that passive smoking accounts for ~3,000 lung cancer deaths per year in the USA [17].

Since these conclusions were reached, several major studies have been carried out to further characterise the association of passive smoking with lung cancer, while taking into account some of the limitations of earlier studies, particularly small sample sizes, exposure misclassification and omission of some potential confounding factors [105, 106].

Passive smoking is more weakly associated with lung cancer than is active smoking, as expected given the generally lower doses of carcinogens passively received by the lung of the nonsmoker compared with the doses received by the active smoker. Because of broad societal implications, the conclusion that this association is causal has generated controversy, some driven by the tobacco industry's effort to maintain continued questioning of the evidence [107, 108]. Questions have been raised about the methodology of the epidemiological studies, including confounding and misclassification of exposure to ETS. Review groups have nonetheless concluded that the association between ETS and lung cancer cannot be attributed to methodological limitations of epidemiological data [16, 17, 105, 109].

Studies have been directed at the specific venues where nonsmokers are exposed to tobacco smoke, including the home, workplaces and public places. Much of the literature has focused on the increased risk associated with being married to a smoker, an exposure variable that can be readily ascertained. Meta-analyses have been conducted periodically to summarise the evidence from the epidemiological studies. A 2002 meta-analysis by BOFFETTA [110] found a 25% increased risk associated with marriage to a smoker; this excess risk appeared to be due to exposure to passive smoking since it could not be explained by confounding or misclassification. This finding was consistent with the 29% estimated increased risk among females whose husbands smoked in the meta-analysis of TAYLOR *et al.* [111], who observed that the association was consistent across study designs and in Western and non-Western nations. Workplace exposure to SHS was associated with a 17% increase in lung cancer risk in the meta-analysis of BOFFETTA [110].

The studies of passive smoking provide further evidence documenting the dose–response relationship between cigarette smoke and lung cancer. The doses extend to far lower levels than those of active smoking and increased risk is observed, suggesting that there is no threshold for tobacco carcinogenesis [16].

Lung cancer histopathology. Notable shifts have taken place in the incidence rates of lung cancer by histological type [112]. After steadily increasing occurrence during the period 1973–1987, adenocarcinoma supplanted squamous cell carcinoma as the most frequent form of lung cancer in the USA [112]. Adenocarcinoma increased markedly in all race/sex subgroups [112].

Lung cancer occurs in multiple histological types as classified by conventional light microscopy. The four major types include squamous cell carcinoma, adenocarcinoma, large cell carcinoma and small cell undifferentiated carcinoma; together these four types of lung cancer account for over 90% of lung cancer cases in the USA [113]. In spite of extensive research, the mechanisms leading to these different types of lung cancer remain uncertain. Hypotheses have focused on the cells of origin of lung cancers and on pathways of differentiation of malignant cells [113]. Smoking has been shown to cause each of the major histological types, although the dose–response relationship with number of cigarettes smoked varies across the types, being steepest for small cell undifferentiated carcinoma [114]. There are a few suggestive links of histological type with occupational agents: small cell lung cancer has been reported to be in excess in workers exposed to chloromethyl ethers and in underground miners exposed to radon progeny [113].

In the initial decades of the smoking-caused epidemic of lung cancer, squamous cell carcinoma was the most frequent type of lung cancer observed in the population among smokers and small cell carcinoma was the next most frequent. In the late 1970s, the first evidence of a shift towards a predominance of adenocarcinoma was noted [113, 115, 116], and now adenocarcinoma of the lung is the most common histologial type [111]. The decline in lung cancer rates has been more rapid for squamous cell and small cell carcinomas than for adenocarcinoma, which is just beginning to show a lower incidence rate [112]. In females, the Surveillance, Epidemiology and End Results (SEER) Program data for 1973–1996 indicate that the incidence rates of squamous cell, small cell and large cell carcinomas have at least reached a plateau, while the rate for adenocarcinoma is still rising [5].

While changing patterns of diagnosis and classification of lung cancers could have led to these changes over time, most observers have set aside an artefactual change [113, 116]. Beginning in the 1970s, new techniques for the diagnosis of lung cancer became available, including the fibreoptic bronchoscope and thin-needle aspiration [117]; improved stains for mucin, the hallmark of adenocarcinoma, were also introduced. Using data from the Connecticut Tumour Registry, Thun *et al.* [117] showed that the rise in adenocarcinoma antedated these diagnostic innovations.

Hypotheses concerning the shift in histopathology have focused on the potential role of changes in the characteristics of cigarettes and consequent changes in the doses of carcinogens inhaled [118]. Puff volume has probably increased over recent decades, with the possibility that patterns of deposition in the lung have changed, tending towards enhanced deposition of tobacco smoke in the peripheral airways and alveoli [118]. Nitrate levels in tobacco smoke have also increased, which enhances the combustion of tobacco smoke. While more complete combustion decreases the concentrations of polycyclic aromatic hydrocarbons, the increased production of nitrogen oxides contributes to increased formation of tobacco-specific nitrosamines. An increase in dose of the potent tobacco-specific nitrosamine, 4-(methylnitrosamino)-1-(3-pyridyl)-1-

butanone (NNK), has been postulated as one factor leading to the increase in adenocarcinoma [118, 119]. NNK induces lung carcinomas, predominantly adenomas and adenocarcinomas, in mice, regardless of route of administration [119, 120].

Few studies can provide data to test these hypotheses because of the need for longitudinal observation of lung cancer risk in relation to the characteristics of the cigarettes smoked over time. THUN *et al.* [117] compared risks for lung cancers of the different histological types among participants in the ACS CPS I and CPS II. They found markedly rising risks associated with smoking for adenocarcinoma of the lung in both males and females over the ~20 yrs separating the two studies. THUN *et al.* [117] concluded that "The increase in lung adenocarcinoma since the 1950s is more consistent with changes in smoking behaviour and cigarette design than with diagnostic advances." In a study that compared tumour location in lung cancer patients, lower-tar cigarettes were associated with a higher likelihood of peripheral than central tumours [121].

Diet.

Overview. Research on diet and lung cancer has now been carried out for nearly three decades. The possible role of diet in modifying the risk of lung cancer has been the focus of intensive investigation, driven initially by the rationale that specific micronutrients might have anti-carcinogenic activity. The most thoroughly investigated dietary factors are also those that at present appear to have the greatest implications for prevention: fruits, vegetables and specific antioxidant micronutrients that are commonly found in fruits and vegetables. Much of the research on diet and lung cancer has been motivated by the hypothesis that diets high in antioxidant nutrients may reduce oxidative DNA damage and thereby protect against cancer [122].

The results of case–control and prospective cohort studies have tended to show that individuals with high dietary intake of fruits or vegetables have a lower risk of lung cancer than those with low fruit or vegetable intake [123]. Evidence from cohort studies published since 2000 has tended to reinforce this notion [124–128]. In the European Prospective Investigation into Cancer and Nutrition (EPIC) study, a strong protective association was observed with fruit, but not vegetable, consumption [129]. A stronger protective association was observed for fruit than vegetable consumption in a pooled analysis of seven cohort studies [130].

To understand better the basis of this protective association, fruits and vegetables have been grouped into classes and also examined individually in relation to lung cancer risk. For example, tomatoes [131–133] and cruciferous vegetables [127, 133] have been associated with a reduced risk of lung cancer in a number of studies, at least for the highest *versus* lowest categories of consumption. These food-based analyses can help to clarify whether it is the complex mixture contained in fruits/vegetables that confers protection against lung cancer, or whether the protection may be due to specific biochemical constituents present in particular fruits and vegetables.

Fruits and vegetables are the major dietary source of antioxidant micronutrients. Two different strategies are used to evaluate the relationship of micronutrients to lung cancer risk in observational epidemiological studies: 1) using data summarised from food-frequency questionnaires to estimate micronutrient intake, and 2) drawing blood samples from study participants and assaying the concentrations of micronutrients in circulation. The former approach provides a better average measure of micronutrient "exposure", whereas the latter approach has the advantage of measuring micronutrient concentrations closer to the cellular level where the postulated biological effect occurs. The differences in measurement approaches may lead to different results in certain situations. A meta-analysis of selenium and lung cancer found that selenium intake as measured by questionnaire showed no association (RR 1.0, 95% confidence interval (CI)

0.8–1.3), whereas associations in the protective direction were observed for selenium concentrations measured in toenails (RR 0.5, 95% CI 0.2–0.9) or serum (RR 0.8, 95% CI 0.6–1.1) [134].

Studies of both dietary intake [135–138] and prediagnostic blood concentrations [139, 140] suggest a protective association between carotenoids and lung cancer. The evidence for vitamin C is scant but suggestive of a protective association, whereas the data on vitamin A has yielded null findings [141]. Reports from recent cohort studies have tended to reinforce the previous findings of protective associations with intake of a variety of carotenoids [126, 133, 142] or a higher antioxidant index [138]. However, a pooled analysis of seven cohort studies did not find strong protective associations with any carotenoids other than β-cryptoxanthin [137].

More recently, studies have examined phytochemicals such as flavonoids and isothiocyanates in relation to lung cancer risk. Phytochemicals are low molecular weight molecules produced by plants. Of the many classes of phytochemicals, those studied in relation to lung cancer include phyto-oestrogens, flavonoids and glucosinoids. The tumour-promoting effects of steroid hormones can be blocked by phyto-oestrogens. Soya beans are a primary source of a specific class of phyto-oestrogens known as isoflavonoids. Flavonoids exhibit potent antioxidant activity. Flavonoid intake has been at least weakly associated with lung cancer in some of the preliminary studies of this topic [143, 144]. Isothiocyanates are metabolites of the class of phytochemicals known as glucosinolates. Isothiocyanates could exert anticancer effects by blocking carcinogens *via* induction of phase II detoxification enzymes, such as glutathione S-transferase (GST). Cruciferous vegetables contain high concentrations of glucosinolates and, hence, consumption leads to higher endogenous isothiocyanate concentrations. As with cruciferous vegetables [145], lung cancer risk is also consistently lower with higher intakes or urinary levels of isothiocyanates [146–148]. When isothiocyanates have been studied in combination with a common polymorphism in the GSTM1 gene, the decreased risk of lung cancer associated with isothiocyanates has been especially pronounced in persons with the GSTM1 null genotype [146–148]. This provides an example of a potential gene–diet interaction that may be relevant to lung carcinogenesis.

Studies of fruits, vegetables and micronutrients have been the centrepiece of studies of diet and lung cancer, but a wide range of dietary and anthropometric factors have been investigated. For example, the results of a meta-analysis showed that alcohol drinking in the highest consumption categories was associated with increased risk of lung cancer [149]. Anthropometric measures have also been studied, indicating a tendency for persons with lower body mass index to have increased lung cancer risk relative to heavier persons [150, 151]. However, effects of both alcohol drinking and low body mass index may be difficult to separate from the concomitant effects of smoking. At present, when considering the possible relationships between lung cancer and factors such as alcohol drinking and lower body mass index, cigarette smoking cannot be dismissed as a possible explanation.

The overwhelming contribution of cigarette smoking as a cause of lung cancer poses a challenge to detecting the role that other lifestyle factors, such as diet, may play in the aetiology of lung cancer. Cigarette smoking is now so closely associated with less healthy lifestyles in the USA and some other countries, such as less healthy diets [152], that it is often difficult to disentangle the dietary factor(s) of interest from the effects of smoking. Cigarette smoke can directly affect circulating concentrations of dietary factors; for example, smokers tend to have lower circulating concentrations of antioxidant micronutrients even after accounting for differences in dietary intake [152]. Additionally, associations between dietary factors and lung cancer risk are likely to be far weaker than the association with active smoking, and diet is measured with much greater error in general than is smoking. Even for a dietary factor such as vegetable consumption, which is fairly consistently associated with a lower risk of lung cancer, the highest exposure category is typically associated with at most a halving in the risk of lung cancer. Thus, in interpreting evidence on diet and lung cancer risk, residual confounding cannot be readily set aside as an explanation for the observed associations between dietary factors and lung cancer [153].

Chemoprevention trials. The experimental rationale for trials of β-carotene and retinoids has been published elsewhere [154]. Experimental data indicated a potential for prevention with these agents, as observational data were supportive of the hypothesis that β-carotene and retinoids might have chemopreventive activity [122]. However, a protective association between β-carotene and lung cancer was not found in three randomised, double-blind, placebo-controlled chemoprevention trials of β-carotene reported during the 1990s [155–157]. In fact, β-carotene supplementation was associated with an increased risk of lung cancer among the high-risk populations of heavy smokers in the α-tocopherol β-carotene (ATBC) cancer prevention study [155] and smokers and asbestos-exposed workers in the β-carotene and retinol efficacy trial (CARET) [157].

In summary, observational evidence suggests that smokers who eat more vegetables are at lower risk of lung cancer than persons who consume fewer vegetables. The evidence is not as consistent for fruit consumption. The specific constituents of vegetables that confer protection are not known. The results of the chemoprevention trials clearly suggest a more complex role for micronutrients than previously proposed.

Physical activity. Several studies have reported that more physically active individuals have a lower risk of lung cancer than those who are more sedentary [158–160], even after adjustment for cigarette smoking. As with the assessment of any lifestyle factor other than smoking with lung cancer risk, potential residual confounding by cigarette smoking needs to be considered as an alternative explanation.

Environmental exposures.

Occupational exposures. Investigations of occupational groups, often heavily exposed over a long time to workplace agents, have provided substantial understanding of the carcinogenicity of a number of chemicals and physical agents. Among cancers that are associated with occupational exposures, cancer of the lung is the most common [161]. Estimates derived from case–control studies of the proportion of lung cancer that is contributed to by occupational exposures (*via* independent or shared causal pathways) have ranged widely, but most point estimates or ranges have included values up to 9–15% [162–168]. While disagreement persists concerning specific estimates [169], the message is clear: in industrialised nations the contribution of occupational exposures to the lung cancer burden is small compared with that of cigarette smoking but large compared with contributions of most other exposure classes. Cigarette smoking potentiates the effect of some known occupational lung carcinogens [41].

Lung cancer has been observed to be associated with many workplace exposures. Workers exposed to tar and soot (which contains benzo[a]pyrene) in concentrations exceeding those present in urban air, such as coke oven workers [170–172], are at increased risk of lung cancer. Occupational exposures to a number of metals, including arsenic, chromium and nickel, are also causes of lung cancer [173]. For many of the worker groups exposed to these agents, there were substantial increments in risk. However, in developed countries these hazards have largely been controlled.

For some other workplace agents, the evidence has been less clear. The results of numerous case–control and cohort studies are compatible with a weak association between exposure to diesel exhaust and the development of lung cancer [174]. Although inadequate control of cigarette smoking limits the inferences that can be drawn from many of these studies, exposure to diesel exhaust remains a likely explanation for these findings [174]. This association remains of public health concern, as the public is exposed to diesel exhaust in urban areas, and in some European countries diesel vehicles are increasingly used [42].

The question of whether silica dust is a risk factor for lung cancer has been controversial [175–177]. A two-fold increase in lung cancer risk was estimated from a meta-analysis of the relationship between silicosis and lung cancer mortality [178]. Effects of smoking have not been well controlled in most of the studies [178]. The evidence on silica exposure, without consideration of silicosis, is less clear [179, 180]. In 1997, the IARC did classify crystalline silica as a human carcinogen [181]; however, some still continue to question its carcinogenicity [180] and the role of silica exposure *versus* that of fibrosis in persons with silicosis [179].

Asbestos. Asbestos, a well-established occupational carcinogen, refers to several forms of fibrous, naturally occurring silicate minerals [182]. The epidemiological evidence dates to the 1950s, although clinical case series had previously led to the hypothesis that asbestos causes lung cancer [183, 184]. In a retrospective cohort study published in 1955, DOLL [185] observed that asbestos textile workers at a factory in the United Kingdom had a 10-fold elevation in lung cancer risk and that the risk was most heavily concentrated during the time frame before regulations were implemented to limit asbestos dust in factories. A seven-fold excess of lung cancer was subsequently observed among insulation workers in the USA [186, 187]. The risk of lung cancer has been noted to increase with increased exposure to asbestos [188] and to be associated with the principal commercial forms of asbestos [189]. Whether asbestos acts directly as a carcinogen or through indirect mechanisms, such as causing chronic inflammation that eventually leads to cancer development, remains uncertain [190, 191].

Asbestos and cigarette smoking are both independent causes of lung cancer, but in combination they act synergistically to increase the risk of lung cancer in a manner that is compatible with a multiplicative effect [192]. Cigarette smoking may increase the lung cancer risk associated with asbestos exposure by enhancing retention of asbestos fibres [193].

Radiation.

Overview. Epidemiological studies of populations exposed to high doses of radiation show that lung cancer is one of the cancers associated with exposure to ionising radiation. However, the risks of low-dose radiation, more relevant to contemporary workers and the general population, have proven difficult to characterise [194]. Assessing the cancer risk associated with low-dose radiation among humans is methodologically difficult because the signal-to-noise ratio is highly unfavourable [195]. Nevertheless, large cohort studies, particularly the study of Japanese atomic bomb survivors, have provided understanding of the risks of low-dose ionising radiation [19, 196, 197].

The following two types of radiation, classified by rate of energy transfer to the tissue, are relevant to lung cancer: low linear energy transfer (LET) radiation (*e.g.* X-rays and gamma rays) and high-LET radiation (*e.g.* neutrons and radon). High-LET radiation produces ionisation of relatively higher density in tissues than low-LET radiation, so in equivalent doses more biological damage is produced by high-LET than low-LET radiation [198]. For both types of radiation, the majority of the epidemiological evidence comes from cohorts exposed at levels substantially greater than those experienced by the general population. Risk assessment methods are then used to estimate risks to the population.

High-LET radiation: radon. Radon is an inert gas that is produced naturally from radium in the decay series of uranium. Two of the decay products of radon emit alpha particles that can, by virtue of their high energy and mass, cause damage to the DNA of cells of the respiratory epithelium. Epidemiological studies of underground miners of uranium and other ores have established exposure to radon daughters as a cause of lung cancer [199, 200]. In the miners exposed to radon in past centuries, very high lung cancer risks were observed; these fell for more recent workers but the recent epidemiological studies still show clear evidence of existing cancer risk [19]. Cigarette smoking and radon decay products synergistically influence lung cancer risk in a manner that is supra-additive but sub-multiplicative [19, 200].

Radon is of broader societal interest because it is a ubiquitous indoor air pollutant, entering buildings in soil gas. On average, indoor exposures to radon for the general population are much less than received by occupational groups such as uranium miners. For example, even the lowest historical radon concentration in a uranium mine is roughly 50–100 times higher than in the average home [200]. Exposure to radon in indoor air is also assumed to cause lung cancer, but the magnitude of the risk is uncertain because of the assumptions underlying the extrapolation of findings from uranium miners to the generally lower exposures indoors. These assumptions relate to dose, dose rate and dosimetry and also reflect the lack of information on risks of exposures of females and children. Strengthening biological evidence supports the assumption that a single hit to a cell by an alpha particle causes permanent cellular change, an assumption leading to a nonthreshold dose–response relationship.

The assumptions made by the US Environmental Protection Agency and the Biological Effects of Ionizing Radiation (BEIR) IV and VI Committees of the National Research Council (Washington, DC, USA) lead to estimates that ~15,000–20,000 lung cancer deaths per year in the USA are caused by radon [201]. Case–control studies concerning indoor exposure to radon as a risk factor for lung cancer, undertaken to directly assess risks, have produced findings that are generally consistent with downward extrapolation of risk models based on the underground miners [202, 203]. This coherence lends support to using extrapolation of the miner data to estimate the risk of indoor radon.

Low-LET radiation: X-rays and gamma rays. Epidemiological data relating low-LET radiation to lung cancer stem from three principal populations: the atomic bomb survivors in Japan [204], patients with diseases such as ankylosing spondylitis [205] or tuberculosis [206, 207] who received multiple radiation treatments, and occupational groups in professions exposed to radiation [208]. The single, high-dose exposure of the atomic bomb survivors was associated with significant lung cancer risk [204]. Regardless of their age when the atomic bombs were dropped, the excess of lung cancer did not occur until the survivors reached the older ages when cancer usually occurs [204], and a consideration of radiation and smoking together suggests an additional relationship [197].

The risks associated with exposure to lower doses of low-LET radiation have been estimated in two ways. Statistical models have been used to extrapolate from the atomic bomb survivors' data to lower doses. Tuberculosis patients who received radiation therapy have also been studied; they were intermittently exposed to radiation. Such intermittent, low-dose exposures may be most pertinent for the general population because this exposure pattern is the most common in technologically advanced societies. Studies of tuberculosis patients suggest that if there is any risk of lung cancer associated with this exposure pattern, it is small [206, 207], implying that the assumptions upon which the higher risk estimates obtained from the atomic bomb survivors' data are based may in actual fact not hold [207].

Low-LET radiation therefore appears to be associated with higher lung cancer risk when exposure occurs at a higher dose rate [207]. These results contrast with those for high-LET radiation, suggesting that the two types of radiation have different dose-rate relationships [207].

Air pollution.
Overview. During a typical day, the average adult inhales about 10,000 L of air [209]. Consequently, even the carcinogens present in the air at low concentrations are of concern as a risk factor for lung cancer. Extrapolation of the risks associated with occupational exposures to the lower concentration of carcinogens in polluted ambient air leads to the conclusion that a small proportion of lung cancer cases could be due to air pollution [161, 210].

Atmospheric air pollution. Carcinogens generated by combustion of fossil fuels include polycyclic aromatic hydrocarbons and metals such as arsenic, nickel and chromium [173]. In considering respiratory carcinogenesis, the constituents of "air pollution" will vary by locale and over time depending on the pollution sources [211]. Consequently, epidemiological investigations of air pollution and lung cancer have been limited by the difficulty of estimating exposure. Nevertheless, descriptive evidence is consistent with a role for air pollution in causing lung cancer. Urbanisation and lung cancer mortality are linked [212–214]. This association could arise from differences in the distributions of other lung cancer risk factors, such as smoking and occupational exposures, by degree of urbanisation. Adjustment for these factors may considerably attenuate the effect of urban location [215, 216], but an urban effect persists in a number of studies [42].

Air pollution has been assessed as a risk factor for lung cancer in both case–control and cohort studies. Whereas early evidence from case–control and cohort studies was found wanting, more recently the evidence supports a causal role for air pollution [217].

Two prospective cohort studies that partially address weaknesses of earlier studies add evidence that suggests air pollution is weakly associated with the risk of lung cancer [218, 219]. By prospectively studying air pollution levels in relation to risk of lung cancer and by controlling for possible confounders such as age, smoking and socioeconomic status at the individual level, these studies surmount some shortcomings noted of much previous research [220]. In a study of six cities in the USA, the adjusted risk of lung cancer mortality in the city with the highest concentration of fine particles was 1.4 times (95% CI 0.8–2.4) higher than in the least polluted city [218]. Using data from the ACS CPS II, Pope *et al.* [219] observed that, compared with the least polluted areas, residence in areas with high sulphate concentrations was associated with an increased risk of lung cancer (adjusted RR 1.4, 95% CI 1.1–1.7) after adjustment for occupational exposures and the aforementioned factors [219]. However, unlike in the six-cities study, fine particulate concentration was not associated with lung cancer risk [219]. In a subsequent updating of this report, follow-up was extended to 1998 [221]. In this report, the risk of lung cancer was observed to increase by 14% for each 10 $\mu g \cdot m^{-3}$ increase in concentration of fine particles [221].

By contrast, in the ACS CPS I cohort, air pollution was not associated with lung cancer risk; in this study males were stratified according to exposures in the workplace, but exposure assessment for air pollution was based on proxy, less specific measures of air pollution [220]. Some case–control studies have reported indices of air pollution to be modestly associated with elevated risks of lung cancer [222–224], but others have reported no association [225].

Another research approach to evaluate the risk of air pollution has been to investigate populations residing around point sources of pollution, such as factories and smelters.

Proximity of residence to the pollution source can be used as a proxy for exposure. Many industries have been studied using this approach. Areas surrounding nonferrous smelters, which emit arsenic, have been of particular interest. An ecological study reported by BLOT and FRAUMENI [36] in 1975 suggested that excess lung cancer occurred in counties of the USA with copper, lead or zinc smelting and refining industries. The results of several subsequent case–control studies lend support to this hypothesis by showing that the risk of lung cancer increased the nearer persons lived to nonferrous smelters, after accounting for personal cigarette smoking and employment at the smelter [226–228]. Other case–control studies did not replicate this finding but were also limited by their failure to account for smoking and employment at the smelter [229, 230].

DOLL and PETO [161], in their 1981 review of the causes of cancer, estimated that perhaps 1–2% of lung cancer was related to air pollution. Even in light of recent findings, this appears to remain a reasonable estimate [231]. The body of evidence linking air pollution to lung cancer is solidifying [217], but the public health impact of this exposure is small relative to cigarette smoking, at least in developed country settings where research has been carried out. This is to be expected, given that respiratory doses of carcinogens from active smoking are significantly greater than those received from the inhalation of atmospheric contaminants.

Indoor air pollution. An individual's total exposure to air pollution depends on indoor as well as outdoor exposures. Indoor air quality has large potential health implications because people may spend substantial amounts of time indoors. Indoor air pollution may stem from incoming outdoor air or originate indoors from tobacco smoking, building materials, soil gases, household products and combustion from heating and cooking [232]. A trade-off exists between energy efficiency and indoor air quality, as ventilation allows heated/cooled air to escape but improves indoor air quality [233].

As already discussed, in more developed countries, two of the most important indoor pollutants most strongly increasing lung cancer risk in never-smokers are passive smoking [16] and radon [201]. Asbestos exposure may pose a risk to building occupants, but concentrations are generally very low [182]. Of major concern in the developing world is the indoor air contamination resulting from the use of unprocessed solid fuels, notably coal, for cooking and space heating [234]. MUMFORD *et al.* [235] inferred that smoky coal was likely to be a major determinant of the geographical distribution of lung cancer in Xuan Wei, China, a finding corroborated by an animal model [236]. Evidence supporting a causal association was strengthened by the results of a retrospective cohort study, which showed that switching from use of unvented firepits to stoves with chimneys almost halved the risk of lung cancer [237].

Host factors

Overview. Genetic susceptibility to lung cancer has long been postulated. Environmental agents, even cigarette smoking, cause lung cancer in only a minority of exposed persons, leading to the hypothesis that susceptibility is inherently determined. Epidemiological studies showing that a family history of lung cancer predicts increased risk further support a genetic basis for lung cancer susceptibility. This long-postulated hypothesis is now being actively addressed using the approach of molecular epidemiology. Full coverage of this topic is beyond the scope of this chapter; aspects of genetic susceptibility for lung cancer have been previously reviewed [238–242].

Familial aggregation of lung cancer has been primarily demonstrated in both case–control and cohort studies [243]. In these studies, a family history of lung cancer tended to be associated with increased risk of lung cancer; most of the studies controlled for smoking, which is known to aggregate in families. In a large study in Louisiana (USA), segregation analysis suggested that lung cancer inheritance was consistent with a Mendelian co-dominant autosomal gene determining early onset of disease [244]. Conversely, the largest study of lung cancer in twins reported to date did not provide evidence indicating a genetic basis for susceptibility [245]. Follow-up of 15,924 male twin pairs in the USA did not show greater concordance in monozygotic compared with dizygotic twins and death rates from lung cancer were similar by zygosity group in surviving twins whose siblings died of lung cancer. The results of a linkage analysis based on 52 extended pedigrees indicated that a locus on chromosome 6q23–25 was associated with a major susceptibility to lung cancer [246].

In a genetic epidemiology study of lung cancer in nonsmokers in Detroit (MI, USA), SCHWARTZ *et al.* [247] explored familial risk for lung cancer. In nonsmokers, they found an association between risk and a history of lung cancer in a first-degree relative (odds ratio 1.4, 95% CI 0.8–2.5). The association was much stronger in those aged 40–59 yrs at diagnosis compared with older persons. This pattern of risk with age suggests that genetic factors may be more important at younger ages. This general finding was confirmed by a subsequent, complex segregation analysis of the same data [248].

Research findings on the genetic basis of lung cancer. With application of the new and powerful tools of modern molecular and cell biology, research findings are now characterising the changes in cells that are caused by exposure to tobacco smoke and providing a framework for understanding the genetic and epigenetic basis of lung cancer risk. Figure 2, proposed by HECHT [119], presents a general schema for the process of carcinogenesis by tobacco smoking. Viewed in the framework set by this type of model, research findings mirror the predictions of the multistage model in many respects and are enhancing understanding of the mechanisms by which smoking causes cancers of the lung and other organs. A rapidly expanding literature addresses dosimetry and metabolism of tobacco carcinogens at the cellular and molecular levels, genetic determinants of susceptibility, and patterns of genetic changes in the tissues of smokers and in the cancers that the tissues develop [119, 240]. Much of the research carried out to date has been based in case–control studies that compare the genotypes of lung cancer cases with those of controls. Studies have also been carried out using cohort designs with affected and nonaffected persons sampled from the cohort and biological samples analysed for the markers of interest.

The understanding of the epigenetic changes that may be involved in the causal pathway to lung cancer is advancing rapidly. For example, there is increasing evidence that methylation of cytosine in the DNA, leading to hypermethylation of promoter regions, is frequent in most types of cancers, including lung cancer [249]. Promoter

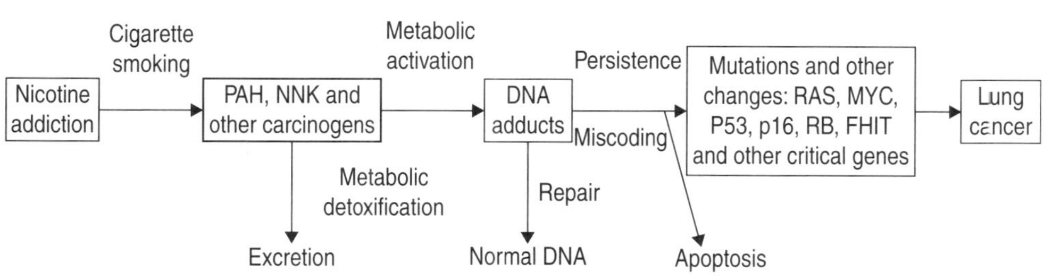

Fig. 2. – Scheme linking nicotine addiction and lung cancer *via* tobacco smoke carcinogens and their induction of multiple mutations in critical genes. Reproduced from [119] with permission from the publisher. PAH: polycyclic aromatic hydrocarbon; NNK: 4-(methylnitrosamino)-1-(3-pyridyl)-1-butanone; RB: retinoblastoma; FHIT: fragile histidine triad.

regions of many human genes have loci rich in CpG dinucleotides, regions referred as CpG islands [249, 250]. Hypermethylation of the CpG islands can be detected by PCR methods. Cells with abnormal methylation of genes have been detected in sputum before the diagnosis of lung cancer, suggesting that hypermethylation could be a useful marker for early detection [251, 252].

In a general formulation of determinants of cancer risk, the risk depends on carcinogen exposure and the factors which determine host susceptibility, including genetic predisposition [253]. For tobacco smoking and lung and other cancers, the elements of this paradigm are all topics of inquiry, using the combination of laboratory- and population-based studies. Biomarkers are central to the molecular epidemiology approach; the term refers to making measurements of indicators of exposure and dose, susceptibility and response in biological materials, including tissue samples, blood, urine and saliva [254]. As research evolves within this paradigm, a more complete biological understanding of the specific events underlying the multistage model, originally proposed on a conceptual basis, can be anticipated.

This framework indicates multiple points where genetically determined host characteristics might be important: carcinogen metabolism and activation, and DNA repair capacity, for example. Reviews have been published previously [239, 255–257] and the evidence has expanded and deepened our understanding of how smoking injures cells and causes cancer and indicates potential approaches to identification of high-risk individuals and molecular screening.

The metabolism of toxic agents, including carcinogens, generally proceeds through two phases [258]. In phase I, unreactive nonpolar compounds are converted, usually by oxidative reactions, to highly reactive intermediates. These intermediates are then able to form complexes with conjugating molecules in phase II conjugation reactions, which are usually less reactive and more easily excreted. However, the intermediate metabolite may react with other cellular components, such as DNA, before conjugation occurs. This binding to DNA may be the first step in the initiation of the carcinogenic process [258].

Many carcinogenic compounds in tobacco smoke, *e.g.* polycyclic aromatic hydrocarbons, undergo metabolic activation by phase I enzymes of the cytochrome p450 system to form reactive intermediates that bind to DNA and cause genetic injury. Several of these enzymes have been investigated with regard to lung cancer risk, including CYP1A1. For CYP1A1, the current evidence suggests that two specific polymorphisms, the MspI polymorphism [259] and a polymorphism in exon 7 [260], are associated with increased risks of lung cancer.

GST is a phase II enzyme that detoxifies reactive metabolites of polycyclic aromatic hydrocarbons. There are at least four genetically distinct classes of the GSTs: μ, α, π and θ. The risk estimates from a meta-analysis indicate that individuals with the GSTM1 null genotype have a higher risk of lung cancer than those with the GSTM1 present genotype, but a pooled analysis of data from 21 case–control studies did not indicate that this susceptibility was stronger among cigarette smokers than among nonsmokers [261]. The importance of interactions between genes is highlighted by the joint assessment of the CYP1A1 Ile462Val and GSTM1 null polymorphisms in nonsmokers, which indicated that the combination of the two variant genotypes was associated with greater than four-fold increased likelihood of lung cancer compared with the combination of the two nonvariant genotypes [262].

There are other candidates for determinants of susceptibility to lung cancer in smokers, including oncogenes, suppressor genes and DNA repair capacity [238]. One gene of particular interest for lung cancer is p53, a tumour suppressor gene [253, 257]. This gene has been described as "at the crossroads" for multiple cellular response pathways considered relevant to carcinogenesis [257]. The gene is frequently mutated in lung cancers, over 90% of small cell cancers and more than 50% of nonsmall cell cancers. The spectrum of mutations in smokers appears to be different from that in nonsmokers [253, 257]. In fact, DENISSENKO *et al.* [263] showed binding of an activated metabolite of benzo[a]pyrene to the same p53 codons where mutations are commonly observed in lung cancers in smokers. However, to date, epidemiological studies of common polymorphisms in the p53 gene have not shown strong associations with lung cancer risk [264].

Substantial research has been directed at DNA repair and susceptibility in lung cancer and other tumours [256, 265]. Persons with specific rare, recessive traits, *e.g.* xeroderma pigmentosa, have long been known to be at increased risk for cancer. DNA repair capacity has now been examined as a specific risk factor for lung cancer, with the underlying hypothesis that lesser capacity would lead to greater lung cancer risk from the multiple DNA-damaging components of tobacco smoke. While much research remains to be done to clarify the association between variation in DNA repair capacity and lung cancer risk, the evidence to date suggests that this is a promising lead [240]. There are a variety of phenotypic assays for susceptibility to DNA damage. Individuals with a less proficient DNA repair capacity phenotype, as measured by a nonspecific mutagen sensitivity assay, have been shown to have an increased risk of lung cancer in some studies [266, 267]. Studies of DNA repair genes have been conducted, including studies of xeroderma pigmentosum complementation groups A and D (*XPA* and *XPD*), X-ray repair complementation groups 1 and 3 (*XRCC1* and *XRCC3*), excision repair cross complementation group 1 (*ERCC1*) and human 8-oxoguanine DNA glycosylase (*hOGG1*). One of the most extensively studied DNA repair genes to date is the nucleotide excision repair gene *ERCC2/XPD* [268, 269]. The evidence to date has not yet revealed a consistent pattern of associations for the Asp312Asn or Lys751Gln polymorphisms of the *ERCC2/XPD* gene [270]. The findings of a review of polymorphisms in three genes in the base excision repair pathway (*hOGG1, APE1/APEX1* nuclease and *XRCC1*) showed that for the *hOGG1* Ser326Cys polymorphism, individuals with the Cys/Cys genotype had an elevated risk of lung cancer (summary odds 1.24, 95% CI 1.01–1.53) [271].

Presence of acquired lung disease

In addition to hereditary factors, increased susceptibility to lung cancer may result from underlying lung disease. Such acquired lung diseases assume two major forms: 1) those that obstruct airflow, such as chronic obstructive pulmonary disease (COPD), and 2) fibrotic disorders that restrict lung capacity, such as pneumoconiosis [272]. Associations between lung cancer and both types of acquired lung disease have been noted but, as will be mentioned in this section, this topic is complex and many issues await resolution, even after debate for over 60 yrs [273].

A substantial body of evidence suggests that COPD or impaired lung function is associated with the occurrence of lung cancer [274]. Cigarette smoking is the principal cause of both COPD [275] and lung cancer, being so strongly causally associated with both of these illnesses that presuming that statistical adjustment procedures "remove" the effect of cigarette smoking may not be well founded. Thus, clarifying the relevance of COPD to the development of lung cancer awaits further proof that this association is not accounted for by cigarette smoking. One potential mechanism hypothesised to link COPD with lung cancer is α_1-antitrypsin (α_1-AT) deficiency, and evidence to support this notion includes the observation that the prevalence of α_1-AT deficiency carriers was higher in lung cancer patients than the general population and higher in lung cancer patients who had never smoked [248]. Alternatively, the presence of COPD may indicate that the affected individual has received a greater dose of tobacco carcinogens than the typical unaffected individual. Regardless of mechanism, the presence of COPD is a clinically useful risk indicator.

Several studies found inverse associations between asthma and lung cancer [276–279]. However, a meta-analysis that rigorously controlled for smoking revealed a positive association between asthma and the risk of lung cancer, especially non-adenoma lung cancer [280]. Subsequently, asthma was found to be associated with lung cancer mortality in the National Health and Nutrition Examination Survey (NHANES) II Mortality Study (1976–1992) [281]. Several potential mechanisms have been proposed to explain this association, including: 1) mucociliary dysfunction leading to accumulation of toxicants, such as lung carcinogens, in the airway; 2) free radical damage to DNA, as a result of imbalance between oxidants and antioxidants; and 3) chronic inflammation leading to chronic mitogenesis and increased likelihood of conversion of endogenous DNA damage into mutations [280]. Appropriately designed studies are needed in order to establish whether and how asthma might increase the risk of lung cancer.

Clarifying the possible relationship between pneumoconioses and lung cancer poses particularly vexing challenges. Even for asbestos exposure, which is clearly established as a potent cause of lung cancer [189], whether lung cancer results from asbestos *per se* or from asbestosis remains controversial [190]. Asbestos is likely to cause lung cancer *via* multiple mechanistic pathways [282, 283]. For other mineral fibres, the situation is murkier. For example, determining whether silica exposure or silicosis mediates the increased lung cancer risk in silica-exposed persons has proven difficult [284, 285]. The presence of silicosis is associated with an increased risk of lung cancer [178]. Understanding the basis of this association will entail isolating the independent effects of silica exposure and lung fibrosis while taking exposure to smoking and other lung carcinogens into account [176, 191].

Such differences in the pattern of associations between pneumoconioses and lung cancer emphasise that "fibrosis" is not a homogeneous exposure but one dependent upon the properties of the specific mineral fibre or other environmental agent. Properties of the agent, such as its size, shape and durability, and the effects of other exposures, such as cigarette smoking, are important considerations in assessing its potential harmfulness [282].

– *End of reproduced excerpt [1]* –

THE EPIDEMIOLOGY OF MESOTHELIOMA

Pleural mesothelioma is unique among respiratory tumours in the specificity of its causation by asbestos and related fibrous materials. As mentioned earlier, asbestos refers to a group of fibrous minerals that includes amphiboles (crocidolite, tremolite, amosite and anthophyllite) and the serpentine form, chrysotile. The possible link between occupation and mesothelial tumours was noted in early case reports [286], and the association with asbestos was made clear in the 33 cases in South Africa reported by WAGNER *et al.* [287] in 1960. After this clinical report, epidemiological studies of the case–control and cohort designs soon provided further and definitive evidence for a causal association of asbestos exposure with mesothelioma; the RR estimates tended to be quite high since a substantial majority of cases appear to be caused by asbestos. Case reports also showed that "para-occupational" asbestos exposures in the families of workers who wore contaminated clothing into their homes could cause mesothelioma in spouses and others [288]. In one region of Turkey, naturally occurring exposure to fibrous eronite was also found to cause mesothelioma [289], and similar observations have subsequently been made elsewhere [290]. Exposures of the general population to asbestos may also take place in indoor environments from fibres released from building materials and in outdoor environments from fibres from brake linings and various industrial sources. In the USA, there was substantial controversy around asbestos-containing materials in buildings, particularly with regard to whether potential health risks are best managed by removal or leaving the materials in place [291].

The epidemiology of mesothelioma and other diseases caused by asbestos has been extensively reviewed previously [292–295]. This section provides an overview and addresses several issues that still remain controversial: the risk of mesothelioma in relation to fibre type, risks associated with environmental exposures and the potential role of other factors in causing mesothelioma, including simian virus (SV)40.

Incidence and mortality trends

Given the highly specific association of asbestos with mesothelioma occurrence, patterns of incidence and mortality should reflect patterns of occupational exposure, within the limitation of diagnostic misclassification. Unfortunately, survival for persons diagnosed with mesothelioma is poor, about 8.4% 5-yr survival [296]. Consequently, the mortality rate for mesothelioma is a useful indication of incidence, *i.e.* new cases. Given occupational exposure patterns, rates for males tend to be much greater than for females; in Britain for 1987–1991, the male annual mortality rate was 4.4 per 100,000 while the female rate was 0.6 per 100,000. Worldwide, incidence rates vary from less than one per 100,000 males in much of the world to a high of 6.4 per 100,000 males in the Trieste region of Italy [297], and in the USA between 2,000 and 3,000 die from malignant mesothelioma each year [298]. Generally, time trends of mesothelioma rates reflect the temporal profile of exposures across the last century, with the heaviest exposures sustained by developed country workers before the 1970s. In the USA, mesothelioma incidence reached a plateau by the 1990s (fig. 3) [299], while the peak is anticipated several decades later in Britain [300].

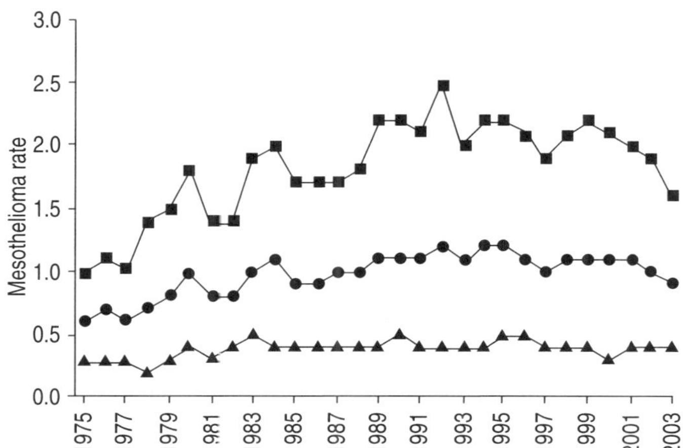

Fig. 3. – Mesothelioma incidence, showing age-adjusted rates. Data taken from the Surveillance, Epidemiology and End Results (SEER) Program, nine registries, 1973–2003, all races and ages. Reproduced from [299], an open-source publication. ■: males; ▲: females; ●: males and females.

LIN *et al.* [301] quantified the relationship between mesothelioma and other asbestos-related diseases and historical consumption of asbestos. The outcome measures were mortality rates for 2000–2004, while the indicator of use was the average of consumption in 1960 and 1970 in relation to population. For all mesotheliomas and for pleural mesotheliomas, a strong and linear relationship was found between mesothelioma mortality and asbestos consumption (fig. 4). For males, the adjusted R^2 for a linear regression model was 0.74; the estimated slope indicated that an increment in national consumption of 1 kg·person^{-1} was associated with a 2.4-fold increase. For females, the relationship was weaker. Nonetheless, this analysis indicates the dominant role of asbestos in determining the frequency of mesothelioma.

In a 2007 review, BECKLAKE *et al.* [293] profiled trends in mesothelioma occurrence in countries that have been major producers and users. Not surprisingly, descriptive trends

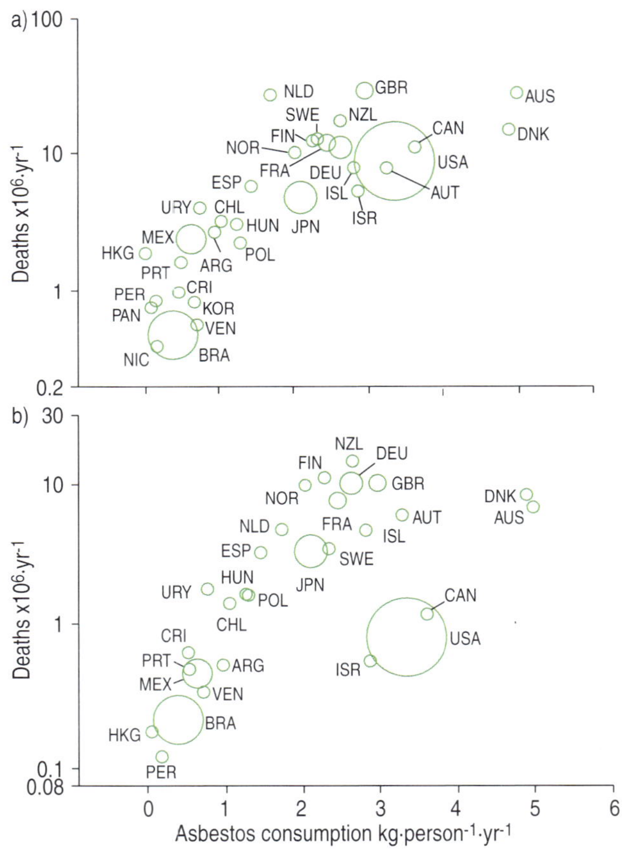

Fig. 4. – Ecological relationships between current mortality rates of mesothelioma (total and pleural; yearly mean for 2000–2004) and historical asbestos consumption (yearly mean for 1960–1969), weighted by the size of sex-specific national populations. Reproduced from [301] with permission from the publisher. a) All mesothelioma (males, n=32). b) Pleural mesothelioma (males, n=29). Circles are proportional to the size of the sex-specific national populations; countries with <20 million sex-specific national populations are drawn to the size of 20 million. ARG: Argentina; AUS: Australia; AUT: Austria; BRA: Brazil; CAN: Canada; CHL: Chile; CRI: Costa Rica; DEU: Germany; DNK: Denmark; ESP: Spain; FIN: Finland; FRA: France; GBR: United Kingdom; HKG: Hong Kong; HUN: Hungary; ISL: Iceland; ISR: Israel; JPN: Japan; KOR: South Korea; MEX: Mexico; NIC: Nicaragua; NLD: The Netherlands; NOR: Norway; NZL: New Zealand; PAN: Panama; PER: Peru; POL: Poland; PRT: Portugal; SWE: Sweden; URY: Uruguay; USA: United States; VEN: Venezuela.

of occurrence follow patterns of use. Production and utilisation continue. For 2005, Russia produced 875,000 tons, over a third of the world's production of 2,200,000 tons. Other major producers were China, Kazakhstan, Canada, Brazil and Zimbabwe.

Risk of mesothelioma

The risk of mesothelioma increases with the fibre burden in the lung, rises with time since exposure and varies across fibre types [182, 302]. Various occupational groups have differing levels of risk, depending on the levels of workplace exposures. Because other causal agents have not been identified for mesothelioma, RRs in occupationally exposed individuals compared with unexposed workers or with the general population are extraordinarily high. For example, in an early report on New York/New Jersey insulation workers, SELIKOFF *et al.* [303] reported 10 mesothelioma deaths out of 307 total deaths. They commented that there were only three deaths from mesothelioma among 31,652 deaths in a general population cohort study carried out by the ACS.

The occurrence of asbestos-associated mesothelioma cases in persons not occupationally exposed has long been documented. These reports have described increased risk associated with naturally occurring fibrous materials, *e.g.* erionite in Turkey, and in communities where asbestos is mined and milled or where production facilities are present. These descriptive reports are significant for documenting that nonoccupational exposures can be sufficient to cause mesothelioma and provide a strong public health rationale for limiting exposures. They also indicate that community exposures carry risks, although without insight into the actual doses of fibres received in community settings.

Several recent reports are illustrative. Two studies addressed risks in communities containing manufacturing facilities: one in Italy and the other in Japan. MAGNANI *et al.* [304] conducted a case–control study in a town in Italy that had the largest asbestos cement factory in the country. Residence in the community was associated with greatly increased risk; a model showed that risk declined to background at residences located at least 15 km from the plant. Findings from a study in Amagasaki City, Japan, also the site of an asbestos cement facility, were quite similar [305]. Among residents of Wittenoom, Western Australia, incidence of mesothelioma was greatly increased among the non-miners [306]. A descriptive analysis for the state of California, USA, found an association between residence location and proximity to naturally occurring asbestos [307].

For the purpose of risk assessment, mathematical models have been developed, using epidemiological data from studies of workers, to describe variation in risk with exposure and time since exposure [182, 308]. These models tend to give great weight to time elapsed since exposure [309]. For example, DE KLERK *et al.* [310] developed a model for mesothelioma mortality among workers at Wittenoom Gorge, Western Australia. The risk increased steeply with time since first employment (RR of 24.9 per log yr since first exposure), but varied little with estimated exposure concentration.

The risks of lower levels of asbestos exposure have also been estimated by directly extending risks in occupational groups exposed at high levels to workers or the general population exposed at lower levels. This approach was used to estimate the potential mesothelioma burden from exposure of the general public to asbestos in public and commercial buildings; the resulting low figure moved policies in the USA towards maintaining asbestos already in place [182].

One of the most controversial issues related to the epidemiology of mesothelioma has been the extent to which risk varies by fibre type. In worker cohorts, those exposed primarily to chrysotile asbestos have substantially lower risk for mesothelioma than those exposed to the amphiboles [182, 302]. The hypothesis has been advanced that chrysotile exposure may not increase risk for mesothelioma and that the mesotheliomas occurring in the Canadian chrysotile miners reflect the tremolite present in the ore. The possibility that risk may vary by fibre type has a potential biological basis, as the chemical and physical properties of the main types are different [311]. The hypothesis of STANTON *et al.* [312] proposes that longer, thinner fibres carry greater risk. Both qualitative and quantitative analyses of epidemiological studies of workers indicate lesser risk for those exposed primarily to chrysotile, although the magnitude of the difference cannot be quantified precisely [302]. Several analyses suggest a risk difference per unit exposure that is two orders of magnitude lower for chrysotile in comparison with crocidolite [302, 313]. One additional line of evidence comes from studies of fibres in lungs of persons with mesothelioma: there tends to be a predominance of amphiboles but the chrysotile fibres have a far shorter half-life [314, 315].

While the comparative toxicity of various fibre types is highly controversial, in part because of litigation, the available evidence neither documents that there is no risk associated with chrysotile or a threshold below which malignant mesothelioma does not develop; the data are insufficient to establish either possibility. Besides asbestos, other agents have not been causally linked to mesothelioma. The possibility that SV40, an oncogenic virus, contributes to the development of asbestos remains under investigation [316]. The hypothesis has been advanced that widespread exposure of humans to SV40 occurred through use of contaminated vaccines during the 1950s and 1960s [317]. Central to this debate is the identification of SV40 DNA sequences in mesothelioma tissues. This is a technically difficult assay and findings have been mixed and controversial [317, 318]. The possibility of genetic susceptibility to asbestos has also been proposed [319].

CONCLUSIONS

The path to preventing lung cancer is charted by the identification of numerous exposures causally associated with lung cancer. For mesothelioma, a single predominant cause has been identified. If steps can be taken to reduce or eliminate the population's exposure to smoking and asbestos, these cancers could be largely controlled. Preventive strategies can be pursued in the public policy arena and in public health interventions directed at individual behaviour. Cigarette smoking provides a useful example to illustrate the multiple levels that can form the basis of preventive strategies. In the legislative/regulatory arena, examples of tobacco control strategies include legislation that limits cigarette advertising, reduces children's access to cigarettes and prohibits smoking in the workplace. Litigation against cigarette manufacturers has also proven to be a productive component of tobacco control strategies, as exemplified by the settlement between states and the tobacco industry. Behavioural interventions to prevent children and adolescents from starting to smoke cigarettes and behavioural/pharmacological interventions to promote smoking cessation are individual-level approaches that, if successful, could be expected to reduce the occurrence of lung cancer. The Framework Convention on Tobacco Control sets a global approach.

In developing lung cancer prevention strategies, certain groups warrant particular attention. Steps need to be taken towards the goal of reducing the very high lung cancer incidence rates in African-American males [320]. Lung cancer is a major female health issue. Due to historical cigarette smoking patterns, the epidemic of lung cancer started later in females than males but, in contrast to the situation in males, lung cancer incidence rates in females have not yet begun to consistently decrease [26]. Although lung cancer remains a critical public health problem, the decrease in the overall lung cancer burden that is at present occurring in the USA, as in much of the developed world, reflects the successes of preventive strategies. A critical global priority is to prevent the uptake of cigarette smoking in developing countries where smoking prevalence is still low, in order to prevent the increase in morbidity and mortality from lung cancer that is certain to follow an increase in smoking prevalence. Similarly, use of asbestos needs to be carefully regulated and controlled to protect workers and communities.

A consideration of the epidemiology of lung cancer consistently reinforces one major theme: the pandemic of lung cancer is a consequence of the tragic and widespread addiction to cigarettes throughout the world. Curtailing the pandemic of lung cancer will require preventing youths from starting to smoke cigarettes and effectively promoting smoking cessation among addicted smokers. There are other causes also needing control, but fortunately there have been successes in reducing exposures to occupational carcinogens in countries of the developed world.

Summary

In the USA, lung cancer remains the leading cause of cancer death in both males and females, even though an extensive list of modifiable risk factors has long been identified. The predominant cause of lung cancer is exposure to tobacco smoke, with active smoking causing most cases but passive smoking also contributing to the lung cancer burden. The reductions in smoking prevalence in males that occurred in the late 1960s until the 1980s will continue to drive lung cancer mortality rates downward in males during the first portion of this century, but rates in females have not yet begun to decrease. Asbestos has been identified as responsible for the great majority of mesothelioma cases. Fortunately, exposures to major occupational respiratory carcinogens have largely been controlled, but the population is still exposed to environmental causes of lung cancer, including radon, the second leading cause of lung cancer death. Mesothelioma incidence has begun to reflect limitations on use of asbestos implemented decades ago and should continue to fall if asbestos use is limited and workers are protected.

Keywords: Asbestos, cigarette smoking, epidemiology, lung cancer, mesothelioma, passive smoking.

Statement of interest
None declared.

References

1. Alberg AJ, Ford JG, Samet JM. Epidemiology of lung cancer: ACCP evidence-based clinical practice guidelines (2nd edition). *Chest* 2007; 132: Suppl. 3, 29S–55S.
2. White C. Research on smoking and lung cancer: a landmark in the history of chronic disease epidemiology. *Yale J Biol Med* 1990; 63: 29–46.
3. Doll R, Hill AB. The mortality of doctors in relation to their smoking habits: a preliminary report. *Br Med J* 1954; 1: 1451–1455.

4. Doll R, Hill AB. Lung cancer and other causes of death in relation to smoking: a second report on the mortality of British doctors. *Br Med J* 1956; 2: 1071–1081.
5. Wingo PA, Ries LA, Giovino GA, *et al.* Annual report to the nation on the status of cancer, 1973–1996, with a special section on lung cancer and tobacco smoking. *J Natl Cancer Inst* 1999; 91: 675–690.
6. International Agency for Research on Cancer (IARC). Tobacco Smoke and Involuntary Smoking. IARC monograph 83. Lyon, IARC, 2004.
7. US Dept of Health and Human Services. The Health Effects of Active Smoking: A Report of the Surgeon General. Washington, US Government Printing Office, 2004.
8. Rosen G. A History of Public Health. Baltimore, Johns Hopkins University Press, 1993.
9. US Dept of Health and Human Services. Reducing the Health Consequences of Smoking. 25 Years of Progress. A Report of the Surgeon General. Washington, US Government Printing Office, 1989.
10. Proctor RN. The Nazi War on Cancer. Princeton, Princeton University Press, 1999.
11. Doll R, Hill AB. Smoking and carcinoma of the lung: preliminary report. *Br Med J* 1950; 2: 739–748.
12. Levin ML, Goldstein H, Gerhardt PR. Cancer and tobacco smoking. A preliminary report. *JAMA* 1950; 143: 336–338.
13. Wynder EL, Graham EA. Tobacco smoking as a possible etiologic factor in bronchiogenic carcinoma. A study of 684 proved cases. *JAMA* 1950; 143: 329–336.
14. US Dept of Health Education and Welfare (DHEW). Smoking and Health. Report of the Advisory Committee to the Surgeon General. DHEW Publication No. (PHS) 1103 Edn. Washington, US Government Printing Office, 1964.
15. Royal College of Physicians of London. Smoking and Health. Summary of a report of the Royal College of Physicians of London on smoking in relation to cancer of the lung and other diseases. London, Pitman Medical Publishing Co., 1962; pp. S2–S70.
16. US Dept of Health and Human Services (DHHS). The health consequences of involuntary smoking. A Report of the Surgeon General. DHHS Publication No. (CDC) 87-8398 Edn. Washington, US Government Printing Office, 1986.
17. US Environmental Protection Agency (EPA). Respiratory Health Effects of Passive Smoking: Lung Cancer and Other Disorders. EPA/600/006F Edn. Washington, US Government Printing Office, 1992.
18. Samet JM. Radon and lung cancer. *J Natl Cancer Inst* 1989; 81: 745–757.
19. National Research Council, Committee on Health Risks of Exposure to Radon, Board on Radiation Effects Research, *et al.* Health Effects of Exposure to Radon (BEIR VI). Washington, National Academy Press, 1999.
20. Coultas DB, Samet JM. Occupational lung cancer. *Clin Chest Med* 1992; 13: 341–354.
21. Ries LAG, Eisner MP, Kosary CL, *et al.* SEER Cancer Statistics Review, 1975–2002. Bethesda, National Cancer Institute, 2005. Available from http://seer.cancer.gov/csr/1975_2002/
22. American Cancer Society. Cancer Facts and Figures 2006. Atlanta, American Cancer Society, 2006.
23. Jemal A, Travis WD, Tarone RE, *et al.* Lung cancer rates convergence in young men and women in the United States: analysis by birth cohort and histologic type. *Int J Cancer* 2003; 105: 101–107.
24. Kazerouni N, Alverson CJ, Redd SC, *et al.* Sex differences in COPD and lung cancer mortality trends – United States, 1968–1999. *J Womens Health (Larchmt)* 2004; 13: 17–23.
25. Haiman CA, Stram DO, Wilkens LR, *et al.* Ethnic and racial differences in the smoking-related risk of lung cancer. *N Engl J Med* 2006; 354: 333–342.
26. Edwards BK, Brown ML, Wingo PA, *et al.* Annual report to the nation on the status of cancer, 1975–2002, featuring population-based trends in cancer treatment. *J Natl Cancer Inst* 2005; 97: 1407–1427.
27. Mao Y, Hu J, Ugnat AM, *et al.* Socioeconomic status and lung cancer risk in Canada. *Int J Epidemiol* 2001; 30: 809–817.

28. Li K, Yu S. Economic status, smoking, occupational exposure to rubber, and lung cancer: a case–cohort study. *J Environ Sci Health C Environ Carcinog Ecotoxicol Rev* 2002; 20: 21–28.
29. van Loon AJ, Goldbohm RA, Kant IJ, *et al.* Socioeconomic status and lung cancer incidence in men in the Netherlands: is there a role for occupational exposure? *J Epidemiol Community Health* 1997; 51: 24–29.
30. Schwartz KL, Crossley-May H, Vigneau FD, *et al.* Race, socioeconomic status and stage at diagnosis for five common malignancies. *Cancer Causes Control* 2003; 14: 761–766.
31. World Health Organization, International Agency for Research on Cancer (IARC). World Cancer Report. Lyon, IARC Press, 2003.
32. International Agency for Research on Cancer (IARC). GLOBOCAN 2002. Lyon, IARC, 2002. Available from http://www-dep.iarc.fr
33. Parkin DM, Pisani P, Lopez AD, *et al.* At least one in seven cases of cancer is caused by smoking. Global estimates for 1995. *Int J Cancer* 1994; 59: 494–504.
34. Gordon T, Crittenden M, Haenszel W. End results and mortality trends in cancer. II. Cancer mortality trends in the United States, 1930–1955. *Natl Cancer Inst Monogr* 1961; 6: 133–350.
35. Stocks P, Campbell JM. Lung cancer death rates among non-smokers and pipe and cigarette smokers. An evaluation in relation to air pollution by benzo[a]pyrene and other substances. *Br Med J* 1955; 2: 923–929.
36. Blot WJ, Fraumeni JF Jr. Arsenical air pollution and lung cancer. *Lancet* 1975; 2: 142–144.
37. Blot WJ, Fraumeni JF Jr. Geographic patterns of lung cancer: industrial correlations. *Am J Epidemiol* 1976; 103: 539–550.
38. Mason TJ, Mckay FW. US Cancer Mortality by County: 1950–1969. USDHEW 74-615 Edn. Washington, US Government Printing Office, 1973.
39. Blot WJ, Fraumeni JF. Cancer among shipyard workers. *In*: Peto R, Schneiderman M, eds. Banbury Report 9. Quantification of Occupational Cancer. New York, Cold Spring Harbor Laboratory, 1981.
40. Blot WJ, Fraumeni JF Jr. Changing patterns of lung cancer in the United States. *Am J Epidemiol* 1982; 115: 664–673.
41. Saracci R, Boffetta P. Interactions of tobacco smoking and other causes of lung cancer. *In*: Samet JM, ed. Epidemiology of Lung Cancer. New York, Marcel Dekker, Inc., 1994; pp. 465–493.
42. Samet JM, Cohen AJ. Air pollution and lung cancer. *In*: Holgate ST, Samet JM, Koren HS, *et al.*, eds. Air Pollution and Health. San Diego, Academic Press, 1999; pp. 841–864.
43. Willett WC. Diet, nutrition, and avoidable cancer. *Environ Health Perspect* 1995; 103: Suppl. 8, 165–170.
44. Peto R, Lopez AD, Boreham J, *et al.* Mortality from Smoking in Developed Countries 1950–2000. Indirect Estimates from National Vital Statistics. Oxford, Oxford University Press, 1994.
45. Samet JM. Lung cancer. *In*: Greenwald P, Kramer BS, Weed DL, eds. Cancer Prevention and Control. New York, Marcel Dekker, Inc., 1995; pp. 561–584.
46. Zaridze D, Peto R. Tobacco: A Major International Health Hazard. Lyon, International Agency for Research on Cancer, 1986.
47. Peto R, Chen ZM, Boreham J. Tobacco – the growing epidemic. *Nat Med* 1999; 5: 15–17
48. Liu BQ, Peto R, Chen ZM, *et al.* Emerging tobacco hazards in China: 1. Retrospective proportional mortality study of one million deaths. *BMJ* 1998; 317: 1411–1422.
49. National Institutes of Health (NIH), National Cancer Institute. Smoking and Tobacco Control Monograph 9. Cigars: Health Effects and Trends. NIH Publication No. 98-4302 Edn. Bethesda, US Dept of Health and Human Services, 1998.
50. Boffetta P, Pershagen G, Jockel KH, *et al.* Cigar and pipe smoking and lung cancer risk: a multicenter study from Europe. *J Natl Cancer Inst* 1999; 91: 697–701.
51. Doll R, Peto R. Cigarette smoking and bronchial carcinoma: dose and time relationships among regular smokers and lifelong non-smokers. *J Epidemiol Community Health* 1978; 32: 303–313.
52. Peto R. Influence of dose and duration of smoking on lung cancer rates. *In*: Zaridze D, Peto R, eds. Tobacco: a Major International Health Hazard; Proceedings of an International Meeting,

June 4–6, 1985, Moscow. International Agency for Research on Cancer (IARC) Science Publication 74. Lyon, World Health Organization, IARC, 1986; pp. 23–33.

53. US Dept of Health and Human Services. Smoking and Health: A National Status Report. Washington, US Government Printing Office, 1987.
54. US Dept of Health and Human Services. The Health Benefits of Smoking Cessation. A Report of the Surgeon General. Washington, US Government Printing Office, 1990.
55. Hrubec Z, McLaughlin JK. Former cigarette smoking and mortality among US veterans: a 26-year follow-up, 1954–1980. *In*: Burns DM, Garfinkel L, Samet JM, eds. Changes in Cigarette-Related Disease Risks and Their Implication for Prevention and Control. Bethesda, US Government Printing Office, 1997; pp. 501–530.
56. Wu-Williams AH, Samet JM. Lung cancer and cigarette smoking. *In*: Samet JM, ed. Epidemiology of Lung Cancer. New York, Marcel Dekker, Inc., 1994; pp. 71–108.
57. Hoffmann D, Hoffmann I, El-Bayoumy K. The less harmful cigarette: a controversial issue. A tribute to Ernst L. Wynder. *Chem Res Toxicol* 2001; 14: 767–790.
58. US Dept of Health and Human Services. The Health Consequences of Smoking – the Changing Cigarette. A Report of the Surgeon General. Washington, US Government Printing Office, 1981.
59. National Cancer Institute. The FTC Cigarette Test Method for Determining Tar, Nicotine, and Carbon Monoxide Yields of US Cigarettes. Bethesda, National Institutes of Health, 1996.
60. Coultas DB, Howard CA, Peake GT, *et al.* Discrepancies between self-reported and validated cigarette smoking in a community survey of New Mexico Hispanics. *Am Rev Respir Dis* 1988; 88: 810–814.
61. Djordjevic MV, Stellman SD, Zang E. Doses of nicotine and lung carcinogens delivered to cigarette smokers. *J Natl Cancer Inst* 2000; 92: 106–111.
62. US Dept of Health and Human Services, National Cancer Institute. Risks Associated with Smoking Cigarettes with Low Machine-Measured Yields of Tar and Nicotine. Bethesda, National Institutes of Health, 2001.
63. Samet JM. The changing cigarette and disease risk: current status of the evidence. The FTC Cigarette Test Method for Determining Tar, Nicotine, and Carbon Monoxide Yields of US Cigarettes. Report of the NCI Expert Committee. NIH Publication No. 96-2789 Edn. US Dept of Human Services, Public Health Service, National Institutes of Heath, National Cancer Institute, 1996; pp. 77–92.
64. Bross IDJ, Gibson R. Risks of lung cancer in smokers who switch to filter cigarettes. *Am J Public Health* 1968; 58: 1396–1403.
65. Wynder EL, Mabuchi K, Beattie EJ Jr. The epidemiology of lung cancer. Recent trends. *JAMA* 1970; 213: 2221–2228.
66. Lubin JH, Blot WJ, Berrino F, *et al.* Patterns of lung cancer risk according to type of cigarette smoked. *Int J Cancer* 1984; 33: 569–576.
67. Garfinkel L, Stellman SD. Smoking and lung cancer in women: findings in a prospective study. *Cancer Res* 1988; 48: 6951–6955.
68. Sidney S, Tekawa IS, Friedman GD. A prospective study of cigarette tar yield and lung cancer. *Cancer Causes Control* 1993; 4: 3–10.
69. Hammond EC, Garfinkel L, Seidman H, *et al.* "Tar" and nicotine content of cigarette smoke in relation to death rates. *Environ Res* 1976; 12: 263–274.
70. Stellman SD, Garfinkel L. Lung cancer risk is proportional to cigarette tar yield: evidence from a prospective study. *Prev Med* 1989; 18: 518–525.
71. Burns DM, Garfinkel L, Samet JM, eds. US Dept of Health and Human Services, Public Health Service, National Cancer Institute. Changes in Cigarette-Related Disease Risks and Their Implication for Prevention and Control. NIH Publication No. 97-4213. Bethesda, US Government Printing Office, 1997.
72. Thun MJ, Day-Lally CA, Calle EE, *et al.* Excess mortality among cigarette smokers: changes in a 20-year interval. *Am J Public Health* 1995; 85: 1223–1230.

73. Thun MJ, Day-Lally C, Myers DG, *et al.* Trends in tobacco smoking and mortality from cigarette use in Cancer Prevention Studies I (1959–1965) and II (1982–1988). *In*: Burns DM, Garfinkel L, Samet JM, eds. Changes in Cigarette-Related Disease Risks and Their Implication for Prevention and Control. NIH Publication No. 97-4213. Bethesda, US Government Printing Office, 1997; pp. 305–382.
74. Doll R, Peto R, Wheatley K, *et al.* Mortality in relation to smoking: 40 years' observations on male British doctors. *BMJ* 1994; 309: 901–911.
75. Doll R, Peto R, Boreham J, *et al.* Mortality in relation to smoking: 50 years' observations on male British doctors. *BMJ* 2004; 328: 1519–1527.
76. Peto R, Darby S, Deo H, *et al.* Smoking, smoking cessation, and lung cancer in the UK since 1950: combination of national statistics with two case–control studies. *BMJ* 2000; 321: 323–329.
77. Stratton K, Shetty P, Wallace R, *et al.* Clearing the Smoke: Assessing the Science Base for Tobacco Harm Reduction. Washington, National Academy Press, 2001.
78. Risch HA, Howe GR, Jain M, *et al.* Are female smokers at higher risk for lung cancer than male smokers? A case–control analysis by histologic type. *Am J Epidemiol* 1993; 138: 281–293.
79. Zang EA, Wynder EL. Differences in lung cancer risk between men and women: examination of the evidence. *J Natl Cancer Inst* 1996; 88: 183–192.
80. Perneger TV. Sex, smoking, and cancer: a reappraisal. *J Natl Cancer Inst* 2001; 93: 1600–1602.
81. Bain C, Feskanich D, Speizer FE, *et al.* Lung cancer rates in men and women with comparable histories of smoking. *J Natl Cancer Inst* 2004; 96: 826–834.
82. Cummings KM, Giovino G, Mendicino AJ. Cigarette advertising and black-white differences in brand preference. *Public Health Rep* 1987; 102: 698–701.
83. Gardiner PS. The African Americanization of menthol cigarette use in the United States. *Nicotine Tob Res* 2004; 6: Suppl. 1, S55–S65.
84. Giovino GA, Sidney S, Gfroerer JC, *et al.* Epidemiology of menthol cigarette use. *Nicotine Tob Res* 2004; 6: Suppl. 1, S67–S81.
85. Ferris WG, Connolly GN. Application, function, and effects of menthol in cigarettes: a survey of tobacco industry documents. *Nicotine Tob Res* 2004; 6: Suppl. 1, S43–S54.
86. Celebucki CC, Wayne GF, Connolly GN, *et al.* Characterization of measured menthol in 48 US cigarette sub-brands. *Nicotine Tob Res* 2005; 7: 523–531.
87. McCarthy WJ, Caskey NH, Jarvik ME, *et al.* Menthol *vs* nonmenthol cigarettes: effects on smoking behavior. *Am J Public Health* 1995; 85: 67–72.
88. Malaiyandi V, Sellers EM, Tyndale RF. Implications of CYP2A6 genetic variation for smoking behaviors and nicotine dependence. *Clin Pharmacol Ther* 2005; 77: 145–158.
89. Green MD, Belanger G, Hum DW, *et al.* Glucuronidation of opioids, carboxylic acid-containing drugs, and hydroxylated xenobiotics catalyzed by expressed monkey UDP-glucuronosyltransferase 2B9 protein. *Drug Metab Dispos* 1997; 25: 1389–1394.
90. Ahijevych KL, Tyndale RF, Dhatt RK, *et al.* Factors influencing cotinine half-life during smoking abstinence in African American and Caucasian women. *Nicotine Tob Res* 2002; 4: 423–431.
91. MacDougall JM, Fandrick K, Zhang X, *et al.* Inhibition of human liver microsomal [S]-nicotine oxidation by [-]-menthol and analogues. *Chem Res Toxicol* 2003; 16: 988–993.
92. Benowitz NL, Herrera B, Jacob P III. Mentholated cigarette smoking inhibits nicotine metabolism. *J Pharmacol Exp Ther* 2004; 310: 1208–1215.
93. Mustonen TK, Spencer SM, Hoskinson RA, *et al.* The influence of gender, race, and menthol content on tobacco exposure measures. *Nicotine Tob Res* 2005; 7: 581–590.
94. Kabat GC, Hebert JR. Use of mentholated cigarettes and lung cancer risk. *Cancer Res* 1991; 51: 6510–6513.
95. Muscat JE, Richie JP Jr, Stellman SD. Mentholated cigarettes and smoking habits in whites and blacks. *Tob Control* 2002; 11: 368–371.
96. Stellman SD, Chen Y, Muscat JE, *et al.* Lung cancer risk in white and black Americans. *Ann Epidemiol* 2003; 13: 294–302.

97. Brooks DR, Palmer JR, Strom BL, *et al.* Menthol cigarettes and risk of lung cancer. *Am J Epidemiol* 2003; 158: 609–616.
98. Carpenter CL, Jarvik ME, Morgenstern H, *et al.* Mentholated cigarette smoking and lung-cancer risk. *Ann Epidemiol* 1999; 9: 114–120.
99. Sidney S, Tekawa IS, Friedman GD, *et al.* Mentholated cigarette use and lung cancer. *Arch Intern Med* 1995; 155: 727–732.
100. Yang CP, Gallagher RP, Weiss NS, *et al.* Differences in incidence rates of cancers of the respiratory tract by anatomic subsite and histologic type: an etiologic implication. *J Natl Cancer Inst* 1989; 81: 1828–1831.
101. Hebert JR. Menthol cigarettes and risk of lung cancer. *Am J Epidemiol* 2003; 158: 617–620.
102. Hirayama T. Non-smoking wives of heavy smokers have a higher risk of lung cancer: a study from Japan. *Br Med J (Clin Res Ed)* 1981; 282: 183–185.
103. Trichopoulos D, Kalandidi A, Sparros L, *et al.* Lung cancer and passive smoking. *Int J Cancer* 1981; 27: 1–4.
104. National Research Council, Committee on Passive Smoking. Environmental Tobacco Smoke: Measuring Exposures and Assessing Health Effects. Washington, National Academy Press, 1986.
105. Fontham ETH, Correa P, Reynolds P, *et al.* Environmental tobacco smoke and lung cancer in nonsmoking women: a multicenter study. *JAMA* 1994; 271: 1752–1759.
106. Boffetta P, Agudo A, Ahrens W, *et al.* Multicenter case–control study of exposure to environmental tobacco smoke and lung cancer in Europe. *J Natl Cancer Inst* 1998; 90: 1440–1450.
107. Muggli ME, Forster JL, Hurt RD, *et al.* The smoke you don't see: uncovering tobacco industry scientific strategies aimed against environmental tobacco smoke policies. *Am J Public Health* 2001; 91: 1419–1423.
108. Drope J, Chapman S. Tobacco industry efforts at discrediting scientific knowledge of environmental tobacco smoke: a review of internal industry documents. *J Epidemiol Community Health* 2001; 55: 588–594.
109. California Environmental Protection Agency (Cal EPA), Air Resources Board. Proposed Identification of Environmental Tobacco Smoke as a Toxic Air Contaminant. Sacramento, Cal EPA, 2005.
110. Boffetta P. Involuntary smoking and lung cancer. *Scand J Work Environ Health* 2002; 28: Suppl. 2, 30–40.
111. Taylor R, Cumming R, Woodward A, *et al.* Passive smoking and lung cancer: a cumulative meta-analysis. *Aust NZ J Public Health* 2001; 25: 203–211.
112. Travis WD, Travis LB, Devesa SS. Lung cancer. *Cancer* 1995; 75: Suppl. 1, 191–202.
113. Churg A. Lung cancer cell type and occupational exposure. *In*: Samet JM, ed. Epidemiology of Lung Cancer. New York, Marcel Dekker, Inc., 1994; pp. 413–436.
114. Khuder SA. Effect of cigarette smoking on major histological types of lung cancer: a meta-analysis. *Lung Cancer* 2001; 31: 139–148.
115. Vincent RG, Pickren JW, Lane WW, *et al.* The changing histopathology of lung cancer: a review of 1682 cases. *Cancer* 1977; 39: 1647–1655.
116. Charloux A, Quoix E, Wolkove N, *et al.* The increasing incidence of lung adenocarcinoma: reality or artefact? A review of the epidemiology of lung adenocarcinoma. *Int J Epidemiol* 1997; 26: 14–23.
117. Thun MJ, Lally CA, Flannery JT, *et al.* Cigarette smoking and changes in the histopathology of lung cancer. *J Natl Cancer Inst* 1997; 89: 1580–1586.
118. Hoffmann D, Hoffmann I. The changing cigarette, 1950–1995. *J Toxicol Environ Health* 1997; 50: 307–364.
119. Hecht SS. Tobacco smoke carcinogens and lung cancer. *J Natl Cancer Inst* 1999; 91: 1194–1210.
120. Hecht SS. Cigarette smoking and lung cancer: chemical mechanisms and approaches to prevention. *Lancet Oncol* 2002; 3: 461–469.
121. Brooks DR, Austin JH, Heelan RT, *et al.* Influence of type of cigarette on peripheral *versus* central lung cancer. *Cancer Epidemiol Biomarkers Prev* 2005; 14: 576–581.

122. Peto R, Doll R, Buckley JD, *et al.* Can dietary beta-carotene materially reduce human cancer rates? *Nature* 1981; 290: 201–208.
123. Alberg AJ, Samet JM. Epidemiology of lung cancer. *In*: Sadler MJ, Caballero B, Strain JJ, eds. Encyclopedia of Human Nutrition. London, Academic Press, 2005.
124. Skuladottir H, Tjoenneland A, Overvad K, *et al.* Does insufficient adjustment for smoking explain the preventive effects of fruit and vegetables on lung cancer? *Lung Cancer* 2004; 45: 1–10.
125. Wright ME, Mayne ST, Swanson CA, *et al.* Dietary carotenoids, vegetables, and lung cancer risk in women: the Missouri women's health study (United States). *Cancer Causes Control* 2003; 14: 85–96.
126. Holick CN, Michaud DS, Stolzenberg-Solomon R, *et al.* Dietary carotenoids, serum beta-carotene, and retinol and risk of lung cancer in the alpha-tocopherol, beta-carotene cohort study. *Am J Epidemiol* 2002; 156: 536–547.
127. Neuhouser ML, Patterson RE, Thornquist MD, *et al.* Fruits and vegetables are associated with lower lung cancer risk only in the placebo arm of the beta-carotene and retinol efficacy trial (CARET). *Cancer Epidemiol Biomarkers Prev* 2003; 12: 350–358.
128. Feskanich D, Ziegler RG, Michaud DS, *et al.* Prospective study of fruit and vegetable consumption and risk of lung cancer among men and women. *J Natl Cancer Inst* 2000; 92: 1812–1823.
129. Miller AB, Altenburg HP, Bueno-de-Mesquita B, *et al.* Fruits and vegetables and lung cancer: findings from the European Prospective Investigation into Cancer and Nutrition. *Int J Cancer* 2004; 108: 269–276.
130. Smith-Warner SA, Spiegelman D, Yaun SS, *et al.* Fruits, vegetables and lung cancer: a pooled analysis of cohort studies. *Int J Cancer* 2003; 107: 1001–1011.
131. Bond GG, Thompson FE, Cook RR. Dietary vitamin A and lung cancer: results of a case–control study among chemical workers. *Nutr Cancer* 1987; 9: 109–121.
132. Brennan P, Fortes C, Butler J, *et al.* A multicenter case–control study of diet and lung cancer among non-smokers. *Cancer Causes Control* 2000; 11: 49–58.
133. Hu J, Mao Y, Dryer D, *et al.* Risk factors for lung cancer among Canadian women who have never smoked. *Cancer Detect Prev* 2002; 26: 129–138.
134. Zhuo H, Smith AH, Steinmaus C. Selenium and lung cancer: a quantitative analysis of heterogeneity in the current epidemiological literature. *Cancer Epidemiol Biomarkers Prev* 2004; 13: 771–778.
135. De Stefani E, Brennan P, Boffetta P, *et al.* Diet and adenocarcinoma of the lung: a case–control study in Uruguay. *Lung Cancer* 2002; 35: 43–51.
136. Knekt P, Jarvinen R, Teppo L, *et al.* Role of various carotenoids in lung cancer prevention. *J Natl Cancer Inst* 1999; 91: 182–184.
137. Mannisto S, Smith-Warner SA, Spiegelman D, *et al.* Dietary carotenoids and risk of lung cancer in a pooled analysis of seven cohort studies. *Cancer Epidemiol Biomarkers Prev* 2004; 13: 40–48.
138. Wright ME, Mayne ST, Stolzenberg-Solomon RZ, *et al.* Development of a comprehensive dietary antioxidant index and application to lung cancer risk in a cohort of male smokers. *Am J Epidemiol* 2004; 160: 68–76.
139. Comstock GW, Alberg AJ, Huang HY, *et al.* The risk of developing lung cancer associated with antioxidants in the blood: ascorbic acid, carotenoids, alpha-tocopherol, selenium, and total peroxyl radical absorbing capacity. *Cancer Epidemiol Biomarkers Prev* 1997; 6: 907–916.
140. Yuan JM, Ross RK, Chu XD, *et al.* Prediagnostic levels of serum beta-cryptoxanthin and retinol predict smoking-related lung cancer risk in Shanghai, China. *Cancer Epidemiol Biomarkers Prev* 2001; 10: 767–773.
141. World Cancer Research Fund, American Institute for Cancer Research. Food, Nutrition, and the Prevention of Cancer: a Global Perspective. Washington, American Institute for Cancer Research, 1997.
142. Michaud DS, Feskanich D, Rimm EB, *et al.* Intake of specific carotenoids and risk of lung cancer in 2 prospective US cohorts. *Am J Clin Nutr* 2000; 72: 990–997.

143. Le Marchand L, Murphy SP, Hankin JH, *et al.* Intake of flavonoids and lung cancer. *J Natl Cancer Inst* 2000; 92: 154–160.
144. Knekt P, Jarvinen R, Seppanen R, *et al.* Dietary flavonoids and the risk of lung cancer and other malignant neoplasms. *Am J Epidemiol* 1997; 146: 223–230.
145. Neuhouser ML. Dietary flavonoids and cancer risk: evidence from human population studies. *Nutr Cancer* 2004; 50: 1–7.
146. Spitz MR, Duphorne CM, Detry MA, *et al.* Dietary intake of isothiocyanates: evidence of a joint effect with glutathione S-transferase polymorphisms in lung cancer risk. *Cancer Epidemiol Biomarkers Prev* 2000; 9: 1017–1020.
147. Zhao B, Seow A, Lee EJ, *et al.* Dietary isothiocyanates, glutathione S-transferase-M1, -T1 polymorphisms and lung cancer risk among Chinese women in Singapore. *Cancer Epidemiol Biomarkers Prev* 2001; 10: 1063–1067.
148. London SJ, Yuan JM, Chung FL, *et al.* Isothiocyanates, glutathione S-transferase M1 and T1 polymorphisms, and lung-cancer risk: a prospective study of men in Shanghai, China. *Lancet* 2000; 356: 724–729.
149. Korte JE, Brennan P, Henley SJ, *et al.* Dose-specific meta-analysis and sensitivity analysis of the relation between alcohol consumption and lung cancer risk. *Am J Epidemiol* 2002; 155: 496–506.
150. Knekt P, Heliovaara M, Rissanen A, *et al.* Leanness and lung cancer risk. *Int J Cancer* 1991; 49: 208–213.
151. Olson JE, Yang P, Schmitz K, *et al.* Differential association of body mass index and fat distribution with three major histologic types of lung cancer: evidence from a cohort of older women. *Am J Epidemiol* 2002; 156: 606–615.
152. Alberg A. The influence of cigarette smoking on circulating concentrations of antioxidant micronutrients. *Toxicology* 2002; 180: 121–137.
153. Fontham ET. Protective dietary factors and lung cancer. *Int J Epidemiol* 1990; 19: Suppl. 1, S32–S42.
154. Gray J, Mao JT, Szabo E, *et al.* Lung cancer chemoprevention: ACCP evidence-based clinical practice guidelines (2nd Edition). *Chest* 2007; 132: Suppl. 3, 56S–68S.
155. The effect of vitamin E and beta-carotene on the incidence of lung cancer and other cancers in male smokers. The Alpha-Tocopheral, Beta-Carotene Cancer Prevention Study Group. *N Engl J Med* 1994; 330: 1029–1035.
156. Hennekens CH, Buring JE, Manson JE, *et al.* Lack of effect of long-term supplementation with beta-carotene on the incidence of malignant neoplasms and cardiovascular disease. *N Engl J Med* 1996; 334: 1145–1149.
157. Omenn GS, Goodman GE, Thornquist MD, *et al.* Effects of a combination of beta-carotene and vitamin A on lung cancer and cardiovascular disease. *N Engl J Med* 1996; 334: 1150–1155.
158. Lee IM, Sesso HD, Paffenbarger RS Jr. Physical activity and risk of lung cancer. *Int J Epidemiol* 1999; 28: 620–625.
159. Mao Y, Pan S, Wen SW, *et al.* Physical activity and the risk of lung cancer in Canada. *Am J Epidemiol* 2003; 158: 564–575.
160. Thune I, Lund E. The influence of physical activity on lung-cancer risk: a prospective study of 81,516 men and women. *Int J Cancer* 1997; 70: 57–62.
161. Doll R, Peto R. The causes of cancer: quantitative estimates of avoidable risks of cancer in the United States today. *J Natl Cancer Inst* 1981; 66: 1191–1308.
162. Dave SK, Edling C, Jacobsson P, *et al.* Occupation, smoking, and lung cancer. *Br J Ind Med* 1988; 45: 790–792.
163. Kvale G, Bjelke E, Heuch I. Occupational exposure and lung cancer risk. *Int J Cancer* 1986; 37: 185–193.
164. Damber LA, Larsson LG. Occupation and male lung cancer: a case–control study in northern Sweden. *Br J Ind Med* 1987; 44: 446–453.
165. Lerchen ML, Wiggins CL, Samet JM. Lung cancer and occupation in New Mexico. *J Natl Cancer Inst* 1987; 79: 639–645.

166. Schoenberg JB, Stemhagen A, Mason TJ, *et al.* Occupation and lung cancer risk among New Jersey white males. *J Natl Cancer Inst* 1987; 79: 13–21.
167. Vineis P, Thomas T, Hayes RB, *et al.* Proportion of lung cancers in males, due to occupation, in different areas of the USA. *Int J Cancer* 1988; 42: 851–856.
168. Siemiatycki J. Risk Factors for Cancer in the Workplace. Boston, CRC Press, 1991.
169. Samet JM, Lerchen ML. Proportion of lung cancer caused by occupation: a critical review. *In*: Bernard J, Gee L, Keith W, *et al.*, eds. Occupational Lung Disease. New York, Raven Press, 1984; pp. 55–67.
170. Doll R, Fisher REW, Gammon EJ, *et al.* Mortality of gas workers with special reference to cancers of the lung and bladder, chronic bronchitis, and pneumoconiosis. *Br J Ind Med* 1965; 22: 1–12.
171. Lloyd JW. Long-term mortality of steelworkers. V. Respiratory cancer in coke plant workers. *J Occup Med* 1971; 13: 53–68.
172. Lawther PJ, Commins BT, Waller RE. A study of the concentrations of polycyclic aromatic hydrocarbons in gas works retort houses. *Br J Ind Med* 1965; 22: 13–20.
173. Alberg AJ, Yung R, Strickland PT, *et al.* Respiratory cancer and exposure to arsenic, chromium, nickel, and polycyclic aromatic hydrocarbons. *Clin Occup Environ Med* 2002; 2: 779–801.
174. Cohen AJ, Higgins MWP. Health Effects of Diesel Exhaust: Epidemiology. Diesel Exhaust: A Critical Analysis of Emissions, Exposure, and Health Effects. A Special Report of the Institute's Working Group. Cambridge, Health Effects Institute, 1995; pp. 251–292.
175. Goldsmith DF, Guidotti TL, Johnston DR. Does occupational exposure to silica cause lung cancer? *Am J Ind Med* 1982; 3: 423–440.
176. Heppleston AG. Silica, pneumoconiosis, and carcinoma of the lung. *Am J Ind Med* 1985; 7: 285–294.
177. McDonald JC. Silica, silicosis, and lung cancer. *Br J Ind Med* 1989; 46: 289–291.
178. Smith AH, Lopipero PA, Barroga VR. Meta-analysis of studies of lung cancer among silicotics. *Epidemiology* 1995; 6: 617–624
179. Checkoway H, Franzblau A. Is silicosis required for silica-associated lung cancer? *Am J Ind Med* 2000; 37: 252–259.
180. Hessel PA, Gamble JF, Gee JB, *et al.* Silica, silicosis, and lung cancer: a response to a recent working group report. *J Occup Environ Med* 2000; 42: 704–720.
181. International Agency for Research on Cancer (IARC). IARC Monographs on the evaluation of carcinogenic risks to humans. Volume 68. Silica, some silicates, coal dust and para-aramid fibrils. Lyon, World Health Organization, IARC, 1997.
182. Health Effects Institute, Asbestos Research Committee, Literature Review Panel. Asbestos in public and commercial buildings: a literature review and a synthesis of current knowledge. Cambridge, Health Effects Institute, 1991.
183. Wedler HW. Asbestose und Lungenkrebs [Asbestosis and pulmonary carcinoma]. *Dtsch Med Wochenschr* 1943; 69: 575–576.
184. Lynch KM, Smith WA. Pulmonary asbestosis. V. A report of bronchial carcinoma and epithelial metaplasia. *Am J Cancer* 1939; 36: 567–573.
185. Doll R. Mortality from lung cancer in asbestos workers. *Br J Ind Med* 1955; 12: 81–86.
186. Selikoff IJ, Churg J, Hammond EC. Asbestos exposure and neoplasia. *JAMA* 1964; 188: 22–26.
187. Selikoff IJ, Hammond EC, Seidman H. Mortality experience of insulation workers in the United States and Canada. *Ann NY Acad Sci* 1979; 330: 91–116.
188. Newhouse ML, Berry G. Patterns of mortality in asbestos factory workers in London. *Ann NY Acad Sci* 1979; 330: 53–60.
189. Lemen RA, Dement JM, Wagoner JK. Epidemiology of asbestos-related diseases. *Environ Health Perspect* 1980; 34: 1–11.
190. Mossman BT, Churg A. Mechanisms in the pathogenesis of asbestosis and silicosis. *Am J Respir Crit Care Med* 1998; 157: 1666–1680.

191. Samet JM. Does idiopathic pulmonary fibrosis increase lung cancer risk? *Am J Respir Crit Care Med* 2000; 161: 1–2.
192. Hammond EC, Selikoff IJ, Seidman H. Asbestos exposure, cigarette smoking and death rates. *Ann NY Acad Sci* 1979; 330: 473–490.
193. Churg A, Stevens B. Enhanced retention of asbestos fibers in the airways of human smokers. *Am J Respir Crit Care Med* 1995; 151: 1409–1413.
194. Boice JD Jr. Studies of atomic bomb survivors. Understanding radiation effects. *JAMA* 1990; 264: 622–623.
195. MacMahon B. Some recent issues in low-exposure radiation epidemiology. *Environ Health Perspect* 1989; 81: 131–135.
196. Preston DL, Shimizu Y, Pierce DA, *et al.* Studies of mortality of atomic bomb survivors. Report 13. Solid cancer and noncancer disease mortality: 1950–1997. *Radiat Res* 2003; 160: 381–407.
197. Pierce DA, Sharp GB, Mabuchi K. Joint effects of radiation and smoking on lung cancer risk among atomic bomb survivors. *Radiat Res* 2003; 159: 511–520.
198. Hendee WR. Estimation of radiation risks. BEIR V and its significance for medicine. *JAMA* 1992; 92: 620–624.
199. National Research Council, Committee on the Biological Effects of Ionizing Radiation. Health Risks of Radon and Other Internally Deposited Alpha-Emitters: BEIR IV. Washington, National Academy Press, 1988.
200. Lubin JH, Boice JD Jr, Edling C, *et al.* Lung cancer in radon-exposed miners and estimation of risk from indoor exposure. *J Natl Cancer Inst* 1995; 87: 817–827.
201. US Environmental Protection Agency. Technical Support Document for the 1992 Citizen's Guide to Radon. Washington, US Government Printing Office, 1992.
202. Krewski D, Lubin JH, Zielinski JM, *et al.* Residential radon and risk of lung cancer: a combined analysis of 7 North American case–control studies. *Epidemiology* 2005; 16: 137–145.
203. Darby S, Hill D, Auvinen A, *et al.* Radon in homes and risk of lung cancer: collaborative analysis of individual data from 13 European case–control studies. *BMJ* 2005; 330: 223.
204. Shimizu Y, Kato H, Schull WJ. Studies of the mortality of A-bomb survivors. 9. Mortality, 1950–1985: Part 2. Cancer mortality based on the recently revised doses (DS86). *Radiat Res* 1990; 90: 120–141.
205. Darby SC, Doll R, Gill SK, *et al.* Long term mortality after a single treatment course with X-rays in patients treated for ankylosing spondylitis. *Br J Cancer* 1987; 87: 179–190.
206. Davis FG, Boice JD Jr, Hrubec Z, *et al.* Cancer mortality in radiation-exposed cohort of Massachusetts tuberculosis patients. *Cancer Res* 1989; 49: 6130–6136.
207. Howe GR. Lung cancer mortality between 1950 and 1987 after exposure to fractionated moderate-dose-rate ionizing radiation in the Canadian Fluoroscopy Cohort Study and a comparison with mortality in Atomic Bomb Survivors Study. *Radiat Res* 1995; 142: 295–304.
208. Gilbert ES, Cragle DL, Wiggs LD. Updated analyses of combined mortality data for workers at the Hanford Site, Oak Ridge National Laboratory, and Rocky Flats Weapons Plant. *Radiat Res* 1993; 136: 408–421.
209. National Research Council, Commission on Life Sciences, Board on Toxicology and Environmental Health Hazards, *et al.* Epidemiology and Air Pollution. Washington, National Academy Press, 1985; pp. 1–224.
210. Doll R. Atmospheric pollution and lung cancer. *Environ Health Perspect* 1978; 22: 23–31.
211. Pershagen G. Air pollution and cancer. *In*: Vainio H, Sorsa M, McMichael AJ, eds. Complex Mixtures and Cancer Risk. Lyon, International Agency for Research on Cancer, 1990; pp. 240–251.
212. Buffler PA, Cooper SP, Stinnett S, *et al.* Air pollution and lung cancer mortality in Harris County, Texas, 1979–1981. *Am J Epidemiol* 1988; 128: 683–699.
213. Nasca PC, Burnett WS, Greenwald P, *et al.* Population density as an indicator of urban–rural differences in cancer incidence, upstate New York, 1968–1972. *Am J Epidemiol* 1980; 112: 362–375.

214. Stocks P. Recent epidemiological studies of lung cancer mortality, cigarette smoking and air pollution, with discussion of a new hypothesis of causation. *Br J Cancer* 1966; 20: 596–623.
215. Shannon HS, Hertzman C, Julian JA, *et al.* Lung cancer and air pollution in an industrial city – a geographical analysis. *Can J Public Health* 1988; 79: 255–259.
216. Weinberg GB, Kuller LH, Redmond CK. The relationship between the geographic distribution of lung cancer incidence and cigarette smoking in Allegheny County, Pennsylvania. *Am J Epidemiol* 1982; 115: 40–58.
217. Vineis P, Forastiere F, Hoek G, *et al.* Outdoor air pollution and lung cancer: recent epidemiologic evidence. *Int J Cancer* 2004; 111: 647–652.
218. Dockery DW, Pope CA III, Xu X, *et al.* An association between air pollution and mortality in six US cities. *N Engl J Med* 1993; 329: 1753–1759.
219. Pope CA III, Thun MJ, Namboodiri MM, *et al.* Particulate air pollution as a predictor of mortality in a prospective study of US adults. *Am J Respir Crit Care Med* 1995; 151: 669–674.
220. Speizer FE. Assessment of the epidemiological data relating lung cancer to air pollution. *Environ Health Perspect* 1983; 47: 33–42.
221. Pope CA III, Burnett RT, Thun MJ, *et al.* Lung cancer, cardiopulmonary mortality, and long-term exposure to fine particulate air pollution. *JAMA* 2002; 287: 1132–1141.
222. Barbone F, Bovenzi M, Cavalleri F, *et al.* Air pollution and lung cancer in Trieste, Italy. *Am J Epidemiol* 1995; 141: 1161–1169.
223. Jedrychowski W, Becher H, Wahrendorf J, *et al.* A case–control study of lung cancer with special reference to the effect of air pollution in Poland. *J Epidemiol Community Health* 1990; 44: 114–120.
224. Vena JE. Air pollution as a risk factor in lung cancer. *Am J Epidemiol* 1982; 116: 42–56.
225. Samet JM, Humble CG, Skipper BE, *et al.* History of residence and lung cancer risk in New Mexico. *Am J Epidemiol* 1987; 125: 800–811.
226. Brown LM, Pottern LM, Blot WJ. Lung cancer in relation to environmental pollutants emitted from industrial sources. *Environ Res* 1984; 34: 250–261.
227. Pershagen G. Lung cancer mortality among men living near an arsenic-emitting smelter. *Am J Epidemiol* 1985; 122: 684–694.
228. Xu Z-Y, Blot WJ, Xiao HP, *et al.* Smoking, air pollution and the high rates of lung cancer in Shenyang, China. *J Natl Cancer Inst* 1989; 81: 1800–1806.
229. Greaves WW, Rom WN, Lyon JL, *et al.* Relationship between lung cancer and distance of residence from nonferrous smelter stack effluent. *Am J Ind Med* 1981; 2: 15–23.
230. Rom WN, Varley G, Lyon JL, *et al.* Lung cancer mortality among residents living near the El Paso smelter. *Br J Ind Med* 1982; 39: 269–272.
231. Cohen AJ, Ross AH, Ostro B, *et al.* The global burden of disease due to outdoor air pollution. *J Toxicol Environ Health A* 2005; 68: 1301–1307.
232. Spengler JD. Sources and concentrations of indoor air pollution. *In*: Samet JM, Spengler JD, eds. Indoor Air Pollution. A Health Perspective. Baltimore, Johns Hopkins University Press, 1991; pp. 33–67.
233. Harrje DT. Building dynamics and indoor air quality. *In*: Samet JM, Spengler JD, eds. Indoor Air Pollution. A Health Perspective. Baltimore, Johns Hopkins University Press, 1991; pp. 68–81.
234. Chen BH, Hong CJ, Pandey MR, *et al.* Indoor air pollution in developing countries. *World Health Stat Q* 1990; 43: 127–138.
235. Mumford JL, He XZ, Chapman RS, *et al.* Lung cancer and indoor air pollution in Xuan Wei, China. *Science* 1987; 235: 217–220.
236. Mumford JL, Helmes CT, Lee XM, *et al.* Mouse skin tumorigenicity studies of indoor coal and wood combustion emissions from homes of residents in Xuan Wei, China with high lung cancer mortality. *Carcinogenesis* 1990; 11: 397–403.
237. Lan Q, Chapman RS, Schreinemachers DM, *et al.* Household stove improvement and risk of lung cancer in Xuanwei, China. *J Natl Cancer Inst* 2002; 94: 826–835.

238. Vineis P, Caporaso N. Tobacco and cancer: epidemiology and the laboratory. *Environ Health Perspect* 1995; 103: 156–160.
239. Shields PG. Molecular epidemiology of smoking and lung cancer. *Oncogene* 2002; 21: 6870–6876.
240. Spitz MR, Wei Q, Dong Q, *et al.* Genetic susceptibility to lung cancer: the role of DNA damage and repair. *Cancer Epidemiol Biomarkers Prev* 2003; 12: 689–698.
241. Schwartz AG. Genetic predisposition to lung cancer. *Chest* 2004; 125: 86S–89S.
242. Liu G, Zhou W, Christiani DC. Molecular epidemiology of non-small cell lung cancer. *Semin Respir Crit Care Med* 2005; 26: 265–272.
243. Matakidou A, Eisen T, Houlston RS. Systematic review of the relationship between family history and lung cancer risk. *Br J Cancer* 2005; 93: 825–833.
244. Sellers TA, Bailey-Wilson JE, Elston RC, *et al.* Evidence for Mendelian inheritance in the pathogenesis of lung cancer. *J Natl Cancer Inst* 1990; 82: 1272–1279.
245. Braun MM, Caporaso NE, Page WF, *et al.* Genetic component of lung cancer: cohort study of twins. *Lancet* 1994; 344: 440–443.
246. Bailey-Wilson JE, Amos CI, Pinney SM, *et al.* A major lung cancer susceptibility locus maps to chromosome 6q23-25. *Am J Hum Genet* 2004; 75: 460–474.
247. Schwartz AG, Yang P, Swanson GM. Familial risk of lung cancer among nonsmokers and their relatives. *Am J Epidemiol* 1996; 144: 554–562.
248. Yang P, Schwartz AG, McAllister AE, *et al.* Lung cancer risk in families of nonsmoking probands: heterogeneity by age at diagnosis. *Genet Epidemiol* 1999; 17: 253–273.
249. Jones PA, Baylin SB. The fundamental role of epigenetic events in cancer. *Nat Rev Genet* 2002; 3: 415–428.
250. Herman JG, Baylin SB. Gene silencing in cancer in association with promoter hypermethylation. *N Engl J Med* 2003; 349: 2042–2054.
251. Belinsky SA, Nikula KJ, Palmisano WA, *et al.* Aberrant methylation of $p16^{\mathrm{ink4a}}$ is an early event in lung cancer and a potential biomarker for early diagnosis. *Proc Natl Acad Sci USA* 1998; 95: 11891–11896.
252. Palmisano WA, Divine KK, Saccomanno G, *et al.* Predicting lung cancer by detecting aberrant promoter methylation in sputum. *Cancer Res* 2000; 60: 5954–5958.
253. Hussain SP, Harris CC. Molecular epidemiology of human cancer: contribution of mutation spectra studies of tumor suppressor genes. *Cancer Res* 1998; 58: 4023–4037.
254. International Agency for Research on Cancer (IARC). IARC Monographs on the Evaluation of the Carcinogenic Risk of Chemicals to Humans: Tobacco Smoking. Lyon, World Health Organization, IARC, 1986.
255. Bergen AW, Caporaso N. Cigarette smoking. *J Natl Cancer Inst* 1999; 91: 1365–1375.
256. Berwick M, Vineis P. Markers of DNA repair and susceptibility to cancer in humans: an epidemiologic review. *J Natl Cancer Inst* 2000; 92: 874–897.
257. Robles AI, Linke SP, Harris CC. The p53 network in lung carcinogenesis. *Oncogene* 2002; 21: 6898–6907.
258. Garte S, Zocchetti C, Taioli E. Gene–environment interactions in the application of biomarkers of cancer susceptibility in epidemiology. *IARC Sci Publ* 1997; 142: 251–264.
259. Vineis P, Veglia F, Benhamou S, *et al.* CYP1A1 T3801 C polymorphism and lung cancer: a pooled analysis of 2451 cases and 3358 controls. *Int J Cancer* 2003; 104: 650–657.
260. Le Marchand L, Guo C, Benhamou S, *et al.* Pooled analysis of the CYP1A1 exon 7 polymorphism and lung cancer (United States). *Cancer Causes Control* 2003; 14: 339–346.
261. Benhamou S, Lee WJ, Alexandrie AK, *et al.* Meta- and pooled analyses of the effects of glutathione S-transferase M1 polymorphisms and smoking on lung cancer risk. *Carcinogenesis* 2002; 23: 1343–1350.
262. Hung RJ, Boffetta P, Brockmoller J, *et al.* CYP1A1 and GSTM1 genetic polymorphisms and lung cancer risk in Caucasian non-smokers: a pooled analysis. *Carcinogenesis* 2003; 24: 875–882.
263. Denissenko MF, Pao A, Tang M, *et al.* Preferential formation of benzo[a]pyrene adducts at lung cancer mutational hotspots in P53. *Science* 1996; 274: 430–432.

264. Matakidou A, Eisen T, Houlston RS. TP53 polymorphisms and lung cancer risk: a systematic review and meta-analysis. *Mutagenesis* 2003; 18: 377–385.
265. Goode EL, Ulrich CM, Potter JD. Polymorphisms in DNA repair genes and associations with cancer risk. *Cancer Epidemiol Biomarkers Prev* 2002; 11: 1513–1530.
266. Wei Q, Cheng L, Amos CI, *et al.* Repair of tobacco carcinogen-induced DNA adducts and lung cancer risk: a molecular epidemiologic study. *J Natl Cancer Inst* 2000; 92: 1764–1772.
267. Zheng YL, Loffredo CA. Bleomycin-induced chromosome breaks as a risk marker for lung cancer: a case–control study with population and hospital controls. *Carcinogenesis* 2003; 24: 269–274.
268. Gao WM, Romkes M, Day RD, *et al.* Association of the DNA repair gene XPD Asp312Asn polymorphism with p53 gene mutations in tobacco-related non-small cell lung cancer. *Carcinogenesis* 2003; 24: 1671–1676.
269. Liang G, Xing D, Miao X, *et al.* Sequence variations in the DNA repair gene XPD and risk of lung cancer in a Chinese population. *Int J Cancer* 2003; 105: 669–673.
270. Benhamou S, Sarasin A. ERCC2/XPD gene polymorphisms and lung cancer: a HuGE review. *Am J Epidemiol* 2005; 161: 1–14.
271. Hung RJ, Hall J, Brennan P, *et al.* Genetic polymorphisms in the base excision repair pathway and cancer risk: a HuGE review. *Am J Epidemiol* 2005; 162: 925–942.
272. Cotran RS, Kumar V, Robbins SL. Robbins Pathologic Basis of Disease. Philadelphia, WB Saunders, 1994.
273. Macklin MT, Macklin CC. Does chronic irritation cause primary carcinoma of the human lung? *Arch Pathol* 1940; 30: 924–955.
274. Tockman MS. Other host factors and lung cancer susceptibility. *In*: Samet JM, ed. Epidemiology of Lung Cancer. New York, Marcel Dekker, Inc., 1994; pp. 397–412.
275. US Dept of Health and Human Services. The Health Consequences of Smoking – Chronic Obstructive Lung Disease. A Report of the Surgeon General. Washington, US Government Printing Office, 1984.
276. Gabriel R, Dudley BM, Alexander WD. Lung cancer and allergy. *Br J Clin Pract* 1972; 26 202–204.
277. Alderson M. Mortality from malignant disease in patients with asthma. *Lancet* 1974; 2: 1475–1477.
278. Markowe HL, Bulpitt CJ, Shipley MJ, *et al.* Prognosis in adult asthma: a national study. *Br Med J (Clin Res Ed)* 1987; 295: 949–952.
279. Eriksson NE, Holmen A, Hogstedt B, *et al.* A prospective study of cancer incidence in a cohort examined for allergy. *Allergy* 1995; 50: 718–722.
280. Santillan AA, Camargo CA Jr, Colditz GA. A meta-analysis of asthma and risk of lung cancer (United States). *Cancer Causes Control* 2003; 14: 327–334.
281. Brown DW, Young KE, Anda RF, *et al.* Asthma and risk of death from lung cancer: NHANES II mortality study. *J Asthma* 2005; 42: 597–600.
282. Barrett JC, Lamb PW, Wiseman RW. Multiple mechanisms for the carcinogenic effects of asbestos and other mineral fibers. *Environ Health Perspect* 1989; 81: 81–89.
283. Rom WN, Travis WD, Brody AR. Cellular and molecular basis of the asbestos-related diseases. *Am Rev Respir Dis* 1991; 143: 408–422.
284. Ng TP. Silica and lung cancer: a continuing controversy. *Ann Acad Med Singapore* 1994; 23: 752–755.
285. Pairon JC, Brochard P, Jaurand MC, *et al.* Silica and lung cancer: a controversial issue. *Eur Respir J* 1991; 4: 730–744.
286. McDonald JC, McDonald AD. The epidemiology of mesothelioma in historical context. *Eur Respir J* 1996; 9: 1932–1942.
287. Wagner IC, Sleggs CA, Marchand P. Diffuse pleural mesothelioma and asbestos exposure in the North Western Cape Province. *Br J Ind Med* 1960; 17: 260–271.

288. Newhouse ML, Thompson H. Epidemiology of mesothelial tumors in the London area. *Ann NY Acad Sci* 1965; 132: 579–588.

289. Baris YI, Artvinli M, Sahin AA. Environmental mesothelioma in Turkey. *Ann NY Acad Sci* 1979; 330: 423–432.

290. Goldberg M, Luce D. Can exposure to very low levels of asbestos induce pleural mesothelioma? *Am J Respir Crit Care Med* 2005; 172: 939–940.

291. Spengler JD, Samet JM, McCarthy JF, *et al.* Indoor Air Quality Handbook. New York, McGraw-Hill, 2000.

292. Cugell DW, Kamp DW. Asbestos and the pleura: a review. *Chest* 2004; 125: 1103–1117.

293. Becklake MR, Bagatin E, Neder JA. Asbestos-related diseases of the lungs and pleura: uses, trends and management over the last century. *Int J Tuberc Lung Dis* 2007; 11: 356–369.

294. Nelson D, Robinson C, Dunham MA, *et al.* Malignant mesothelioma. *In*: Rom WM, ed. Environmental and Occupational Medicine. 4th Edn. Philadelphia, Lippincott William & Wilkins, 2007; pp. 318–327.

295. Robinson BW, Musk AW, Lake RA. Malignant mesothelioma. *Lancet* 2005; 366: 397–408.

296. Caporaso NE, Dodd KW, Tucker MA. New malignancies following cancer of the respiratory tract. *In*: Curtis RE, Freedman DM, Ron E, *et al.*, eds. New Malignancies Among Cancer Survivors: SEER Cancer Registries, 1973–2000. NIH Publication No. 05-5302. Bethesda, National Cancer Institute, 2006; pp. 145–180.

297. International Agency for Research on Cancer (IARC). Cancer incidence in five continents. Vol VII. 143 Edn. Lyon, IARC Press, 1997.

298. Centers for Disease Control and Prevention. Deaths from selected occupational diseases for persons 15 years of age and over: United States, selected years 1980–2005, 2008. Available at http://www.cdc.gov/nchs/data/hus/hus08.pdf Date last updated: April 2, 2009.

299. National Cancer Institute (NCI). The Surveillance, Epidemiology, and End Results (SEER) Program. Available at http://seer.cancer.gov/faststats/index.php Date last updated: April 15, 2009.

300. Peto J, Hodgson JT, Matthews FE, *et al.* Continuing increase in mesothelioma mortality in Britain. *Lancet* 1995; 345: 535–539.

301. Lin RT, Takahashi K, Karjalainen A, *et al.* Ecological association between asbestos-related diseases and historical asbestos consumption: an international analysis. *Lancet* 2007; 369: 844–849.

302. Hodgson JT, Darnton A. The quantitative risks of mesothelioma and lung cancer in relation to asbestos exposure. *Ann Occup Hyg* 2000; 44: 565–601.

303. Selikoff IJ, Churg J, Hammond EC. Relation between exposure to asbestos and mesothelioma. *N Engl J Med* 1965; 272: 560–565.

304. Magnani C, Dalmasso P, Biggeri A, *et al.* Increased risk of malignant mesothelioma of the pleura after residential or domestic exposure to asbestos: a case–control study in Casale Monferrato, Italy. *Environ Health Perspect* 2001; 109: 915–919.

305. Kurumatani N, Kumagai S. Mapping the risk of mesothelioma due to neighborhood asbestos exposure. *Am J Respir Crit Care Med* 2008; 178: 624–629.

306. Reid A, Berry G, de Klerk N, *et al.* Age and sex differences in malignant mesothelioma after residential exposure to blue asbestos (crocidolite). *Chest* 2007; 131: 376–382.

307. Pan XL, Day HW, Wang W, *et al.* Residential proximity to naturally occurring asbestos and mesothelioma risk in California. *Am J Respir Crit Care Med* 2005; 172: 1019–1025.

308. Doll R, Peto J. Asbestos: Effects on Health of Exposure to Asbestos. Health and Safety Commission. London, Her Majesty's Stationery Office, 1985.

309. Hillerdal G. Mesothelioma: cases associated with non-occupational and low dose exposures. *Occup Environ Med* 1999; 56: 505–513.

310. De Klerk NH, English DR, Armstong BK. A review of the effects of random measurement error on relative risk estimates in epidemiological studies. *Int J Epidemiol* 1989; 18: 705–712.

311. Institute of Medicine, Committee on Asbestos, Selected Health Effects. Asbestos. Selected Cancers. Washington, National Academies Press, 2006.
312. Stanton MF, Layard M, Tegeris A, *et al.* Relation of particle dimension to carcinogenicity in amphibole asbestos and other fibrous minerals. *J Natl Cancer Inst* 1981; 67: 965–975.
313. Berman DW, Crump KS. A meta-analysis of asbestos-related cancer risk that addresses fiber size and mineral type. *Crit Rev Toxicol* 2008; 38: Suppl. 1, 49–73.
314. Smith AH, Wright CC. Chrysotile asbestos is the main cause of pleural mesothelioma. *Am J Ind Med* 1996; 30: 252–266.
315. Roggli VL, Vollmer RT. Twenty-five years of fiber analysis: what have we learned? *Hum Pathol* 2008; 39: 307–315.
316. Strickler HD, Goedert JJ, Devesa SS, *et al.* Trends in US pleural mesothelioma incidence rates following simian virus 40 contamination of early poliovirus vaccines. *J Natl Cancer Inst* 2003; 95: 38–45.
317. Carbone M, Pass HI, Miele L, *et al.* New developments about the association of SV40 with human mesothelioma. *Oncogene* 2003; 22: 5173–5180.
318. Lopez-Rios F, Illei PB, Rusch V, *et al.* Evidence against a role for SV40 infection in human mesotheliomas and high risk of false-positive PCR results owing to presence of SV40 sequences in common laboratory plasmids. *Lancet* 2004; 364: 1157–1166.
319. Neri M, Ugolini D, Dianzani I, *et al.* Genetic susceptibility to malignant pleural mesothelioma and other asbestos-associated diseases. *Mutat Res* 2008; 659: 126–136.
320. US Dept of Health and Human Services. Tobacco Use Among US Racial/Ethnic Minority Groups: African Americans, American Indians and Alaska Natives, Asian Americans and Pacific Islanders, Hispanics. A Report of the Surgeon General. Washington, US Government Printing Office, 1998.

CHAPTER 22

Diagnosis and staging of mesothelioma

A. Scherpereel

Correspondence: A. Scherpereel, Service de Pneumologie et d'Oncologie Thoracique, Hôpital Calmette, CHRU de Lille, 59037 Lille Cedex, France. Fax: 33 320445611; E-mail: a-scherpereel@chru-lille.fr

Malignant mesothelioma is a highly aggressive tumour with a poor survival rate, which arises from the surface cells of the pleura (in 90% of cases), more rarely involving the peritoneum and/or the pericardium. Previously considered as a rare tumour, malignant pleural mesothelioma (MPM) has become a very important public health issue because of its increasing incidence worldwide. This incidence is expected to continue to increase for at least the next 10 yrs [1]. Occupational asbestos exposure has been clearly established as the main factor involved in MPM pathogenesis [2]. However, the screening and diagnosis of MPM in asbestos-exposed subjects are difficult because, first, the disease may occur up to 30–40 yrs after exposure and, secondly, the differential diagnosis on pleural biopsies between MPM and pleural benign disease, also frequently induced by asbestos exposure, or pleural metastasis of adenocarcinoma may be difficult in some cases even using immunohistochemistry [3]. Management of patients with MPM also remains problematic because the patients are often diagnosed late in the evolution of the disease, only very few are candidates for radical surgery, and MPM exhibits a high resistance to chemotherapy. New therapeutic strategies, including multimodal treatment (radical surgery, chemotherapy and radiotherapy), gene or cell therapy and targeted drugs such as angiogenesis inhibitors or histone deacetylase inhibitors, are still on clinical trial [4, 5]. Accurate initial staging is essential to provide both prognostic information and guidance on the most appropriate therapeutic options, and also to allow recruitment of homogeneous groups of MPM patients into clinical trials. Since 1995, the International Mesothelioma Interest Group (IMIG) classification, based on computed tomography (CT) scanning, has been the most frequently used classification [6–8]. Although the current classification has been only validated with patients who have been surgically treated, a small minority of cases in practice, use of the IMIG classification is recommended until a new system of classification, better adapted to MPM, has been set up [9, 10]. Thus, clinical staging is based on a chest CT scan, coupled or not coupled with a positron emission tomography (PET) scan. However, the conversion of such images into "tumour, node, metastasis" (TNM) stages is often inconclusive and very tricky. Finally, there is no validated biological marker yet to help MPM diagnosis or to predict response to treatment or prognosis [11].

Diagnosis

Clinical signs

The clinical manifestations of MPM are unspecific and usually appear late at an advanced stage in the course of the disease. Clinical signs suggesting a diagnosis of

Eur Respir Mon, 2009, 44, 392–406. Printed in UK - all rights reserved. Copyright ERS Journals Ltd 2009; European Respiratory Monograph; ISSN 1025-448x.

MPM may include chest pain, thoracic "shrinkage", and/or a unilateral pleural effusion or thoracic mass, in a patient with a past history of (professional) asbestos exposure. Therefore, occupational history must be obtained for each MPM patient. However, it has been noticed that an asbestos exposure is found only in <50% of female cases of MPM *versus* about 90% in males. It is not possible to establish an exhaustive list of occupations or work sectors associated with an increased risk of MPM. Nevertheless, several occupations are clearly associated with a reproducible relative risk of MPM: plumbers/pipe fitters, electricians, carpenters, cabinet makers and other occupations in the construction industry. In addition, several other work sectors have been associated with an increased risk of mesothelioma in several studies. These include shipyards, industries producing and manufacturing articles made of asbestos and the construction industry in general. However, the list of risk situations should not be restricted to these occupations or work sectors. Weight loss, asthenia, peritoneal effusion and very rare extra-thoracic metastasis usually appear even later, with tumour progression [12, 13]. Therefore, a diagnosis of MPM should not be based on clinical criteria [10].

Imaging

Chest radiographs (fig. 1) and CT scans (fig. 2) usually show a nonspecific, unilateral (in 95% of cases) pleural effusion with or without mediastinal shift, in MPM patients. More rarely, a pleural thickening or mass, without pleurisy, may be observed [10, 12]. In the literature, about 20% of patients exhibit the association of pulmonary interstitial fibrosis due to asbestos, whereas pleural plugs are very common (70% of cases) [14]. Although chest radiography is relatively cheap, its diagnostic accuracy (sensitivity and specificity) is poor. Therefore chest radiographs should not be used to assess the diagnosis of MPM. Chest high-resolution CT scanning is a key imaging procedure for the diagnosis of MPM. It does not provide a definitive diagnosis, but certain features, such as the presence of diffuse pleural thickening or mass with thickening of interlobular fissures, are highly suggestive of MPM (fig. 2a–c). However, the value of CT scans in patients with an abundant pleural effusion is poor (showing nonspecific features). CT scanning is also relevant, before a thoracoscopy, for the evaluation of tumour extension to the chest wall, pericardium, diaphragm, mediastinal structures or locoregional lymph nodes, and the detection of infra-diaphragmatic invasion or metastases. Therefore, it is recommended that follow-up be carried out,

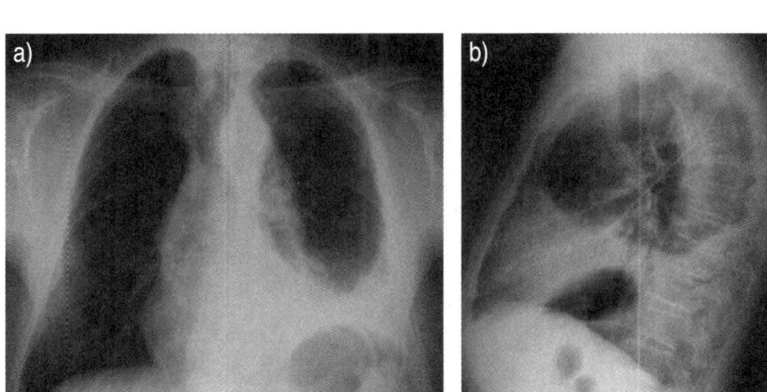

Fig. 1. – Patient with left malignant pleural mesothelioma (MPM). a) Postero-anterior and b) lateral angles. In patients with MPM, chest radiography usually shows unilateral features, such as pleural effusion and/or thickening, with or without mediastinal shift by hemithoracic "shrinkage" (reflected by the elevation of the left hemidiaphragm).

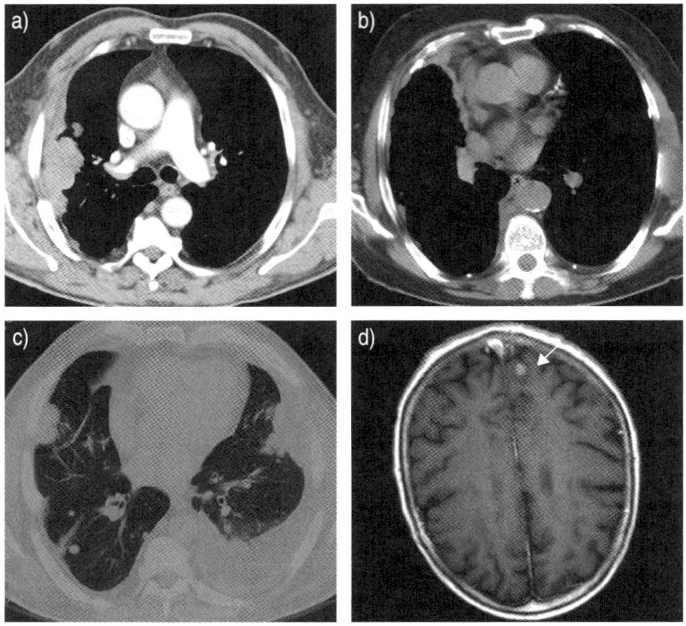

Fig. 2. – On computed tomography scanning, a–c) a pleural diffuse thickening or mass with thickening of interlobular fissures are highly suggestive of malignant pleural mesothelioma (MPM). a and b) Pleural thickening or mass without pleural effusion may be observed. b) Pleural plugs are very common (70% of cases). c) Bilateral MPM is rare but may be observed, mostly at a later stage of disease when tumour spreads in the chest. Much more rarely, distant metastasis may be detected c) in the lung or d) in extrathoracic organs such as the brain (arrow).

after removal of pleural fluid, by a chest and abdominal multidetector CT scan with multiplaner reformation, for diagnosis and staging of MPM [10].

In contrast to CT scanning, magnetic resonance imaging (MRI) is not systematically performed because it is not relevant for the diagnosis of mesothelioma. However, MRI can be helpful for the determination of the extent of the tumour to the local organs (diaphragm, mediastinum or chest wall), mostly for patients who are candidates for radical surgery [15].

18-Fluorodeoxyglucose (^{18}FDG)-PET usually shows a hypermetabolism of pleural mesothelioma, metastatic adenopathy and metastasis (fig. 3). The diagnostic relevance of these features is considered poor. PET, with or without combination with CT scanning, currently appears not to be useful for the diagnosis of mesothelioma, even if it seems quite sensitive for some of the tumours, but sensitivity and specificity varies in the literature. Sensitivity of 91% and specificity of 100% have been measured when using PET to differentiate MPM from benign pleural lesions (BPL) in asbestos-exposed subjects. Patients with BPL (benign pleural effusion and/or thickening) had a low hypermetabolism or no hypermetabolism at all when performing ^{18}FDG-PET [15, 16]. The standard uptake value was significantly increased in MPM compared with BPL. PET-CT scanning may be helpful for MPM staging in the search for contralateral mediastinal adenopathy (stage N3) and distant metastasis, whereas its value in the assessment of locoregional invasion is poor [15, 17]. Metastases may be found in MPM, usually at the same sites as lung cancer (lung, brain, liver, *etc.*; fig. 2c and d), but are quite rare in clinics compared with their incidence (up to 50%) previously reported from necropsy studies [18, 19]. The metastatic spread happens through mediastinal and hilar lymph nodes and the

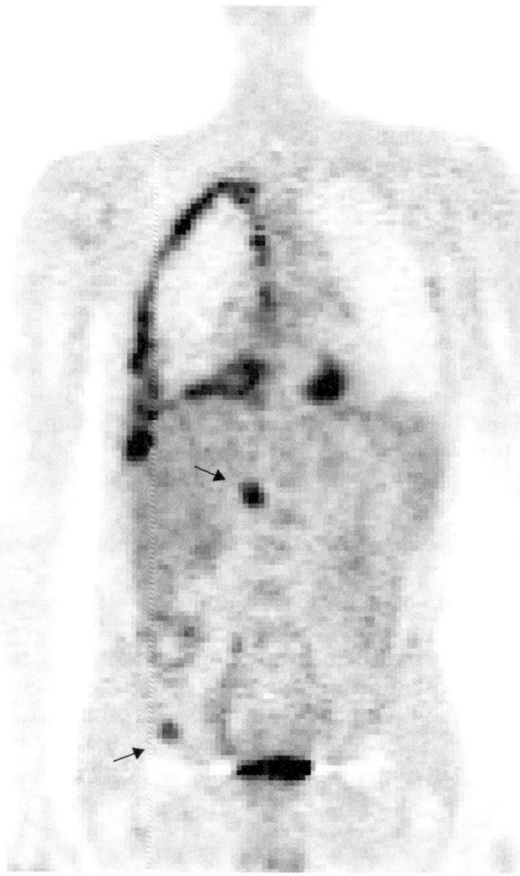

Fig. 3. – 18-Fluorodeoxyglucose positron emission tomography (PET) scanning usually shows a hypermetabolism of malignant pleural mesothelioma (MPM), metastatic adenopathy and metastasis (arrows). PET scanning is useful for MPM staging, mostly to assess N3 and M1 status.

visceral pleura to the opposite lung. MPM can also directly spread to the peritoneum through the diaphragm. Finally, PET assessment should be performed before talc pleurodesis because the talc induces nonspecific inflammation responsible for an intense hypermetabolism. In conclusion, PET should not currently be performed for the diagnosis of MPM [10].

Pathology and diagnostic procedures

The accurate diagnosis of mesothelioma is made on histopathological examination. However, this diagnosis can be extremely difficult because mesothelioma can show various misleading histopathological pitfalls. Moreover, the pleural cavity is a common site for metastases of various tumours, mostly lung and breast cancers, which are much more frequent than mesothelioma (about one MPM per 50 cases of pleural metastases in the USA).

The macroscopic appearance of mesothelioma depends on when in its natural history the tumour is first observed. As a mesothelioma grows, the gross appearance becomes more suggestive of MPM to some extent, although other malignant tumours (thymomas, carcinomas, lymphomas and angiosarcomas) can appear with a pseudomesotheliomatous aspect [19]. The microscopic appearances of MPM are well defined in the international classification of pleural tumours (table 1) [20]. This classification provides a comparative basis for diagnosis, prognosis and patient management. Two groups of MPM are described, a diffuse type and a localised type, which are divided into four histological subtypes: epithelioid, sarcomatoid, desmoplastic (very fibrous with rare fusiform cells) and biphasic (mixed epithelioid and sarcomatoid MPM) subtypes [19].

Thus, MPMs have varied and deceptive appearances in a high percentage of cases and may mimic pleural metastatic lesions. Diagnostic problems also occur with benign inflammatory or reactive lesions of the pleura. These very frequent lesions occur often in patients of the same age group as mesothelioma (pleural effusion during cardiac failure, collagen disease, pneumonia or cirrhosis), and they may lead to atypical mesothelial hyperplasia, which can result in diagnostic error. In the French National Program of Mesothelioma Survey (1998–2007), such errors represented 13% of initially diagnosed cases of MPM [10, 21].

Which specimens for which clinical presentation? As pleural effusion is usually the first clinical sign of MPM, a pleural puncture is often the first procedure to be carried out. However, a diagnosis of mesothelioma should not be based on cytology alone because of the high risk of error [10, 12]. In fact, when malignant mesothelial cells are well differentiated, they are very difficult to distinguish from reactive mesothelial cells. MPM cells may also have a pseudocarcinomatous aspect that could be confused with metastases of carcinoma. Finally, pleural cytology is completely inappropriate in sarcomatoid subtypes of MPM because they do not desquamate [19]. Pleural effusion analysis usually shows an exudate with high levels of proteins, lactate dehydrogenase

Table 1. – World Health Organization international histological classification of tumours of the pleura

Mesothelial tumours
Diffuse malignant mesothelioma
Epithelioid mesothelioma
Sarcomatoid mesothelioma
Desmoplastic mesothelioma
Biphasic mesothelioma
Localised malignant mesothelioma
Other tumours of mesothelial origin
Well-differentiated papillary mesothelioma
Adenomatoid tumour
Mesenchymal tumours
Epithelioid haemangioendothelioma
Angiosarcoma
Synovial sarcoma
Monophasic
Biphasic
Solitary fibrous tumour
Calcifying tumour of the pleura
Desmoplastic round cell tumour
Lymphoproliferative disorders
Primary effusion lymphoma
Pyothorax-associated lymphoma

Data taken from [20].

(LDH) and hyaluronic acid. However, all these features are nonspecific and insufficient for the unequivocal diagnosis of MPM (see also the section of this chapter about biological markers).

Diagnosis of mesothelioma from fine needle biopsies (Abrams or Castelain needles) is associated with the same problems as cytology. A conclusive diagnosis can only be made if the material is representative of the tumour and in sufficient quantity to allow immunohistochemical characterisation. Thus, sensitivity for the diagnosis of mesothelioma using fine needle biopsies is low (around 30%) [22]. This sensitivity goes up to 40% when using both pleural fluid analysis and transthoracic pleural biopsy, and may be improved if the biopsies are guided by ultrasound or CT scan but mostly at later stages of the disease when the pleural lesions are much more important and therefore the treatment is probably less efficient. Thus, transparietal biopsies with or without CT scan or ultrasound guidance are not recommended for the diagnosis of MPM except in patients for whom thoracoscopy is contraindicated [10].

The histopathology can be confusing between MPM and lymphatic drainage of normal mesothelial cells originating from a pleural effusion. In a very few cases, a diagnosis of MPM can be obtained by a biopsy of superficial adenopathy. However, it is crucial not to base a diagnosis of MPM on lymph node biopsies without validation by a panel of pathologist, experts in mesothelioma [10].

Medical thoracoscopy (pleuroscopy) or surgical thoracoscopy (video-assisted thoracoscopic surgery (VATS)) is the best method to obtain the diagnosis of MPM when suspected on clinical or radiological data. Diagnostic accuracy is greater than 90% and complications occur in less than 10% of cases [23]. Investigation of exudative pleural effusion in asbestos-exposed patients represents one of the main targets of thoracoscopy. During the thoracoscopy (fig. 4), a complete visual examination of the pleura is recommended before multiple pleural guided biopsies of potential tumour lesions and/or biopsies in the form of pleural scrapes when facing uniformly thick pleura. Pleural plugs are very common in MPM patients (fig. 4a), evoking a previous exposure to asbestos, but, to our best knowledge, there is no proof that plugs may be considered as pre-neoplasic lesions. However, MPM may start next to the pleural plugs. Therefore, we proposed making biopsies at these sites during thoracoscopy if there are no evident lesions [10]. In fact, MPM may exhibit many macroscopic and mostly nonspecific aspects. Most of the time, MPM will appear as nodules or masses of various diameter (fig. 4b); more rarely (10–15% of cases), a typical grape-like aspect

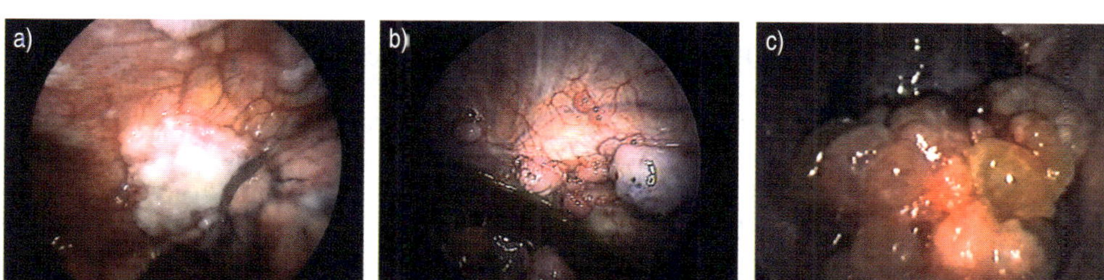

Fig. 4. – Thoracoscopy (pleuroscopy or video-assisted thoracoscopic surgery) is the best method of obtaining the diagnosis of malignant pleural mesothelioma (MPM) and is helpful for tumour staging. During the thoracoscopy in MPM patients, various macroscopic and mostly nonspecific aspects may be observed. a) Pleural plugs are very common in MPM patients next to tumour lesions, evoking a previous exposure to asbestos. b) Most of the time, MPM will appear as nodules or masses of various diameter. c) Less often (10–15% of cases), a typical grape-like aspect may be found.

may be found (fig. 4c). Other abnormalities, such as diffuse pleural thickening nonspecific inflammation or lymphangitis, may be observed in association with nodules or alone. Thus, a pleuroscopy is essential for MPM management because it has several benefits. 1) Its sensitivity and specificity are higher than other diagnostic methods, and its cost/efficiency ratio is better than surgery. 2) Pleuroscopy may show the tumour extension to the visceral pleura, a bad prognostic factor. 3) During pleuroscopy, it may also be realised whether it would be possible for therapeutic instillations of talc to achieve a pleurodesis in cases of recurrent pleural effusion, or other potential intrapleural antitumour treatments that have been evaluated in clinical trials [10].

Direct access to the pleura by mini-thoracotomy enables tissue biopsies to be obtained for histological examination, notably in the absence of pleural effusion. However, this technique should be reserved for cases where thoracoscopy has failed and pleurodesis is still to be attempted [10].

In conclusion, when a mesothelioma is suspected on clinical or radiological data, thoracoscopy is the best method to obtain the diagnosis. Therefore, except in the case of pre-operative contraindication or previous pleurodesis, it is recommended to perform thoracoscopy for the diagnosis of MPM [10]. The 2008 European Respiratory Society (ERS)/European Society of Thoracic Surgeons (ESTS) experts on MPM recommend the same approach for diagnosis of MPM [24].

What are the role and the technical requirements of immunohistochemical examination in the diagnosis of mesothelioma? In accordance with the International Mesothelioma Panel, a diagnosis of MPM must always be based on immunohistochemical examination. It is recommended to use two markers with positive diagnostic value for mesothelioma (nuclear markers such as anti-calretinin and anti-WT1 or the membrane marker anti-EMA or, for epithelioid mesothelioma, anti-CK5/6) and two markers with negative diagnostic value to validate the diagnosis (such as anti-Ber-EP4 (a membrane marker), anti-TTF1 (a nuclear marker) or monoclonal anti-CEA (cytoplasmic staining)). For sarcomatoid forms, it is recommended to use two broad-spectrum anti-cytokeratin antibodies (negative immunostaining with a single antibody does not exclude the diagnosis, according to the advice of experts), and two markers with negative predictive value to confirm the diagnosis (such as anti-CD34 and anti-BCL2, anti-desmin or anti-S100) [10, 19].

Should other diagnostic examination be performed? Electron microscopy is not routinely needed to confirm the diagnosis of mesothelioma. However, this technique is of value for epithelial tumours when immunohistochemical results are discordant, and in some sarcomatoid tumours. The presence of long, thin microvilli is highly suggestive of mesothelioma. Currently, there are no diagnostic reasons for freezing pleural tumour tissue, but MPM tissue material should be frozen for research purposes.

Finally, due to the histological difficulties described, it seems logical to recommend asking a panel of independent and experienced pathologists to confirm a diagnosis of mesothelioma when the result is doubtful or for patients recruited in randomised clinical trials.

Blood and pleural biological markers

Biomarkers have been searched in an attempt to obtain an early and reliable diagnosis of MPM, and to help the management of patients. However, this search is extremely challenging due to the biological features of mesothelioma and the need to differentiate

MPM from the more frequent diagnoses such as benign pleural diseases and metastatic pleural malignancies [25].

Mesothelin is a glycoprotein expressed on the cell surface of normal mesothelial cells, highly overexpressed in mesothelioma and various carcinomas. Soluble mesothelin (SM; or SM-related peptides (SMRP)) has emerged as a promising potential biomarker for MPM [26]. SM levels were greatly increased in the serum and in the pleural effusions of patients with MPM compared with healthy asbestos-exposed subjects or patients with BPL or pleural metastasis. Serum and pleural fluid SM showed excellent sensitivity (70–80%) and specificity (80–100%) as diagnostic markers for MPM [25–27]. However, SM does not capture sarcomatoid (and some biphasic) mesotheliomas. This fact hampers using SM as a sole diagnostic marker [26, 27]. Combining other potential MPM markers such as osteopontin or CA125 assessment with SM was not helpful in this goal [28, 29].

In asbestos-exposed subjects, it has been suggested that elevated serum SM may predict the later development of MPM [26], reflecting the presence of undetectable small foci of mesothelioma and preceding clinical disease presentation. The association of pleural abnormalities and high SMRP level in these subjects should be "aggressively" managed to exclude mesothelioma or metastatic malignancies, or at least attempt "early" identification. Such a strategy would need to be validated by prospective trials. At present, mesothelioma cannot meet the essential criteria for cancer screening programmes: there is no validated screening tool or effective cure for MPM, and no evidence that early detection alters outcome [25]. However, detecting mesothelioma years before its clinical presentation may allow testing of new therapeutic approaches in early-stage patients. Thus, studies assessing SM alone or combined with other potential biomarkers for MPM diagnosis or screening are ongoing. Currently, SM remains the best candidate biomarker for MPM diagnosis [30].

In conclusion, there is not enough evidence yet to justify clinical applications of serum or pleural effusion SM assessment in MPM. SM alone has insufficient specificity and sensitivity for MPM screening, but may help clinicians with the diagnosis of epithelioid MPM, even if histopathological diagnosis remains the "gold standard", taking account of the important therapeutic and medicolegal implications of mesothelioma.

Table 2. – Summary of "tumour, node, metastasis" (TNM) classification in malignant pleural mesothelioma

Stage	TNM	Tumour involvement
Ia	T1a N0 M0	Ipsilateral parietal pleura (no visceral pleura)
Ib	T1b N0 M0	Ipsilateral parietal pleura and visceral pleura
II	T2 N0 M0	Ipsilateral lung, diaphragm, confluent involvement of visceral pleura
III	Any T3 M0	Endothoracic fascia, mediastinal fat, focal chest wall, nontransmural pericardium
	Any N1 M0	Ipsilateral bronchopulmonary or hilar lymph node
	Any N2 M0	Subcarinal or ipsilateral mediastinal lymph node
IV	Any T4	Contralateral pleura, peritoneum, rib, extensive chest wall or mediastinal invasion, myocardium, brachial plexus, spine, transmural pericardium, malignant pericardial effusion (locally advanced, technically unresectable tumour)
	Any N3	Contralateral mediastinal, internal mammary, hilar, ipsilateral/contralateral supraclavicular, scalene lymph node
	Any M1	Extrathoracic metastasis

Data taken from [6–8].

Staging and pre-therapeutic assessment

Which staging classification should we use?

There are several staging systems available in MPM, describing the anatomical extent of the tumour. The latest one (summarised in table 2) was proposed in 1995 by members of the IMIG and approved by the Union Internationale Contre le Cancer (UICC) [6–8]. The main weakness of the classifications is the inaccuracy in describing T- and N-extent by current imaging techniques. In particular, the present and most frequently used classification (IMIG) is based on CT scanning and has only been validated in patients who have been surgically treated. Thus, there is a clear need for the development of a new robust and uniform clinical staging system that should be prospectively validated, TNM-based, and include the existing surgical-pathological staging systems. However, in the absence of this validated staging system, the 2008 ERS/ESTS experts on MPM advocate the use of the most recent TNM-based UICC/IMIG classification until a new system of classification better adapted to MPM has been set up [24]. An updated classification from the IMIG is expected in 2009.

At this time, one should note that only performance status of the patient and histological subtype of the tumour (epithelioid MPM have a "better" survival than other subtypes) are recognised as prognostic factors for the management of MPM in the clinical practice. The TNM stage and other potential prognostic parameters from the Cancer and Leukemia Group B (CALGB) and the European Organisation for Research and Treatment of Cancer (EORTC) [31–33], such as age, certain symptoms (*e.g.* chest pain) and blood parameters (haemoglobin, platelet count and LDH), are mostly useful for analysis of clinical trial results but not in routine practice.

Minimal pre-treatment staging investigations from the 2008 ERS/ESTS guidelines for MPM management

An optimal pre-treatment assessment protocol should be simple and widely applicable, sequential and logical, not unnecessarily invasive and identify candidates for appropriate treatment. Based on empirical observation, good clinical practice and the fact that the treatment intent differs between patients, the 2008 ERS/ESTS experts on MPM propose a pre-treatment assessment, empirically split into three steps, which are to some degree overlapping [34]. Step I is to be considered in all patients at presentation or diagnosis. Step II is to be considered in patients who are candidates for any kind of active treatment (table 3). Step III is the final process of patient selection for combined modality or radical locoregional treatment (table 4). This step

Table 3. – Investigations to perform in patients likely to receive any kind of active treatment

Investigations	Details
CT scan of chest and upper abdomen	Spiral technique, with injection of contrast material, after removal of pleural fluid
Pulmonary function tests	Forced vital capacity, forced expiratory volume in 1 s
Bone scan	Not routine, to be considered on clinical suspicion only;
Brain CT/MRI	CT/MRI to confirm doubtful findings

From the 2008 European Respiratory Society/European Society of Thoracic Surgeons guidelines for malignant pleural mesothelioma management [24]. CT: computed tomography; MRI: magnetic resonance imaging.

Table 4. – Investigations to be considered in patients who are candidates for radical treatment

Area	Investigation	Patient group	Confirmatory tests
Primary tumour	Adequate biopsy for histological subtyping	Every patient considered for radical treatment	
Diaphragm	Chest radiograph, inspiration and expiration	Every patient considered for radical treatment	Fluoroscopy
Extrathoracic, excluding "occult" M1	Full-ring ^{18}FDG-PET scan or PET-CT scan	Every patient considered for radical treatment	Biopsy of suspected extrathoracic lesions
	Laparoscopy	According to institutional practice	
Mediastinum, excluding T4, N2/3 involvement	Cervical mediastinoscopy	According to institutional practice	
	Thoracoscopy, contralateral thoracoscopy	According to institutional practice	
	Thoraco-abdominal CT scan with *i.v.* contrast and reconstructions, or MRI of the chest, gadolinium-enhanced	According to institutional practice	
	E(B)US-FNA	Investigational	

From the 2008 European Respiratory Society/European Society of Thoracic Surgeons guidelines for malignant pleural mesothelioma management [24]. ^{18}FDG: 18-fluorodeoxyglucose; PET: positron emission tomography; CT: computed tomography; MRI: magnetic resonance imaging; E(B)US-FNA: endoscopic/endobronchial ultrasound fine needle aspiration.

III would occur only in a small minority (≤10%) of patients with MPM, explaining the lack of experience of most of the centres and the low level of evidence in the literature.

It is essential that patients proceeding to step II or beyond should have a confidently established diagnosis of mesothelioma. Of course, the interval within which the pre-treatment assessment has to be finalised should be as short as possible, and recent (<1-month-old) imaging studies should be available prior to invasive procedures. In the absence of comparative trials, the 2008 ERS/ESTS experts could not give any formal advice regarding the respective efficacy of the different investigations (MRI or PET scan) or intrathoracic techniques (mediastinoscopy, pleuroscopy, VATS or endoscopic ultrasound/endobronchial ultrasound (EBUS) fine needle aspiration).

Step I: assessment in patients at presentation or diagnosis of MPM. A minimum assessment should include a clinical examination, collecting data such as demographics (age, sex, asbestos exposure history), performance status, presence/absence of chest pain, dyspnoea and hemithoracic "shrinkage", change in body weight or body mass index, a chest radiograph (before and after pleural effusion removal, if applicable), and blood tests including prognostic parameters proposed by CALGB/EORTC (haemoglobin, leucocytes, platelets and basic biochemistry).

This proposal is similar to the one from the experts of the Pulmonary Society of French Language (SPLF) 2006 guidelines on MPM [9, 10]. For research purposes, the SPLF experts proposed also to assess potential biological markers such as SMRP and osteopontin.

Step II: investigations to perform in patients likely to receive any kind of active treatment. These investigations are reported in table 3. Patients are often referred to pulmonary physicians already with a chest CT scan but it is necessary to perform another CT scan of the chest and upper abdomen (with injection of contrast material) after removal of pleural fluid (if applicable) to optimise the staging of the patient before any active treatment is considered. With the same goal, a thoracoscopy with exhaustive and standardised report is helpful to establish the TNM status of the MPM and to guide the treatment [9, 10].

Step III: investigations to be considered in patient candidates for radical treatment. These investigations, detailed in table 4, aim to select MPM patients who may be candidates for radical treatment according to criteria from the literature as summarised in the 2008 European Society of Medical Oncology recommendations for MPM: good Eastern Cooperative Oncology Group performance status, early-stage disease without mediastinal lymph node involvement, epithelioid histology and adequate pulmonary function to withstand a pneumonectomy [12]. Potential radical treatment means extrapleural pneumonectomy, an approach generally combined with chemotherapy and/or adjuvant radiotherapy, with the exception of pleurectomy in very rare stage Ia (T1a N0 M0) [9, 10, 12, 24]. This multimodal approach is not validated yet and must be considered only by experienced multidisciplinary teams, preferably in a randomised multicentre clinical trial. Pre-surgical assessment should also include at least lung function, pulmonary scintigraphy and a cardiac ultrasound [9, 10].

Figure 5 summarises a proposal for MPM management.

Conclusion

Several scientific societies have proposed guidelines for MPM management, underlining the increasing interest of the medical community in this disease with increasing incidence worldwide [35, 36]. The level of recommendation for many of these guidelines is quite low, due to scanty literature on MPM with a high level of proof. However, there is currently a coming together of international collaborators and studies in the field of mesothelioma, raising new hopes for our patients and ourselves. New tools, such as PET-CT scan, EBUS and soluble biomarkers, or therapeutic approaches, including multimodal treatments and targeted therapies, seem promising for management even if they still need to be validated. Optimising the diagnosis and staging of MPM patients is a crucial step towards enhancing the treatments of MPM and improving the patients' outcome through randomised multicentre trials.

Key messages

Key messages from this chapter can be summarised as follows. 1) The diagnosis of MPM should not be based on clinical criteria or chest radiography, which could be suggestive but are usually nonspecific. 2) After removal of pleural effusion, chest (and abdominal) CT scan with multiplaner reformation is the key investigation for diagnosis and staging of MPM. The value of PET combined with CT scan in the diagnosis and the staging of MPM requires further evaluation. 3) A diagnosis of MPM should not be based on pleural cytology alone, because of the high risk of error, or on the analysis of pleural or serum markers, even if SM seems promising, because no marker has been validated yet in routine practice. 4) Diagnosis must always be based on histology with immunohistochemical examination, using the international World Health Organization 2004 classification: "tissue is the issue"! 5) Due to their

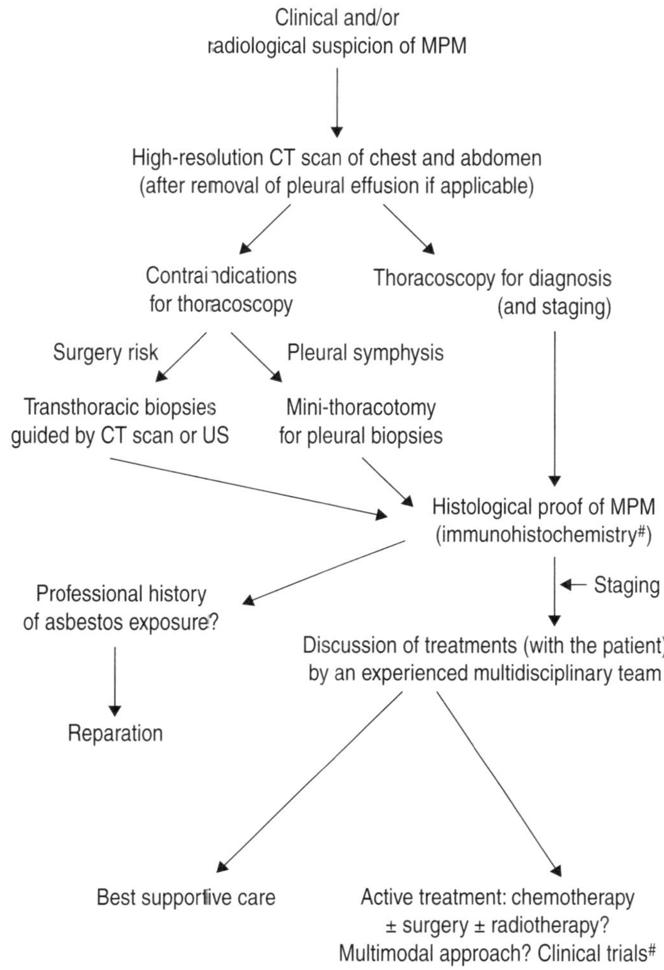

Fig. 5. – General proposal for malignant pleural mesothelioma (MPM) management. CT: computed tomography; US: ultrasound. #: recommended.

low sensitivity (~30%), fine needle transparietal biopsies with or without CT scan or ultrasound guidance are not recommended for the diagnosis of MPM except in patients for whom thoracoscopy is contraindicated. 6) Thoracoscopy is the best method to obtain the diagnosis of MPM when suspected from clinical or radiological data. Diagnostic accuracy is greater than 90% and complications occur in less than 10% of cases. Mini-thoracotomy should be reserved for patients with potential pleural symphysis leading to the failure of the thoracoscopy procedure. 7) Although there are limitations to the current classification, the IMIG staging system should be used until a new system of classification better adapted to MPM has been set up. 8) The 2008 ERS/ESTS experts on MPM recommend a three-step process for the pre-therapeutic assessment of patients.

Summary

Malignant pleural mesothelioma (MPM) is a previously rare cancer with an increasing incidence worldwide linked to asbestos, its main aetiological factor. Moreover, MPM patients have a poor prognosis despite recent improvements in disease management. Most patients are diagnosed late in the course of the disease when radical treatment is no longer an option. Therefore, an earlier diagnosis of MPM is needed to potentially increase the survival of patients.

To date, a firm and reliable diagnosis of mesothelioma is based on histology, usually obtained by biopsies during a thoracoscopy, the key procedure for MPM, and using international 2004 World Health Organization classification and guidelines from pathologists. Several soluble markers assessed in blood or pleural effusions, including soluble mesothelin and osteopontin, have been previously proposed for MPM diagnosis but none has been validated yet. Soluble mesothelin, the most promising candidate, has good diagnostic and prognostic values but is quite specific for the epithelioid subtype, the most frequent type of mesothelioma, thus restraining its usefulness in practice. Other potential markers, such as osteopontin, are of little interest for MPM diagnosis because of their low specificity.

Imaging, such as computed tomography (CT) scanning and positron emission tomography, separately or better when coupled, may help MPM diagnosis and staging, but present data do not justify their use for MPM screening among asbestos-exposed subjects. Current international "tumour, node, metastasis" classification for MPM staging is of limited use in routine practice, because it is based on CT scans and has only been validated with patients who have been surgically treated, quite rare in clinical practice.

Optimising early diagnosis and staging of MPM, along with developing new treatments for patients through large and randomised clinical trials, must be our main goals in improving the outcome of patients.

Keywords: Asbestos, cancer, diagnosis, mesothelioma, pleura, staging.

Statement of interest

A. Scherpereel's laboratory has received a research grant from CisBio International. A. Scherpereel has also received a fee for speaking at the 2008 IMIG Congress from CisBio and his travel to this meeting was funded by the same company.

References

1. Robinson BW, Musk AW, Lake RA. Malignant mesothelioma. *Lancet* 2005; 366: 397–408.
2. Pass HI, Vogelzang N, Hahn S, *et al.* Malignant pleural mesothelioma. *Curr Probl Cancer* 2004; 28: 93–174.
3. Ordóñez NG. The immunohistochemical diagnosis of mesothelioma: a comparative study of epithelioid mesothelioma and lung adenocarcinoma. *Am J Surg Pathol* 2003; 27: 1031–1051.
4. Weder W, Stahel RA, Bernhard J, *et al.* Multicenter trial of neo-adjuvant chemotherapy followed by extrapleural pneumonectomy in malignant pleural mesothelioma. *Ann Oncol* 2007; 18: 1196–1202.
5. Fennell DA, Gaudino G, O'Byrne KJ, *et al.* Advances in the systemic therapy of malignant pleural mesothelioma. *Nat Clin Pract Oncol* 2008; 5: 136–147.

6. Rusch VW. A proposed new international TNM staging system for malignant pleural mesothelioma. From the International Mesothelioma Interest Group. *Chest* 1995; 108: 1122–1128.
7. Greene FL, Page DL, Fleming ID, *et al.*, eds, American Joint Committee on Cancer. Cancer Staging Handbook. 6th Edn. New York, Springer, 2002; p. 6.
8. Wittekind C, Greene FL, Hutter RVP, Klimpfinger M, Sobin LH, eds. Union Internationale Contre le Cancer. TNM Atlas. 5th Edn. Berlin, Springer, 2004; pp. 169–176.
9. Société de Pneumologie de Langue Française. [The French Language Society of Pneumology guidelines on the pleural mesothelioma]. *Rev Mal Respir* 2006; 23: Suppl. 3, 6S80–6S92.
10. Scherpereel A, French Speaking Society for Chest Medicine (SPLF) Experts Group. Guidelines of the French Speaking Society for Chest Medicine for management of malignant pleural mesothelioma. *Respir Med* 2007; 101: 1265–1276.
11. Grigoriu BD, Chahine B, Vachani A, *et al.* Kinetics of soluble mesothelin in patients with malignant pleural mesothelioma during treatment. *Am J Respir Crit Care Med* 2009; [Epub ahead of print PMID: 19201924].
12. Stahel RA, Weder W, Felip E, ESMO Guidelines Working Group. Malignant pleural mesothelioma: ESMO clinical recommendations for diagnosis, treatment and follow-up. *Ann Oncol* 2008; 19: Suppl. 2, ii43–ii44.
13. British Thoracic Society Standards of Care Committee. BTS statement on malignant mesothelioma in the UK, 2007. *Thorax* 2007; 62: Suppl. 2, ii1–ii19.
14. Roggli VL, Oury TD, Sporn TA, eds, Pathology of Asbestos-Associated Diseases. 2nd Edn. New York, Springer, 2004.
15. Wang ZJ, Reddy GP, Gotway MB, *et al.* Malignant pleural mesothelioma: evaluation with CT, MR imaging, and PET. *Radiographics* 2004; 24: 105–119.
16. Duysinx BC, Larock MP, Nguyen D, *et al.* 18F-FDG PET imaging in assessing exudative pleural effusions. *Nucl Med Commun* 2006; 27: 971–976.
17. Flores RM, Akhurst T, Gonen M, *et al.* Positron emission tomography defines metastatic disease but not locoregional disease in patients with malignant pleural mesothelioma. *J Thorac Cardiovasc Surg* 2003; 126: 11–16.
18. Roggli VL, Sharma A, Butnor KJ, *et al.* Malignant mesothelioma and occupational exposure to asbestos: a clinicopathological correlation of 1445 cases. *Ultrastruct Pathol* 2002; 26: 55–65.
19. Galateau-Sallé F, ed. Pathology of Malignant Mesothelioma. 1st Edn. New York, Springer, 2005.
20. Travis WD, Brambilla E, Müller-Hermelink HK, Harris CC, eds. World Health Organization Classification of Tumours. Pathology and Genetics of Tumours of the Lung, Pleura, Thymus and Heart. Lyon, International Agency for Research on Cancer, 2004.
21. Goldberg M, Imbernon E, Rolland P, *et al.* The French National Mesothelioma Surveillance Program. *Occup Environ Med* 2006; 63: 390–395.
22. Maskell NA, Gleeson FV, Davies RJ. Standard pleural biopsy *versus* CT-guided cutting-needle biopsy for diagnosis of malignant disease in pleural effusions: a randomised controlled trial. *Lancet* 2003; 361: 1326–1330.
23. Blanc FX, Atassi K, Bignon J, *et al.* Diagnostic value of medical thoracoscopy in pleural disease: a 6-year retrospective study. *Chest* 2002; 121: 1677–1683.
24. Scherpereel A, Astoul P, Baas P, *et al.* Guidelines of the European Respiratory Society and the European Society of Thoracic Surgeons for management of Malignant Pleural Mesothelioma. *Eur Respir J* 2009; (in press).
25. Scherpereel A, Lee YCG. Biomarkers for mesothelioma. *Curr Opin Pulm Med* 2007; 13: 339–343.
26. Robinson BW, Creaney J, Lake R, *et al.* Mesothelin-family proteins and diagnosis of mesothelioma. *Lancet* 2003; 362: 1612–1616.
27. Scherpereel A, Grigoriu B, Conti M, *et al.* Soluble mesothelin-related peptides in the diagnosis of malignant pleural mesothelioma. *Am J Respir Crit Care Med* 2006; 173: 1155–1160.
28. Grigoriu BD, Scherpereel A, Devos P, *et al.* Utility of osteopontin and serum mesothelin in malignant pleural mesothelioma diagnosis and prognosis assessment. *Clin Cancer Res* 2007; 13: 2928–2935.

29. Creaney J, van Bruggen I, Hof M, *et al.* Combined CA125 and mesothelin levels for the diagnosis of malignant mesothelioma. *Chest* 2007; 132: 1239–1246.
30. Creaney J, Yeoman D, Demelker Y, *et al.* Comparison of osteopontin, megakaryocyte potentiating factor, and mesothelin proteins as markers in the serum of patients with malignant mesothelioma. *J Thorac Oncol* 2008; 3: 851–857.
31. Herndon JE, Green MR, Chahinian AP, *et al.* Factors predictive of survival among 337 patients with mesothelioma treated between 1984 and 1994 by the Cancer and Leukemia Group B. *Chest* 1998; 113: 723–731.
32. Curran D, Sahmoud T, Therasse P, *et al.* Prognostic factors in patients with pleural mesothelioma: the European Organization for Research and Treatment of Cancer experience. *J Clin Oncol* 1998; 16: 145–152.
33. van Meerbeeck JP, Gaafar R, Manegold C, *et al.* Randomized phase III study of cisplatin with or without raltitrexed in patients with malignant pleural mesothelioma: an intergroup study of the European Organisation for Research and Treatment of Cancer Lung Cancer Group and the National Cancer Institute of Canada. *J Clin Oncol* 2005; 23: 6881–6889.
34. van Meerbeeck JP, Boyer M. Consensus report: pretreatment minimal staging and treatment of potentially resectable malignant pleural mesothelioma. *Lung Cancer* 2005; 49: Suppl. 1, S123–S127.
35. Pelucchi C, Malvezzi M, La Vecchia C, *et al.* The mesothelioma epidemic in Western Europe: an update. *Br J Cancer* 2004; 90: 1022–1024.
36. Astoul P. Introduction: Mésothéliome pleural. *In*: Astoul P, ed. Mésothéliome Pleural. Paris, Elsevier SAS, 2005; pp. 1–2.

CHAPTER 23

Surgery and multimodality treatment for malignant pleural mesothelioma

W. Weder, I. Opitz, R. Stahel

Thoracic Surgery and Medical Oncology, University Hospital Zurich, Zurich, Switzerland.

Correspondence: W. Weder, Division of Thoracic Surgery, University Hospital Zurich, Rämistrasse 100, 8091 Zurich, Switzerland. E-mail: walter.weder@usz.ch

Surgery for malignant pleural mesothelioma (MPM) encompasses diagnostic, palliative and potentially curative procedures. For diagnosis, an open or, preferentially, video-assisted thoracoscopic surgery (VATS) approach can be chosen for full thickness pleural biopsy. Talc pleurodesis or pleurectomy to relieve dyspnoea aims to palliate the patient's symptoms. For eradication of the tumour, two aggressive surgical treatments of resectable tumours are used such as cytoreductive debulking procedures (pleurectomy/decortication (P/D)) and radical resection (extrapleural pneumonectomy (EPP)). During EPP, which is the most radical and demanding approach, the entire (tumour containing) parietal and visceral pleura are resected *en bloc* with the underlying lung, ipsilateral pericardium and diaphragm. It is performed on patients with adequate performance and lung function status. A less radical cytoreductive procedure is P/D, where the parietal pleura is resected and the underlying lung is decorticated from the visceral pleura, so that the lung can expand and fill the pleural cavity. P/D is therefore also an option for palliation when standard treatments, such as chemical pleurodesis, have failed. In early cases, it can be performed using a VATS approach.

The aggressiveness of the MPM and the limited effect of single-modality therapies have led to the treatment of MPM patients using more than one modality, including chemotherapy or radiotherapy beside surgery. To a certain extent, the choice of operation should also be determined by the type of adjuvant therapy planned (*e.g.* high-dose irradiation after EPP). The availability of more effective chemotherapy drugs and documented survival benefits of neoadjuvant chemotherapy in the context of locally advanced nonsmall cell lung cancer have changed treatment dogmas over the last decades.

Evidence

Surgery

The role of surgery in pleural mesothelioma continues to be a matter of debate. A systematic review based on the literature from 1985 to 2004 could not determine whether the use of EPP improves survival or effectively palliates symptoms of pleural mesothelioma [1]. There are no randomised controlled trials comparing EPP with P/D, but there are several prospective, noncontrolled case-series reporting on both procedures. The difficulty in interpreting the results arises from the fact that different

Eur Respir Mon, 2009, 44, 407–418. Printed in UK - all rights reserved. Copyright ERS Journals Ltd 2009; European Respiratory Monograph; ISSN 1025-448x.

staging systems are used, the patient's selection including histology and stage is variable, and often other treatment modalities are added. Furthermore EPP and its perioperative management is demanding and requires the experience of a dedicated and specialised surgical team. Not surprisingly, perioperative mortality and morbidity varies significantly between different reports.

Palliative surgery

At present, there are no randomised trials supporting debulking surgery but there is a national study ongoing in the UK comparing VATS debulking with chemical pleurodesis (MesoVATS). Retrospective studies provide low-grade evidence for debulking pleurectomy, but the reported median survival rates of 14–17 months and morbidity rates of 16–22% are good arguments for this approach as it may provide symptom control (table 1) [2–5]. The associated morbidity due to thoracotomy can be eliminated by a VATS approach, which seems to be superior [6]; however, this procedure is applicable only in an early stage of the disease.

Radical surgery. While the published results and reviews so far are suggestive that radical surgery within a multimodality concept may indeed be associated with a longer survival than chemotherapy alone, final proof of this concept will only come from a randomised study. These data may be forthcoming from the Mesothelioma and Radical Surgery (MARS) trial initiated in the UK; although this trial is only at a pilot stage with 50 patients entered. In this study, patients are randomised after three cycles induction chemotherapy to either have or not have EPP, followed by radiotherapy. Again, a difficulty may be the role of the surgeon performing EPP. Since this operation is relatively rarely performed but needs good experience, mortality, morbidity and local radicality (*i.e.* extent of resection) may vary in different centres.

Prospective, noncontrolled studies as well as retrospective studies involving both P/D and EPP are summarised in table 2. Only those reports which contained survival data are included. In most of the studies, a variety of treatments in addition to surgery were applied (*e.g.* chemotherapy, radiotherapy, intrapleural therapy, photodynamic therapy).

PASS *et al.* [10] reported a statistically better survival after P/D compared with EPP, however, patients undergoing EPP had a significantly larger tumour volume compared with patients undertaking P/D; an indicator that the two patient groups were not comparable. Similar results were reported by RUSCH *et al.* [7] with the same biases, as EPP was performed in patients with more advanced disease and P/D was reserved for patients with minimal tumour involvement of the visceral pleura. A retrospective study from a case series of 111 patients showed no significant differences in survival between P/D and EPP [19] when P/D was offered to patients with locally advanced disease.

Table 1. – Current surgical data for palliative pleurectomy/decortication (P/D) of malignant pleural mesothelioma

First author [ref.]	Design	Procedure	Mortality %	Morbidity %	Median survival months
MARTIN-UCAR [6]	Prospective	VATS P/D (n=51)	7.8	13.7	7.2
HALSTEAD [2]	Prospective	P/D (n=51), biopsy (n=28)	2.5	NR	13.8
BRANCATISANO [5]	Retrospective	P/D (n=45)	2	16	16
SOYSAL [4]	Retrospective	P/D (n=100)	1	22	17

VATS: video-assisted thoracoscopic surgery; NR: not reported.

Table 2. – Current data including extrapleural pneumonectomy (EPP) and pleurectomy/decortication (P/D) for surgical treatment of malignant pleural mesothelioma

First author [ref.]	Year	Design	Procedure	Combined modality	Mortality %	Median survival months
Rusch [7]	1991	Prospective	EPP (n=20)	Adjuvant CTX	15	OS 10
			Limited/no resection (n=63)		3	
Rusch [8]	1999	Prospective	EPP (n=115)	Adjuvant CTX and/or RT	5	14.7
			P/D (n=59)		3	18.5
Rusch [9]	2001	Prospective	EPP (n=62)	Adjuvant RT	11.2	17
			P/D (n=5)		0	
Pass [10]	1997	Prospective	EPP (n=39)	PDT/CTX	NR	9.4*
			P/D (n=39)		NR	14.5*
			Total n=95		2	
Pass [11]	1998	Prospective	EPP (n=25)	PDT/ICTX	Overall 2.1	11
			P/D (n=23)			22
Rice [12]	1994	Prospective	EPP (n=10)	ip-CTX and adjuvant CTX	Overall 5	OS 13
			P/D (n=9)			
Moskal [13]	1998	Prospective	EPP (n=7)	PDT	14	OS 15
			P/D (n=28)		0	
			Total			
Maggi [14]	2001	Prospective	EPP (n=23)	Adjuvant CTX and/or RT	Overall 6	OS 9.5
			P/D (n=9)			
Calavreszos [15]	1988	Prospective	57 CM (including surgery)	Yes	NR	13
			75 SC			5–7
Rosenzweig [16]	2005	Prospective	EPP (n=7)	HDR-IORT	14.3	Study closed
			P/D (n=6)		16.7	
Antmann [17]	1988	Retrospective	EPP (n=16)	Adjuvant CTX and RT	NR	18
		Prospective	P/D (n=NR)			
			EPP and CTX (n=68)			
Branscheid [18]	1991	Retrospective	EPP (n=76)	Adjuvant CTX	11.8	9.3
			P/D (n=82) palliative		2.4	10.4
Aziz [19]	2002	Retrospective	EPP (n=23)	Adjuvant CTX	9.1	13
			P/D (n=47) palliative		0	14
			EPP and CTX (n=51)			35
Chailleux [20]	1988	Retrospective	EPP (n=4)	Adjuvant CTX and/or RT	NR	OS 13
			P/D (n=14)		NR	
			Partial P/D (n=25)		NR	
Ruffie [21]	1989	Retrospective	EPP (n=23)	Adjuvant CTX and RT	13	9.3
			P/D (n=63)		NR	9.8
Schipper [22]	2008	Retrospective	EPP (n=73)	(Neo)adjuvant CTX and/or adjuvant RT	8.2	16
			Subtotal P/D (n=34)		2.9	8
			Radical P/D (n=10)		0	17.2
Harvey [23]	1990	Retrospective	EPP (n=7)	CTX and RT	NR	18
			P/D (n=9)		0	
Allen [24]	1994	Retrospective	EPP (n=40)	Adjuvant CTX and RT	7.5	13.3
			P/D (n=56)		5.4	9
Lampl [25]	1999	Retrospective	EPP (n=23)	No	4.2	16
			P/D (n=19)		0	14

Table 2. – Continued

First author [ref.]	Year	Design	Procedure	Combined modality	Mortality %	Median survival months
DE VRIES [26]	2003	Retrospective	EPP (n=15) P/D (n=29) palliative	Adjuvant CTX and/or RT	5.8 3.8	12 9
HUNCHAREK [27]	1996	Retrospective	EPP (n=3) P/D (n=17) CM (n=21)	Adjuvant CTX and/or RT	NR NR	NR NR 23.9
ACHATZY [28]	1989	Retrospective	Radical P/D (n=46) Palliative P/D (n=72)	Adjuvant CTX and RT	4.3 11.1	OS 9.2
FLORES [29]	2008	Retrospective	EPP (n=385) P/D (n=278)	Adjuvant CTX and/or RT	7 4	12* 16*
NAKAS [3]	2008	Retrospective, age 65 yrs	EPP (n=13) P/D (n=8) VATS P/D palliative (n=42)	Adjuvant CTX and/or RT	23 12.5 7.1	11.5 12.4 14

CTX: chemotherapy; OS: overall survival; RT: radiotherapy; PDT: photodynamic therapy; NR: not reported; ICTX: immunochemotherapy; ip: intrapleural; CM: combined modality; SC: supportive care; HDR-IORT: high-dose rate intraoperative radiotherapy; VATS: video-assisted thoracoscopic surgery. *: $p<0.05$.

Combining the experience of three large centres in the USA, the outcome of 663 patients, treated between 1990 and 2006, was analysed retrospectively [29]. The median survival for the entire group was 14 months, with a significant advantage for P/D (16 months) compared with EPP (12 months). Operative mortality was 7% for EPP and 4% for P/D. A difference was noted in the site of first recurrence. Local recurrence occurred in 33% and distant recurrence in 66% after EPP compared with 65% and 35%, respectively, after P/D. Thus, because of biases in patient selection for a certain procedure according to the tumour stage and the retrospective nature of the analysis, no firm conclusions can be drawn regarding the optimal surgical procedure for patients with MPM.

Other retrospective studies provide low level of evidence because data were mostly collected over extended time periods ranging up to 20 yrs. Again, all studies included some form of adjuvant treatment. None of the studies reported a significant difference in median survival for EPP compared with P/D [20, 21, 23–27].

Some centres advise P/D for patients with compromised cardiac or pulmonary function, advanced age or certain disease distributions, in particular with early disease mainly located on the parietal pleura only, in order to remove the tumour while sparing lung function. When comparing results of EPP with VATS P/D in patients aged >65 yrs, the group in Leicester documented a reduced 30-day mortality using the VATS procedure with a similar survival outcome (11.5 months for EPP and 14 months for VATS P/D) [3]. However, in experienced centres, the perioperative mortality is low with 3.8% after EPP, as reported by the Boston group [30]. In a Swiss multicentre study, a perioperative mortality of 2.2% compares favourably and was achieved even after neoadjuvant chemotherapy [31].

Combined modality

With regard to the role of surgery, results from randomised controlled trials evaluating the effectiveness of adjuvant or neodadjuvant chemotherapy, or post-operative radiotherapy are not available; however, a randomised controlled trial is

Table 3. – Current data for multimodality treatment of malignant pleural mesothelioma

First author [ref.]	Year	Design	Procedure	Combined modality	Mortality %	Median survival months
EPP and adjuvant CTX						
SUGARBAKER [30]	1999	Retrospective	EPP (n=183)	Adjuvant CTX and RT	3.8	19
BALDINI [32]	1997	Retrospective	EPP (n=49)	Adjuvant CTX and RT	4	22
EPP and neoadjuvant CTX						
LWEDER [33]	2004	Prospective	EPP (n=19)	Neoadjuvant CTX and adjuvant RT	0	23
WEDER [31]	2007	Prospective	EPP (n=61)	Neoadjuvant CTX and adjuvant RT	2.2	23
REA [34]	2007	Prospective	EPP (n=21)	Neoadjuvant CTX and adjuvant RT	0	25.5
FLORES [35]	2006	Prospective	EPP (n=8)	Neoadjuvant CTX and adjuvant RT	0	33.5
DE PERROT [36]	2009	Retrospective	EPP (n=45)	Neoadjuvant CTX and adjuvant RT	6.7	59#
KRUG [37]	2009	Retrospective	EPP (n=54)	Neoadjuvant CTX and adjuvant RT	3.7	29.1
OPITZ [38]	2009	Prospective	EPP (n=105)	Neoadjuvant CTX and adjuvant RT	4.8	22
Surgery and RT						
RUSCH [9]	2001	Prospective	EPP (n=62) P/D (n=5)	Adjuvant RT	11 0	17
RICE [39]	2007	Prospective	EPP (n=37) EPP and IMRT (n=63)	Neoadjuvant CTX and adjuvant IMRT	8	10.2 14.2
ROSENZWEIG [16]	2005	Prospective	EPP (n=7) P/D (n=6)	HDR-IORT	14.3 16.7	Study closed
HILARIS [40]	1984	Retrospective	P/D	Intraoperative BT	0	21
GUPTA [41]	2005	Retrospective	P/D (n=123)	Adjuvant RT and (neo)adjuvant CTX, BT	3.3	13.5

EPP: extrapleural pneumonectomy; CTX: chemotherapy; RT: radiotherapy; P/D: pleurectomy/decortication; IMRT: intensity-modulated radiation therapy; HDR-IORT: high-dose rate intraoperative radiotherapy BT: brachytherapy. #: without mediastinal lymph node.

currently ongoing in Switzerland studying the role of hemithoracic radiotherapy after EPP. The studies available in the literature are summarised in table 3. A retrospective multi-institutional analysis by FLORES *et al.* [29] of 663 consecutive patients undergoing either P/D or EPP suggested a survival impact by using multimodality approach compared with surgery alone.

Surgery and adjuvant chemotherapy. The largest published report, with a total of 183 patients treated trimodally with EPP followed by adjuvant chemotherapy and radiotherapy (30 Gy) is reported by SUGARBAKER *et al.* [30] with a median survival of 19 months and a perioperative mortality of 3.8% (figs 1 and 2). These survival data are confirmed in further reports from this group [32]. Another retrospective series on multimodality treatment was reported by the Mayo Clinic with a median survival of 16 months after EPP (n=73) plus (neo)adjuvant and/or adjuvant radiotherapy [22]. The longest survival rate in this therapy setting was reported in a retrospective study by AZIZ *et al.* [19] with a median survival of 35 months after EPP and adjuvant platin-based systemic chemotherapy.

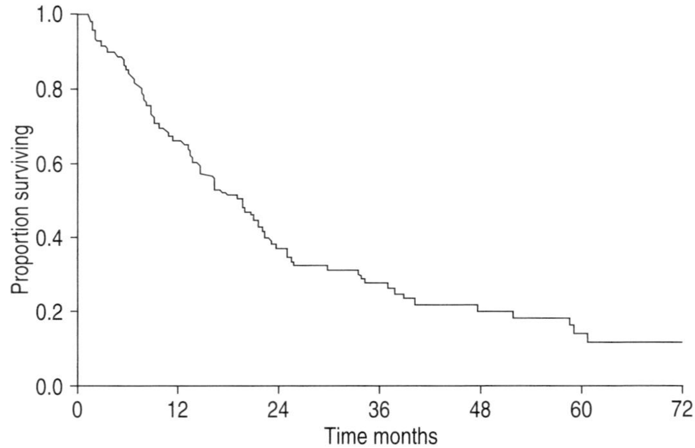

Patients at risk

176	94	41	22	12	7	6

Fig. 1. – Kaplan–Meier survival curve for all patients surviving surgery (n=176). Reproduced from [30] with permission from the publisher.

Surgery and neoadjuvant chemotherapy. In a Swiss pilot study on 19 patients, response to neoadjuvant cisplatin and gemcitabine was 31% and 16 patients underwent EPP with no perioperative mortality. The overall median survival of patients was 23 months, and two of those patients remained disease free for $\geq$6 yrs after surgery [33]. These results were confirmed in a prospective multicenter phase II trial enrolling 61 patients with T1–T3 and N0–N2 disease and including all histologies who received three cycles of neoadjuvant cisplatin and gemcitabine [31]. A total of 45 patients received EPP (74%) with an operative mortality of 2.2% and median survival of 23 months (fig. 3).

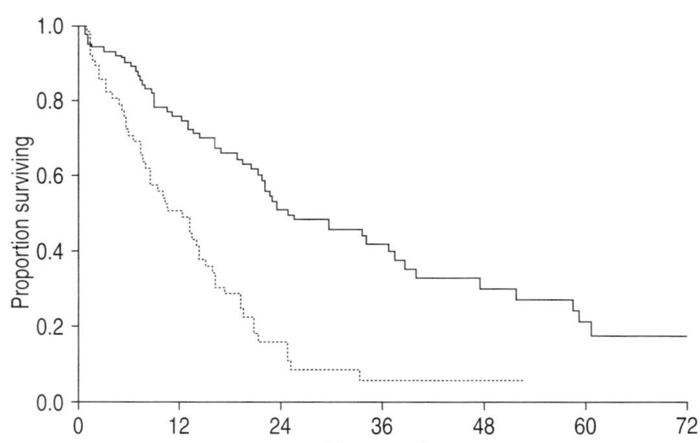

Patients at risk

E	103	65	34	20	11	7	6
SM	73	29	7	2	1	0	0

Fig. 2. – Kaplan–Meier survival curves for patients with epithelial (E; ——) *versus* sarcomatous and mixed (SM; ······) disease. n=176; p<0.0001. Reproduced from [30] with permission from the publisher.

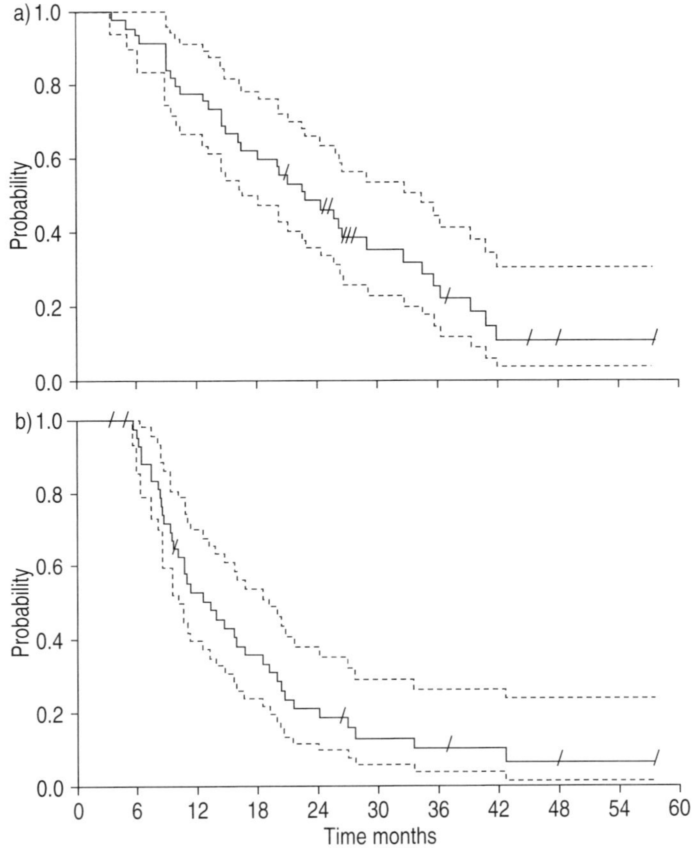

Fig. 3. – a) Survival and b) time to recurrence of the 45 patients undergoing extrapleural pneumonectomy (EPP). a) For the 45 patients undergoing EPP, estimated median survival was 23 months (95% confidence intervals (CI) 16.6–32.9). b) Tumour recurrence after EPP was observed in 38 patients with a median time to recurrence of 13.5 months (95% CI 10.2–18.8). Reproduced from [31] with permission from the publisher. Slashes represent events. -----: 95% CI.

FLORES *et al.* [35] reported a 35.5 months median survival for eight patients receiving four cycles of cisplatin and gemcitabine followed by EPP and radiotherapy, in a phase II trial. A median survival of 25.5 months for patients undergoing EPP after neoadjuvant chemotherapy followed by adjuvant chemotherapy, confirmed the results of this concept [34]. Several groups have demonstrated that perioperative morbidity and mortality is not increased when chemotherapy is performed before EPP [42, 43]. Recently, two studies (a multicentre study from the USA and a single centre study from Canada) confirmed these results and reported median survival time of 29 months [37]. A subgroup analysis performed in the Canadian cohort reported even 59 months for patients without mediastinal lymph node involvement [36]. Our current experiences of over 100 patients who underwent EPP after induction chemotherapy included all histological subtypes and mediastinal lymph node involvement and the median survival time remains close to 2 yrs [38].

Based on the results of a prospective randomised trial demonstrating the survival benefit of combination chemotherapy of cisplatin with pemetrexed over cisplatin alone, this combination or the combination of cisplatin with pemetrexed has been adopted for a neoadjuvant approach by most centres [44].

Surgery and radiotherapy. In 2001, a phase II trial using EPP followed by high-dose external-beam radiotherapy (54 Gy) was conducted in 54 patients, with a median survival of 33 months for stage I and stage II tumours [9]. GUPTA *et al.* [41] reported a retrospective review of 123 patients treated with P/D plus adjuvant radiotherapy and intraoperative brachytherapy in half of the patients, with a median overall survival of 13.5 months. Although earlier studies with intraoperative brachytherapy were optimistic [40], a pilot trial conducted by ROSENZWEIG *et al.* [16] evaluating high-dose intraoperative radiotherapy after EPP or P/D showed that the treatment was prohibitively toxic and was therefore abandoned. The group from the MD Anderson Cancer Centre (University of Texas, Houston, TX, USA) published results from 63 patients with a median survival of 14 months after EPP, and intensity-modulated radiotherapy (IMRT; median dose 45 Gy); however, six patients died within 6 months after IMRT due to pulmonary toxicity [39]. A series studying 13 patients, treated in Boston, reported the development of fatal pneumonitis in six patients, the most likely explanation being dose–volume effects on the contralateral lung [45]. The role of radiotherapy after neoadjuvant chemotherapy and EPP is currently being evaluated in a prospective randomised study in Switzerland jointly with several other European centres.

Surgery and intrapleural therapy. Several intrapleural or local therapies were designed to attack microscopic residual disease after surgery. Photodynamic therapy (PDT) is light-activated sensitisation of malignant cells with a photosensitiser and was assessed in small case series by several investigators [46–51]. A phase II study of 31 patients undergoing surgery and intracavitary photodynamic therapy reported an overall survival of 12 months [51], which is comparable to other reports [48]. A phase III study was performed on 63 patients undergoing surgery, with or without intraoperative PDT, followed by post-operative immunochemotherapy [49] but could not prove a difference in median survival. Hyperthermic intrapleural chemotherapy was reported by RICHARDS *et al.* [52] in a phase I dose-escalating study administering hyperthermic cisplatin intrapleurally after P/D in 44 patients. Median survival was 13 months but operative mortality was high with 11% [52]. Other studies, prospectively investigating the effect of intrapleural chemotherapy after P/D, showed median survivals of 9 [53] and 11.5 months [54, 55]. Earlier studies, with intrapleural application of cisplatin and mitomycin after P/D in 28 patients, showed a median survival of 17 months and also reported serious toxicity [56], so these approaches need to be further refined. Immunotherapy for mesothelioma was most recently reported by LUCCHI *et al.* [57] with a regimen consisting of intrapleural preoperative interleukin (IL)-2, P/D, intrapleural post-operative epidoxorubicin, IL-2, adjuvant radiotherapy (30 Gy), systemic chemotherapy (cisplatin and gemcitabine) and long-term application of subcutaneous IL-2 with a median survival of 26 months.

Conclusion

P/D should not be proposed as a curative procedure; however, it can be considered either in patients for obtaining symptom control, especially symptomatic patients with entrapped lung syndrome who cannot benefit from chemical pleurodesis, or in patients in whom a pneumonectomy is not recommended because of comorbidities or mesothelioma located mainly at the parietal pleura. The VATS approach is preferred if it is possible.

A multimodality approach has demonstrated favourable results but the optimum combination has yet to be defined. EPP as part of a multimodality concept should be performed in experienced centres.

Although not proven by a randomised study, neoadjuvant chemotherapy followed by EPP may be superior to an adjuvant chemotherapy treatment. Cisplatin and antifolates (pemetrexed/ralitrexed) or gemcitabine are the cytotoxic agents of choice.

The risk/benefit ratio of hemithoracic radiotherapy, especially its effect on quality of life, needs to be assessed and should therefore be performed in clinical trials only.

Intrapleural chemotherapy, as well as photodynamic therapy, needs to be further refined.

There is still a lack of information as to the real value of these invasive procedures, as the relative paucity of cases makes multicentre randomised controlled trials essential, and hardly any have been performed.

Summary

Over the past 10 yrs, there have been several achievements in the management of malignant pleural mesothelioma (MPM), including a better insight into the tumour biology, more effective chemotherapy with pemetrexed or gemcitabine in combination with cisplatin, and extrapleural pneumonectomy (EPP) within a multimodality treatment. Nevertheless, the choice of the best treatment remains a matter of debate. A systematic review of the value of surgery remains highly critical as to the quality of the studies and the lack of randomised studies. Pleurectomy/decortication (P/D) has proven its effectiveness as a palliative procedure for symptom control such as relief of dyspnoea due to control of pleural effusion and freeing a tumour-entrapped lung but it is limited to good performance status patients. P/D provides the advantage of avoiding a pneumonectomy and may be indicated for patients with reduced cardiopulmonary capacity or mesotheliomas located mainly at the parietal pleura. However, P/D is, by intent, less radical than EPP. Furthermore, the application of full adjuvant hemithoracic radiotherapy is not possible because of the risk of damage to the remaining lung. The best long-term results may be achieved by multidisciplinary concepts including EPP together with neo- or adjuvant chemotherapy and a median survival time of about 2 yrs has been reported by several studies. Hemithoracic radiotherapy after EPP has been suggested to decrease the rate of local relapse; however, it is a complex procedure associated with additional morbidity and mortality.

Diagnosis and treatment of MPM remains a challenge and is best performed in a specialised centre by a multidisciplinary team, in order to balance treatment related morbidity with potential treatment benefit. Proper randomised trials are still needed to answer these basic questions.

Keywords: Extrapleural pneumonectomy, intrapleural therapy, multimodality treatment, neoadjuvant chemotherapy, pleurectomy/decortication, radiotherapy.

Statement of interest

W. Weder was an invited speaker on mesothelioma treatment at various meetings. The multicentre study on neoadjuvant chemotherapy followed by surgery was organised/financed by SAKK.

References

1. Maziak DE, Gagliardi A, Haynes AE, *et al.* Surgical management of malignant pleural mesothelioma: a systematic review and evidence summary. *Lung Cancer* 2005; 48: 157–169.
2. Halstead JC, Lim E, Venkateswaran RM, *et al.* Improved survival with VATS pleurectomy-decortication in advanced malignant mesothelioma. *Eur J Surg Oncol* 2005; 31: 314–320.
3. Nakas A, Martin Ucar AE, Edwards JG, *et al.* The role of video assisted thoracoscopic pleurectomy/decortication in the therapeutic management of malignant pleural mesothelioma. *Eur J Cardiothorac Surg* 2008; 33: 83–88.
4. Soysal O, Karaoğlanoğlu N, Demiracan S, *et al.* Pleurectomy/decortication for palliation in malignant pleural mesothelioma: results of surgery. *Eur J Cardiothorac Surg* 1997; 11: 210–213.
5. Brancatisano RP, Joseph MG, McCaughan BC. Pleurectomy for mesothelioma. *Med J Aust* 1991; 154: 455–457.
6. Martin-Ucar AE, Edwards JG, Rengajaran A, *et al.* Palliative surgical debulking in malignant mesothelioma. Predictors of survival and symptom control. *Eur J Cardiothorac Surg* 2001; 20: 1117–1121.
7. Rusch VW, Piantadosi S, Holmes EC. The role of extrapleural pneumonectomy in malignant pleural mesothelioma. A Lung Cancer Study Group trial. *J Thorac Cardiovasc Surg* 1991; 102: 1–9.
8. Rusch VW, Venkatraman ES. Important prognostic factors in patients with malignant pleural mesothelioma, managed surgically. *Ann Thorac Surg* 1999; 68: 1799–1804.
9. Rusch VW, Rosenzweig K, Venkatraman E, *et al.* A phase II trial of surgical resection and adjuvant high-dose hemithoracic radiation for malignant pleural mesothelioma. *J Thorac Cardiovasc Surg* 2001; 122: 788–795.
10. Pass HI, Kranda K, Temeck BK, *et al.* Surgically debulked malignant pleural mesothelioma: results and prognostic factors. *Ann Surg Oncol* 1997; 4: 215–222.
11. Pass HI, Temeck BK, Kranda K, *et al.* Preoperative tumor volume is associated with outcome in malignant pleural mesothelioma. *J Thorac Cardiovasc Surg* 1998; 115: 310–318.
12. Rice TW, Adelstein DJ, Kirby TJ, *et al.* Aggressive multimodality therapy for malignant pleural mesothelioma. *Ann Thorac Surg* 1994; 58: 24–29.
13. Moskal TL, Dougherty TJ, Urschel JD, *et al.* Operation and photodynamic therapy for pleural mesothelioma: 6-year follow-up. *Ann Thorac Surg* 1998; 66: 1128–1133.
14. Maggi G, Casadio C, Cianci R, *et al.* Trimodality management of malignant pleural mesothelioma. *Eur J Cardiothorac Surg* 2001; 19: 346–350.
15. Calavrezos A, Koschel G, Hüsselmann H, *et al.* Malignant mesothelioma of the pleura. A prospective therapeutic study of 132 patients from 1981–1985. *Klin Wochenschr* 1988; 66: 607–613.
16. Rosenzweig KE, Fox JL, Zelefsky MJ, *et al.* A pilot trial of high-dose-rate intraoperative radiation therapy for malignant pleural mesothelioma. *Brachytherapy* 2005; 4: 30–33.
17. Antman K, Shemin R, Ryan L, *et al.* Malignant mesothelioma: prognostic variables in a registry of 180 patients, the Dana-Farber Cancer Institute and Brigham and Women's Hospital experience over two decades, 1965–1985. *J Clin Oncol* 1988; 6: 147–153.
18. Branscheid D, Krysa S, Bauer E, *et al.* Diagnostic and therapeutic strategy in malignant pleural mesothelioma. *Eur J Cardiothorac Surg* 1991; 5: 466–473.
19. Aziz T, Jilaihawi A, Prakash D. The management of malignant pleural mesothelioma; single centre experience in 10 years. *Eur J Cardiothorac Surg* 2002; 22: 298–305.
20. Chailleux E, Dabouis G, Pioche D, *et al.* Prognostic factors in diffuse malignant pleural mesothelioma. A study of 167 patients. *Chest* 1988; 93: 159–162.
21. Ruffie P, Feld R, Minkin S, *et al.* Diffuse malignant mesothelioma of the pleura in Ontario and Quebec: a retrospective study of 332 patients. *J Clin Oncol* 1989; 7: 1157–1168.
22. Schipper PH, Nichols FC, Thomse KM, *et al.* Malignant pleural mesothelioma: surgical management in 285 patients. *Ann Thorac Surg* 2008; 85: 257–264.

23. Harvey JC, Fleischman EH, Kagan AR, *et al.* Malignant pleural mesothelioma: a survival study. *J Surg Oncol* 1990; 45: 40–42.
24. Allen KB, Faber LP, Warren WH. Malignant pleural mesothelioma. Extrapleural pneumonectomy and pleurectomy. *Chest Surg Clin N Am* 1994; 4: 113–126.
25. Lampl L, Jakob R. How should we treat malignant pleural mesothelioma (MPM)? *Acta Chir Hung* 1999; 38: 87–90.
26. de Vries WJ, Long MA. Treatment of mesothelioma in Bloemfontein, South Africa. *Eur J Cardiothorac Surg* 2003; 24: 434–440.
27. Huncharek M, Kelsey K, Mark EJ, *et al.* Treatment and survival in diffuse malignant pleural mesothelioma; a study of 83 cases from the Massachusetts General Hospital. *Anticancer Res* 1996; 16: 1265–1268.
28. Achatzy R, Beba W, Ritschler R, *et al.* The diagnosis, therapy and prognosis of diffuse malignant mesothelioma. *Eur J Cardiothorac Surg* 1989; 3: 445–448.
29. Flores RM, Pass HI, Seshan VE, *et al.* Extrapleural pneumonectomy *versus* pleurectomy/decortication in the surgical management of malignant pleural mesothelioma: results in 663 patients. *J Thorac Cardiovasc Surg* 2008; 135: 620–626.
30. Sugarbaker DJ, Flores RM, Jaklitsch MT, *et al.* Resection margins, extrapleural nodal status, and cell type determine postoperative long-term survival in trimodality therapy of malignant pleural mesothelioma: results in 183 patients. *J Thorac Cardiovasc Surg* 1999; 117: 54–65.
31. Weder W, Stahel RA, Bernhard J, *et al.* Multicenter trial of neo-adjuvant chemotherapy followed by extrapleural pneumonectomy in malignant pleural mesothelioma. *Ann Oncol* 2007; 18: 1196–1202.
32. Baldini EH, Recht A, Strauss GM, *et al.* Patterns of failure after trimodality therapy for malignant pleural mesothelioma. *Ann Thorac Surg* 1997; 63: 334–338.
33. Weder W, Kestenholz P, Taverna C, *et al.* Neoadjuvant chemotherapy followed by extrapleural pneumonectomy in malignant pleural mesothelioma. *J Clin Oncol* 2004; 22: 3451–3457.
34. Rea F, Marulli G, Bortolotti L, *et al.* Induction chemotherapy, extrapleural pneumonectomy (EPP) and adjuvant hemi-thoracic radiation in malignant pleural mesothelioma (MPM): feasibility and results. *Lung Cancer* 2007; 57: 89–95.
35. Flores RM, Krug LM, Rosenzweig KE, *et al.* Induction chemotherapy, extrapleural pneumonectomy, and postoperative high-dose radiotherapy for locally advanced malignant pleural mesothelioma: a phase II trial. *J Thorac Oncol* 2006; 1: 289–295.
36. de Perrot M, Feld R, Cho BC, *et al.* Trimodality therapy with induction chemotherapy followed by extrapleural pneumonectomy and adjuvant high-dose hemithoracic radiation for malignant pleural mesothelioma. *J Clin Oncol* 2009; 27: 1413–1418.
37. Krug LM, Pass HI, Rusch VW, *et al.* Multicenter phase II trial of neoadjuvant pemetrexed plus cisplatin followed by extrapleural pneumonectomy and radiation for malignant pleural mesothelioma. *J Clin Oncol* 2009; [Epub ahead of print PMID: 19364962].
38. Opitz I, Schramm A, Kestenholz P, *et al.* A 10 year follow-up of a single centre experience with induction chemotherapy followed by extrapleural pneumonectomy for malignant pleural mesothelioma. *Lung Cancer* 2009; 64: Suppl. 1, S63–S64.
39. Rice DC, Stevens CW, Correa AM, *et al.* Outcomes after extrapleural pneumonectomy and intensity-modulated radiation therapy for malignant pleural mesothelioma. *Ann Thorac Surg* 2007; 84: 1685–1692.
40. Hilaris BS, Nori D, Kwong E, *et al.* Pleurectomy and intraoperative brachytherapy and postoperative radiation in the treatment of malignant pleural mesothelioma. *Int J Radiat Oncol Biol Phys* 1984; 10: 325–331.
41. Gupta V, Mychalczak B, Krug L, *et al.* Hemithoracic radiation therapy after pleurectomy/decortication for malignant pleural mesothelioma. *Int J Radiat Oncol Biol Phys* 2005; 63: 1045–1052.
42. Opitz I, Kestenholz P, Lardinois D, *et al.* Incidence and management of complications after neoadjuvant chemotherapy followed by extrapleural pneumonectomy for malignant pleural mesothelioma. *Eur J Cardiothorac Surg* 2006; 29: 579–584.

43. Stewart DJ, Martin-Ucar AE, Edwards JG, *et al.* Extra-pleural pneumonectomy for malignant pleural mesothelioma: the risks of induction chemotherapy, right-sided procedures and prolonged operations. *Eur J Cardiothorac Surg* 2005; 27: 373–378.
44. Vogelzang NJ, Rusthoven JJ, Symanowski J, *et al.* Phase III study of pemetrexed in combination with cisplatin *versus* cisplatin alone in patients with malignant pleural mesothelioma. *J Clin Oncol* 2003; 21: 2636–2644.
45. Allen AM, Czerminska M, Jänne PA, *et al.* Fatal pneumonitis associated with intensity-modulated radiation therapy for mesothelioma. *Int J Radiat Oncol Biol Phys* 2006; 65: 640–645.
46. Ris HB, Altermatt HJ, Nachbur B, *et al.* Intraoperative photodynamic therapy with m-tetrahydroxyphenylchlorin for chest malignancies. *Lasers Surg Med* 1996; 18: 39–45.
47. Ris HB, Altermatt HJ, Inderbitzi R, *et al.* Photodynamic therapy with chlorins for diffuse malignant mesothelioma: initial clinical results. *Br J Cancer* 1991; 64: 1116–1120.
48. Schouwink H, Rutgers ET, van der Sijp J, *et al.* Intraoperative photodynamic therapy after pleuropneumonectomy in patients with malignant pleural mesothelioma: dose finding and toxicity results. *Chest* 2001; 120: 1167–1174.
49. Pass HI, Temeck BK, Kranda K, *et al.* Phase III randomized trial of surgery with or without intraoperative photodynamic therapy and postoperative immunochemotherapy for malignant pleural mesothelioma. *Ann Surg Oncol* 1997; 4: 628–633.
50. Baas P, Murrer L, Zoetmulder FA, *et al.* Photodynamic therapy as adjuvant therapy in surgically treated pleural malignancies. *Br J Cancer* 1997; 76: 819–826.
51. Takita H, Dougherty TJ. Intracavitary photodynamic therapy for malignant pleural mesothelioma. *Sem Surg Oncol* 1995; 11: 368–371.
52. Richards WG, Zellos L, Bueno R, *et al.* Phase I to II study of pleurectomy/decortication and intraoperative intracavitary hyperthermic cisplatin lavage for mesothelioma. *J Clin Oncol* 2006; 24: 1561–1567.
53. Sauter ER, Langer C, Coia LR, *et al.* Optimal management of malignant mesothelioma after subtotal pleurectomy: revisiting the role of intrapleural chemotherapy and postoperative radiation. *J Surg Oncol* 1995; 60: 100–105.
54. Lee JD, Perez S, Wang HJ, *et al.* Intrapleural chemotherapy for patients with incompletely resected malignant mesothelioma: the UCLA experience. *J Clin Oncol* 1995; 60: 262–267.
55. Colleoni M, Sartori F, Calabro F, *et al.* Surgery followed by intracavitary plus systemic chemotherapy in malignant pleural mesothelioma. *Tumori* 1996; 82: 53–56.
56. Rusch V, Saltz L, Venkatraman E, *et al.* A phase II trial of pleurectomy/decortication followed by intrapleural and systemic chemotherapy for malignant pleural mesothelioma. *J Clin Oncol* 1994; 12: 1156–1163.
57. Lucchi M, Chella A, Melfi F, *et al.* A phase II study of intrapleural immuno-chemotherapy, pleurectomy/decortication, radiotherapy, systemic chemotherapy and long-term sub-cutaneous IL-2 in stage II–III malignant pleural mesothelioma. *Eur J Cardiothorac Surg* 2007; 31: 529–534.

CHAPTER 24

Systemic treatment of malignant mesothelioma

R.M. Rudd

Correspondence: R.M. Rudd, London Lung Cancer Group, Barts Mesothelioma Research, 54 New Cavendish Street, London, UK. E-mail: robin@robinrudd.com

Most patients with malignant pleural mesothelioma have disease which is not suitable for radical surgery in the form of extra-pleural pneumonectomy. Palliative surgery may help to deal with a recurrent pleural effusion and radiotherapy may alleviate pain or reduce chest-wall masses but the only type of treatment demonstrated by randomised trials to prolong survival is systemic chemotherapy. Biological targeted therapies have been used with disappointing results so far, although many new agents are under investigation. Immunotherapy and gene therapy displayed initial promise but now appear unlikely to make a major impact.

Chemotherapy

Until quite recently there had been no large-scale randomised trials of chemotherapy in mesothelioma. Such evidence as was available was derived from small-scale phase II trials. These had established that a number of single agents had useful activity in mesothelioma, as assessed by radiographic evidence of tumour response. Survival duration was very variable, probably owing more to variable entry criteria and prognostic factors than any effect of treatment. Little evidence had been gathered about the effect of chemotherapy on symptom control and quality of life (QoL). Interpretation of results was complicated by various factors. Patients tended to be younger and of better performance status (PS) than average. Staging of the disease was often reported but this is of limited prognostic value in mesothelioma and often there was inadequate information about known prognostic factors. There was no evidence that any chemotherapy prolonged survival. In the last few years, three randomised phase III trials have provided important information. Before discussion of these and other studies, it is worth considering some general points concerning chemotherapy trials in mesothelioma.

Response to chemotherapy

It is important to appreciate what is meant by "response" to treatment in mesothelioma. In older studies this was a purely radiological criterion. In most of the studies in the literature, the criteria used were the World Health Organization (WHO) response criteria, which were always difficult to apply to mesothelioma. They were designed for solid tumours whose diameters in two dimensions were readily measurable by imaging. The criteria are difficult and sometimes impossible to apply by CT scan and

Eur Respir Mon, 2009, 44, 419–434. Printed in UK - all rights reserved. Copyright ERS Journals Ltd 2009; European Respiratory Monograph; ISSN 1025-448x.

usually impossible to apply reproducibly on plain chest radiograph, which was relied upon for response assessment in older chemotherapy studies.

The WHO criteria have largely been replaced by Response Evaluation Criteria in Solid Tumors (RECIST) criteria which allow use of unidimensional measurements as an alternative to bidimensional measurements [1]. RECIST is based on the assumption that tumours are generally spherical and that a maximal unidimensional measurement correlates well with an overall reduction in tumour size. Mesothelioma tends to grow as a rind around the chest wall so a maximal tumour measurement is impossible to obtain. Changes in tumour bulk are often manifested as changes in tumour thickness perpendicular to the chest wall. Discrepancies between tumour measurement in mesothelioma using the WHO and RECIST criteria have been reported [2]. RECIST criteria have been modified specifically for pleural mesothelioma [3]. Tumour thickness is measured perpendicular to the chest wall at two points at three levels on a CT scan (fig. 1). The sum of the measurements is taken as the baseline and partial response is defined as a reduction of 30% in the sum of the measurements maintained for $\geq$4 weeks. Importantly, response assessed in this way correlated with increase in forced vital capacity during treatment, and predicted longer survival.

A complicating factor is that pleurodesis causes an inflammatory response and this may lead to an increase in pleural thickening. It is therefore important that a baseline computed tomography (CT) scan for the purpose of subsequent response assessment is performed following pleurodesis and prior to chemotherapy.

Despite improvements in response assessment in some patients, because of the configuration of disease it is still very difficult to assess response according to RECIST criteria. It may be that radiological response assessment is not actually very important. There is evidence that partial response may not be the most important prognostic feature in predicting the outcome after chemotherapy. Time to progression, which is easier to assess radiologically, may be a better surrogate for survival than partial response [5].

There is also interest in the possibility of using other means of assessing response to therapy. Sometimes there is little or no assessable disease present, particularly if treatment is started soon after diagnosis. A reduction of fludeoxyglucose uptake by the tumour on positron emission tomography (PET) scan may prove to be a better indicator

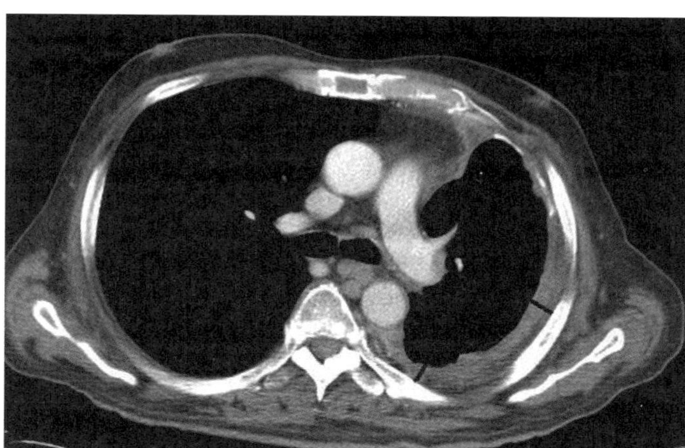

Fig. 1. – Black lines demonstrate measurement of tumour thickness perpendicular to the chest wall at two points for the purpose of assessment of response using the modified Response Evaluation Criteria in Solid Tumors (RECIST) criteria [3].

of response in such cases and perhaps this could be used more generally. Levels of mesothelin in the blood correlate with tumour bulk and it may be that tumour response could be assessed by monitoring blood levels. Further studies are needed to determine the correlation between various methods of assessing response and, more importantly, the relationship between response as assessed by each method and subsequent survival.

Of more importance to the patient than radiological response are the efficacy of the treatment in alleviating symptoms of the disease, toxicity, and the effect of treatment on QoL. Systematic reporting of these outcomes was uncommon in the older studies but has been incorporated into recent studies.

Earlier phase II studies

Early phase II studies established that several agents produced partial responses of up to 20%. A meta-analysis of older studies found that cisplatin was the most active single agent and cisplatin with doxorubicin was the most active combination with an estimated response rate of 28.5% [5]. However, a relatively large phase II trial of cisplatin with epirubicin in 69 patients, which used CT scans for response assessment, found a partial response rate of only 19% [6]. Cisplatin containing regimes were significantly more active than those containing carboplatin.

Recent phase II studies

Two phase II studies subsequently led to the development of a large-scale randomised phase III study in the UK. A study of the combination of mitomycin, vinblastine and cisplatin (MVP) administered 3-weekly to 39 patients, reported a partial response in eight (20%) patients and relief of symptoms reported to be present initially in 24 (62%) [7]. Median survival was disappointing at 6 months. In an extended series of 150 patients, the partial response rate was lower at 15% with a similar median survival of 7 months [8].

A study of single agent vinorelbine administered to 29 patients on an out-patient basis in cycles of 6-weekly injections reported partial response in seven (24%) with symptomatic benefit as assessed by Rotterdam symptom checklist in around half the patients [9]. The regimen was generally well tolerated with no treatment-related deaths. Median survival was 10.6 months.

Phase III randomised trials of chemotherapy

Chemotherapy versus *active supportive care*

The phase II studies of MVP and vinorelbine formed the basis for the development of a phase III, three-arm randomised trial known as MSO-1 in which patients were allocated to active symptom control (ASC) alone or with one of these two chemotherapy regimens [10]. At the time that the trial was devised, there was no consensus on the role of chemotherapy because of the low response rates and the lack of randomised trial evidence of efficacy. The essential elements of ASC were defined as regular follow-up in a specialist clinic, structured physical, psychological and social assessments at every clinic visit, rapid involvement of additional specialists, and parallel nursing support. Patients could receive, as required, steroids, analgesics, appetite stimulants, bronchodilators and palliative radiotherapy. In the two chemotherapy arms, patients received, in addition to ASC, either four cycles of MVP, *i.e.* mitomycin 6 $mg{\cdot}m^{-2}$, vinblastine

6 mg·m^{-2} (maximum 10 mg) and cisplatin 50 mg·m^{-2}, all given on day 1 of a 21-day cycle, or vinorelbine 30 mg·m^{-2} (maximum 60 mg) weekly by injection for 12 weeks with a 2-week gap between cycles 6 and 7. Clinicians were free to give nonprotocol treatment at any stage if was felt to be in the patient's best interest, although such patients remained in the trial for follow-up and analysis.

Tumour response was formally assessed by CT scan at 15 weeks using modified RECIST criteria. Patients were asked to complete QoL questionnaires at baseline (pre-randomisation) and at every subsequent assessment. As one of the main aims of treatment was the control of common presenting symptoms (particularly chest pain, breathlessness, malaise and sweating) and, as the EORTC questionnaires did not include an item on sweating, this additional question was added.

The initial aim was to recruit 840 patients into the three arms over 4 yrs. However, after 3 yrs accrual only, 232 patients had been entered, and it was clear that the target of 840 patients was not going to be reached in a timely fashion. There were two main reasons for slow accrual. First, some patients did not want any chemotherapy, an observation confirmed by a study in Leeds (UK), which audited all referred mesothelioma cases between 2002 and 2005 and indicated that of 54 patients who were fit for, and offered, chemotherapy, only 25 (46%) accepted it [11]. Secondly, the results of a large randomised trial, showing a survival advantage for cisplatin/pemetrexed was presented at the American Society of Clinical Oncology (ASCO) Annual Meeting in 2002 and subsequently published [12]. After that, many UK patients who were fit for chemotherapy received this combination. The trial design was therefore changed to a two-arm comparison by combining the two chemotherapy arms, although the three-way randomisation was retained to allow some exploratory analyses of those arms. The two-arm design aimed for a total of 420 patients (140 ASC, 280 ASC and chemotherapy) and eventually closed with 409 patients recruited.

Assessment of tumour response in peripheral centres proved problematic and reliable data were not obtained. There was no clear benefit from either type of chemotherapy in relief of symptoms of mesothelioma and patients who had received chemotherapy experienced more lethargy and alopecia with both regimes during treatment but not after it ended. Chemotherapy had no significant effect on QoL.

There was a small nonsignificant survival advantage for patients who were in the chemotherapy arm (hazard ratio (HR) 0.89, 95% confidence interval (CI) 0.72–1.12; p=0.32). The estimated median and 1-yr survival rate for patients in the ASC group were 7.6 months and 30% respectively, and 8.5 months and 37% respectively for the chemotherapy patient group. Exploratory analyses showed that patients on vinorelbine had longer survival than ASC patients (HR 0.81, 95% CI 0.63–1.05; p=0.11), median 9.4 months but there was no suggestion of any survival benefit with MVP (HR 0.98, 95% CI 0.76–1.28; p=0.91).

Pemetrexed (Alimta®)

Pemetrexed (Alimta®), a multi-targeted antifolate agent, has excited considerable interest. As a single agent, the response rate among 64 patients was 14% with a median survival of 10.7 months [13]. Activity was higher in combination with cisplatin [14].

The largest randomised trial of chemotherapy in mesothelioma carried out so far, compared a combination of pemetrexed and cisplatin (PC) with cisplatin (C) alone in patients with mesothelioma [12]. Inclusion criteria included Karnofsky PS ≥70, corresponding to WHO or Eastern Cooperative Oncology Group (ECOG) PS 0–1. Patients were excluded if they had had prior chemotherapy, a second primary malignancy or brain metastases, or if they were unable to interrupt nonsteroidal anti-inflammatory therapy, which is not recommended for simultaneous use with pemetrexed because it may delay pemetrexed clearance. Patients received cisplatin 75 mg·m^{-2} with or without pemetrexed 500 mg·m^{-2} at 3-weekly intervals.

Severe toxicity during the first part of the trial, with three possible treatment related deaths among the first 43 patients treated with pemetrexed, was noted to be associated with high blood levels of homocysteine and methylmalonic acid, linked to reduced levels of folic acid and vitamin B12. Similar evidence from trials in other diseases led to the introduction of folic acid and vitamin B12 supplementation, which was observed to reduce toxicity substantially. The change resulted in three patient subgroups: never supplemented, partially supplemented and fully supplemented. The sample size was substantially increased to ensure adequate statistical power of the fully supplemented subgroup. Dexamethasone was administered as premedication before each cycle of chemotherapy. Dose adjustments could be made if haematological toxicity occurred.

Patients were recruited from 88 centres in 20 countries. 574 patients signed a consent form but only 456 patients were randomised, of whom, eight, who did not receive chemotherapy, were excluded from analysis. Median age was 61 yrs in the PC arm and 60 yrs in the C arm. In both arms, 68% had epithelioid sub-type. Patients on the PC arm received a median of six cycles while those on the C arm received a median of four cycles. Never supplemented patients received a median of two cycles on each arm. Survival and time to progression are shown in table 1.

The survival advantage for the two drug regimes did not quite reach statistical significance in the fully supplemented patients; however, the size of the difference between the arms was similar to that in the whole group and time to progression remained significantly longer. The slightly longer survival in the supplemented group may have reflected the higher number of cycles administered because of less toxicity. Interestingly survival improved with vitamin supplementation in both arms.

The investigators reported a tumour partial response rate of 41% in the PC arm and 17% with C. However, a review of the data by the Food and Drug Administration (FDA) confirmed only half of the partial responses originally reported [15].

The PC arm showed higher rates of severe leucopenia, anaemia, thrombocytopenia, nausea, vomiting, diarrhoea, constipation, anorexia and mucositis, but the frequency of toxicity was substantially reduced by vitamin supplementation. In the fully and partially supplemented patients, grade 3–4 toxicities with PC were: neutropenia 23%, nausea 12%, vomiting 10% and fatigue 9% of patients.

An abstract of QoL data presented at the ASCO Annual Meeting in 2003 reported a significant sustained improvement in QoL and symptom relief when compared with cisplatin alone [16]. This differentiation in QoL and symptoms was reported to have occurred within the first three cycles and had reached statistical significance in most variables (global QoL, pain, dyspnoea, fatigue, anorexia and cough) by week 15, all in

Table 1 – Time to progression and survival in the pemetrexed/cisplatin *versus* cisplatin trial [12]

	All patients			Fully vitamin supplemented		
	Pemetrexed and cisplatin	Cisplatin	p-value (log-rank)	Pemetrexed and cisplatin	Cisplatin	p-value (log-rank)
Patients n	226	222		168	163	
Median survival months	12.1	9.3	0.02	13.2	10.0	0 051
Median time to progression months	5.7	3.9	0.001	6.1	3.9	0 008

favour of the combination regimen. A more detailed account of QoL was promised but has so far not appeared.

Large proportions of patients in both arms received second-line treatment, 37% in the PC arm and 47% in the C arm. Patients who received second-line therapy survived significantly longer than those who did not [17]. However, the greater proportion of patients receiving second-line therapy in the control arm might reasonably be supposed to have been likely to diminish rather than augment the difference between the trial arms.

There are several reasons for caution in interpretation of the study. Patients were on average younger and with better PS than mesothelioma patients presenting to the clinic. No explanation was offered as to why 118 patients, who signed consent forms, were not randomised. Eight randomised patients were excluded from the survival analysis because they did not receive chemotherapy, so it was not a true intention to treat analysis which would be conventional in a study of this type. The survival advantage in the fully vitamin supplemented patients was not quite statistically significant. The control arm, *i.e.* moderately high-dose single agent cisplatin, is not standard therapy for mesothelioma and few clinicians would consider this regime, with low efficacy and substantial toxicity, to be a worthwhile treatment option outside a clinical trial. Patients randomised to cisplatin received an average of four cycles compared with six cycles in the combination arm and this may have contributed to the difference between the arms. Because a nonstandard chemotherapy arm was chosen as a control arm, the survival difference between what was in practice standard treatment outside the USA, *i.e.* supportive care, and the combination of pemetrexed and a platinum agent remains unknown.

Finally, for many mesothelioma patients, a small increase in life expectancy may not be the primary aim for either the patient or the clinician. Symptom control and QoL are very important and, with the full QoL data from the pemetrexed study remaining unpublished 5-yrs after the main study was reported, it remains unclear how QoL balances with any change in the duration of survival. QoL differences will remain difficult to evaluate in this study even when data are published because the control arm consisted of relatively high-dose cisplatin, which is fairly toxic and relatively ineffective treatment. It is possible that QoL advantages for pemetrexed may be at least partially a result of toxicity without relief of disease symptoms in the control arm.

Nevertheless, on the basis of this study the US FDA approved pemetrexed for the treatment of mesothelioma and it has also been licensed for this indication in Europe and many other countries. Belatedly, it was approved in 2008 by the National Institute for Clinical Excellence (NICE) in the UK for use by the National Health Service.

Raltitrexed

Support for the efficacy of antifolates is provided by similar results from a smaller randomised phase III trial of raltitrexed in 250 patients with mesothelioma [18]. An important difference from the pemetrexed study was that PS-2 patients were eligible and formed 13% of the total. Median age was 58 yrs. Patients were treated with cisplatin (C) 80 $mg \cdot m^{-2}$ with or without raltitrexed (RC) 3 $mg \cdot m^{-2}$ 3-weekly. Median overall and 1-yr survival for C *versus* RC were 8.8 (CI 7.8–10.8) *versus* 11.4 (CI 10.1–15) months and 40% *versus* 46%, respectively ($p=0.048$). There was no detriment to QoL from raltitrexed. Overall, the results were very similar to those of the pemetrexed study.

The message from the pemetrexed and raltitrexed studies was that, unless cisplatin alone actually shortens survival, which seems unlikely, these drugs probably do confer a small median survival advantage and, as with any chemotherapy, patients whose tumours respond well to therapy are likely to gain more than average in terms of survival. The effects on QoL are as yet not fully evaluated but at least do not appear to be detrimental.

Other aspects of chemotherapy

Further pemetrexed studies

The substitution of carboplatin for cisplatin is associated with reduced symptomatic toxicity, particularly with regard to nausea and vomiting, and increased ease of administration with less need for prolonged hydration with intravenous fluids. An initial small phase II study in 25 patients suggested that efficacy may be approximately similar when carboplatin in a dose of AUC 5 is used instead of cisplatin in combination with pemetrexed [19]. Another phase II study in which 102 patients received pemetrexed 500 $mg \cdot m^{-2}$ with carboplatin AUC 5 $mg \cdot mL^{-1} \cdot min^{-1}$ 3-weekly, reported a response rate of 18.6% [20], only maginally lower than the response rate with cisplatin and pemetrexed as verified by the FDA, *i.e.* 20% [15]. Median survival was 12.7 months, almost the same as with the pemetrexed and cisplatin combination. Grade 3–4 neutropenia occurred in <10% of treatment cycles and nonhaematological toxicity was described as negligible [20].

A nonrandomised case series from the International Expanded Access Program for Pemetrexed included 843 patients who received cisplatin and 861 who received carboplatin [21]. The response rates were 26.3% for pemetrexed with cisplatin and 21.7% with carboplatin. However, median time to progression (7.0 *versus* 6.9 months, respectively) and 1-yr survival (63 *versus* 64%, respectively) were virtually identical. Patients on cisplatin received a median of five cycles *versus* six on carboplatin. Grade 3–4 neutropenia occurred in 24% with cisplatin and 36% with carboplatin. It therefore seems that efficacy may be the same and symptomatic toxicity less if pemetrexed is used with carboplatin rather than with cisplatin, although a randomised study to confirm this is so far unavailable.

Alternative chemotherapy regimens

A study of 21 patients treated with gemcitabine and cisplatin reported a high partial response rate of 47.6% and median survival of 9.5 months, and patients were reported to have benefited symptomatically [22]. However, further studies of this regime have shown lower response rates between 16 and 33% with median survivals between 9.6 and 13 months [23–25]. Carboplatin is as effective as cisplatin in combination with gemcitabine, with a partial response rate of 26% and median survival of 15 months [26]. However, there are no large randomised trials of gemcitabine regimes demonstrating improvement in survival.

Irinotecan in combination with cisplatin and mitomycin has conferred a response rate of 35% in previously untreated patients and 30% in patients who had previously received chemotherapy [27].

Whether regimens, which appear to have useful activity in mesothelioma, such as the combination of gemcitabine with a platinum agent and single agent vinorelbine, might have similar beneficial effects on survival to those achieved with the combination of pemetrexed with a platinum agent is unknown as no randomised trials have been performed. As it is very unlikely that other regimes would be better than those including pemetrexed, the only interest in such trials would be that other drugs are cheaper and, by the time a large phase III trial could be completed, it is likely that pemetrexed would be off patent so relative cost would no longer be important.

Duration of chemotherapy

In the pivotal trial of pemetrexed and cisplatin, the median number of cycles administered was six and the maximum 12 [12]. In clinical practice, many patients receive only four because, by analogy with nonsmall cell lung cancer (NSCLC), clinicians doubt that administration of more than four cycles to patients who are becoming increasingly tired and intolerant of chemotherapy will confer significant benefit. However, there is no clear evidence available upon which to base a decision as to the duration of treatment.

A small phase II study investigated the toxicity and effectiveness of pemetrexed maintenance therapy in 13 patients who had not experienced disease progression after six cycles of induction therapy including pemetrexed [28]. Maintenance pemetrexed 500 $mg \cdot m^{-2}$ 3-weekly was continued until disease progression or unacceptable toxicity. The median number of cycles was four (range two to 14). No grade 4 toxicity was observed. Grade 3 toxicities were fatigue in 15%, neutropenia in 15% and anaemia in 8%. During maintenance therapy, three (23%) patients, who had stable disease after induction therapy achieved partial response. These promising results have led to the design of larger randomised trials of maintenance therapy.

Timing of chemotherapy

In some patients, especially those with the epithelioid sub-type, mesothelioma progresses slowly and there may be a period of months or even a year or more of relative freedom from symptoms and good QoL, without treatment, after the diagnosis has been established and any pleural effusion effectively dealt with by drainage and pleurodesis. Should such patients be offered chemotherapy as soon as the diagnosis has been made or is it acceptable to adopt a "watch and wait" policy with a view to initiation of chemotherapy when symptoms worsen and chemotherapy may be used with the dual aims of alleviating symptoms as well as prolonging survival? The latter policy is widely adopted in practice but experience shows that often the transition from "too well for chemotherapy" to "too ill for chemotherapy" is more rapid than expected and the patient dies without ever receiving chemotherapy from which they might have benefited.

One small randomised study sought to address this question [29]. A total of 43 patients were randomised to receive MVP or carboplatin, either at diagnosis or at the time of symptomatic disease progression. Median time to symptomatic progression was 25 weeks in the early group compared with 11 weeks for the delayed group ($p=0.1$). Median survival was 14 months (1-yr survival 66%) for the early group compared with 10 months (1-yr survival 36%) for the delayed group ($p=0.1$). QoL was in general better maintained for early treatment and the health resources use was similar in both arms. However, the study was difficult to interpret as the recent randomised phase III trial showed that MVP confers no survival advantage compared with supportive care [10]. It is difficult to see how administration of ineffective chemotherapy earlier rather than later would confer a survival advantage unless perhaps late administration to debilitated patients actually shortened survival. A larger randomised study employing more modern effective chemotherapy is required to address this important question.

Second-line chemotherapy

Evidence is accumulating for the value of second-line chemotherapy in mesothelioma. A phase III study randomised 243 patients to best supportive care (BSC) with or without pemetrexed 500 mg·m^{-2} 3-weekly [30]. Partial response occurred in 19% with pemetrexed and 2% without. Median time to progression was 3.7 months in the chemotherapy arm, significantly longer than 1.5 months in the BSC arm (p=0.0002). Post-protocol chemotherapy of various types including pemetrexed was used in 52% in the BSC arm, significantly more frequently than 29% in the pemetrexed arm and it was used significantly earlier in the BSC arm. These factors may well account for the failure to demonstrate a survival advantage from the trial chemotherapy. Median survival was 8.4 months with pemetrexed and 9.7 months without (nonsignificant). Chemotherapy was generally well tolerated with grade 3–4 toxicity as follows: haematological 7%, nausea 2.5% and vomiting 2.5%. There was no significant difference between the arms in QoL as assessed by the Lung Cancer Symptom Scale, though data collection was incomplete.

Retreatment with a pemetrexed-based regime can produce second responses in patients whose tumours initially responded well [31]. Alternatively, other agents can be used.

In a phase II study of 63 patients with relapsed disease after first-line chemotherapy which did not include vinorelbine single agent vinorelbine 30 mg·m^{-2} was administered by weekly intravenous injection with a 2-week break after every sixth injection [32]. The median number of drug administrations was 11. The partial response rate was 16% and median survival was 9.6 months. Treatment was generally well tolerated. The main grade 3–4 toxicity was neutropenia which occurred at some time in 55% of patients but there were no treatment-related deaths.

In a phase II study, irinotecan in combination with cisplatin and mitomycin conferred a response rate of 30% in patients who had previously received other chemotherapy, a little less than 37% in previously untreated patients [27]. In the second-line setting, median survival from initiation of second-line therapy was 7.3 months.

Conclusions: the current role for chemotherapy for pleural mesothelioma

Despite the need for caution in interpretation of the data, pemetrexed is an agent with demonstrable clinical efficacy in treatment of mesothelioma. It has some advantages over alternatives in terms of lesser toxicity, particularly when used with carboplatin rather than cisplatin, and ease of administration, with a 3-weekly out-patient treatment schedule. As the only drug licensed for treatment of this disease on the basis of randomised trial evidence, pemetrexed should be considered the first choice of drug, used in combination with cisplatin or carboplatin or as a single agent in patients unfit for platinum therapy. Unfortunately raltitrexed is not being licensed or marketed for the treatment of mesothelioma. Other agents with useful activity include vinorelbine, gemcitabine, and irinotecan with mitomycin and cisplatin but none has been shown to confer a survival advantage in a randomised trial. It is reasonable to use these agents if cost constraints prevent use of pemetrexed first line or in the second-line setting of disease progression after pemetrexed.

New agents for systemic treatment of mesothelioma

Cytotoxic therapy relies, in part, on the induction of programmed cell death or apoptosis for efficacy. Anti-cancer activity is typically limited by intrinsic apoptosis resistance in incurable, metastatic solid tumours. Mesothelioma typically exhibits significant insensitivity to induction of apoptosis but the molecular basis of this phenotype has not been fully elucidated.

Increasing knowledge of carcinogenesis has led to the discovery of many ways in which tumour cells differ from normal cells and "targeted therapies" try to exploit these to inhibit and kill tumour cells without damaging normal cells.

Angiogenesis inhibitors

Angiogenesis is essential for the growth of all tumours including mesothelioma. Various agents have been developed which can interfere with angiogenesis and hence retard or arrest tumour growth.

Vascular endothelial growth factor (VEGF) is an important mediator of angiogenesis. VEGF binds to receptors on endothelial cells and initiates a signalling cascade that stimulates new blood vessel formation. Mesothelioma patients have high circulating VEGF levels and VEGF expression in mesothelioma correlates with microvessel density which, in turn, correlates with poor survival [33]. There was therefore good reason to hope that interference with the action of VEGF might have therapeutic potential for mesothelioma.

Bevacizumab is a recombinant monoclonal antibody to VEGF, which has proved useful in treatment of colonic, lung and breast cancer and is under investigation for treatment of many other cancers. Addition of bevacizumab to standard chemotherapy improved response rate, progression free survival and overall survival in patients with advanced nonsquamous NSCLC, in which high VEGF levels also predict poor prognosis [34]. Unfortunately, a randomised phase II trial did not suggest any survival advantage when bevacizumab was added to gemcitabine plus cisplatin for treatment of pleural mesothelioma, although interestingly among patients treated with bevacizumab, those with lower VEGF levels survived longer [35]. Further studies combining bevacizumab with pemetrexed and platinum agents are in progress.

Vatalanib inhibits all VEGF receptor tyrosine kinases as well as platelet-derived growth factor receptor β (PDGFRβ). A phase II study in which 47 previously untreated patients were included reported a partial response in 5 (11%) and a best response of stable disease in 32 (66%) with a median progression free survival of 4.1 months [36].

Sunitinib is an oral, small-molecule, multi-targeted receptor tyrosine kinase inhibitor which has useful activity in renal carcinoma. Preliminary results from a continuing study of sunitinib in previously treated mesothelioma patients showed partial response on CT scan in three (15%) out of 22 patients, and three out of the 10 assessable patients showed a reduction in metabolic rate on PET scan [37].

Thalidomide inhibits angiogenesis by multiple pathways mediated by VEGF and basic fibroblast growth factors. Thalidomide has been demonstrated to have synergistic activity when combined with cytotoxic agents for the treatment of various tumour types. Thalidomide also has benefical anticachexia, and immunomodulatory properties, which might be hoped to reduce the disease-related and treatment-induced cachexia frequently seen in advanced mesothelioma. Disappointingly, two large randomised studies of thalidomide added to chemotherapy found no beneficial effect on survival or QoL in patients with small cell lung cancer or advanced NSCLC, but it did increase the risk of thrombotic events [38].

Thalidomide has been used in patients with mesothelioma. A phase II trial in 40 patients with pleural mesothelioma, 20 of whom had previously received chemotherapy, found disease stabilisation for 6 months or more as the best response in 11 (27.5%) patients with no partial or complete tumour responses [39]. The authors considered that the proportion of patients with prolonged disease stabilisation merited further studies of thalidomide in mesothelioma. Australian investigators have previously studied thalidomide in combination with cisplatin and gemcitabine but preliminary observations on tolerability from a small number of patients were presented only in abstract form [40]. The Australasian Lung Cancer Trials Group and a Dutch Group (NVALT 5 study) [41] have each embarked upon further studies of thalidomide maintenance therapy in patients with pleural mesothelioma after initial chemotherapy including pemetrexed.

Cell survival pathway inhibitors

Apoptosis is programmed cell death which occurs normally in all living tissues. In malignant cells regulation of apoptosis is deficient resulting in their survival and proliferation [42]. The poor response of mesothelioma to radiotherapy and chemotherapy reflects a defect in apoptosis. Malignant cells commonly depend upon signalling pathways that are not present or not important in normal cells for their survival. Treatment may be directed at interrupting these pathways, theoretically killing tumour cells without seriously harming normal cells.

Platelet-derived growth factor (PDGF) A and B are important in mesothelioma cell growth. A high level of expression of PDGFRβ was seen in mesothelioma cells but not in normal human mesothelial cells. Expression of PDGF A and B was detected at higher levels in mesothelioma cells than in normal mesothelial cells and a significant reduction in mesothelioma cell growth or migration was observed by blocking PDGF A and B [43]. Expression of c-Kit in mesothelioma cells is associated with chemoresistance [44]. These receptors activate the PI3K-Akt pathway which is important in resistance to apoptosis in mesothelioma cells.

These observations have led to the investigation of imatinib in mesothelioma. Imatinib is a specific inhibitor of a number of tyrosine kinase enzymes. It has proved useful in treatment of chronic myeloid leukaemia and has activity against other tumour types. Imatinib suppresses PDGF by inhibiting PDGFRβ and this leads to indirect inhibition of Akt which has been shown to increase sensitivity of mesothelioma cells to chemotherapy [45]. There was therefore reason to hope imatinib might be active against mesothelioma. Unfortunately, two clinical pilot studies of imatinib in treatment of pleural mesothelioma found no useful activity [46, 47]. However, it is still possible that imatinib may have some activity if used in combination with chemotherapy to which it may increase sensitivity. Synergy between imatinib and gemcitabine or pemetrexed in inducing cell death has been demonstrated in the laboratory. These observations are being followed up by the authors in a phase II clinical trial using gemcitabine with imatinib.

Sorafenib is an inhibitor of both VEGF receptor 2 and PDGFRβ which inhibits angiogenesis and cell proliferation. It has proved useful in treatment of renal carcinoma. A phase II study evaluated its efficacy in patients with pleural mesothelioma [48]. They treated 51 patients who had previously received pemetrexed. Two (4%) partial responses were observed and 28 (60%) patients had stable disease. Median time to progression of disease was 3.6 months. The level of activity was disappointing but the authors plan to study expression of various factors by the tumour which might help to predict which patients might benefit from the drug.

Bortezomib is a proteasome inhibitor that has been shown to increase apoptosis in mesothelioma cell lines. Bortezomib also increased the cytotoxicity of cisplatin and pemetrexed in a concentration-dependent manner when administered prior to either [49]. Trials of bortezomib as a single agent and in combination with chemotherapy are currently in progress.

Epidermal growth factor receptor (EGFR) is overexpressed in the cells of certain types of human cancers, including lung and breast. This leads to inappropriate activation of the antiapoptotic Ras signal transduction cascade, eventually leading to uncontrolled cell proliferation. Inhibitors of the EGFR tyrosine kinase such as gefitinib (Iressa®) and erlotinib (Tarceva®) have antitumour activity in these cancers. Expression of the EGFR in mesothelioma encouraged investigation of inhibitors of this receptor. In the laboratory, gefitinib inhibits mesothelioma but unfortunately these agents have proven to have no useful antitumour activity in clinical trials in mesothelioma [50, 51].

Suberoylanilide hydroxamic acid (SAHA) is a potent inhibitor of histone deacetylases and other proteins involved in the regulation of gene expression and cell cycle progression. It induces differentiation and/or apoptosis in certain transformed cells in culture and it is a potent inhibitor of mesothelioma cell growth. 13 patients with mesothelioma, 12 previously treated with chemotherapy, were included in a phase I trial of oral SAHA and there were two (15%) partial responses [52]. A placebo-controlled, randomised phase III study of oral SAHA is now open for patients with mesothelioma in whom treatment with pemetrexed has failed.

Argininosuccinate synthetase is a rate-limiting enzyme in arginine production which is reduced or deficient in more than half of mesotheliomas, offering the possibility of treating mesothelioma by arginine depletion which normal cells but not tumour cells will be able to survive [53]. ADI-PEG 20 is a pegylated form of the enzyme arginine deiminase derived from the bacterium, *Mycoplasma hominus*, which degrades arginine, an essential amino acid for the growth of tumour cells that lack expression of argininosuccinate synthetase (AS). AS-negative tumours undergo apoptosis following withdrawl of arginine. Preclinical and phase I/II clinical studies in hepatocellular cancer and metastatic melanoma have demonstrated significant activity of single agent ADI-PEG 20. A phase II clinical trial in mesothelioma is expected to start in the UK in the near future.

Immunotherapy

Immunotherapy with agents including interleukin-2 and interferon, which have some limited activity against mesothelioma, has proved disappointing [54] and appears less likely to be valuable with the emergence of newer targeted agents.

Gene therapy

Gene therapy remains an attractive concept but so far has no practical use outside small clinical trials [55]. It seems clear that a single transgene is never likely to be able to eradicate a solid tumour like mesothelioma which is diagnosed late in its natural history and any role is likely to be as part of multimodality therapy.

Conclusion

There is now reasonably well tolerated chemotherapy available for mesothelioma which has been demonstrated by randomised trial to prolong median survival. In the current state of knowledge all patients who would be fit enough to receive chemotherapy, including all PS 0–1 and some PS2 patients, should be given accurate information about chemotherapy and should have the opportunity to discuss it with a specialist experienced in use of chemotherapy for mesothelioma. Patients who prefer to receive chemotherapy after a discussion of the pros and cons of this form of treatment, should be offered it. The era of nihilism in which it was acceptable for respiratory physicians to tell patients simply that there is no useful treatment available for mesothelioma has ended.

Increasing knowledge of pathways involved in mesothelioma carcinogenesis has resulted in the discovery of many new approaches to treatment. None has yet led to a major breakthrough in the form of clinically effective treatment but research continues with justified optimism.

Summary

Systemic chemotherapy is the only type of treatment for malignant pleural mesothelioma, which has been demonstrated by randomised trial to confer prolongation of survival without detrimental effect on quality of life. The combination of pemetrexed with cisplatin prolongs survival by a median of ~3 months. Carboplatin can probably be substituted for cisplatin for greater tolerability without significant loss of efficacy. Pemetrexed with a platinum agent should be regarded as first choice therapy in the current state of knowledge. The combination of gemcitabine with a platinum agent and single agent vinorelbine are other regimes which have useful antitumour activity, although they have not been demonstrated by randomised trial to prolong survival. The optimal timing and duration of chemotherapy have not yet been determined. There is some evidence to support the use of second-line chemotherapy in selected patients. Patients who are fit enough to receive chemotherapy should be given full information about it by a clinician experienced in treating mesothelioma with chemotherapy, so they can decide whether they wish to receive it. It is no longer acceptable for respiratory physicians to tell patients that there is no treatment available for mesothelioma. Many new targeted agents have been utilised for treatment of mesothelioma. Epithelial growth factor receptor inhibitors have proved to be of no value. Additionally, to date, results with angiogenesis inhibitors have been disappointing although trials of various agents of this type and other cell-cycle pathway inhibitors are in progress.

Keywords: Chemotherapy, mesothelioma, pemetrexed, pleural, targeted, therapy.

Statement of interest
None declared.

References

1. Therasse P, Arbuck SG, Eisenhauer EA, *et al.* New guidelines to evaluate the response to treatment in solid tumours. *J Natl Cancer Inst* 2000; 92: 205–216.
2. van Klaveren RJ, Aerts JG, de Bruin H, *et al.* Inadequacy of the RECIST criteria for response evaluation in patients with malignant pleural mesothelioma. *Lung Cancer* 2004; 43: 63–69.
3. Byrne MJ, Nowak AK. Modified RECIST criteria for assessment of response in malignant pleural mesothelioma. *Ann Oncol* 2004; 15: 257–260.
4. Fennell DA, Parmar A, Shamash J, *et al.* Statistical Validation of the EORTC prognostic model for malignant pleural mesothelioma based on three consecutive phase II trials. *J Clin Oncol* 2005; 23: 184–189.

5. Berghmans T, Paesmans M, Lalami Y, *et al.* Activity of chemotherapy and immunotherapy on malignant mesothelioma: a systematic review of the literature with meta-analysis. *Lung Cancer* 2002; 38: 111–121.
6. Berghmans T, Lafitte JJ, Paesmans M, *et al.* A phase II study evaluating the cisplatin and epirubicin combination in patients with unresectable malignant pleural mesothelioma. *Lung Cancer* 2005; 50: 75–82.
7. Middleton GW, Smith IE, O'Brien ME, *et al.* Good symptom relief with palliative MVP (mitomycin-C, vinblastine and cisplatin) chemotherapy in malignant mesothelioma. *Ann Oncol* 1998; 9: 269–273.
8. Andreopoulou E, Ross PJ, O'Brien ME, *et al.* The palliative benefits of MVP (mitomycin C, vinblastine and cisplatin) chemotherapy in patients with malignant mesothelioma. *Ann Oncol* 2004; 15: 1406–1412.
9. Steele JPC, Shamash J, Evans M, *et al.* Phase II study of vinorelbine in patients with malignant pleural mesothelioma. *J Clin Oncol* 2000; 18: 3912–3917.
10. Muers MF, Stephens RJ, Fisher P, *et al.* Active symptom control with or without chemotherapy in the treatment of patients with malignant pleural mesothelioma (MS01): a multicentre randomised trial. *Lancet* 2008; 371: 1685–1694.
11. Chapman A, Mulrennan S, Ladd B, *et al.* Population based epidemiology and prognosis of mesothelioma in Leeds, UK. *Thorax* 2008; 63: 435–439.
12. Vogelzang NJ, Rusthoven JJ, Symanowski J, *et al.* Phase III study of pemetrexed in combination with cisplatin *versus* cisplatin alone in patients with malignant pleural mesothelioma. *J Clin Oncol* 2003; 21: 2636–2644.
13. Scagliotti GV, Shin DM, Kindler HL, *et al.* Phase II study of single agent pemetrexed with and without folic acid and vitamin B12 as front-line therapy in malignant pleural mesothelioma. *J Clin Oncol* 2003; 21: 1556–1561.
14. Thödtmann R, Depenbrock H, Dumez H, *et al.* Clinical and pharmacokinetic phase I study of multitargeted antifolate (LY231514) in combination with cisplatin. *J Clin Oncol* 1999; 17: 3009–3016.
15. Hazarika M, White RM Jr, Booth BP, *et al.* Pemetrexed in malignant pleural mesothelioma. *Clin Cancer Res* 2005; 11: 982–992.
16. Gralla RJ, Hollen PJ, Liepa AM, *et al.* Improving quality of life in patients with malignant pleural mesothelioma: Results of the randomized pemetrexed + cisplatin *vs.* cisplatin trial using the LCSS-meso instrument. *Proc Am Soc Clin Oncol* 2003; 22: 2496.
17. Manegold C, Symanowski J, Gatzemeier U, *et al.* Second-line (post-study) chemotherapy received by patients treated in the phase III trial of pemetrexed plus cisplatin *versus* cisplatin alone in malignant pleural mesothelioma. *Ann Oncol* 2005; 16: 923–927.
18. Van Meerbeeck JP, Gaafar R, Manegold C, *et al.* Randomized phase III study of cisplatin with or without raltitrexed in patients with malignant pleural mesothelioma: an intergroup study of the European Organisation for Research and Treatment of Cancer Lung Cancer Group and the National Cancer Institute of Canada. *J Clin Oncol* 2005; 23: 6881–6889.
19. Hughes A, Calvert P, Azzabi A, *et al.* Phase I clinical and pharmacokinetic study of pemetrexed and carboplatin in patients with malignant pleural mesothelioma. *J Clin Oncol* 2002; 20: 3533–3544.
20. Ceresoli GL, Zucali PA, Favaretto AG, *et al.* Phase II Study of pemetrexed plus carboplatin in malignant pleural mesothelioma. *J Clin Oncol* 2006; 24: 1443–1448.
21. Santoro A, O'Brien ME, Stahel RA, *et al.* Pemetrexed plus cisplatin or pemetrexed plus carboplatin for chemonaïve patients with malignant pleural mesothelioma: results of the International Expanded Access Program. *J Thorac Oncol* 2008; 3: 756–763.
22. Byrne MJ, Davidson JA, Musk AW, *et al.* Cisplatin and gemcitabine treatment for malignant mesothelioma: a phase II study. *J Clin Oncol* 1999; 17: 25–30.
23. Nowak AK, Byrne MJ, Williamson R, *et al.* A multicentre phase II study of cisplatin and gemcitabine for malignant mesothelioma. *Br J Cancer* 2002; 87: 491–496.

24. van Haarst JM, Baas P, Manegold C, *et al.* Multicentre phase II study of gemcitabine and cisplatin in malignant pleural mesothelioma. *Br J Cancer* 2002; 86: 342–345.
25. Castagneto B, Zai S, Dongiovanni D, *et al.* Cisplatin and gemcitabine in malignant pleural mesothelioma: a phase II study. *Am J Clin Oncol* 2005; 28: 223–226.
26. Favaretto AG, Aversa SM, Paccagnella A, *et al.* Gemcitabine combined with carboplatin in patients with malignant pleural mesothelioma: a multicentric phase II study. *Cancer* 2003 97: 2791–2797.
27. Fennell DA, Steele JP, Shamash J, *et al.* Efficacy and safety of first- or second-line irinotecan, cisplatin and mitomycin in mesothelioma. *Cancer* 2007; 109: 93–99.
28. van den Bogaert DP, Pouw EM, van Wijhe G, *et al.* Pemetrexed maintenance therapy in patients with malignant pleural mesothelioma. *J Thorac Oncol* 2006; 1: 25–30.
29. O'Brien ME, Watkins D, Ryan DC, *et al.* A randomised trial in malignant mesothelioma (M) of early (E) *versus* delayed (D) chemotherapy in symptomatically stable patients: the MED trial. *Ann Oncol* 2006; 17: 270–275.
30. Jassem J, Ramlau R, Santoro A, *et al.* Phase III trial of pemetrexed plus best supportive care compared with best supportive care in previously treated patients with advanced malignant pleural mesothelioma. *J Clin Oncol* 2008; 26: 1698–1704.
31. Razak AR, Chatten KJ, Hughes AN. Retreatment with pemetrexed-based chemotherapy in malignant pleural mesothelioma (MPM): a second line treatment option. *Lung Cancer* 2008; 60: 294–297.
32. Stebbing J, Powles T, McPherson K, *et al.* The efficacy and safety of weekly vinorelbine in relapsed malignant pleural mesothelioma. *Lung Cancer* 2009; 63: 94–97.
33. Edwards JG, Swinson DE, Jones JL, *et al.* Tumor necrosis correlates with angiogenesis and is a predictor of poor prognosis in malignant mesothelioma. *Chest* 2003; 124: 1916–1923.
34. Sandler A, Gray R, Perry MC, *et al.* Paclitaxel-carboplatin alone or with bevacizumab for non-small-cell lung cancer. *N Engl J Med* 2006; 355: 2542–2550.
35. Karrison T, Kindler HL, Gandara DR, *et al.* Final analysis of a multi-center, double-blind, placebo-controlled, randomized phase II trial of gemcitabine/cisplatin (GC) plus bevacizumab (B) or placebo (P) in patients (pts) with malignant mesothelioma (MM). *J Clin Oncol* 2007; 25: Suppl. 18, 7526.
36. Jahan TM, Gu L, Wang X, *et al.* Vatalanib (V) for patients with previously untreated advanced malignant mesothelioma (MM): a phase II study by the Cancer and Leukemia Group B (CALGB 30107). *Proc Am Soc Clin Oncol* 2007; 25: Suppl. 18, 7081.
37. Nowak AK, Millward MJ, Francis R, *et al.* Phase II study of sunitinib as second-line therapy in malignant pleural mesothelioma (MPM). *Proc Am Soc Clin Oncol* 2008; 26: Suppl. 20, 8063.
38. Lee S, Rudd RM, Woll PJ, *et al.* Two randomised phase III, double blind, placebo controlled trials of thalidomide in patients with advanced non-small cell lung cancer (NSCLC) and small cell lung cancer (SCLC). *Proc Am Soc Clin Oncol* 2008; 26: Suppl. 20, 8045.
39. Baas P, Boogerd W, Dalesio O, *et al.* Thalidomide in patients with malignant pleural mesothelioma. *Lung Cancer* 2005; 48: 291–296.
40. Pavlakis N, Williams G, Harvey R, *et al.* Thalidomide alone and in combination with cisplatin/gemcitabine chemotherapy for malignant mesothelioma (MM): preliminary results from two phase II studies. *Proc Am Soc Clin Oncol* 2002; 21: 1885.
41. NVALT5 study: Phase III trial of the antiangiogenic agent thalidomide in patients with malignant pleural mesothelioma after the first line chemotherapy. www.ikcnet.nl/trials/index.php?id=177 Date last accessed: September 29, 2008.
42. Fennell DA, Rudd RM. Defective core-apoptosis signalling in diffuse malignant pleural mesothelioma: opportunities for effective drug development. *Lancet Oncol* 2004; 5: 354–362.
43. Pogrebniak HW, Lubensky IA, Pass HI. Differential expression of platelet derived growth factor-β in malignant mesothelioma: a clue to future therapies? *Surg Oncol* 1993; 2: 235–240.
44. Catalano A, Rodilossi S, Rippo MR, *et al.* Induction of stem cell factor/c-Kit/slug signal transduction in multidrug-resistant malignant mesothelioma cells. *J Biol Chem* 2004; 279: 46706–46714.

45. Bertino P, Porta C, Barbone D, *et al.* Preliminary data suggestive of a novel translational approach to mesothelioma treatment: imatinib mesylate with gemcitabine or pemetrexed. *Thorax* 2007; 62: 690–695.
46. Mathy A, Baas P, Dalesio O, *et al.* Limited efficacy of imatinib mesylate in malignant mesothelioma: a phase II trial. *Lung Cancer* 2005; 50: 83–86.
47. Porta C, Mutti L, Tassi G. Negative results of an Italian Group for Mesothelioma (G.I.Me.) pilot study of single-agent imatinib mesylate in malignant pleural mesothelioma. *Cancer Chemother Pharmacol* 2007; 59: 149–150.
48. Janne PA, Wang XF, Krug LM, *et al.* Sorafenib in malignant mesothelioma (MM): A phase II trial of the Cancer and Leukemia Group B (CALGB 30307). *Proc Am Soc Clin Oncol* 2007; 25: Suppl. 18, 7707.
49. Gordon GJ, Mani M, Maulik G, *et al.* Preclinical studies of the proteasome inhibitor bortezomib in malignant pleural mesothelioma. *Cancer Chemother Pharmacol* 2008; 61: 549–558.
50. Garland LL, Randkin C, Gandara DR, *et al.* Phase II study of erlotinib in patients with malignant pleural mesothelioma: a Southwest Oncology Group study. *J Clin Oncol* 2007; 25: 2406–2413.
51. Govindan R, Kratzke RA, Herndon JE 2nd, *et al.* Gefitinib in patients with malignant mesothelioma: a phase II trial by the Cancer and Leukemia Group B. *Clin Cancer Res* 2005; 11: 2300–2304.
52. Krug LM, Curley T, Schwartz L, *et al.* Potential role of histone deacetylase inhibitors in mesothelioma: clinical experience with suberoylanilide hydroxamic acid. *Clin Lung Cancer* 2006; 7: 257–261.
53. Szlosarek PW, Klabatsa A, Pallaska A, *et al.* *In vivo* loss of expression of argininosuccinate synthetase in malignant pleural mesothelioma is a biomarker for susceptibility to arginine depletion. *Clin Cancer Res* 2006; 12: 7126–7131.
54. Robinson BW, Musk AW, Lake RA. Malignant mesothelioma. *Lancet* 2005; 366: 397–408.
55. van der Most RG, Robinson BW, Nelson DJ. Gene therapy for malignant mesothelioma: beyond the infant years. *Cancer Gene Ther* 2006; 13: 897–904.

Statements of interest

S.M. Bentzen. None declared. (*Author of chapter 17*)

C.T. Bolliger. None declared. (*Author of chapter 10*)

E. Brambilla. None declared. (*Author of chapter 2*)

H.E. Davies. None declared. (*Author of chapter 19*)

D. De Ruysscher. None declared. (*Author of chapter 17*)

M. Edelmann. None declared. (*Author of chapter 14*)

T. Eisen has received reimbursement for attending symposia from AstraZeneca and Roche; a speaker's fee from Roche; a fee for organising education from Boehringer Ingelheim; research funding from Bayer and Pfizer; and consulting fees from AstraZeneca, Roche, Bayer, Pfizer, Boehringer Ingelheim and Wyeth. (*Author of chapter 6*)

U. Gatzemeier received honoraria and reimbursement for attending conferences from Roche, AstraZeneca, Bayer, Merck and Lilly. He received speakers' honoraria from Novartis, GlaxoSmithKline, Lilly, Roche, AstraZeneca, Bayer and Pierre Fabre, and consulting fees from Roche, Lilly, Novartis, Merck and AstraZeneca. (*Author of chapter 16*)

D. Gilligan has received lecture fees, funding to attend international meetings and consultancy fees from Pierre-Fabre, Eli Lilly, AstraZeneca and Roche Pharmaceuticals. (*Author of chapter 13*)

H.J.M. Groen has received funds for translational research from Pfizer and Roche. (*Author of chapter 17*)

M.Q.F. Hatton. None declared. (*Author of chapter 12*)

D.F. Heigener received speaking fees from Roche, manufacturer of some targeted therapies mentioned in this chapter. (*Author of chapter 16*)

F.J.F. Herth has received travel support to the ERS congress from the ERS, and anhonorarium to speak at the PG courses (*Author of chapter 20*)

F.R. Hirsch. None declared. (*Author of chapter 3*)

R.M. Huber performed various trials in radiochemotherapy partly with support from Sanofi Aventis, Pierre Fabre and Bristol Myers Squibb. (*Author of the introduction and chapter 14*)

S.M. Janes. None declared. (*Author of the introduction and chapters 8 and 11*)

J.R. Jett. None declared. (*Author of chapter 4*)

C.F.N. Koegelenberg. None declared. (*Author of chapter 10*)

S. Lantuejoul. None declared. (*Author of chapter 2*)

M.H. Lawson. None declared. (*Author of chapter 6*)

Y.C.G. Lee was the lead investigator of a project involving mesothelin. All ELISAs were provided by CisBio Ltd for free. Y.C.G. Lee is a co-investigator of the multi-centre intrapleural sepsis trial-2, which is funded in part by a unrestricted education grant from Roche UK Ltd. Y.C.G. Lee did not receive any personal benefits from these studies. (*Author of chapter 19*)

J. Martin. None declared. (*Author of chapter 12*)

D.T. Merrick has previously participated in and received a fee for speaking at a symposium sponsored by AstraZeneca (*Author of chapter 3*)

D.E. Midthun. None declared. (*Author of chapter 4*)

E. Mishra. None declared. (*Author of chapter 19*)

M. Mukesh. None declared. (*Author of chapter 13*)

N. Navani. None declared. (*Author of chapters 5 and 8*)

I. Opitz. None declared. (*Author of chapter 23*)

D. Plekker. None declared. (*Author of chapter 10*)

P.E. Postmus. None declared. (*Author of chapter 18*)

C. Pöttgen. None declared. (*Author of chapter 17*)

E. Potton. None declared. (*Author of chapter 11*)

E. Quoix has been appointed during the last 2 years onto advisory boards (Roche for tarceva and avastin, BMS for ixabepilone, and Boehringer Ingelheim for new targeted therapies). She has also been invited to the American Society of Clinical Oncology annual meeting by Lilly (with a symposium on pemetrexed) and by Merck to the world lung cancer conference in 2007 (with a symposium on vorinostat). (*Author of chapter 15*)

M. Reck received honoraria and reimbursement for attending conferences from Roche, Lilly and Pierre Fabre. He received speakers' honoraria from Roche, Lilly, Merck, Pfizer and AstraZeneca, and consulting fees from Roche, Lilly, Pfizer, Merck and AstraZeneca. (*Author of chapter 16*)

R.M. Rudd. None declared. (*Author of chapter 24*)

J.M. Samet. None declared. (*Author of chapter 21*)

A. Scherpereel has received a research grant from CisBio International® for his laboratory. He has received a fee for speaking at the 2008 IMIG congress from CisBio® and his travel to this meeting was funded by the same company. (*Author of chapter 22*)

J-P. Sculier. None declared. (*Author of chapter 9*)

P. Shaw. None declared. (*Author of chapter 7*)

E.F. Smit. None declared. (*Author of chapter 18*)

S.G. Spiro. None declared. (*Author of the introduction, chapters 5 and 11*)

R. Stahel. None declared. (*Author of chapter 23*)

M.N. Taylor. None declared. (*Author of chapter 7*)

N. van Zandwijk. None declared. (*Author of chapter 1)*

W. Weder was an invited speaker on mesothelioma treatment at various meetings. The multi-centre study on neoadjuvant chemotherapy followed by surgery was organised/financed by SAKK. (*Author of chapter 23*)

Previously published in the European Respiratory Monograph Series:

Respiratory Diseases in the Elderly, Monograph 43
Edited by V. Bellia and R. Antonelli Incalzi (2009)

Smoking Cessation, Monograph 42
Edited by S. Nardini (2008)

Noninvasive Ventilation, Second Edition, Monograph 41
Edited by J-F. Muir, N. Ambrosino and A.K. Simonds (2008)

Clinical Exercise Testing, Monograph 40
Edited by S.A. Ward, P. Palange (2007)

Pathology of the Lung, Monograph 39
Edited by W Timens, H H Popper (2007)

Management of Chronic Obstructive Pulmonary Disease, Monograph 38
Edited by N M Siafakas (2006)

Respiratory Diseases in Infants and Children, Monograph 37
Edited by U Frey, J Gerritsen (2006)

Respiratory Emergencies, Monograph 36
Edited by S Nava, T Welte (2006)

Cystic Fibrosis, Monograph 35
Edited by A K Webb, F A Ratjen (2006)

Pulmonary Manifestations of Systemic Diseases, Monograph 34
Edited by G M Verleden, M G Demedts, R Westhovens, M Thomer (2005)

Diagnosis, Prevention and Treatment of Exercise-Related Asthma, Respiratory and Allergic Disorders in Sports, Monograph 33
Edited by K-H Carlsen, L Delgado, S Del Giacco (2005)

Sarcoidosis, Monograph 32
Edited by M Drent, U Costabel (2005)

Lung Function Testing, Monograph 31
Edited by R Gosselink, H Stam (2005)

Imaging, Monograph 30
Edited by A Bankier, P A Gevenosis (2004)

Surgery for Non-Neoplastic Disorders of the Chest: a Clinical Update, Monograph 29
Edited by G M Verleden, D Van Raemdonck, T Lerut, M Demedts (2004)

Antibiotics and the Lung, Monograph 28
Edited by M Cazzola, F Blasi, S Ewig (2004)

Pulmonary Vascular Pathology: A Clinical Update, Monograph 27
Edited by M Demedts, M Delcroix, R Verhaeghe, G M Verleden (2004)

Lung Transplantation, Monograph 26
Edited by J Boe, M Estenne, W Weder (2003)

Respiratory Diseases in Women, Monograph 25
Edited by C Mapp, S Buist (2003)

Nutrition and Metabolism in Respiratory Disease, Monograph 24
Edited by J Boe, M Estenne, W Weder (2003)

Asthma, Monograph 23
Edited by F Chung, L M Fabbri (2003)

Pleural Diseases, Monograph 22
Edited by R Loddenkemper, V B Antony (2002)

The Impact of Air Pollution on Respiratory Health, Monograph 21
Edited by G D'Amato, S T Holgate (2002)

ARDS, Monograph 20
Edited by T W Evans, M J D Griffiths, B F Keogh (2002)

Growing up with Lung Disease: The Lung in Transition to Adult Life, Monograph 19
Edited by A Bush, K-H Carlsen, M S Zach (2002)

The Nose and Lung Diseases, Monograph 18
Edited by B Wallaërt, P Chanex, P Godard (2001)

Lung Cancer, Monograph 17
Edited by S G Spiro (2001)

Noninvasive Mechanical Ventilation, Monograph 16
Edited by J-F Muir, N Ambrosino, A K Simonds (2001)